Visit our website

to find out about other books from W. B. Saunders
and our sister companies in Harcourt Health Sciences

Register free at
www.harcourt-international.com

and you will get

- the latest information on new books, journals and electronic products in your chosen subject areas

- the choice of e-mail or post alerts or both, when there are any new books in your chosen areas

- news of special offers and promotions

- information about products from all Harcourt Health Sciences' companies including Baillière Tindall, Churchill Livingstone, Mosby and W. B. Saunders

You will also find an easily searchable catalogue, online ordering, information on our extensive list of journals...and much more!

Visit the Harcourt Health Sciences' website today!

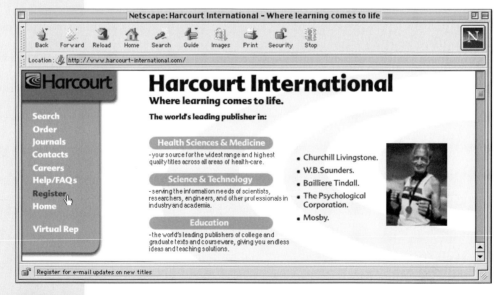

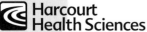

Carotid Artery Surgery

A Problem Based Approach

Commissioning Editor: Sue Hodgson
Project Manager: Ian Stoneham
Production Supervisor: Helen Sofio

Carotid Artery Surgery
A Problem Based Approach

Edited by

A Ross Naylor MD FRCS
Consultant Vascular Surgeon and
Honorary Senior Lecturer,
Department of Surgery,
Leicester Royal Infirmary,
Leicester, UK

and

William C Mackey MD
Professor of Surgery,
Tufts University School of Medicine;
Chief of Vascular Surgery,
New England Medical Center Hospital,
Boston, MA, USA

W. B. SAUNDERS

London • Edinburgh • New York • Philadelphia • St Louis • Sydney • Toronto • 2000

WB SAUNDERS
An imprint of Harcourt Publishers Limited

© Harcourt Publishers Limited 2000

 is a registered trademark of Harcourt Publishers Limited

The right of A R Naylor and W C Mackey to be identified as the
editors of this work has been asserted by them in accordance
with the Copyright, Designs and Patents Act 1988.

First published 2000

ISBN 0 7020 2432 5

British Library Cataloguing in Publication Data
A catalogue record for this book is available from the British
Library

Library of Congress Cataloging in Publication Data
A catalog record for this book is available from the Library of
Congress

Note
Medical knowledge is constantly changing. As new information
becomes available, changes in treatment, procedures,
equipment and the use of drugs become necessary. The
contributors and the publishers have taken care to ensure that
the information given in this text is accurate and up to date.
However, readers are strongly advised to confirm that the
information, especially with regard to drug usage, complies
with the latest legislation and standards of practice.

The
publisher's
policy is to use
**paper manufactured
from sustainable forests**

Printed in China

Contents

Contributors   **vii**   Preface (A Ross Naylor, William C Mackey)   **xiii**

Foreword   **xi**

Part One Patient Selection

1 The randomized trials for symptomatic carotid disease: how should they influence my clinical practice? (Europe: Peter RD Humphrey; USA: Wesley S Moore)   **3**

2 The randomized trials for asymptomatic carotid disease: how should they influence my clinical practice? (Europe: Dafydd Thomas; USA: Jerry Goldstone)   **15**

3 Is there a role for emergency or urgent carotid endarterectomy? (Europe: Roger M Greenhalgh; USA: Jonathan P Gertler, William M Abbott)   **25**

4 When should I perform carotid endarterectomy after a completed stroke? (Europe: Jens Allenberg, Hans H Eckstein; USA: Mark W Sebastian, Anthony D Whittemore)   **36**

5 In patients with combined carotid and coronary artery disease, should I perform a staged or synchronous procedure? (Europe: Peter RF Bell; USA: William C Mackey)   **46**

6 Is there a role for carotid artery surgery in patients with non-hemispheric or vertebrobasilar symptoms? (Europe: Roger M Greenhalgh; USA: John Ricotta, Kara Kvilekval)   **57**

7 Should cost-effectiveness influence patient selection for carotid surgery? (Europe: A Ross Naylor, Peter Rothwell USA: Jack L Cronenwett, John D Birkmeyer)   **66l**

Part Two Evaluation and Preoperative Management

8 Is duplex ultrasound alone sufficient for preoperative imaging? (Europe: Peter R Taylor; USA: Andrew H Schulick, Richard P Cambria)   **85**

9 Is there a role for preoperative magnetic resonance angiography? (Europe: Peter RD Humphrey; USA: Sheela T Patel, K Craig Kent)   **99**

10 Which patients should undergo contrast angiography? (Europe: Torben V Schroeder, Niels Levi, Henrik H Sillesen; USA: Patrick J Lamparello)   **118**

11 Does routine preoperative CT scanning alter patient management? (Europe: Dafydd Thomas; USA: Magruder C Donaldson)   **129**

12 Which patients require preoperative assessment by a neurologist? (Europe: Dafydd Thomas; USA: James M Estes)   **139**

13 Which non-cardiac medical conditions alter the operative risk? (Europe: Jonathan P Thompson; USA: Allen D Hamdan, Frank B Pomposelli Jr)   **149**

14 When is preoperative cardiac evaluation advisable? (Europe: Jonathan P Thompson; USA: Michael Belkin, Mark W Sebastian)   **164**

15 What does optimal medical management really entail? (Europe: Peter RD Humphrey; USA: Louis R Caplan, Brian Silver)   **180**

Part Three Operative Care

16 What evidence is there that regional anaesthesia confers any benefit over general anaesthesia? (Europe: Michael Horrocks; USA: Caron B Rockman, Thomas S Riles)   **193**

17 What steps can I take to minimize inadvertent cranial nerve injury? (Europe: Torben V Schroeder, Niels Levi; USA: James M Estes)   **206**

18 What practical steps can I take if I (a) know preoperatively that the lesion extends very high or (b) unexpectedly encounter a high lesion during operation? (Europe: Peter RF Bell; USA: Alexander D Shepard, Peter S Dovgan)   **219**

19 What is the optimal perioperative antithrombotic regimen? (Europe: David Bergqvist; USA: Mark W Sebastian, Michael S Conte)   **230**

Contents

20 Should all patients be shunted? If not, how can I predict which patients will require a shunt? (Europe: Jonathan D Beard; USA: Allen D Hamdan, Frank W LoGerfo) **244**

21 How can I achieve the optimal flow surface and distal end-point following carotid endarterectomy? (Europe: Nicholas JM London; USA: Joseph P Archie Jr) **255**

22 Should all patients be patched? If not, how should I select which patients to patch? (Europe: Hakan Parsson, David Bergqvist; USA: Hugh A Gelabert) **273**

23 When should I abandon a planned endarterectomy? (Europe: Nicholas JM London; USA: Jonathan P Gertler) **286**

24 Is there any evidence that perioperative monitoring and quality control assessment alter clinical outcome? (Europe: A Ross Naylor; USA: D Preston Flanigan) **298**

25 Is there a role for carotid angioplasty or stenting? (Europe: Jonathan D Beard; USA: Robert W Hobson II) **315**

Part Four **Postoperative Management**

26 How should I manage the patient who suffers a perioperative neurological deficit? (Europe: A Ross Naylor; USA: David Rosenthal) **333**

27 How can I balance patient safety and cost-effectiveness in planning early postoperative care and hospital discharge? (Europe: Peter R Taylor; USA: Paul E Collier) **350**

28 Does serial postoperative clincal or duplex surveillance reduce the long-term stroke risk? (Europe: Jonathan D Beard; USA: William C Mackey) **360**

29 When should I reoperate for recurrent carotid stenosis? (Europe: Michael Horrocks; USA: G Patrick Clagett) **371**

30 How should I manage a patient with an infected prosthetic patch? (Europe: Peter RF Bell; USA: Bruce A Perler) **384**

Index **397**

Contributors

William M Abbott MD
Professor of Surgery, Harvard Medical School; Chief of Vascular Surgery, Massachusetts General Hospital, Boston, MA, USA

Jens R Allenberg MD
Professor of Vascular Surgery,
Chief of Department of Vascular Surgery,
University of Heidelberg, Heidelberg, Germany

Joseph P Archie Jr PhD, MD
Carolina Cardiovascular Surgical Associates; Clinical Professor of Surgery, University of North Carolina, Chapel Hill; Adjunct Professor of Mechanical and Aerospace Engineering, NC State University, Raleigh, NC, USA

Jonathan D Beard MB BS, BSc, ChM, FRCS
Consultant Vascular Surgeon, Sheffield Vascular Institute, Northern General Hospital, Sheffield, UK

Michael Belkin MD
Associate Professor of Surgery, Harvard Medical School Attending Surgeon, Brigham and Women's Hospital, Boston, MA, USA

Peter RF Bell MD, FRCS, MB ChB
Professor of Surgery, Department of Surgery, Leicester Royal Infirmary, Leicester, UK

David Bergqvist MD, PhD
Professor of Vascular Surgery, Department of Surgery, University Hospital, Uppsala, Sweden

John D Birkmeyer MD
Assistant Professor of Surgery, Dartmouth-Hitchcock Medical Center and The Center for Evaluative Clinical Sciences, Dartmouth Medical School, Lebanon, NH, USA

Richard P Cambria MD
Professor of Surgery, Harvard Medical School Visiting Surgeon, Massachusetts General Hospital, Boston, MA, USA

Louis R Caplan MD
Professor of Neurology, Harvard Medical School; Chief, Stroke Service, Beth Israel Deaconess Medical Center, Boston, MA, USA

G Patrick Clagett MD
Chairman, Division of Vascular Surgery, Professor of Surgery, University of Texas Southwestern Medical Center Dallas, TX, USA

Paul E Collier MD, FACS
Staff Surgeon and Director, Non-invasive Vascular Lab, Sewickley Valley Hospital, Sewickley, PA, USA

Michael S Conte MD
Assistant Professor of Surgery, Harvard Medical School Attending Surgeon, Brigham and Women's Hospital, Boston, MA, USA

Jack L Cronenwett MD
Professor of Surgery, Dartmouth Medical School; Chief, Section of Vascular Surgery, Dartmouth-Hitchcock Medical Center, Lebanon, NH, USA

Magruder C Donaldson MD
Associate Professor of Surgery, Harvard Medical School Attending Surgeon, Brigham and Women's Hospital, Boston, MA, USA

Peter S Dovgan MD
Assistant Professor, Division of Vascular Surgery, Department of Surgery, University of Florida, Jacksonville, Florida, USA

Hans H Eckstein MD
Lecturer in Surgery, Department of Vascular Surgery, University of Heidelberg, Heidelberg, Germany

James M Estes MD
Attending Surgeon, New England Medical Center; Assistant Professor, Tufts University Medical School, Boston, MA, USA

D Preston Flanigan MD
Clinical Professor of Surgery, University of California, Irvine, Orange, CA, USA

Hugh A Gelabert MD
Associate Professor of Surgery, Division of Vascular Surgery, University of California, Los Angeles School of Medicine, Los Angeles, CA, USA

Jonathan P Gertler MD
Associate Professor of Surgery, Harvard Medical School; Associate Visiting Surgeon, Associate Director, Vascular Laboratory, Massachusetts General Hospital, Boston, MA, USA

Jerry Goldstone MD
Professor and Chief, Division of Vascular Surgery, Case Western Reserve University, University Hospitals of Cleveland, Cleveland, Ohio, USA

Roger M Greenhalgh MA, MD, MChir, FRCS
Professor of Surgery, Head of Department of Vascular Surgery, Imperial College School of Medicine, Charing Cross Hospital, London, UK

Contributors

Allen D Hamdan MD
Instructor in Surgery, Harvard Medical School; Attending Surgeon, Division of Vascular Surgery, Beth Israel Deaconess Medical Center, Boston, MA, USA

Robert W Hobson II MD
Professor of Surgery and Physiology, Director, Division of Vascular Surgery, University of Medicine and Dentistry of New Jersey, New Jersey Medical School, Newark, NJ, USA

Michael Horrocks MRCS, LRCP, MBBS, FRCS, MS
Professor of Surgery, Department of Surgery, Royal United Hospital, Bath, UK

Peter RD Humphrey MA, BMBCh, DM, FRCP
Consultant Neurologist, Walton Center for Neurology and Neurosurgery NHS Trust, Liverpool, UK

K Craig Kent MD
Chief, Division of Vascular Surgery, Director of Vascular Center, New York Presbyterian Hospital, Weill Medical College of Cornell University, New York, NY, USA

Kara Kvilekval MD, FACS
Attending Vascular Surgery, Vascular Associates of Long Island, Stony Brook, NY, USA

Patrick J Lamparello MD
Associate Professor of Surgery and Director of Vascular Surgery, New York University School of Medicine, New York, NY, USA

Niels Levi MD
Senior Registrar in Surgery, Department of Vascular Surgery, Rigshospitalet 3111, University of Copenhagen, Copenhagen, Denmark

Frank W LoGerfo MD
Professor of Surgery, Harvard Medical School; Chief of Vascular Surgery, Beth Israel Deaconess Medical Center, Boston, MA, USA

Nicholas JM London MB ChB, FRCP (Ed), MD, FRCS
Professor of Surgery and Honorary Consultant Vascular Surgeon, Department of Surgery, Leicester Royal Infirmary, Leicester, UK

William C Mackey MD
Professor of Surgery, Tufts University School of Medicine; Chief of Vascular Surgery, New England Medical Center Hospital, Boston, MA, USA

Wesley S Moore MD, FACS
Professor of Surgery, Division of Vascular Surgery, University of California, Los Angeles School of Medicine, Los Angeles, CA, USA

A Ross Naylor MD FRCS
Consultant Vascular Surgeon and Honorary Senior Lecturer, Department of Surgery, Leicester Royal Infirmary, Leicester, UK

Hakan Parsson MD, PhD
Associate Professor of Vascular Surgery, Department of Surgery, University Hospital, Uppsala, Sweden

Sheela T Patel MD
Research Fellow, The New York Hospital Cornell Medical Center, New York, NY, USA

Bruce A Perler MD
Professor of Surgery, Johns Hopkins University School of Medicine; Director of the Vascular Surgery Fellowship and Non-invasive Vascular Laboratory, The Johns Hopkins Hospital, Baltimore, MD, USA

Frank B Pomposelli Jr MD
Associate Professor of Surgery, Harvard Medical School; Clinical Chief, Division of Vascular Surgery, Beth Israel Deaconess Medical Center, Boston, MA, USA

John J Ricotta MD
Professor and Chairman, Department of Surgery, SUNY at Stony Brook, New York, NY, USA

Thomas S Riles MD
Professor of Surgery, New York University School of Medicine; Chief of Vascular Surgery, New York University Medical Center, New York, NY, USA

Caron B Rockman MD
Assistant Professor of Surgery, Department of Surgery, Division of Vascular Surgery, New York University Medical Center, New York, NY, USA

David Rosenthal MD
Department of Vascular Surgery, Atlanta Medical Center, Atlanta, Georgia, Clinical Professor of Vascular Surgery, Medical College of Georgia, Augusta, Georgia, USA

Peter M Rothwell MD, PhD
MRC Senior Clinical Fellow, Department of Clinical Neurology, Radcliffe Infirmary, Woodstock Road, Oxford, UK

Torben V Schroeder MD, DMSc
Professor of Surgery, Consultant Vascular Surgeon, Department of Vascular Surgery RK, Rigshospitalet 3111, University of Copenhagen, Copenhagen, Denmark

Andrew H Schulick MD
Assistant Professor of Surgery, Division of Vascular
Surgery, Weill Cornell Medical College, New York, NY,
USA

Mark W Sebastian MD
Assistant Professor of Surgery, Duke University School of
Medicine, Durham, NC, USA

Alexander D Shepard MD
Senior Staff Surgeon, Director Vascular Laboratory, Henry
Ford Hospital, Detroit, MI, USA

Henrik H Sillesen MD, DMSc
Consultant, Vascular Surgery, Head of Department,
Gentofte University Hospital, Hellerup, Denmark

Brian Silver MD
Fellow, Department of Neurology, Beth Israel Deaconess
Medical Center, Boston, MA, USA

Peter R Taylor MA, MChir, FRCS
Consultant Vascular Surgeon, Department of Surgery,
Guy's and St Thomas' Hospital Trust, London, UK

Dafydd Thomas MA, MD, FRCP
Consultant Neurologist, Department of Neurology, St
Mary's Hospital, London, UK

Jonathan P Thompson BSc, MB ChB, FRCA
Senior Lecturer and Honorary Consultant in Anaesthesia,
Department of Anaesthesia, Leicester Royal Infirmary,
Leicester, UK

Anthony D Whittemore MD
Chief Medical Officer, Chief, Division of Vascular Surgery,
Brigham and Women's Hospital; Professor of Surgery,
Harvard Medical School, Boston, MA, USA

Foreword

Carotid artery surgery should be straight forward; right? All the trials have settled issues regarding indications for operating upon symptomatic and asymptomatic patients, and the technique of carotid endarterectomy (CEA) has been pretty well standardized. Wrong! The contents of this problem-based book exposes this fallacy, but what makes it so suitable for the vascular surgeon in practice and in training, and even for those of us who are looked upon to educate them, is that it poses all the right questions. It then answers them, using evidence-based information wherever possible, with discussions of each of the controversial issues by recognized experts from both sides of the Atlantic. "Twenty Questions" was a popular television show for many years. I predict that the "thirty questions" posed and answered in this book will make it a popular reference for many years to come. The questions reflect upon just about every decision one needs to make in today's practice and the answers reflect the best current knowledge.

The section on "Patient selection" not only discusses residual issues from the trials on elective CEA, but identifies indications for emergency operation, for operations for non-hemispheric and vertebrobasilar disease and for staging of CEA when indicated in association with coronary revascularization. The section on "Preoperative evaluation and management" covers when to use duplex scanning, magnetic resonance angiography and contrast arteriography, when to get a preoperative brain scan, and several aspects of preoperative preparation of high risk patients. The section on "Operative care" tackles choice of anesthesia, use of adjunctive antithrombotic drugs and such technical issues as shunting, patching, avoiding nerve injury, distal endpoint management, methods for assessing technical adequacy, and exposing the high carotid lesion. Finally, the section on "Postoperative management" deals with proper management of patients developing a neurologic deficit, prosthetic patch infection, and the issue of patient safety versus methods of cutting costs and achieving early discharge. It not only scrutinizes the value of long-term surveillance for recurrent stenosis, but when to operate if it is found. The role of carotid angioplasty is not overlooked and many of the issues mentioned above are discussed from the basis of cost-effectiveness, which is becoming increasingly important in today's practice.

Indeed, every nuance of carotid surgery is covered. It is *the* book for those who don't yet know all the questions; those who know the questions but who are unsure of many of the answers; and even for the attending surgeons who ask these questions on rounds, and would like to be sure to cover every consideration in giving definitive advice.

Robert B Rutherford MD, FACS, FRCS (Glasg)

Preface

There can be few operations that have been subjected to more scientific scrutiny than carotid endarterectomy (CEA). Since its introduction in 1953, millions of CEAs have been performed worldwide with the seemingly simple aim of preventing ischaemic stroke. Since 1980, it has become the single most commonly performed arterial procedure in most vascular units. The rationale underlying CEA is attractively simple. Yet, the paradox will always remain that the very operation which is performed to prevent stroke in the long term will itself be directly responsible for causing a stroke in a small but significant proportion of patients. It is a sobering fact that, since its introduction, about 100 000 patients have suffered a stroke as a direct consequence of the operation. In the 1980s this paradox led a number of doctors to question the overall value of CEA, particularly as the number of operations increased each year, with apparently little regard for either the appropriateness of the indications or the parallel improvements in the medical management of risk factors.

The randomized trials have now, however, clearly demonstrated that CEA has a role in the management of selected patients with carotid artery disease. As a result, the trial organizers and collaborators have not only clarified the role of CEA but have also established level 1 evidence-based studies as the 'gold standard' against which local or national outcomes should be compared. Yet, despite the fact that CEA confers an unequivocal benefit in selected patients, there are growing concerns that one cannot generalize from the results of the randomized trials to routine clinical practice. The international trials used highly selected surgeons, and most patients were assessed independently by neurologists and all underwent preoperative contrast angiography. However, many of these basic criteria are no longer applied in current clinical practice. Moreover, there is a growing perception that the trials have been used by some surgeons as a 'green light' to proceed with impunity, with a tendency to use the trial data to justify clinical practice without ever quoting – or perhaps even knowing – their own individual patients' operative risk.

The annual number of operations is once again increasing rapidly, with more than 90% of CEAs in the USA currently being performed in non-trial centres. A significant proportion are not evaluated by neurologists and there is an increasing trend towards non-invasive assessment, thereby avoiding the risks (and occasional benefits) of carotid angiography. Perhaps most worrisome is growing evidence in both Europe and North America that the 30-day operative risk of death and/or stroke may be significantly higher than that reported in the international trials and that outcome may, indeed, be related to volume and experience. In parallel with this ongoing debate, there have been further improvements in risk factor management and the emergence of angioplasty as an alternative to CEA.

Thus, surgeons once again find that CEA is facing a potential credibility issue. Many might feel this to be unfair, and possibly even inappropriate, but it is important that surgeons continually review all aspects of their practice in order to remain cognizant of ongoing developments, optimize patient selection, rationalize investigations and ensure that the overall results (especially the initial operative risk) are as good as, if not better than, the randomized trial results.

With the plethora of published information on CEA, one might reasonably ask whether there is a need for another text on the subject. The editors feel that, at a time of increasing CEA frequency and the increasing controversy about outcome, a focused text oriented towards the practical issues of patient selection, investigation, operative management and perioperative care has a clear role. It is our hope that this book will enable colleagues to achieve results equivalent or superior to those achieved in the randomized trials. In choosing the subjects for debate we have tried to anticipate many of the common and not so common decision points that surgeons and trainees will inevitably face and that might influence patient outcome. It is clear that surgeons bear the sole responsibility for patient outcome. Patient selection and especially operative technique are the critical factors in determining success or failure.

This book is based on a series of practical questions, such as 'How should I manage the patient with an infected prosthetic patch?' Each question has been addressed by two clinicians – one from Europe and one from North America – in order to give as balanced and pragmatic a viewpoint as possible. Each was asked to provide supporting published evidence where available as well as relevant details of personal experience. At the conclusion of each chapter, the editors have compiled key points together with a commentary on areas of consensus and ongoing controversy. Because of this format, some duplication is inevitable, but the editors have found the frequent transatlantic similarities in practice to be reassuring and worth documenting. More often than not, however, one of the pair of contributors has tended to concentrate more on the

practical, clinical aspects of the question while the other has focused attention on supportive data. The rationale underlying the inclusion of authors from both Europe and North America was not to highlight potential areas of disagreement but to provide as balanced and representative a viewpoint as possible, so that surgeons from both sides of the Atlantic can understand and benefit from the experience of their transatlantic colleagues.

A Ross Naylor
William C Mackey
2000

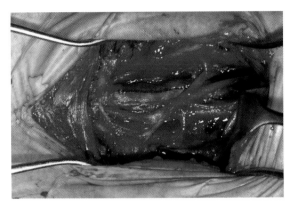

Fig. 17.3
Operative view of a completed endarterectomy in a patient with an abnormal pattern of cranial nerves traversing the bifurcation.

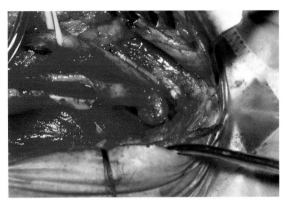

Fig. 24.1
Shunt malfunction can occur due to impaction of the shunt lumen against a distal coil in the internal carotid artery. In this case, the coil was readily exposed and the shunt repositioned but, in the absence of some form of monitoring, this would otherwise pass undetected.

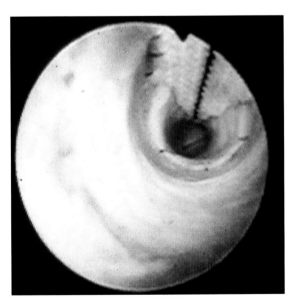

Fig. 24.4
Normal angioscopic examination of the distal endarterectomy zone and internal carotid artery. Reproduced with permission from Lennard *et al.*[30]

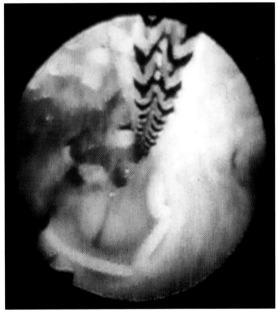

Fig. 24.5
Angioscopy of the proximal intimal step of the common carotid artery. There is an adherent thrombus present: its source was bleeding from an underlying vasa vasorum. The thrombus retrieved in this case is shown in Figure 24.6. Reproduced with permission from Lennard *et al.*[30]

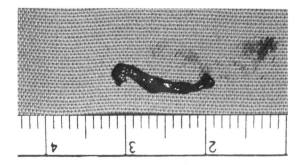

Fig. 24.6
Thrombus retrieved from the proximal common carotid artery intimal step. The angioscopic image is presented in Figure 24.5.

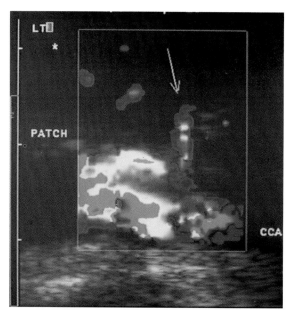

Fig. 30.1
Duplex examination showing a small jet of blood (arrow) into a false aneurysm, suggesting an impending dehiscence of the carotid patch.

Part One

Patient Selection

1.1

The randomized trials for asymptomatic carotid disease: how should they influence my clinical practice?

Peter RD Humphrey (Europe)

INTRODUCTION

The first successful surgical reconstruction of the carotid artery was described in 1954 but, in spite of many interim publications, it took 37 years before the true value of carotid endarterectomy (CEA) was conclusively demonstrated. Thus, 1991 was a landmark year in the management of carotid stenosis with the publication of both the European Carotid Surgery Trial (ECST) and the North American Symptomatic Carotid Endarterectomy Trial (NASCET).[1,2]

THE EUROPEAN CAROTID SURGERY TRIAL

The ECST published data about the risk of stroke in symptomatic patients with mild (0–29%), moderate (30–69%) and severe (70–99%) carotid stenoses. For those with a minor or moderate stenosis, CEA did not confer significant benefit over best medical therapy alone and is not indicated in the treatment of

these patients.[1,3] Figure 1.1 summarizes the annual risk of any major stroke in patients treated by best medical therapy alone relative to the degree of stenosis. As can be seen, the annual risk of stroke in patients with a symptomatic stenosis of 0–49% never exceeds 3%. For those with a 50–69% stenosis, the annual risk of any major stroke does not exceed 5%. Irrespective of the initial degree of stenosis, the annual risk of stroke never exceeds 5% after 3 years of treatment have elapsed.

For the 778 patients randomized in the severe stenosis group, surgery virtually abolished the risk of ipsilateral ischaemic stroke during follow-up. Table 1.1 details the average annual risk of ipsilateral ischaemic stroke following a successful endarterectomy.

Overall, the 3-year risk of stroke in patients with a severe (70–99%) stenosis was 21.9% in medically treated patients and 12.3% in patients treated with

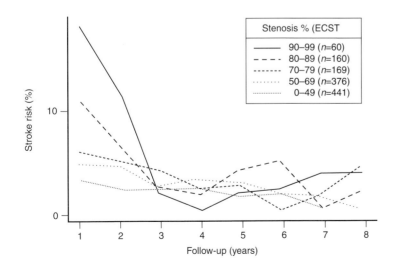

Stroke risk (%) / Follow-up (years)

Stenosis % (ECST
— 90–99 (*n*=60)
– – – 80–89 (*n*=160)
------ 70–79 (*n*=169)
·········· 50–69 (*n*=376)
·········· 0–49 (*n*=441)

Fig 1.1
Risk of any major stroke (first and subsequent) in control patients in the European Carotid Surgery Trial by severity of stenosis and in each of the 8 years after randomization. Adapted from European Carotid Surgery Trialists' Collaborative Group[4] with permission.

3

surgery. This equates to a 9.6% absolute risk reduction and a 56% relative risk reduction. Figure 1.1 and Table 1.2 clearly indicate that the 3-year risk of stroke in symptomatic patients with severe carotid disease is directly related to the degree of stenosis. For patients with a symptomatic stenosis of 90–99% who are treated medically, the risk of stroke is about 18% in the first year, 14% in the second year and 6% in the third year, which gives an approximate 3-year stroke risk of 35%. For those with a 70–79% stenosis, the corresponding figures are 6% in the first year, 6% in the second year and 5% in the third year.

Table 1.1
Average annual risk of ipsilateral ischaemic stroke following successful carotid endarterectomy

Carotid stenosis (%)	Annual risk of ipsilateral ischaemic stroke (%)
0–19	2.6
20–29	2.7
30–39	2.7
40–49	1.9
50–59	1.7
60–69	2.0
70–79	1.9
80–89	1.7
90–99	1.6

Adapted from European Carotid Surgery Trialists' Collaborative Group[4] with permission.

THE NORTH AMERICAN SYMPTOMATIC CAROTID ENDARTERECTOMY TRIAL
The NASCET randomized symptomatic patients with moderate (30–69%) or severe (70–99%) stenoses to receive CEA plus best medical therapy versus best medical therapy alone.[2,5] Overall, CEA was definitely beneficial in symptomatic patients with severe stenoses (Table 1.3). Patients with a moderate stenosis (50–69%) achieved a small but statistically significant benefit, whilst CEA was of no benefit in patients with milder stenosis (30–49%). As was observed in the ECST, the operative risk was lower in patients undergoing CEA for severe internal carotid artery disease (5.8%) as opposed to moderate disease (6.7%). NASCET calculated the degree of stenosis differently from ECST, so that a 85–99% stenosis by ECST was broadly equivalent to an 70–99% stenosis by the NASCET method.

Implications for clinical practice
In practical terms, the ECST and NASCET results mean that for centres with an operative death/any stroke rate <5%, it would probably be reasonable to consider CEA in symptomatic patients with a 70–99% stenosis using the ECST method or a 50–99% stenosis using the NASCET method.[6] For those units with a higher complication rate, CEA should probably be restricted to symptomatic patients with an 80–99% stenosis (ECST) or 70–99% stenosis (NASCET).

TIMING OF SURGERY
Figure 1.1 summarizes the natural history of stroke with respect to the degree of stenosis in the

Table 1.2
Three-year risk of stroke in medically treated patients with a severe carotid stenosis

Carotid stenosis (%)	Annual risk of stroke (%)			Three-year risk (%)
	1st year	2nd year	3rd year	
70–79	6	6	5	17
80–89	11	6	3	20
90–99	18	14	3	35

Adapted from European Carotid Surgery Trialists' Collaborative Group[4] with permission.

Table 1.3
Effect of carotid endarterectomy on reducing stroke or death in the North American Symptomatic Carotid Endarterectomy Trial

Degree of stenosis	Mean follow-up	Stroke/death (surgery)	Stroke/death (medical)	Absolute risk reduction	Relative risk reduction	P
30–49%	5 years	14.9%	18.7%	3.8%	20.3%	0.16
50–69%	5 years	15.7%	22.2%	6.5%	29.8%	0.045
70–99%	2 years	9.0%	26.0%	17%	65.4%	<0.001

Adapted from North American Symptomatic Carotid Endarterectomy Trial Collaborators[2] and Barnett et al.[5] with permission.

medically treated group in the ECST.[4] The 3-year stroke risk for those with a 90–99% stenosis was around 35%, for those with an 80–89% stenosis it was about 20%, while for those with a 70–79% stenosis it was less than 20%. The greatest overall benefit was therefore observed in those patients with the tightest stenoses. However, 3 years after onset of symptoms there is little difference in the natural history risk of stroke between those with 0–49% stenoses and those with 90–99% stenoses. These findings are remarkably similar to those presented in the final NASCET data.[5]

Both trials have also shown that the risk of stroke in patients with an 80–99% stenosis remains high for 1–2 years after their initial presenting symptoms. Although the ECST and NASCET only operated upon patients who presented within 6 months of their most recent symptoms, my personal practice would now be to extend this time period to 12 months.

Thus, patients with transient ischaemic attacks (TIAs) or minor stroke need to be seen, investigated and referred for surgery as soon as possible. This requires rapid clinical assessment and immediate ultrasound, followed by angiography (either digital subtraction angiography or magnetic resonance angiography) if this is deemed appropriate. Any delay beyond 2 weeks should not be accepted, even though this is unfortunately commonplace in the UK.

If the patient has suffered a stroke, it is generally accepted that surgery is probably best delayed for 6 weeks,[7] although this arbitrary time limit is currently under review. It does, however, allow the area of infarction to stabilize (possibly reducing the risk of haemorrhagic transformation); the ischaemic penumbra may be reduced and delay may reduce the risk of perioperative stroke. Any delay must, however, be balanced against the increased risk of stroke that is inevitably present during the first 8 weeks after presentation. The question of early versus delayed CEA is debated elsewhere in this book.

PATIENT SELECTION

Clinical presentation
Emboli may pass into the ipsilateral eye causing amaurosis fugax (transient monocular blindness) or central retinal artery occlusion. If emboli pass into the ipsilateral cerebral hemisphere, then dysphasia, hemiparesis or hemisensory attacks may occur. Sometimes the degree of sensory or motor impairment can be very focal with just the face, foot or fingers being affected. Thus, it may occasionally be difficult to be sure whether one is dealing with a cortical or peripheral nerve event and the input of a specialist neurologist may be important.

The natural history risk of stroke is greatest if there is an ipsilateral localized carotid bruit, increasing frequency of TIAs in the previous 3 months, male sex, coexisting peripheral vascular disease and hemispheric (rather than ocular) TIA.[8] These patients require the most urgent assessment. Carotid stenoses are much more likely to be found in those with combined ocular and hemispheric symptoms and in those with increasing numbers of vascular risk factors. The presence of ulceration and irregularity of the stenosis may also increase the risk of stroke.[9]

It is important to emphasize that, while a localized bruit is the most useful indicator of an underlying stenosis, it is only of predictive value in about 50% of cases.[10,11] Paradoxically, the tightest stenoses often have no bruit. False-positive bruits may occur with moderate degrees of internal carotid stenoses, external carotid stenoses and even with contralateral and ipsilateral carotid occlusions. In the latter situations, the bruit is partly due to increased collateral flow through the remaining patent vessels. As a result, I no longer listen for a bruit when looking for a carotid stenosis. In the presence of carotid territory symptoms, I would perform an immediate Doppler/duplex ultrasound.

Patients who have mild or moderate degrees of stenosis are best treated medically.[3] I see no indication to operate on patients with a stenosis of less than 70%. The natural history for these patients is excellent and symptoms can nearly always be managed medically. Those with a severe stenosis but with a major persisting neurological deficit or with serious comorbidity are probably best treated medically. Fitness for carotid endarterectomy is biological, not chronological. We operate on patients up to their mid-80s if they are fit. The life expectancy at age 80 is approximately 8 years.

Sometimes the patients in the ECST and NASCET are criticized as not being typical of the population in general. In the ECST, each randomizing centre was free to enter patients in their 'grey' area – if the clinician was not sure what to do in that particular situation. For some centres, this may have meant only randomizing those with mild or moderate stenoses, while for some it included all symptomatic patients. The range of patients in both studies therefore crossed all degrees of stenoses and the trial results are as representative as is possible.

Perioperative complications

The risk of stroke or death in the ECST was 7% and in the NASCET, 6%. However, does this transpose to the community in general? The

answer is, unfortunately, no. Whilst those in the ECST and NASCET had 30-day complication rates of 5–7%, those in the Medicare system fared less well.[12]

Wong *et al.* have presented data which suggest that the complication rate in local hospitals exceeded the published data and the accompanying editorial emphasizes the need for independent audit.[13] Furthermore, 20% of patients were felt to have been operated on inappropriately, 33% appropriately and 49% for uncertain reasons. This reinforces my view that the investigation of these patients should be by a multidisciplinary team, preferably with neurological input, even though it is clear that the surgeon performing the operation retains the final decision regarding surgery.

In addition, trials in which the end-points are reported by neurologists tend to have the highest operative complication rates while those from single-author surgeons have the lowest.[14] Series with complication rates of 1% are well described in the literature but, unless they are independently audited, I am afraid the reader must retain some degree of scepticism. It is manifestly obvious, therefore, that all surgeons must quote their *own* complication rate (preferably independently audited), although it is accepted that this may be difficult until sufficient numbers of operations have been performed. The benefit of the surgery is lost if the operative complication rate exceeds 10%. All units should aim for a stroke/death rate of under 5%.

In the ECST the confidence limits for the complication rate after CEA for all of the different participating centres overlapped, except for one. The stroke/death rates varied between 0 and 25%; the number of operations performed in these different centres varied from 1 to 90. This demonstrates how difficult it can be to obtain reliable, statistically valid information from individual surgeons.

Evidence suggests that patients are more likely to suffer a perioperative stroke or death if they are female, aged over 75 years, have systolic hypertension, peripheral vascular disease, occlusion of the contralateral internal carotid artery, stenosis of the ipsilateral external carotid artery, carotid syphon or if the patient has had cerebral events rather than ocular symptoms.[15] There is, however, no consensus about whether coexisting carotid syphon stenosis should alter the management of carotid bifurcation stenosis in the neck. Our policy is usually to proceed with routine carotid endarterectomy.

Thus, the information from the international trials now allows clinicians carefully to advise and plan optimal care with their patients. For example, when discussing the rationale of CEA with my patients, I give them three pieces of information:

1   the predicted natural history risk of stroke over the next 3 years based on their presenting symptoms and degree of stenosis, e.g. a 35% risk of stroke for patients with a hemispheric TIA and a 95% stenosis;
2   the natural history risk of stroke in the next 3 years assuming successful surgery – approximately 5%;
3   the local institution complication rate for carotid endarterectomy; which in our case is 3%.

I then leave the patient to decide what he or she wants to do. Most patients will make up their own minds and it is especially helpful if there is a friend or relative to help them interpret what can otherwise be a bewildering array of statistics. In this respect, it is important to remember that many patients will have a poor recollection of the quoted risks, which could undermine the principle of informed consent.[16] A few ask me what I would do and I usually say that the lower risk is to undergo the operation. I prefer, however, to give patients the options and leave them to decide for themselves. This is what I would want if and when I had to make a decision regarding any surgery for myself. It is how most of us behave when buying a car, house or pension!

HOW BIG IS THE PROBLEM?

Each general practitioner will see, on average, one TIA and four stroke cases each year. Thus, in a population of 200 000, there will be approximately 168 TIAs or non-disabling strokes occurring annually.[17] Of these, only 18 will be found to have a carotid stenosis in excess of 70%. This compares with approximately 1500 people in the same community who will have an asymptomatic carotid stenosis. The risk of inappropriate surgery is clear. In the UK, there is the potential for approximately 5000 carotid endarterectomies for symptomatic disease each year which might be expected to prevent 800 strokes during the next 2 years.

Intuitively, experience and interest must be important factors in obtaining good surgical results. Leaving the carotid endarterectomy site as smooth and clean as possible must be important in preventing emboli forming on the endarterectomy site. In the ECST, the highest complication rate was observed with those surgeons who did the operation quickest (in less than 30 minutes). Thus, it seems that for CEA to be performed with maximum benefit, it should probably be performed in a limited number of designated centres within each region so that each surgeon obtains a minimum of experience (25 cases per surgeon per year seems to me an acceptable number). I appreciate that there are few hard data to support this statement, but all physicians and surgeons know that experience is of paramount importance.

Some have argued that health authorities should not fund carotid endarterectomy, as the overall number of strokes prevented per annum is low in comparison to the annual total number of strokes. However, stroke is a multifactorial illness and no single treatment will have more than a small effect. For example, aspirin reduces the overall incidence of stroke by 1–2% and even treating all hypertensives would only reduce stroke mortality by 15%.[18]

Carotid endarterectomy is of proven value and could reduce the individual's risk of stroke by 70%. What is really needed is for health authorities to fund cost-effective, low-risk carotid endarterectomy. In the UK it is estimated that each operation costs approximately £3000, although there is the additional cost of investigating the other patients who do not require surgery in terms of hospital time and ultrasonography. However, this remains relatively small when compared to the total cost of one stroke, which has been estimated to be of the order of £45 000.[19] Similar calculations have been made in North America.[20]

REFERENCES

1 European Carotid Surgery Trialists' Collaborative Group. MRC European Carotid Surgery Trial: interim results for symptomatic patients with severe (70–99%) or with mild (0–29%) carotid stenosis. *Lancet* 1991; **337**: 1235–1243.

2 North American Symptomatic Carotid Endarterectomy Trial Collaborators. Beneficial effect of carotid endarterectomy in symptomatic patients with high grade carotid stenosis. *New England Journal of Medicine* 1991; **325**: 445–453.

3 European Carotid Surgery Trialists' Collaborative Group. Endarterectomy for moderate symptomatic carotid stenosis: interim results from the MRC European Carotid Surgery Trial. *Lancet* 1996; **347**: 1591–1593.

4 European Carotid Surgery Trialists' Collaborative Group. Randomised trial of endarterectomy for recently symptomatic carotid stenosis: final results of the MRC European Carotid Surgery Trial (ECST). *Lancet* 1998; **351**: 1379–1387.

5 Barnett HJM, Taylor DW, Eliasziw M *et al*. Benefit of carotid endarterectomy in patients with symptomatic moderate or severe stenosis. *New England Journal of Medicine* 1998; **331**: 1415–1425.

6 Donnan GA, Davis SM, Chambers BR, Gates PC. Surgery for prevention of stroke. *Lancet* 1998; **351**: 1372–1373.

7 Pritz MB. Timing of carotid endarterectomy after stroke. *Stroke* 1997; **28**: 2563–2567.

8 Hankey GJ, Slattery JM, Warlow CP. Transient ischaemic attacks: which patients are at high (and low) risk of serious vascular events. *Journal of Neurology, Neurosurgery and Psychiatry* 1992; **55**: 640–652.

9 Rothwell PM, Salinas R, Ferrando LA, Slattery J, Warlow CP. Does the angiographic appearance of a carotid stenosis predict the risk of stroke independently of the degree of stenosis? *Clinical Radiology* 1995; **50**: 830–833.

10 Davies KN, Humphrey PRD. Do carotid bruits predict disease of the internal carotid artery? *Postgraduate Medical Journal* 1994; **70**: 433–435.

11 Mead GE, Wardlaw J, Lewis SC, McDowell M, Dennis MS. Can simple clinical features be used to identify patients with severe carotid stenosis on Doppler ultrasound? *Journal of Neurology, Neurosurgery and Psychiatry* 1999; **66**: 16–19.

12 Stukenborg GJ. Comparison of carotid endarterectomy. Outcomes for randomised controlled trials and Medicare administrative databases. *Archives of Neurology* 1997; **54**: 826–832.

13 Wong JH, Findlay JM, Suarez-Almazor ME. Regional performance of carotid endarterectomy. Appropriateness, outcomes and risk factors for complications. *Stroke* 1997; **28**: 889–898.

14 Rothwell PM, Slattery J, Warlow CP. A systematic review of the risks of stroke and death due to endarterectomy for symptomatic carotid stenosis. *Stroke* 1996; **27**: 260–265.

15 Rothwell PM, Slattery J, Warlow CP. Clinical and angiographic predictors of stroke and death from carotid endarterectomy: systematic review. *British Medical Journal* 1997; **315**: 1571–1577.

16 Lloyd AJ, Hayes PD, London NJM, Bell PRF, Naylor AR. Patients' ability to recall risk associated with treatment options. *Lancet* 1999; **353**: 645.

17 Brown MM, Humphrey PRD on behalf of the Association of British Neurologists. Carotid endarterectomy: recommendations for management of transient ischaemic attack and ischaemic stroke. *British Medical Journal* 1992; **305**: 1071–1074.

18 Dennis M, Warlow C. Strategy for stroke. *British Medical Journal* 1991; **303**: 636–638.

19 Bamford J. The cost of care. Seminar on district stroke services. London: Stroke Association 1993: 5

20 Nussbaum ES, Heros RC, Erickson DL. Cost effectiveness of carotid endarterectomy. *Neurosurgery* 1996; **38**: 237–244.

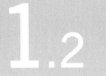

1.2 The randomized trials for symptomatic carotid disease: how should they influence my daily practice?

Wesley S Moore (USA)

RANDOMIZED TRIALS VERSUS RETROSPECTIVE OR COMPARATIVE STUDIES

Beginning in the 1960s, retrospective reviews of results from multiple institutions following carotid endarterectomy were published. Reports from single authors or from centers of excellence described good results with respect to operative stroke morbidity, mortality, and stroke-free survival in relatively small series of patients. It was not clear whether these data would be applicable to the average patient in the community. Furthermore, the critics of carotid endarterectomy were suspicious about the objectivity of these reports since the accuracy of the complication rates was determined by the surgeon reporting the series. For that reason, these retrospective reviews were considered to be relatively low level evidence-based medicine. On the other hand, prospective randomized trials would contain a large number of patients from multiple institutions and multiple surgeons. In addition, patients treated in institutions participating in a prospective randomized trial would be examined by several individuals other than the surgeon performing the operation. For that reason, it was believed that the stroke morbidity and mortality would be more accurately reported. The results of prospective randomized trials are considered to be the highest level of evidence. Therefore, if a surgeon can match the parameters reported in a prospective randomized trial, it is reasonable to assume that indications for operation defined within the context of a trial are appropriate for the individual patient and surgeon.

MEASUREMENT OF CAROTID STENOSIS

It has now been shown that the risk of stroke morbidity and mortality in symptomatic patients will increase as the percentage of stenosis increases. Since the quantitative measurement of the lesion now becomes a critical issue in selecting patients for operation, it is important to discuss the method by which stenosis is calculated. The method of calculating carotid stenosis in North America is quite different from the method used in Europe. A 70% stenosis calculated by the North American method is not the same as a 70% stenosis calculated by the European method. Since prospective randomized trials are being performed in both North America and Europe, and the threshold stenosis for operation is being reported, it is important to recognize the differences in methodology. The North American method has been used in trials beginning with the Extracranial Arterial Occlusive Disease Study of the 1950s and continued with the Veterans' Administration (VA) Asymptomatic Trial, the NASCET trial, and the Asymptomatic Carotid Atherosclerosis Study (ACAS) trial.

The method involves measuring the luminal diameter at the point of tightest stenosis (n) on a contrast angiogram (preferably using cut film) and comparing that to the diameter of the internal carotid artery, distal to the stenosis where the walls of the internal carotid artery become parallel (d). The percent stenosis equals $1 - n/d \times 100$. The calculation of percent stenosis by the European method involves drawing the hypothetical boundaries of the bulb of the internal carotid artery, which is normally considerably larger than the diameter of the distal internal carotid artery. If the bulb of the internal carotid artery is represented by the letter e, then the calculation of percent stenosis is $1 - n/e \times 100$. Because of these differences in measurement, there will be a considerable difference in percent stenosis for the same lesion depending upon whether the European method or the North American method is employed. These differences are most exaggerated at the lower levels of stenosis and become closer as higher percentages of stenosis are reached. These differences are compared in Table 1.4.

Table 1.4
Comparison of carotid stenosis by European and North American methods

European method	North American method
60%	18%
70%	40%
80%	61%
90%	80%

In reviewing the data from Table 1.4, it is apparent that a 70% stenosis in the European method is only a 40% stenosis by the North American method. The importance of these differences will become apparent as we review the results of the North American and European trials.

A report in which symptomatic carotid stenoses in 1001 patients were measured by three different methods, including the European and North American techniques, has been published. The same stenoses, measured by the European method, indicated severe stenosis twice as often as by the North American method.[21]

THE NORTH AMERICAN SYMPTOMATIC CAROTID ENDARTERECTOMY TRIAL

The NASCET study was designed to test the hypothesis that symptomatic patients (hemisphere or monocular TIA or prior mild stroke) with ipsilateral carotid stenosis (30–99% as measured by the North American method) will have fewer fatal and non-fatal strokes following carotid endarterectomy plus best medical management than patients treated with medical management alone, including aspirin. It was planned to enter 3000 patients into a prospective randomized trial and follow them for a period of 5 years. The patients were to be stratified into severe

(70–99%) stenosis and those with moderate (30–69%) stenosis. On 25 February 1991, a clinical alert was issued by the Oversight Committee of the National Institutes of Health indicating that an end-point had been reached in the severe stenosis category (70–99%) in favor of carotid endarterectomy, and that portion of the study was stopped. No end-point had been reached in the 30–69% group, and that portion of the study was to continue. The initial results were published shortly thereafter.[22]

The trial was conducted in 50 clinical centers in the USA and Canada. A total of 659 patients with 70–99% stenoses who had experienced hemispheric or retinal TIA or a non-disabling stroke within 120 days of entry were randomized. All patients received optimum medical therapy, including antiplatelet drugs. Those randomized to surgical treatment underwent carotid endarterectomy. All patients were examined by neurologists at 1, 3, 6, 9, and 12 months following entry, and then every 4 months thereafter.

Life table estimates of cumulative risk of any ipsilateral stroke at 2 years were 26% in 331 patients randomized to medical management, and 9.0% in 328 patients randomized to surgery (including the perioperative surgical risk). This is an absolute risk reduction in favor of surgery of 17%, and a relative risk reduction of 71%. There was also a corresponding lowered mortality rate in the two groups from 12% in the medical group to 5.0% in the surgical group. This was a statistically significant mortality risk reduction of 58% in favor of carotid endarterectomy. This benefit was made possible, in part, by a relatively low risk of operation. Thus, the 30-day neurologic morbidity and mortality in the surgical group was 5.8%. It was also noted that the risk of neurologic morbidity and mortality in the medical group increased with each decile percent stenosis between 70 and 99%. It was further noted that retinal TIAs had a less grave prognosis than hemispheric TIAs in the medical control group. In 59 patients entering NASCET with retinal TIA and randomized to medicine, the likelihood of ipsilateral stroke at 2 years was 17%, in contrast to the 70 patients with hemispheric TIA, in whom the likelihood of stroke at 2 years was 44%.

It was also noted that the presence of a contralateral

occlusion significantly worsened the prognosis of patients in the medical group. At 2-year follow-up, 54.6% of patients with contralateral occlusion and ipsilateral stenosis randomized to medicine experienced stroke or death, compared with 20% in the surgical group.[23] Patients entered in the study with a diagnosis of TIA but who were found to have an infarct on computed tomographic scan had an increased likelihood of ipsilateral stroke during the follow-up. Patients without silent brain infarction had a 13% risk of stroke during follow-up, in contrast to those with silent brain infarction, who had a risk of 26%. In a subsequent publication, the NASCET investigators also noted that the presence of plaque ulceration on arteriography significantly altered the prognosis.

The risk of ipsilateral stroke at 24 months in medically treated patients with ulcerated plaques increased in increments from 26.3% to 73.2% as the degree of stenosis increased from 70% to 99%. Interestingly, for patients without ulceration, the risk of stroke remained constant at 21.3% for all percentages of stenosis. In contrast, the risk of operation in patients with and without ulceration was not significantly altered. Therefore, surgery had an even greater benefit for patients with ulceration as well as benefiting those with smooth stenoses.[24]

In February 1998, at the Joint Conference on Stroke and Cerebral Circulation, the NASCET investigators reported their results with the 30–69% stenosis category. They concluded that, in the 50–69% subset stenosis category, the patients treated with surgery plus best medical management had a better 5-year outcome than those patients treated medically alone. While the difference was statistically significant, it was not as dramatic as in the higher-grade stenosis category. In addition, surgical morbidity and mortality were higher, at 6.7%. This continues to follow the pattern illustrating that the higher the percentage of stenosis, the greater the risk with medical management and the greater the benefit with surgical management.

THE MEDICAL RESEARCH COUNCIL SYMPTOMATIC EUROPEAN CAROTID SURGERY TRIAL

Beginning in 1981, a prospective randomized trial was initiated under the auspices of the Medical Research Council of Great Britain. Eighty centers in 14 European countries were involved. A total of 2518 patients were entered into the study after a carotid territory non-disabling ischemic stroke, hemispheric TIA, or a retinal infarction in which a carotid lesion was identified. The study was stratified into three subsets as a function of percent stenosis: 0–29%, 30–69%, and 70–99%. These percent stenoses were measured by the European method.

In 1991, the investigators reported their preliminary results, corresponding with the results reported from the North American trial. For 374 patients with mild (0–29%) stenosis, the 3-year risk of ipsilateral stroke in the absence of surgery was quite small, and the authors concluded that surgery was not indicated. For the 778 patients with severe (70–99%) stenosis, the benefits were clearly in favor of operation. In spite of a 7.5% 30-day surgical morbidity and mortality, there was a sixfold reduction of ipsilateral stroke in patients treated by carotid endarterectomy. After 3 years of follow-up, the total risk of surgical death, surgical stroke, and ipsilateral stroke or any other stroke was 12.3% in the surgical group and 21.9% in the medical group. This difference was statistically significant, with a P value of 0.01.

In 1996, the European Trialists reported their results with the intermediate (30–69%) carotid stenosis group. They found no benefit of carotid endarterectomy over medical management in this group of patients as measured by the European method.[26] Once again, it should be pointed out that a 69% stenosis as measured by the European method is <40% as measured by the North American method. Likewise, the lower decile of the high-grade stenosis category in the European group, 70%, is equivalent to a 40% stenosis as measured by the North American method.

THE VETERANS' ADMINISTRATION COOPERATIVE STUDY FOR CAROTID ENDARTERECTOMY IN PATIENTS WITH SYMPTOMATIC CAROTID STENOSIS

In 1986, planning for the VA trial was begun. Thirteen VA medical centers were selected to participate. Patients with symptomatic carotid artery disease who had a 50% or greater stenosis were randomized to carotid endarterectomy plus best medical management versus best medical management alone. The study was halted when the results of the North American and European trials were reported. None the less, the results were consistent with those reported in other major trials. In this study, 193 patients were randomized. After a mean follow-up of 11.9 months, the end-points of ipsilateral stroke or crescendo TIA were 7.7% in the surgery group and 19.4% in the medical group. This difference was statistically significant, at a *P* value of 0.01. It is also of interest that the benefit of surgery, in retrospect, became apparent after only 2 months of randomization. The 30-day perioperative neurologic morbidity was 2.2% and mortality 3.3%, giving a cumulative neurologic morbidity/mortality of 5.5%.[27]

PATIENT SELECTION BASED ON SURGICAL MORBIDITY, MORTALITY, AND ANTICIPATED LONGEVITY

The North American trial, the European trial, and the Veterans Affairs trial, have conclusively demonstrated that patients with 50% carotid stenosis or greater, as measured by the North American method, and having symptoms of hemispheric TIA, retinal TIA, or non-disabling stroke, do significantly better with carotid endarterectomy and medical management than with medical management alone. However, it must be kept in mind that the parameters defined within these studies must be adhered to. The 30-day perioperative neurologic morbidity/mortality in the North American trial ranged from 5.8% to 6.7%; for the European trial it was 7.5%, and for the Veterans Affairs trial it was 5.5%. This is consistent with prior recommendations made by a committee of the American Heart Association in which it was stated that, for the indication of prior stroke, the perioperative neurologic morbidity and mortality

must be 7.0% or less and that the 30-day perioperative neurologic morbidity/mortality for the indication TIA should be 5.0% or less.[28] If an individual surgeon decides to recommend carotid endarterectomy for a specific patient, the surgeon must be able to demonstrate that his or her own personal statistics fit within those parameters.

Patient admission to the randomized trials depended on the patient being in a reasonable state of health, suggesting that the patient's longevity would be from 3 to 5 years or greater. Clearly, if a patient has major comorbidity, that would place that individual at increased risk for morbidity and mortality within the 30-day perioperative interval or would make it less likely for the individual to live long enough to benefit from the results of operation, and this must be taken into consideration. Finally, it should also be noted that it is possible to subcategorize patients depending upon the nature of their symptoms and the lesion. Since patients with retinal TIAs have a better prognosis than those with hemispheric TIA or stroke, this must be considered when balancing the risk/benefit ratio depending upon other associated comorbidity and individual surgeon's risk for operation. Likewise, contralateral carotid occlusion, evidence of ulceration by angiography, and the presence of silent brain infarction on computed tomographic scan all worsen the prognosis of patients treated medically. Therefore, the presence of one or more of these factors would weigh in favor of carotid endarterectomy in spite of increasing comorbidity.

Finally, the definitive information provided by the highest level of medical evidence, the prospective randomized trial, has once and for all closed the controversy concerning the efficacy of carotid endarterectomy that existed in the 1980s, when the best level of evidence was a retrospective review. While the retrospective data suggested that carotid endarterectomy was beneficial for symptomatic patients, it remained for a scientific study to prove it.

REFERENCES

21 Rothwell PM, Gibson RJ, Slattery J, Sellar RJ, Warlow CP. Equivalents of measurements of carotid stenosis. A comparison of three methods on 1001 angiograms.

European Surgery Trialists Collaborative Group. *Stroke* 1994; **25**: 2435–2439.
22 North American Symptomatic Carotid Endarterectomy Trial

Collaborators. Beneficial effect of carotid endarterectomy in symptomatic patients with high-grade carotid stenosis. *New England Journal of Medicine* 1991; **325**: 445–453.

23 Barnett HJM. Prospective randomized trial of symptomatic patients: results from the NASCET study. In: Moore WS (ed.) *Surgery for Cerebrovascular Disease*, 2nd edn, ch. 74, pp. 537–539. WB Saunders, 1996.

24 Eliasziw M, Streifler JY, Fox AJ, Hachinski VC, Ferguson GG, Barnett HJM. Significance of plaque ulceration in symptomatic patients with high-grade carotid stenosis. North American Symptomatic Carotid Endarterectomy Trial. *Stroke* 1994; **25**: 304–308.

25 European Carotid Surgery Trialists' Collaborative Group. MRC European Carotid Surgery Trial: interim results for symptomatic patients with severe (70–99%) or with mild (0–29%) carotid stenosis. *Lancet* 1991; **337**: 1235–1243.

26 European Carotid Surgery Trialists' Collaborative Group. Endarterectomy for moderate symptomatic carotid stenosis: interim results from the MRC European carotid surgery trial. *Lancet* 1996; **347**: 1591–1593.

27 Mayberg MR, Wilson SE, Yatsu F *et al*. Carotid endarterectomy and prevention of cerebral ischemia in symptomatic carotid stenosis. Veterans Affairs Cooperative Studies Program 309 Trialists Group. *Journal of the American Medical Association* 1991; **266**: 3289–3294.

28 Beebe HG, Clagett GP, DeWeese JA *et al*. Assessing risk associated with carotid endarterectomy: a statement for health professionals by an ad hoc committee on carotid surgery standards of the Stroke Council, American Heart Association. *Stroke* 1989; **20**: 314–315; *Circulation* 1989; **79**: 472–473.

1.3 Editorial Comment

KEY POINTS

1 Carotid endarterectomy is of proven value in stroke prevention in selected symptomatic patients.
2 Long-term benefits are inextricably linked to initial operative risk. All surgeons should quote their individual risk, and preferably this should be independently audited.
3 In selecting patients for CEA, surgeons must consider both perioperative risk and anticipated longevity/stroke risk.

Both authors comment on the high level of reliability attributable to randomized clinical trials and their preference for practicing truly evidence-based medicine when making decisions on operative candidacy. Based on the randomized trials for symptomatic carotid disease, there is consensus that patients with hemispheric TIAs, TMB (temporary monocular blindness), or minor stroke with good recovery and with 70% or greater carotid stenosis (by either North American or European criteria) will benefit from surgery with an absolute stroke risk reduction of 17% at 2 years (NASCET) or approximately 10% at 3 years (ECST). In addition, more recent data from NASCET reveal a significant but less impressive benefit for surgery in those with 50–69% stenosis (by North American criteria), while in the ECST there was no benefit for surgery in those with less than 70% stenosis (by European criteria). This difference in findings for the moderate stenosis group is easily explained, as pointed out by both authors, by the difference in the North American and European methods of determininig degree of stenosis, whereby a 70% stenosis by the European method is equivalent to a 40% stenosis by the North American method.

Obviously, as both authors point out, the benefit of endarterectomy depends on maintaining low perioperative stroke morbidity and mortality rates. In addition, the anticipated longevity of the patient must be sufficient so that significant benefit can accrue. Furthermore, the benefit of surgery depends on a hierarchy of risk within medically managed patients. With medical management, stroke risk increased with degree of stenosis, especially in those with ulcerated plaques, with hemispheric as opposed to ocular events, with contralateral occlusion, and with silent infarction on computed tomographic scan. Surgery may impart greater benefit in these settings, despite a slightly higher perioperative risk in some of these subgroups. Similarly, there is a hierarchy of surgical risk that must be considered. Patients with severe inoperable coronary disease, cardiomyopathy, recent significant stroke, and uncontrolled hypertension, may best be managed medically when surgical risk is extreme.

Given the apparently differing conclusions regarding the threshold stenosis for surgery, the following guidelines might apply. For those centers with a perioperative death/stroke rate of <5%, it would be reasonable to consider CEA for symptomatic patients with 70–99% stenosis (ECST) or 50–99% stenosis (NASCET). For those centers where the operative risk is 5–7%, it would be preferable to limit CEA to symptomatic patients with a stenosis in excess of 80% (ECST) or 70% (NASCET). Those centers with an operative risk in excess of 7% should review their patient selection and operative technique.

2.1

The randomized trials for asymptomatic carotid disease: how should they influence my clinical practice?

Dafydd Thomas (Europe)

INTRODUCTION

Results from large multicentre trials may be useful for providing guidelines for general provision of care but they may be less helpful in guiding the management of individual patients.

In the 1980s there was growing concern about the appropriateness of carotid endarterectomy (CEA), particularly in the USA where >100 000 operations were being performed without any clear-cut evidence of benefit from randomized trials. As a consequence of the publication of the results of the North American Symptomatic Carotid Endarterectomy Trial (NASCET), the European Carotid Surgery Trial (ECST) and the Asymptomatic Carotid Atherosclerosis Study (ACAS),[1–4] the number of CEAs performed annually in the USA is now nearing 150 000. One-third of these are currently in patients with asymptomatic disease.

Evidence suggests that at least five symptomatic patients must undergo CEA in order to prevent one stroke. This unsatisfactory state of affairs, where 80% of patients essentially undergo an unnecessary operation, needs to be improved by better patient selection. Similarly (and perhaps more worryingly), the ACAS trial suggests that > 20 asymptomatic patients require an operation to prevent one stroke. The results from the existing trials are therefore not sufficiently convincing to base the whole of the future management of asymptomatic carotid disease upon them.

WHAT IS ASYMPTOMATIC?

Definitions vary. Some would only regard a patient as asymptomatic if he or she had described no cerebral ischaemic symptoms at all and was thereafter found to have a severe carotid stenosis at routine screening. Others might wish to include only patients without any central nervous system symptoms or, more specifically, patients with symptoms that were not attributable to the anterior (carotid) cerebral circulation. Perhaps the most appropriate definition, particularly from the clinical trial viewpoint, would be one that included only patients with no symptoms directly referable to the carotid stenosis of interest.

However, time is also an important consideration. All of the symptomatic trials define patients as being symptomatic if they suffered their last ischaemic event within the last 6 months. Should patients whose most recent event was > 6 months be considered symptomatic or currently asymptomatic?

ARE SYMPTOMS A GOOD GUIDE?

There is increasing concern that a patient's ability to recall a transient ischaemic attack (TIA) or stroke (especially fleeting events) may be a rather poor guide to disease activity. Only 20% of the brain is clinically evocative, i.e. visual, sensory and motor areas will give symptoms if temporarily disturbed. The remaining 80% of the clinically silent brain may not. Furthermore, when one also considers that approximately one-third of life is spent asleep, only 13% of all cerebral ischaemic attacks are likely to be labelled as being symptomatic and 87% will go undetected.

Increasing experience with magnetic resonance imaging (MRI) scanning of the brain has confirmed that there is underreporting of cerebral injury in high-risk patients. MRI is considerably better than computed tomographic (CT) scanning in identifying intracranial ischaemic disease. Not only does it show lesions, but very often it will give some guide to the underlying aetiology. For example, small deeply situated high signal areas are much more likely to be due to small-vessel intracranial disease secondary to hypertension, hyperlipidaemia and diabetes as opposed to thromboembolism. However, cortical infarcts are much more likely to be due to thromboembolic disease. Not only are symptoms a poor guide at initial assessment but they are also a poor guide at predicting new events during follow-up.

Therefore, should a patient with a severe stenosis and no clinical history of symptoms (but who has cortical infarcts of likely thromboembolic origin) be regarded in the same context as a similar patient with a normal MRI scan? Is CEA more or less important in asymptomatic patients with coexistent small-vessel intracranial disease? These important questions remain unanswered.

Similarly, recent advances in transcranial Doppler (TCD) ultrasound now enable us to look for the first time at the potential importance of silent emboli and intracranial flow patterns. The latter may be very relevant when trying to disentangle the pathophysiology in a patient with significant carotid artery disease who presents with symptoms suggestive of a vertebrobasilar aetiology. TCD may, for example, demonstrate flow reversal in the circle of Willis so that the carotid inflow supplies flow through the communicating arteries to the posterior cerebral arteries. In such a patient, occipital lobe symptoms with hemianopic changes are likely to be due to the carotid disease rather than any vertebrobasilar pathology, i.e. the carotid stenoses may not be asymptomatic in this situation.

THE ASYMPTOMATIC CAROTID SURGERY TRIALS

The Veterans' Administration study
The Veterans' Administration (VA) study[5] was performed in a high-risk vascular group of > 400 patients who were predominantly male and heavy smokers. Surgery was of some benefit in reducing the risk of TIA and stroke but the overall value of surgery was lessened somewhat by late deaths, particularly from other vascular disease and myocardial infarction. However, two very important lessons came from this study. First, the carotid artery should not be considered in isolation and, in particular, greater care must be taken in optimizing the management of ischaemic heart disease. Second, patients with a poor general prognosis should not undergo CEA.

The Asymptomatic Carotid Atherosclerosis Study
ACAS was an excellent study for its time – although it is now somewhat out of date – and was based on outcome in 1600 patients with a stenosis in excess of 60%.[4] Overall, the aggregate risk of stroke or death in surgical patients was 5.1% as compared with 11% in medical patients. This equates to a 50% relative risk reduction but only a 5.9% absolute risk reduction. Put another way, CEA reduced the absolute risk of stroke by about 1% per annum.

However, CEA did not prevent disabling stroke and there was little benefit in women. Perhaps most surprisingly, unlike the ECST and NASCET, an inverse correlation was demonstrated between stenosis severity and stroke risk in medically treated patients (Table 2.1). Similarly, there was no association between stroke risk and the number of coexistent risk factors. In NASCET, there was a strong association between the number of risk factors and the incidence of late stroke in symptomatic patients who were treated by optimal

Table 2.1	
5-year stroke risk relative to the degree of stenosis in Asymptomatic Carotid Atherosclerosis Study	
Degree of stenosis	5-year stroke risk
60–69%	11.4%
70–79%	6.7%
80–99%	3.7%

Adapted from Executive Committee for the Asymptomatic Carotid Atherosclerosis Study[4] and Barnett et al.[6] with permission.

medical therapy. A similar, but less dramatic, association was demonstrated in the non-operated (asymptomatic) carotid artery.[1,6] Although one would intuitively have expected a similar trend to be apparent in ACAS, no such data were forthcoming. This is an important area of study for the future as the presence of coexistent risk factors may militate towards surgery in some patients and against surgery in others.

Unfortunately, duplex scanning was not generally available while the study was being performed and most of the ultrasound data were derived from Doppler waveform analysis. Moreover, because the risk of ipsilateral stroke was judged to be lower in asymptomatic patients as opposed to symptomatic patients (3% per annum compared with 5%), strict controls were maintained on the selection of surgeons on the basis of proven low mortality and morbidity rates. Questions therefore remain as to the appropriateness of translating these extremely good results into routine clinical practice.

The ACAS results also have significant clinical and cost-effectiveness implications. Following release of the ACAS alert, there was a 64% increase in the number of CEAs performed in Florida: the additional cost amounting to US$56 million per year.[7] If the findings of ACAS were to be applied uncritically, evidence from Australia suggests that such a policy would prevent only 3% of all strokes,[8] while costing about A$1.5 million per stroke prevented. Moreover, most studies suggest that screening for an asymptomatic stenosis is probably not cost-effective[9,10] and evidence suggests that at least 10 000 patients would have to be screened, with a 20% predicted prevalence of finding a stenosis > 60%, in order to prevent 100 strokes.[11] When the costs of CEA and screening are taken into context with the overall number of strokes prevented, some national bodies have strongly recommended that CEA for asymptomatic disease should not be performed.[12]

Evidence from other trials
Benavente et al.[13] have recently performed an overview of the five randomized trials of patients with an asymptomatic stenosis in excess of 50%. This has again shown a small but significant benefit in favour of CEA but the absolute risk reduction was 2% over 3 years. It should be noted, however, that the stenosis threshold was 50% and it will be more relevant to repeat this meta-analysis in those with more severe disease once the ongoing European Asymptomatic Carotid Surgery Trial has reported its findings.

Further evidence to improve the management of patients with asymptomatic disease has come from ECST and NASCET.[1,14] In the ECST, the risk of stroke in the non-operated asymptomatic hemisphere has been investigated and it appears that there is no significant risk unless the stenosis exceeds 90% and is in combination with other risk factors such as hypertension.[14] In this situation, the annual risk of ipsilateral stroke is approximately 5% (14% over 3 years). The NASCET study also showed that the risk of stroke increased with the degree of stenosis, but that the operative risk approximately doubled if the contralateral artery was occluded. This is an important observation because patients are commonly found to have an asymptomatic severe stenosis and a contralateral occlusion.

The Asymptomatic Carotid Surgery Trial
In the light of many of these problems, the Medical Research Council and the UK Stroke Association have supported a further trial into the role of CEA in patients with asymptomatic disease (the Asymptomatic Carotid Surgery Trial (ACST)). In this study, good-quality duplex as well as Doppler is employed, and this will facilitate plaque characterization and the identification of high-risk subgroups for both perioperative stroke and late stroke. To date, more than 2000 patients have been randomized and recruitment continues.

PROPHYLACTIC CEA AND MAJOR SURGERY
There continues to be considerable uncertainty about the place of prophylactic CEA before cardiac surgery. To date, there is no evidence that CEA should be performed before any other major procedures such as aortic aneurysm repair unless the carotid artery stenosis is symptomatic. In that extremely rare situation, careful deliberation about the merits and risks of a synchronous procedure should be made.

However, although there has been a gratifying reduction in the risk of perioperative cerebral injury following cardiac surgery through the use of pulsatile bypass and improved filtration techniques, there is still an important minority of patients who will suffer major postoperative neurological and cognitive problems. A proportion of these patients will have significant extracranial carotid artery disease. The haemodynamic benefit offered by prophylactic CEA is attractive but as yet unproven in randomized trials. A large trial was recently proposed but funding has not been forthcoming, possibly because of the considerable cardiological interest in carotid angioplasty. The exact risks of carotid angioplasty, with or without stenting, in this context are unknown and the durability of such procedures is open to question. Trial evidence is badly needed.

CONCLUSIONS

In summary, therefore, the available trials suggest that CEA may be associated with a small but significant benefit which amounts to an actual risk reduction of 1% per annum. There is no evidence that CEA prevents late disabling stroke in currently asymptomatic patients. The benefit is, however, inextricably linked to the initial operative risk and disappears if the 30-day risk of death or stroke exceeds 4%. At present, therefore, there is no compelling clinical or cost-based evidence for translating the ACAS results into routine clinical practice and, where possible, patients should be entered into the ACST. Otherwise, asymptomatic patients with a stenosis >90% might be considered for CEA if their general prognosis is good and if the predicted operative risk is less than 3%, particularly if there is CT or MRI evidence of silent infarction or transcranial Doppler evidence of ongoing embolization.

REFERENCES

1 North American Symptomatic Carotid Endarterectomy Trial Collaborators. Beneficial effect of carotid endarterectomy in symptomatic patients with high grade stenosis. *New England Journal of Medicine* 1991; **325**: 445–453.
2 European Carotid Surgery Trialists' Collaborative Group. MRC European Carotid Surgery Trial: interim results for symptomatic patients with severe (70–99%) or with mild (0–29%) stenosis. *Lancet* 1991; **337**: 1235–1241.
3 European Carotid Surgery Trialists' Collaborative Group. Randomised trial of endarterectomy for recently symptomatic carotid stenosis: final results of the MRC European Carotid Surgery Trial (ECST). *Lancet* 1998; **351**: 1379–1387.
4 Executive Committee for the Asymptomatic Carotid Atherosclerosis Study. Endarterectomy for asymptomatic carotid artery stenosis. *Journal of the American Medical Association* 1995; **273**: 1421–1428.
5 Hobson RW, Weiss DG, Fields WS. Veterans' Administration Co-operative Study group. Efficacy of carotid endarterectomy for asymptomatic carotid stenosis. *New England Journal of Medicine* 1993; **328**: 221–227.
6 Barnett HJM, Eliasziw M, Meldrum HE, Taylor DW. Do the facts and figures warrant a tenfold increase in the performance of carotid endarterectomy in asymptomatic patients? *Neurology* 1996; **466**: 603–608.
7 Huber TS, Wheeler KG, Cuddeback JK, Dame DA, Flynn TC, Seeger JM. Effect of the Asymptomatic Carotid Atherosclerosis Study on carotid endarterectomy in Florida. *Stroke* 1998; **29**: 1099–1105.
8 Hankey GJ. Asymptomatic carotid stenosis: how should it be managed? *Medical Journal of Australia* 1995; **163**: 197–200.
9 Yin D, Carpenter JP. Cost-effectiveness of screening for asymptomatic carotid stenosis. *Journal of Vascular Surgery* 1998; **27**: 245–255.
10 Lee TT, Solomon NA, Heidenreich PA, Oehlert J, Garber AM. Cost-effectiveness of screening for carotid stenosis in asymptomatic persons. *Annals of Internal Medicine* 1997; **126**: 337–346.
11 Whitty CJM, Sudlow CLM, Warlow CP. Investigating individual subjects and screening populations for asymptomatic carotid stenosis can be harmful. *Journal of Neurology Neurosurgery and Psychiatry* 1998; **64**: 619–623.
12 Perry JR, Szalai JP, Norris JW for the Canadian Stroke Consortium. Consensus against both endarterectomy and routine screening for asymptomatic carotid artery stenosis. *Archives of Neurology* 1997; **54**: 25–28.
13 Benavente O, Moher D, Pham B. Carotid endarterectomy for asymptomatic carotid stenosis: a meta-analysis. *British Medical Journal* 1998; **317**: 1477–1480.
14 Rothwell PM, Slattery J, Warlow CP. A systematic comparison of the risks of stroke and death due to carotid endarterectomy for symptomatic and asymptomatic stenosis. *Stroke* 1996; **27**: 266–269.

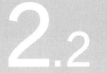

2.2

The randomized trials for asymptomatic carotid disease: how should they influence my clinical practice?

Jerry Goldstone (USA)

As recently as 1985, the indications for performing carotid edarterectomy were generally accepted to be the following;

1 Hemispheric TIAs;
2 Transient monocular visual loss (amaurosis fugax);
3 Vertebrobasilar insufficiency;
4 Global hypoperfusion;
5 Stroke with minimal residual deficit;
6 Lesion or lesion combination predisposing to stroke.

This last indication was, of course, a euphemism for asymptomatic carotid stenosis. Non-stenotic but severely ulcerated carotid bifurcation plaques in both symptomatic and asymptomatic patients were also considered appropriate lesions for surgical treatment by many prominent surgeons. At that time, the evaluation of virtually every patient who was considered a candidate for carotid endarterectomy included conventional angiography, but there were no standards for measuring either percent diameter or percent cross-sectional area reduction. It was widely held that a 50% diameter reduction represented a hemodynamically and therefore clinically significant lesion predisposing to stroke, which was therefore appropriate for surgical removal. In addition, many, if not most, surgeons accepted the premise that the risk of intraoperative hypotension in the presence of carotid stenosis was a particularly dangerous combination. As a result, asymptomatic carotid lesions were looked for and prophylactically repaired in patients scheduled for abdominal aortic or cardiac surgical procedures. With these indications, by 1985, carotid endarterectomy had become the most commonly performed peripheral vascular operation in the USA: over 107 000 were performed in non-federal USA hospitals in that year.[15]

This large and steadily increasing number of operations did not escape the notice of many leading neurologists. Articles began to appear in the literature questioning the safety and efficacy of carotid operations in general and particularly for patients with no symptoms. Several important publications pointed out potential flaws in the thinking that underpinned the generally accepted indications for recommending carotid surgery. First among these was the report of the extracranial to intracranial artery bypass study.[16] In this multi-institutional, randomized, prospective clinical trial, patients with cerebrovascular symptoms and anatomy unsuitable for standard carotid endarterectomy were randomized to receive either an extracranial–intracranial bypass or no surgical treatment at all. In spite of an extremely high technical success rate of this new and sophisticated procedure, there was no statistically significant benefit derived from the operation, contrary to the results of many previously published individual or institutional series. This led several leading neurologists to wonder whether the same might be true for carotid endarterectomy, a popular procedure supported by large numbers of retrospective studies but not subjected to a rigorous, contemporarily designed randomized prospective clinical trial.

The second important publication in this regard was the review by Brott and Thalinger of all carotid endarterectomies performed in Cincinnati, Ohio, in 1984.[17] They found a surprisingly high 9.5% morbidity and mortality, and argued that these

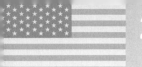

results were likely to be typical of those found in hospitals across the country and, if so, would negate any benefit derived from surgical treatment of carotid bifurcation lesions. Concerns such as these led to the design, initiation, and ultimately the completion of several randomized prospective clinical trials in both symptomatic and asympatomatic patients, comparing carotid endarterectomy with best available medical therapy. These trials were designed to determine whether carotid endarterectomy was as good at stroke prevention as most surgeons believed. The seven major trials conducted in North America and Europe included three in symptomatic patients and four in asymptomatic patients. All of the trials were multicenter, prospective, and randomized but each employed different inclusion and exclusion criteria, different methods for determining the degree of carotid stenosis, and different methods of reporting results. In spite of these differences, there has been substantial agreement about the important outcomes of all of the symptomatic trials and in two of the three asymptomatic trials that have so far been reported. A fourth asymptomatic trial is still ongoing.

The first of the asymptomatic carotid surgery trials to be published was that of the Casanova study group (Carotid Artery Surgery Asymptomatic Narrowing operation vs Aspirin), a European trial directed by AC Diener of Germany which enrolled patients with asymptomatic internal carotid diameter reductions of 50–90%, as determined by angiography.[18] Patients with stenosis > 90% were deemed unsuitable for randomization because of the severity of stenosis and were therefore excluded from randomization and preferentially operated upon. All patients received 330 mg aspirin plus 225 mg dipyridamole per day. A total of 410 patients were randomized and followed for an average of 43 months. With a 6.9% perioperative stroke and death rate in the surgically treated patients, no significant differences were found between the surgical and non-surgical groups after a median follow-up of 42 months (Table 2.2). This led the authors to conclude that endarterectomy was not appropriate for symptom-free patients with internal carotid stenosis < 90%. However, there were serious methodologic flaws in the design of this trial, including the exclusion of patients with the most severe degrees of stenosis (> 90%) and the large number of cross-overs from medical to surgical treatment (118/206, 57%); the events leading to the cross-over were not considered as end-points. Thus, most of the patients in this trial actually underwent endarterectomy. These, and other methodologic problems have caused this trial to be severely criticized and its results have not had a significant impact on clinical care.

The Department of Veterans' Administration ACST,

Table 2.2
Randomized trials of carotid endarterectomy in asymptomatic patients

	CASANOVA[18]	VAACET[19]	ACAS[20]
Patients	410	444	1662
Perioperative stroke/death (%)	6.9	4.3	2.3
Average follow-up (months)	42	48	30
End-points: surgical (%)	10.7	8.0	5.1
End-points: medical (%)	11.3	20.6	11.0
Absolute risk reduction	0.6	12.6	5.9
Relative risk reduction	5.3	38	53

CASANOVA, Carotid Artery Surgery Asymptomatic Narrowing operation vs Aspirin; VAACET Veterans Administration Asymptomatic Control Endarterectomy Trial; ACAS Asymptomatic Carotid Atherosclerosis Study under the direction of Dr Robert W Hobson, was published in 1993, although the trial began in 1982.[19] This trial enrolled 444 men with carotid stenosis > 50% diameter reduction as determined by angiography. All received aspirin 1300 mg/day and were followed for an average of 60 months. Study end-points were hemispheric TIAs (transient monocular blindness) or stroke. The perioperative stroke and death rate was 4.3% and there was a statistically significant reduction in the combined neurologic outcomes of TIA and stroke in the surgical group (8.0%) compared with the medical group (20.6%) (Table 2.2). However, when strokes alone were analyzed, even though the surgically treated group suffered only 50% of the strokes in comparison to the medically treated group (4.7% vs 9.4%), the difference was not statistically significant. This was probably due to the relatively small sample size of this study. Furthermore, when stroke and death were analyzed together, there were virtually no differences in the medically and surgically treated groups. For these reasons, this study has been controversial and not universally accepted as the basis for clinical decision-making.

The third and most recently published study in symptom-free patients was ACAS, which was organized and directed by Dr James Toole.[20] ACAS was a much larger trial than the others: 1662 patients were randomized. All had ≥60% reduction in diameter of the internal carotid artery and all received 325 mg aspirin in addition to risk factor modification counseling. The stenosis was determined by either duplex ultrasound or arteriography, or both, but arteriography was only required in patients selected for endarterectomy. Primary end-points were ipsilateral TIA, stroke, or any perioperative stroke or death. After a median follow-up of 2.7 years, the actuarial risk over 5 years for ipsilateral stroke and any stroke or death was 5.1% for the surgically treated patients and 11% for patients treated medically (Table 2.2). This 5.9% absolute and 53% relative risk reduction was highly statistically significant.

One of the most striking features of this trial was the extremely low perioperative morbidity and mortality rate of 2.3%. In addition, half of this morbidity (1.2%) was the result of the preoperative

angiography. Furthermore, unlike the results of NASCET, ACAS found no differences in surgical benefit related to decrements in percent diameter reduction of the studied carotid artery.

Surprisingly, ACAS was criticized on methodologic grounds, particularly the short median follow-up of 2.7 years and the small number of patients (9%) who completed the full 5 years of follow-up.[21] Nevertheless, this large and well-conducted trial has been acknowledged by the practicing medical community as providing solid evidence in support of the appropriateness of surgical treatment for patients with asymptomatic moderate to severe carotid stenosis.[22] ACAS was not designed to detect gender differences, but men enjoyed a 66% relative risk reduction compared with women, whose relative risk reduction was only 17%. The complete explanation of this difference is not certain but may in part be due to the fact that women had a higher perioperative complication rate than men (3.6% vs 1.7%). It is also interesting that 5 patients (1.2%) randomized to the surgical arm of the study suffered stroke as a complication of their presurgical arteriography, accounting for approximately 50% of the perioperative morbidity in this group. If these perioperative strokes are excluded from the calculations, the perioperative risk for the surgically treated patients is reduced from 2.3% to 1.5%. This exceptionally low operative morbidity and mortality rate must be considered when the results of ACAS are used to make clinical decisions.

The last significant trial comparing the surgical and non-surgical treatment of asymptomatic carotid stenosis is ACST, which is being conducted in Europe.[23] This trial is similar in design to ECST, in that it is based on the uncertainty principal, whereby patients are only eligible for randomization if there is substantial uncertainty whether the patient is better treated by surgery and appropriate medical treatment or by medical treatment alone.[24] This will be the largest of the asymptomatic trials. Over 2000 of the planned 3000 patients have been randomized so far, but no results are available yet.

IMPACT OF RANDOMIZED TRIALS ON CLINICAL PRACTICE
National statistics indicate that the number of carotid

endarterectomies performed in the USA increased at a significant rate from the 1960s until 1985 when there were over 107 000 performed in short-stay, non-federal hospitals.[15,25] With the debate about and subsequent initiation of the randomized clinical trials for both symptomatic and asymptomatic patients in the 1980s, the number of endarterectomies fell dramatically, reaching a low of approximately 70 000 in 1991. This trend was abruptly reversed following release of the data from NASCET in 1991, with a further increase following release of the ACAS data in 1994. Although the rate of carotid endarterectomy varies from one region to another and from one country to another, the trends are similar in several areas where they have been studied (Table 2.3). By 1995, more than 130 000 carotid endarterectomies were performed in the US. A recently published survey from all 172 US VA medical centers revealed a dramatic increase in the volume of carotid endarterectomies performed, despite decreases in numbers of inpatients and numbers of inpatient surgical procedures.[26] How have all of these randomized clinical trials changed the indications for carotid endarterectomy? It is difficult if not impossible to provide an answer to this question for the practice of any individual surgeon or group of surgeons. It is likely that individual surgeons have somewhat modified their indications for carotid endarterectomy to include more asymptomatic patients. However, the greatest impact of these trials has probably been on non-surgeons, who appear to be referring more patients with carotid stenosis for surgical therapy.

So, how have all these data derived from the randomized clinical trials influenced my clinical practice? Actually, they have led me to be more conservative rather than more aggressive. Although in a global sense, ACAS and, to a lesser extent, the VAACET support carotid endarterectomy in asymptomatic patients, another way of looking at ACAS data is that the risk of not having a stroke or dying up to 5 years after discovering a ≥60% carotid stenosis is nearly 89% if endarterectomy is not performed and 94.9% if it is. Although this is a statistically significant difference favoring surgical treatment, it is not, in my opinion, an overwhelming, clinically imperative difference. I have always believed that carotid endarterectomy was appropriate in good-risk patients with high-grade carotid stenosis. But what is a high-grade stenosis? In my opinion, it is ≥80% diameter reduction of the internal carotid artery. This can be determined by duplex sonography performed in a reliable vascular laboratory. Operation is also recommended for some patients with lesions of lesser severity, i.e. 70–80% stenosis, or lesions that have shown rapid progression. The composition of the plaque is an important modifying factor: heterogeneous and sonolucent plaques are probably more dangerous than homogeneous, fibrous plaques.

With increasing clinical risk for elective surgery, there is likely to be decreasing long-term benefit, so these recommendations are modified by patients' comorbid conditions, life expectancy, and other factors. ACAS data do not support the concept that risk of stroke increases with increasing degrees of carotid stenosis, but only 11% of ACAS patients had stenosis of ≥80% and there were very few end-point events. In addition, many retrospective and even some prospective studies have shown a higher stroke risk for patients with high-grade stenosis. I am not convinced that the degree of stenosis doesn't matter, nor am I convinced by the available data that 60–70% stenotic lesions are particularly dangerous in most patients. And I now rarely recommend operation for asymptomatic, non-stenotic ulcerated plaques. The marked reduction in benefit for women compared to men in ACAS has made me more cautious about recommending endarterectomy for asymptomatic women, even

Table 2.3 Changing incidence of carotid endarterectomy			
Location	1984	1989	1995
California, US	126	66	99
New York, US	65	40	96
Ontario, Canada	40	15	38

Rates are operations per 100 000 population. Data from Tu *et al.*[15]

though women have fared equally as well as men in my own experience.

Perhaps the most important lesson to be learned from these trials is that there is a very small margin between the surgical and medical treatment of asymptomatic carotid stenosis and that any events that increase the perioperative morbidity and mortality above 2.3–4% will negate any potential benefit. Patient selection, avoidance of angiography when possible, and meticulous surgical technique are all important factors. Clearly, surgeons cannot just assume that the ACAS results apply to them; they must be aware of their own data and this must be a factor in each and every patient decision.

REFERENCES

15 Tu JV, Hannan EL, Anderson GM *et al.* The fall and rise of carotid endarterectomy in the United States and Canada. *New England Journal of Medicine* 1998; **339**: 1441–1448.

16 EC-IC Bypass Study Group. Failure of extracranial–intracranial arterial bypass to reduce the risk of ischemic stroke. *New England Journal of Medicine* 1985; **313**: 1191–1196.

17 Brott T, Thalinger K. The practice of carotid endarterectomy in a large metropolitan area. *Stroke* 1984; **15**: 950–955.

18 The Casanova Study Group. Carotid surgery vs. medical therapy in asymptomatic carotid stenosis. *Stroke* 1991; **22**: 1229–1235.

19 Hobson RW II, Weiss DG, Fields WS *et al.* Efficacy of carotid endarterectomy for asymptomatic carotid stenosis. *New England Journal of Medicine* 1993; **328**: 221–227.

20 Executive Committee for the ACAS. Endarterectomy for asymptomatic carotid artery stenosis. *Journal of the American Medical Association* 1995; **273**: 1421–1462.

21 Barnett H, Eliasziw M, Meldrum H, Taylor W. Do the facts and figures warrant a 10-fold increase in the performance of carotid endarterectomy on asymptomatic patients? *Neurology* 1996; **46**: 603–608.

22 Biller J, Feinberg WM, Castaldo JE *et al.* Guidelines for carotid endarterectomy. A statement for healthcare professionals from a special writing group of the stroke council, American Heart Association. AHA scientific statement. *Circulation* 1998; **97**: 501–509.

23 Halliday AW, Thomas D, Mansfield A. The Asymptomatic Carotid Surgery Trial (ACST) rationale and design. *European Journal of Vascular Surgery* 1994; **8**: 703–710.

24 Goldstone J. The tribulation of trials: a summary of carotid surgery, 1993. *Cardiovascular Surgery* 1994; **2**: 170–175.

25 Stukenborg GJ. Comparison of carotid endarterectomy outcomes from randomized controlled trials and Medicare administrative databases. *Archives of Neurology* 1997; **54**: 826–832.

26 Huber TS, Durance PW, Kazmers A, Jacobs LA. Effect of Asymptomatic Carotid Atherosclerosis Study on carotid endarterectomy in Veterans Affairs Medical Centers. *Archives of Surgery* 1997; **132**: 1134–1139.

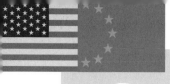

Editorial Comment

2.3

KEY POINTS

1 The randomized trials indicate that CEA is associated with a small but significant stroke prevention benefit in patients with severe stenosis.
2 The average risk reduction is about 1% per year, with greater benefit in men than women.
3 There is no evidence to date that CEA reduces the overall long-term risk of disabling stroke.
4 The benefits of CEA are inextricably linked to the initial operative risk, which was commendably low in ACAS.
5 Because of surgeon selection in ACAS, the results may not be generalizable to all practice settings.

Because the benefit of CEA in asymptomatic patients is so small and so highly dependent on perioperative risk, there is reluctance to translate the ACAS findings into routine clinical practice. The evidence suggests that, while awaiting the results of the ACST, surgeons should remain cautious in selection criteria. Certainly, any surgeon with an operative stroke/death rate > 4% in asymptomatic patients should not perform CEA in this setting.

As with the symptomatic patients, there is a hierarchy of benefit and risk in asymptomatic patients. Assuming longevity > 3 years and operative risk of < 4%, surgeons might consider CEA in asymptomatic patients with:

1 bilateral > 70% stenosis (NASCET) or > 80% (ECST);
2 > 70% stenosis (NASCET) or 80% (ECST) with contralateral occlusion;
3 unilateral severe stenosis (young patients).

There are no clinical or cost/benefit analysis data supporting surgery for asymptomatic patients over 80 years of age. However, physiologic and not chronologic age should be considered.

3.1 Is there a role for emergency or urgent carotid endarterectomy?

Roger M Greenhalgh (Europe)

Carotid endarterectomy has been shown to be beneficial in the treatment of selected patients with transient ischaemic attack (TIA), amaurosis fugax and minor stroke with recovery in both the North American and European trials. The overall benefits increase in proportion to the degree of stenosis in these symptomatic patients. These trials were multicentre and therefore incorporated a variety of surgical skills. However, the entry criteria excluded asymptomatic patients on the one hand and established, progressing and acute strokes as well as crescendo TLA patients on the other hand. There are no randomized controlled trials to guide management decisions in patients with more severe symptoms. However, for years, Dr Jesse Thompson of Dallas has shown that the overall outcomes primarily relate to the severity of the initial presenting symptoms and this is in accordance with my own experience.[1] In short, the operative morbidity and mortality are least in asymptomatic patients, increased for amaurosis fugax, TIA and established stroke and highest following surgery for progressing stroke and crescendo TIA.[1]

PREOPERATIVE ASSESSMENTS

As the outcomes from carotid surgery relate to presenting symptom and patient status, we find it vital that every patient should be seen by a neurologist before surgery is performed. The key investigation is colour duplex scan performed by an experienced vascular technologist who investigates the carotid and the vertebral arteries. It is helpful to have the precise dimensions of the carotid artery and in particular to know the exact length of disease by duplex scan proximal and distal to the carotid bifurcation. This makes the dissection easier and

enables the surgeon at operation to find the end of the arterial stenosis without palpating the artery and disturbing loose atheroma. A transcranial assessment with colour duplex is performed to visualize and locate the site of the middle cerebral artery signal so that this can be monitored during carotid surgery. A computed tomographic (CT) scan is performed to rule out occasional intracranial alternative pathology and also to check for cerebral infarction in both hemispheres. I no longer routinely request preoperative angiography and almost never request selective catheterization of the great vessels. This immediately avoids the morbidity associated with these procedures.

OPERATIVE PROCEDURE

Carotid surgery should only be performed by specialist vascular surgeons with particular training in the procedure. It is not an operation for the occasional surgeon. I know of no other operation in which details of technique and choice of operation relate so obviously to morbidity levels. This effectively means that, in my view, carotid surgery should be performed in regional (usually university) centres. It is particularly helpful if the regional vascular centre is alongside the regional neurological centre, as high-quality neurological input is essential at all times. I use dexamethasone with the premedication and for 48 h after surgery to discourage cerebral oedema which is associated with increased blood flow. The operation takes place under general anaesthetic through a skin-crease incision with transcranial Doppler monitoring. Intravenous heparin 5000 u is used 3 min before cross-clamping. I prefer to use a Javid intraluminal shunt for cerebral protection if the stump pressure is either below 50 mmHg or if the waveform is flat. If the stump pressure is above 50 mmHg and the waveform pulsatile after clamping, this implies that there is satisfactory collateral circulation via the circle of Willis and no shunt is used.[2] Transcranial signal change is noted and, if there is any doubt, a Javid shunt is used. Using these criteria, the shunt is used somewhat more than 50% of the time. A 5 mm Dacron patch is my preference for closing the arteriotomy if the distal internal carotid diameter is < 6 mm diameter.[3] 6–0 Prolene is used. Before restoring blood flow, the internal, external and common carotid arteries are thoroughly flushed of solid material and of air bubbles. After releasing the clamps, the result is checked at once on the table with a Doppler pencil probe and any change in the transcranial signal is noted.

IMMEDIATE POSTOPERATIVE RECOVERY

The patient recovers under careful scrutiny and, if any ipsilateral neurological events occur, then in my experience these are almost always the result of a technical problem, missed at the time of operation. Some minor neurological episodes occurred in 3.4% of our patients in earlier series. The patients were returned to the operating theatre at once and under general anaesthesia the arteriotomy was reopened and the problem corrected. This reduced the 30-day stroke rate from 3.4% to 0.9%.[4]

INDICATIONS FOR URGENT CAROTID SURGERY

These patients are scheduled for the next elective operating session if they have had an attack of amaurosis fugax, TIA or stroke with recovery associated with a tight stenosis of > 95%. They are admitted at once, heparinized intravenously and investigated in the same way as described above. A repeat colour duplex scan is performed immediately before surgery to check that occlusion has not occurred. If it has, the operation is cancelled. Since we have adopted this protocol of immediate admission and heparinization, we have not seen carotid occlusion occur for severe stenoses before urgent carotid surgery has been performed. This is the only indication in my practice for urgent carotid surgery; the other indications require carotid surgery

either immediately and certainly within 24 h, which I define as emergency carotid surgery.

INDICATIONS FOR EMERGENCY CAROTID SURGERY

Acute Stroke (Fig. 3.1)

Since the joint American study in 1970[5] showed that the surgical treatment of acute stroke has results much worse than those of medical treatment, there has been an understandable reluctance to perform surgery for acute stroke. The carotid pioneers performed carotid surgery for carotid occlusion; indeed, Dr Michael DeBakey's first carotid endarterectomy in August 1953 was for an occluded carotid artery. He reported the patient after a follow-up of some 19 years.[6] Nowadays, even he would not perform carotid surgery for carotid occlusion and there remains reluctance to perform any surgery for acute stroke. The early pioneers feared that revascularization would convert the so-called anaemic into a haemorrhagic[5] infarct if performed acutely or too soon after stroke and for years, patients were left for 3 months and, more recently, at least 6 weeks.

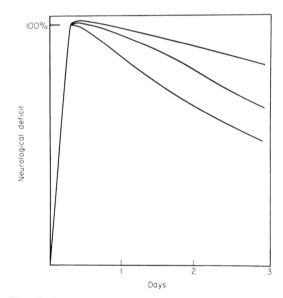

Fig. 3.1
Neurological recovery following acute stroke. Note that the initial deficit is rapidly severe but that the rate of recovery varies amongst individual patients.

I would only consider surgery for acute stroke if the patient occluded a carotid artery whilst in hospital, either following a carotid endarterectomy or following an angiogram.

Transient Stroke and Established Stroke

Using the terminology of the Marseilles classification, by 'transient stroke' is implied a ministroke which lasts longer than 24 h but less than 3 weeks. Beyond 3 weeks, an 'established' stroke is said to occur. This was formerly called a completed or frank stroke. If a patient who has suffered a transient or established stroke with good recovery has a severe stenosis of greater than 70%, I would schedule carotid surgery in less than 6 weeks but not regard this as an indication for emergency or even urgent carotid surgery. I would be disinclined to heparinize the patient after established stroke, particularly in the presence of cerebral infarction, unless the ipsilateral carotid stenosis was very tight. The decision for the timing of carotid surgery[7] is always a balance between perceived risk of too early revascularization and fear of occlusion of the carotid artery. I have tended to schedule the procedure earlier and earlier and usually within a week, and have not found evidence to wait for the 6 weeks, let alone 3 months.

Progressing Stroke

By this, I understand that a neurological deficit progresses relentlessly over at least a 24-h period. For example, a patient develops a neurological deficit in the hand; it extends 24 h later to the forearm and then to the upper arm 24 h after that. Patients to be considered for operation are fully alert, awake, conscious and rational. Generally, a severe stenosis is found but frequently the stump pressure at operation is high, implying that the progressing stroke was caused by repeated embolization.[8]

Carotid surgery has been performed in the two types of progressing stroke, namely 'stroke in evolution' (Fig. 3.2), in which the progression is linear and 'stuttering hemiplegia', in which the progression fluctuates day by day (Fig. 3.3).[1,8] The results of carotid surgery have shown > 90% benefit compared with the awful outcome previously described in patients who had progressing stroke, in whom carotid surgery was not performed.[9]

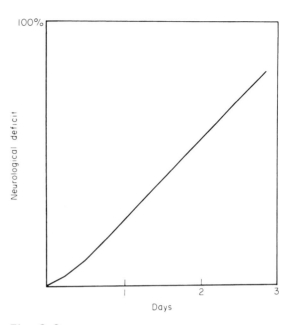

Fig. 3.2
Progressing stroke (stroke in evolution).

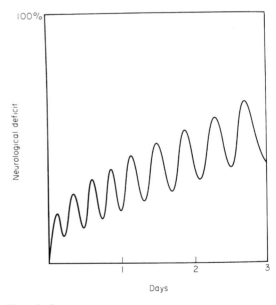

Fig. 3.3
Progressing stroke: fluctuating stroke (stuttering hemiplegia).

Crescendo Transient Ischaemic Attacks

As this is the group in which the highest morbidity and mortality await the carotid surgeon, enthusiasm to intervene for these patients is low. By crescendo TIA, it is understood that the patient has a series of TIAs (each TIA completely recovers between attacks, leaving no deficit whatsoever), with increasing severity of deficit in each attack or a shorter period between attacks (Fig. 3.4). Almost invariably these patients have bilateral severe carotid stenoses and the operative mortality and morbidity have been poorer than for other indications. In retrospect, I suspect that on many occasions the symptoms could have been caused by variations in cardiac output, implying a primary cardiac pathology. My current preference is for these patients to be heparinized and to await stability before considering carotid surgery and thus avoiding emergency carotid surgery in view of our reported poorer operative outcomes. As the operative outcomes for progressing stroke are vastly better, it is logical to attempt to avoid surgical intervention for crescendo TIA patients who by definition completely recover from neurological deficit after each attack.

CONCLUSIONS

Emergency carotid surgery is indicated for progressing stroke and the results are much better than historical natural history reports. Numbers are so small and the literature reports so infrequent for this condition that it is unlikely that a randomised. Controlled trial will prove the benefit of carotid surgery for progressing stroke. There are reservations

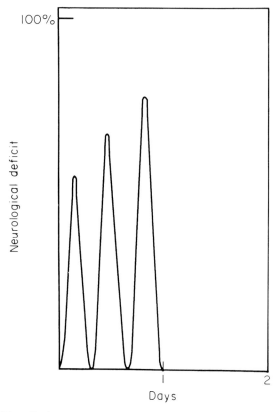

Fig. 3.4
Crescendo transient ischaemic attacks.

for emergency carotid surgery for a crescendo TIA, but there is enthusiasm for immediate intervention for neurological deficit following carotid surgery or angiography.

REFERENCES

1 Golledge J, Cuming R, Beattie DK, Davies AH, Greenhalgh RM. Influence of patient-related variables on the outcome of carotid endarterectomy. *Journal of Vascular Surgery* 1996; **24**: 120–126.

2 Greenhalgh RM. Selective shunting during carotid endarterectomy. In: Greenhalgh RM (ed.) *Vascular and Endovascular Surgical Techniques*, pp. 128–133. London: WB Saunders, 1994.

3 Golledge J, Cuming R, Ellis M, Beattie DK, Davies AH, Greenhalgh RM. Duplex imaging findings predict stenosis after carotid endarterectomy. *Journal of Vascular Surgery* 1997; **26**: 43–48.

4 Cuming R, Blair SD, Powell JT, Greenhalgh RM. The use of duplex scanning to diagnose perioperative carotid occlusions. *European Journal of Vascular Surgery* 1994; **8**: 143–147.

5 Fields WS, Maslevikov V, Meyer JS, Hass WK, Remington RD, Macdonald MC. Joint study of extracranial arterial occlusion. *Journal of the American Medical Association* 1970; **211**: 1993.

6 DeBakey ME. Successful carotid endarterectomy for cerebrovascular insufficiency. *Journal of the American Medical Association* 1975; **233**: 1083–1085.

7 Greenhalgh RM, Meek AC, Kitchen N, Cuming R, McCollum CN. The timing of carotid surgery after documented stroke. In: Veith F (ed.) *Current Critical*

Problems and New Horizons in Vascular Surgery, pp. 505–508. Quality Medical, 1989.

8 Greenhalgh RM, Cuming R, Perkin GD, McCollum CN. Urgent carotid surgery for high risk patients. *European Journal of Vascular Surgery* 1993; **7** (Suppl A): 25–32.

9 Millikan CH. Clinical management of cerebral ischaemia. In: MacDonnell FL, Brennan RW (eds) *Cerebral Vascular Disease – Eighth Conference*, p. 209. New York: Grune & Stratton, 1973.

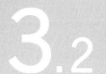

3.2 Is there a role for emergency or urgent carotid endarterectomy?

Jonathan P Gertler (USA)

William M Abbott (USA)

INTRODUCTION

Therapy for acute stroke has changed significantly in the last decade with increasing realization of the value of reperfusion and cerebral tissue protection. The establishment of stroke units in numerous tertiary medical centers has facilitated the study of thrombolytic therapy, and the revolution in brain imaging has allowed for a better understanding of and therapy for the patient with acute neurologic deficit. Carotid endarterectomy (CEA), despite its recent validation as effective elective therapy for the carotid stroke-prone patient, has been utilized in the setting of acute stroke without the prospective validation afforded its elective use. This chapter will attempt to summarize the theoretical basis for and the results of urgent or emergent CEA in the neurologically unstable patient.

Patients with cerebral ischemia caused by extracranial cerebrovascular disease have a wide variety of symptoms. The primary goal of CEA in elective circumstances is stroke prophylaxis. In the neurologically unstable patient, removal of a source of ongoing emboli and/or reperfusion of ischemic but not infarcted areas of brain form the rationale for urgent or emergent CEA.

Randomized controlled trials have validated CEA as effective in preventing stroke in patients with both symptomatic and asymptomatic carotid artery stenosis.[10–12] Since the publication of these trials there has been a marked increase in the referral of patients with asymptomatic and symptomatic carotid artery disease. Among these patients are those with unstable neurologic conditions in whom the outcome is not as well defined as in the elective situation. Because such patients represent a high-risk group not included in the randomized controlled trials, the outcome data from these trials cannot be applied to decision-making in their care.

There are four clinical scenarios in which urgent or emergent CEA might be considered: stroke in evolution (SIE), crescendo transient ischemic attack (CTIA), fluctuating or severe neurologic deficit caused by acute occlusion of the carotid artery (NDAO), and anatomically compelling (AC) findings on cerebral angiography (i.e. free-floating thrombus and atheroma). A variety of series and case reports over the years have addressed patients in these circumstances. Many of these reports predated and none applied the standardized reporting methods advocated by the Subcommittee on Reporting Standards for Cerebral Vascular Disease of the Society for Vascular Surgery and the International Society for Cardiovascular Surgery, North American chapter (SVS/NA-ISCVS).[13]

The lack of modern anesthetic and critical care techniques and the lack of reliable brain imaging studies during the early years of CEA contributed to poor surgical results, especially in patients with acute neurologic presentations. Unsatisfactory neurologic outcome or fatality was the rule rather than the exception in many early studies, and these poor surgical results led to an understandable conservatism in patients with SIE, acute carotid occlusion, CTIA, or anatomically intimidating lesions. More recent series with much better results have tempered this conservatism somewhat. Excellent results have been reported in patients with anatomically compelling lesions or CTIAs and in selected patients with SIE. Fair results have been reported in patients with neurologic instability related to acute occlusion, especially if intervention is carried out within 3 hours of the onset of symptoms

Table 3.1
Collated recent series of emergency carotid endarterectomy

Indication	Outcome		
	Satisfactory	Unsatisfactory	Death
SIE	84%	15%	5%
CTIA	98%	2%	2%
NDAO CEA <3 h	61%	39%	10%
NDAO CEA >3 h	47%	53%	19%
AC	79%	21%	5%

SIE, stroke in evolution; CTIA, crescendo transient ischemic attack; NDAO, neurologic deficit caused by acute occlusion of the carotid artery; CEA, carotid endarterectomy; AC, anatomically compelling findings on cerebral angiography.

(Table 3.1). The poor outcome of these conditions treated medically, and improvements in anesthetic care, perioperative care, and brain imaging have reawakened interest in CEFL in these settings.

REVIEW OF THE MASSACHUSETTS GENERAL HOSPITAL EXPERIENCE

In order to re-evaluate the role of urgent or emergent CEA, we reviewed our 15-year experience with CEA in neurologically unstable patients.[14] We chose this time interval as standardization of endarterectomy techniques, availability of intraoperative electroencephalographic monitoring, improved cardiovascular anesthetic management, improved brain imaging studies, and organized intensive care of neurologically and cardiologically compromised patients became available in this era. Five symptom complexes were identified as indications for CEA in neurologically unstable patients. Group A included patients with tight stenosis and SIE, defined as an acute neurologic deficit that, within hours or days of the initial diagnosis, progressed to a greater deficit after a waxing and waning of signs but without disappearance of the deficit.[15] Group B included NDAO (either as a primary presentation, within several hours of angiography, or in the postoperative period after CEA). Group C included CTIAs that continued despite the administration of heparin. CTIAs were defined as recurrent transient cerebral or retinal events in the distribution of the carotid artery,

characterized by a definite change in pattern: increased frequency or multiple episodes in increased duration, or spread in the distribution of ischemia with greater or new motor sensory, speech, or visual deficits. Group D included CTIAs (above criteria) ceasing with administration of intravenous heparin. Group E included AC situations on cerebral angiography, i.e., string sign representing almost no flow distal to the preocclusive carotid artery stenosis, or an intraluminal filling defect suggesting free-floating thrombosis or loose atheroma.

Sixty-eight patients undergoing 70 CEAs met the clinical criteria defined above. Seventy CEAs were performed in 68 neurologically unstable patients. There were 42 male and 26 female patients, with a median age of 67.5 years (range: 40–84). There were 17 patients in group A, 4 in group B, 14 in group C, 20 in group D, and 13 in group E. There were an additional 16 patients with an intraluminal thrombosis distributed in groups A–D. These cases were evaluated together with group E patients in a separate analysis of all AC findings. These 68 patients represent only 3.9% of the 1734 patients undergoing endarterectomy at out institution during the study period (1/1978–12/1992).

Preoperative and postoperative neurologic impairment was graded using the Neurologic Event Severity Scale (NESS).[13] The NESS classification grades neurologic signs and symptoms and

Table 3.2
Neurologic Event Severity Scale

Severity	Impairment	Neurologic symptoms	Neurologic signs
1	None	Present	Absent
2	None	Absent	Present
3	None	Present	Present
4	Minor* in one or more domains†	Present	Present
5	Major* in only one domain	NA	NA
6	Major in any two domains	NA	NA
7	Major in any three domains	NA	NA
8	Major in any four domains	NA	NA
9	Major in all five domains	NA	NA
10	Reduced level of consciousness	NA	NA
11	Death	NA	NA

*Minor: independence maintained; major: independence lost.
†Domains: swallowing, self-care, ambulation, communication, comprehension.
NA, not applicable.

impairments in the following domains: swallowing, self-care, ambulation, communication, and comprehension. This classification scheme is shown in Table 3.2.

Forty-three percent of patients underwent preoperative CT scanning or magnetic resonance imaging (MRI) of the brain. In more than 50% of these, no disease could be demonstrated, whereas in only 8 cases was an appropriate infarct found (7 from group A and 1 from group C). There was no correlation between CT/MRI findings and early or late neurologic outcome.

Surgery was performed with continuous electroencephalographic monitoring in 56 patients and shunts were placed in 40 of 70 cases. Fourteen arteriotomies were closed with a patch.

Comparison of the pre- and postoperative NESS scores for the five groups is instructive. In group A ($n = 17$), the NESS score of 1 patient fell, while that of another patient rose. The other 15 patients remained in their admission NESS category, although the condition of 10 of these patients improved within the same NESS category.

In group B ($n = 5$), the condition of 1 patient remained unchanged, whereas the condition of 4 patients improved, though in only 1 patient was the improvement reflected by an improved NESS score. Thirteen of the 14 patients from group C had no fixed neurologic finding at the time of surgery, despite repeated TIAs, and all patients had no change in their NESS scores. Eighteen of the 21 cases in group D had only intermittent neurologic findings and no symptoms with administration of heparin. The other 3 patients with neurologic findings had NESS scores ranging from 1 to 3. Twenty of the 21 patients were symptom-free at the time of discharge, but 1 patient had acute occlusion of the left carotid artery immediately after right CEA. This patient, who is also included in group B for the left side, was diagnosed with a neurologic deficit of 10 by NESS criteria and improved to a NESS score of 5 after emergency left CEA. Because NESS scoring does not differentiate between the hemispheres, the right CEA yielded an unsatisfactory result. In the 55 patients in groups A–D, the NESS score stabilized or rose in

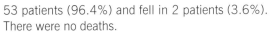
53 patients (96.4%) and fell in 2 patients (3.6%). There were no deaths.

Of the 13 patients in group E (AC findings), the condition of 1 patient deteriorated by NESS criteria and 2 patients died. Analysis of the 16 cases of AC findings, culled from groups A–D, yields a 6.9% postoperative mortality rate and a 3.4% neurologic deterioration rate.

For the entire series, the postoperative mortality rate was 2.9% and the neurologic deterioration rate was 4.3%. Interestingly, there was only one postoperative hemorrhagic infarct. This resulted in massive stroke and death on the first postoperative day.

CONCLUSIONS AND TREATMENT RECOMMENDATIONS

Several salient points emerge from our experience in treating neurologically unstable patients: First, with modern brain imaging studies and our patient selection criteria and monitoring techniques, the risk of converting a bland infarct to a hemorrhagic infarct is very small (1.5%). This risk has been used as an argument against emergency CEA immediately after stroke since the publication of the joint studies of extracranial disease in the early 1960s.[16] Poor preoperative identification of the degree of cerebral injury in the era before CT or MRI and inexact methods of monitoring and treating postoperative hypertension may have been significant contributors to the early incidence of post-reperfusion hemorrhage. However, more modern reports suggest that a significant subgroup of patients will benefit from emergency revascularization in the setting of acute stroke.[17,18] In selected patients with critical carotid lesions and even acute carotid occlusions, active intervention is preferable to anticoagulation or other conservative regimens. Newer radiological technologies, such as single-photon emission computed tomography (SPECT), may further refine patient selection for aggressive surgical therapy by accurately distinguishing infarcted from ischemic but salvageable tissue.[19]

The achievement of satisfactory results in 93% (63/68) of our patients with unstable neurologic conditions and/or compelling arteriographic findings is striking. These outcomes are far better than the natural history of or results of medical therapy for these conditions and lends support to earlier reports supporting a role for emergent CEA. Often, and especially in the setting of an evolving deficit associated with acute carotid occlusion, time is critical and intervention must be carried out within 3 hours of presentation. On the basis of experimental and clinical results, it seems likely that an extended ischemic penumbra exists after carotid artery occlusion and that salvage of significant neurologic function is possible with early intervention, especially if distal embolization is not extensive and there is some pre-existing collateral flow.

It is noteworthy that patients at highest risk for adverse outcomes were those with compelling arteriographic findings, even in the absence of compelling symptoms. Indeed, those with AC findings without an unstable clinical presentation had the worst outcome (15.4%, 2/13 mortality, and 7.7%, 1/13 neurologic deterioration). This finding serves to emphasize the importance of technique in carotid surgery, especially in the patient with intraluminal thrombus or grossly unstable plaque. Careful dissection with minimal handling of the artery and placement of the distal clamp before complete dissection around the bifurcation or allowing the internal carotid to back-bleed prior to clamping are important maneuvers in these patients. Even with impeccable technique, the risk in these patients is high and suboptimal outcomes will occur.

From our experience with neurologically unstable patients, we have developed the following treatment algorithm. After presentation and initial clinical assessment, patients deemed potential candidates for aggressive intervention undergo immediate CT scan to exclude hemorrhage and massive hemispheric infarction with edema, midline shift, etc. In the absence of CT findings contraindicating anticoagulation, heparin is administered. Rapid duplex and, in most cases, angiographic evaluation are then carried out. In patients with symptoms unresponsive to heparin and compelling operable arterial anatomy, emergent endarterectomy is carried out. In patients whose symptoms abate with heparin and in those with compelling arterial anatomy but stable or no symptoms, urgent or expedited surgery with a rested experienced team, dedicated vascular

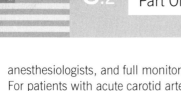
anesthesiologists, and full monitoring is preferred. For patients with acute carotid artery occlusion and a fixed deficit, observation after anticoagulation is preferred, except in selected patients when lytic therapy is immediately available. Rarely, if the occlusion is known to be very recent and the patient is not moribund but has limited or fluctuating neurologic signs consistent with hypoperfusion or ongoing embolization, immediate surgery is indicated. Any patient with acute neurologic deficit related to suspected early post-endarterectomy thrombosis should undergo emergent reoperation.

In conclusion, emergent CEA is appropriate for selected neurologically unstable patients because the results of early surgical intervention are superior to those associated with medical management. In these compelling situations, patient selection and surgical technique determine outcome.

REFERENCES

10 North American Symptomatic Carotid Endarterectomy Trial Collaborators. Beneficial effect of carotid endarterectomy in symptomatic patients with high-grade carotid stenosis. *New England Journal of Medicine* 1991; **325**: 445–453.

11 European Carotid Surgery Trialists' Collaborative Group. MRC European Carotid Surgery Trial; interim results for patients with severe (70–99%) or with mild (0–29%) carotid stenosis. *Lancet* 1991; **337**: 1235–1243.

12 Executive Committee for the Asymptomatic Carotid Atherosclerosis Study. Endarterectomy for asymptomatic carotid artery stenosis. *Journal of the American Medical Association* 1995; **273**: 1421–1428.

13 Baker JD, Rutherford RB, Bernstein EF *et al*. Suggested standards for reports dealing with cerebrovascular disease. Subcommittee on Reporting Standards for Cerebrovascular Disease, Ad Hoc Committee on Reporting Standards, Society for Vascular Surgery/North American Chapter, International Society for Cardiovascular Surgery. *Journal of Vascular Surgery* 1988; **8**: 721–729.

14 Gertler JP, Blankensteijn JD, Brewster DC *et al*. Carotid endarterectomy for unstable and compelling neurologic conditions: do results justify an aggressive approach? *Journal of Vascular Surgery* 1994; **19**: 32–42.

15 Mentzer RM Jr, Finkelmeier BA, Crosby IK, Wellons HA. Emergency carotid endarterectomy for fluctuating neurologic deficits. *Surgery* 1981; **89**: 60–66.

16 Blaisdell WF, Clauss RH, Galbraith JG, Imparto AM, Wylie EJ. Joint study of extracranial arterial occlusion, IV: a review of surgical considerations. *Journal of the American Medical Association* 1969; **209**: 1889–1895.

17 Meyer FB, Sundt TM Jr, Piepgras DG, Sandok BA, Forbes G. Emergency carotid endarterectomy for patients with acute carotid occlusion and profound neurological deficits. *Annals of Surgery* 1986; **203**: 82–89.

18 Goldstone J, Moore WS. Emergency carotid artery surgery in neurologically unstable patients. *Archives of Surgery* 1976; **111**: 1284–1291.

19 Lishmanov Y, Shvera I, Ussov W, Shipulin V. The effect of carotid endarterectomy on cerebral blood flow and cerebral blood volume studied by SPECT. *Journal of Neuroradiology* 1997; **24**: 155–162.

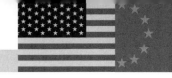

3.3 Editorial Comment

KEY POINTS

1 There are no randomized trials (and unlikely to be any in the future) to provide any evidence base on which to evaluate the role of urgent or emergent CEA.
2 Emergent CEA (immediate) should be considered in patients who:
   - suffer a perioperative thrombotic stroke post-CEA;
   - suffer a carotid thrombosis stroke post-angiography or angioplasty;
   - have a severe stenosis with SIE or CTIAs.
3 Urgent CEA (within 48 h) should be considered in patients whose imaging studies suggest free-floating carotid thrombus.
4 Expedited CEA (< 7 days) should be considered in symptomatic patients with a preocclusive lesion.
5 There is no indication for urgent/emergent surgery in moribund acute stroke patients or in patients with large-volume infarcts.
6 There is no indication for urgent/emergent CEA in patients who present with rapid resolution of a neurologic deficit related to acute carotid thrombosis.

This has always been a controversial area. In practice, however, the evidence presented by the authors suggests that the above criteria for urgent/emergent CEA will only apply to a small, highly select group of patients. It is essential, therefore, that each vascular surgeon collaborates closely with the stroke neurologists to define a strict protocol for expedited investigation and management of these high-risk cases. It seems clear that the best results will be obtained in centers with multidisciplinary input and regular outcome review.

The management of patients with SIE or CTIAs is clearly controversial. This is largely due to the lack of any standard definition for these clinical events. For example, does 3 TIAs per month/week/day qualify for the diagnosis of CTIAs? Alternatively, might this diagnosis also include any pattern of frequent TIAs failing to respond to anticoagulant therapy? Precise definition of these syndromes is necessary for the development of standardized treatment algorithms.

4.1

When should I perform carotid endarterectomy after a completed stroke?

Jens Allenberg (Europe)

Hans H Eckstein (Europe)

INTRODUCTION

The attitude of neurologists towards the prevention of ischaemic stroke has changed over the last decade, primarily as a consequence of international randomized trials.[1,2] Similarly, the treatment of acute stroke has been enhanced by the establishment of stroke units which have been able to take advantage of advances in medical care, notably blood pressure control and thrombolysis. Treatment aimed at early reperfusion may be able to alter the natural history of acute stroke by improving the blood supply to the ischaemic penumbra surrounding the area of infarction. In contrast, the role of prophylaxis is directed towards the prevention of early recurrent stroke.

Although the prevention of recurrent stroke involves careful control of risk factors, one of the enduring controversies has been the timing of carotid endarterectomy (CEA) in patients following stroke who are subsequently found to have significant internal carotid artery (ICA) disease. In short, a balance needs to be struck between avoiding unnecessary operative deaths and the increased risk of early recurrent stroke.

THE NATURAL HISTORY OF ISCHAEMIC STROKE

With the exception of a transient ischaemic attack (TIA), it is often impossible to predict the reversibility of a neurological deficit in the acute stage of stroke. Clinical symptoms can progress (progressing stroke, stroke in evolution, fluctuating stroke, stuttering hemiplegia), stabilize at a distinct level, improve or disappear completely. Otherwise they can reappear as a recurrent stroke.

In order to compare the natural course of stroke with the effect of therapeutic intervention, the modified Rankin scale has proved to be useful: 0 = no deficit, 1 = minimal deficit, 2 = minor deficit, 3 = moderate deficit (walking unaided), 4 = severe deficit (walking but aided), 5 = disabling stroke confined to bed, 6 = mortality. Similarly, a neurological deficit which persists for up to 3 weeks is traditionally considered to be a transient stroke. Where symptoms continue for more than 3 weeks, the term established stroke is usually applied. Unfortunately, it may be impossible to discriminate between the two subgroups at an early stage.

In order to assess the prognosis of stroke in the context of any potential therapeutic intervention, it is important to clarify the severity of the neurological deficit and determine the location and size of any infarct. Additional contributing factors which may influence the reversibility of the neurological deficit include the quality and amount of collaterals and the time period between the onset of ischaemia and reperfusion. Thus, the time frame in which thrombolysis or operation should be considered is not solely dependent on the time interval since the onset of symptoms.

Severe ischaemic stroke

One of the problems in interpreting the role of carotid surgery or medical therapy in patients following acute stroke has been the heterogeneity of presentations, definitions and timing of surgery. In its simplest form, a severe acute ischaemic stroke usually implies the presence of a profound neurological deficit with or without impairment of the conscious level. In a group of 45 patients with severe acute ischaemic stroke, Hafner found that 71% had an underlying ICA occlusion, whilst 29% had an ICA stenosis.[3]

When should I perform carotid endarterectomy after a completed stroke?

4.1

In the Oxfordshire Community Stroke Project, total anterior circulation infarction (the most severe form of acute ischaemic stroke) was specifically defined as the triad of hemiplegia/hemisensory loss, higher cortical dysfunction (aphasia/visuospatial neglect) and homonymous hemianopia.[4] The principal cause of total anterior cerebral infarction (TACI) was major vessel occlusion (i.e. ICA and/or middle cerebral artery (MCA)). TACI was associated with a 30-day mortality of 39% and only 4% of survivors were independent at 30 days (Rankin 0–2).

Non-disabling stroke

The term non-disabling stroke is applied to a neurological deficit of Rankin 0–3 or where the deficit improves markedly within a few days (the neurological plateau phase). In the Oxfordshire Community Stroke Project, this would be equivalent to the partial anterior circulation infarction (defined as one or two components of the TACI clinical triad, but never all three). In contrast to patients with TACI, patients with partial anterior circulation infarction had a 30-day mortality rate of 4% and 56% were independent at 30 days.[4]

Patients with a non-disabling stroke due to extracranial carotid disease are thereafter exposed to a 5–10% risk of recurrent stroke within 30 days of the initial event.[5–7] In the Oxfordshire Community Stroke Project, patients with partial anterior cerebral infarction had a recurrence rate of 17% within 1 year, with the highest risk being within the first few months.[8]

Progressive stroke

The clinical features and outcome of surgery in patients with progressive stroke have been summarized elsewhere. These patients, however, have a gloomier prognosis, with a mortality rate of 14–36% and a long-term disability rate of up to 69%[9,10] due to the risk of ongoing embolization or ischaemia caused by impaired cerebral blood flow. The essential difference with regard to a completed stroke is that, in progressive stroke there remains a higher volume of functionally impaired but non-infarcted brain tissue in the ischaemic penumbra.

Stroke following carotid endarterectomy

The natural history of acute stroke after CEA depends on the mechanism leading to the cerebral injury. Riles et al.[11] showed that 40% of perioperative strokes were caused by immediate or delayed postoperative thrombosis or embolism. Only 15% were related to cerebral ischaemia during surgery, while 20% followed suture line disruption, strokes in other vascular territories or cardiac embolism. Inadvertent technical error remains the commonest single predisposing factor.[11] The role of emergency surgery in patients with a stroke following CEA has been detailed elsewhere.

THE TIMING OF SURGERY AFTER COMPLETED STROKE

The international randomized trials have demonstrated a proven role for CEA in patients with a severe ICA stenosis and who present with a non-disabling stroke.[1,2] However, the optimal time to perform the operation remains controversial. For the last 20 years, most centres have traditionally waited 6–8 weeks before performing CEA, primarily because of the poor results encountered in the 1960s, when haemorrhagic transformation of the infarct was a particular problem.[12,13] However, as will be seen, this conclusion was primarily based on the outcome of emergency surgery in patients with severe neurological deficits secondary to acute carotid occlusion and relatively few studies have concentrated on the timing of CEA after non-disabling stroke.

Carotid surgery in severe acute stroke

In a systematic review of the published literature, Mead et al. showed that the operative mortality following emergency/urgent surgery in patients with acute stroke and a severe neurological deficit was 18%.[14] The highest operative mortality was observed in patients who presented with a severe stroke secondary to acute carotid occlusion, with the commonest cause being haemorrhagic transformation of the infarct.

Only one of these studies was randomized (the Joint Study of Extracranial Artery Occlusion). Within this study, there was a subgroup of 50 patients who underwent CEA within 2 weeks of stroke onset, with an operative mortality rate of 42%. This compares with an operative mortality rate of 17% in patients in whom surgery was deferred for > 2 weeks.[12] This study was, thereafter, largely responsible for surgeons tending to avoid CEA in the first 6–8 weeks after *any* stroke.

Carotid surgery after non-disabling stroke

Patients suffering a non-disabling stroke due to extracranial ICA disease have a better prognosis but are exposed to a 5–10% risk of recurrent stroke within 30 days due to ongoing embolization or carotid occlusion.[5,6,8] Should the patient suffer a recurrent stroke secondary to carotid artery occlusion, 40–69% will be permanently disabled, 16–55% will die and only 2–12% will make a good recovery.[15]

As a consequence, there has been renewed interest in the role of expedited surgery in selected patients with completed stroke.[16] In the North American Symptomatic Carotid Endarterectomy Trial (NASCET), patients who were operated upon within 30 days of suffering a non-disabling stroke (median 16 days, 3–30 days) had a perioperative stroke rate of 4.8% which was no different to the 5.2% rate in patients who underwent CEA after > 30 days had elapsed.[6] In particular, no patient undergoing early endarterectomy suffered an intracranial haemorrhage. A similar finding was observed by Piotrowski *et al.*[17], who deferred CEA until the patient's condition had reached a neurological plateau phase (Fig. 4.1). There was no association between timing of the operation and operative risk and only 1 patient suffered an intracerebral haemorrhage which, in retrospect, was thought to be due to poor blood pressure control in the

perioperative period. Overall, the operative mortality in patients operated upon within 6 weeks (2.4%) was less than the 6.3% mortality observed in patients who had a deferred operation.[17]

In a systematic review of the role of expedited carotid surgery in 1054 patients with a non-disabling stroke, Mead *et al.*[14] showed that the operative mortality rate was only 3.6%. Even allowing for the potentially confounding effects of patient heterogeneity, potential bias and individual selection, these results have led many surgeons and neurologists to question whether the traditional approach of waiting 6–8 weeks is appropriate.

THE HEIDELBERG EXPERIENCE

Hypothesis

Our hypothesis was that early CEA in selected patients with a non-disabling carotid territory stroke was beneficial in terms of preventing early recurrent stroke and was not associated with adverse outcome.

Indications

Since 1980, we have adopted an increasing policy of expedited CEA in selected patients presenting to our institution with completed stroke. Our principal inclusion criteria, which have been developed in conjunction with our neurologists, include:

1   severe carotid stenosis;
2   focal non-disabling neurological deficit in the carotid territory;

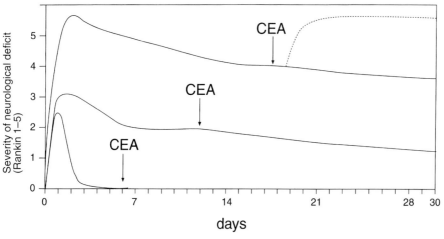

Fig. 4.1
Timing of early carotid endarterectomy after a non-disabling stroke. Interrupted line indicates the onset of a recurrent stroke. Carotid endarterectomy (arrowed) should be performed when the patient's condition reaches the neurological plateau phase, i.e. before a recurrent stroke intervenes.

3 rapid neurological improvement within a few days of onset (the neurological plateau phase).

Specific contraindications for CEA in the early period after stroke include:

1 impaired concious level;
2 significant residual neurological deficit;
3 haemorrhagic infarction on computed tomographic (CT) scan;
4 significant comorbidity (e.g. recent myocardial infarction);
5 patient already confined to bed or wheelchair.

Patient numbers

Between 1980 and 1996, 74 patients with completed stroke underwent CEA within 4 weeks of onset (median 14 days). This represents 3.1% of our overall workload (2213 CEAs) during this period. During the latter years, the proportion of patients steadily increased, from 1.7% between 1980 and 1993, to 8.1% of all CEAs during the period 1994–1996.[18]

All patients were transferred from the department of neurology and were clinically assessed according to the modified Rankin scale in the pre- and postoperative period. Nineteen patients had suffered a stroke with complete recovery, 54 still had a residual minor neurological deficit and 74% had evidence of an ischaemic carotid territory infarction on CT scan.

Operative details

Since 1992, surgery has been performed using somatosensory evoked potential (SSEP) monitoring. Loss of SSEP and/or the presence of minimal or non-pulsatile stump pressure required the insertion of an indwelling shunt. In nearly one-third of our patients, neuromonitoring by SSEPs has not been reliable due to insufficient baseline measurements and the fact that SSEP interpretation is confounded by electrical changes associated with areas of recent infarction.

Since 1995, blood flow velocity in the middle cerebral artery (MCAV) has also been monitored using transcranial Doppler (TCD) ultrasound. The combination of SSEPs and TCD seems to have achieved optimal intraoperative monitoring of cerebral blood flow during clamping. As will be seen, we have observed some deterioration in the pre-existing neurological deficit in about 3% of patients

following surgery. In view of the fact that it is not always easy to be sure who needs a shunt in this situation, we have now decided to employ an intraluminal shunt in all patients undergoing expedited CEA for stroke.

Our preferred operative technique is eversion endarterectomy, which would normally require us to insert the shunt immediately after the endarterectomy was performed. However, if the TCD showed a significant fall in MCAV, we consider rapid shunt insertion to be vital. In this situation, we would perform a transposition of the carotid bifurcation in order to put the shunt in place *before* the endarterectomy was performed (Fig. 4.2). Only in very few cases has a vein graft been necessary (e.g. stenosis plus carotid aneurysm).

In order to minimize the risks of intracranial haemorrhage, careful perioperative blood pressure monitoring is mandatory.

Results

No patient died in the 30-day perioperative period and no disabling stroke occurred. Two of 74 patients

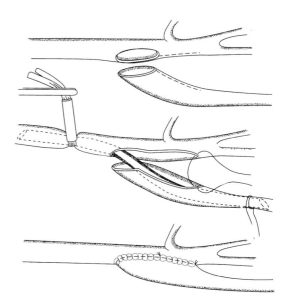

Fig. 4.2
Operative technique showing the method of transposition of the carotid bifurcation. This enables the shunt to be inserted before endarterectomy for those surgeons who prefer to use the eversion endarterectomy method.

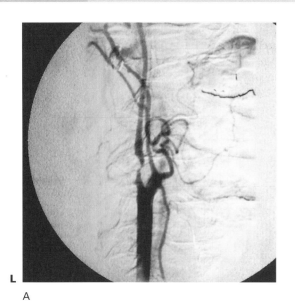

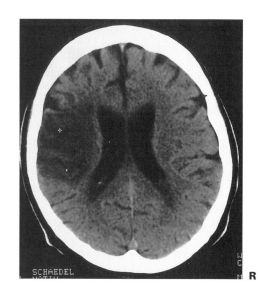

A

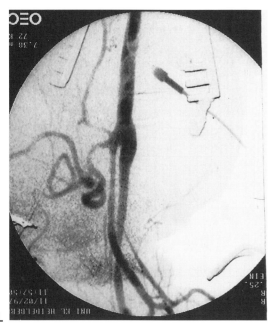

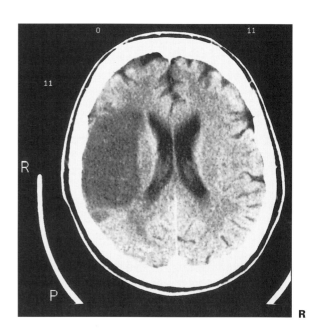

B

Fig. 4.3
A 68-year-old male who underwent carotid endarterectomy 10 days after a completed stroke. (A) Preoperative angiogram (left) and computed tomographic (CT) scan (right). (B) Intraoperative completion angiogram (left). The patient suffered a minor worsening of his pre-existing deficit but a postoperative CT scan showed no change in the area of infarction (right).

suffered a worsening of their pre-existing deficit, resulting in a minor stroke rate of 2.7%. Postoperative CT scanning in these 2 patients showed no evidence of intracranial haemorrhage and no evidence of worsening of the area of ischaemic infarction (Fig. 4.3). Following surgery, most patients continued to improve neurologically and, at 6 months, no patient was classified as Rankin grade 4.

The long-term results are available for the period 1980–1995 ($n = 56$). Using Kaplan Meier life-table analysis, cumulative survival was 95.6% at 1 year, 90.8% at 2 years and 86% at 5 years. No major or fatal ipsilateral stroke occurred during follow-up. Cumulative freedom from any ipsilateral stroke was 94.5% at 5 years. Cumulative freedom from any stroke was 94.5% at 1 year, 90.3% at 2 years and 83.1% at 5 years.[19]

CONCLUSIONS

The traditional recommendation to delay CEA for 6–8 weeks after stroke onset was largely based on experience following CEA in patients with extensive residual neurological deficits and occluded carotid arteries. While we would still not advocate early CEA in these high-risk patients, evidence now suggests that CEA can be performed within 4 weeks of suffering a non-disabling stroke without compromising patient safety. The principal advantage of early operation is the prevention of recurrent stroke.

In Germany, a multicentre observational trial (Carotid Surgery for Ischaemic Stroke (CASIS)) has been implemented to audit the role of expedited CEA in a larger number of patients, using the selection criteria summarized earlier in this chapter.

REFERENCES

1 European Carotid Surgery Trialists' Collaborative Group. MRC European carotid surgery trial: interim results for symptomatic patients with severe (70–99%) or with mild (0–29%) carotid stenosis. *Lancet* 1991; **337**: 1235–1243.

2 North American Symptomatic Carotid Endarterectomy Trial Collaborators. Beneficial effect of carotid endarterectomy in symptomatic patients with high-grade carotid stenosis. *New England Journal of Medicine* 1991; 409, **325**: 445–453.

3 Hafner CD. Totally and nearly occluded extracranial internal carotid arteries. In: Ernst CB, Stanley JC (eds). *Current Therapy in Vascular Surgery*, pp. 46–49. Philadelphia: BC Decker, 1987.

4 Bamford J, Sandercock P, Dennis M, Burn J, Warlow C. Classification and natural history of clinical identifiable subtypes of cerebral infarction. *Lancet* 1991; **337**: 1521–1526.

5 Dosick SM, Whalen RC, Gale SS et al. Carotid endarterectomy in the stroke patient: computerized axial tomography to determine timing. *Journal of Vascular Surgery* 1985; **2**: 214–219.

6 Gasecki AP, Ferguson GG, Eliasziw M et al. Early endarterectomy for severe carotid artery stenosis after a non-disabling stroke: results from the North American Symptomatic Carotid Endarterectomy Trial. *Journal of Vascular Surgery* 1994; **20**: 288–295.

7 Hier DB, Foulkes MA, Swiontoniowski M et al. Stroke recurrence within 2 years after ischaemic infarction. *Stroke* 1991; **22**: 155–161.

8 Burn J, Dennis M, Bamford J et al. Long-term risk of recurrent stroke after a first-ever stroke. The Oxfordshire Community Stroke Project. *Stroke* 1991; **25**: 333–337.

9 Millikan CH, McDowell FH. Treatment of progressive stroke. *Stroke* 1981; **10**: 397–409.

10 Toni D, Fiorelli M, Gentile M et al. Progressing neurological deficit secondary to acute ischaemic stroke. A study on predictability, pathogenesis and prognosis. *Archives of Neurology* 1995; **52**: 670–675.

11 Riles TS, Imparato AM, Jacobowitz GR et al. The cause of perioperative stroke after carotid endarterectomy. *Journal of Vascular Surgery* 1994; **19**: 206–216.

12 Blaisdell WF, Clauss RH, Gailbrath JG, Smith JR. Joint study of extracranial carotid artery occlusion: a review of surgical considerations. *Journal of the American Medical Association* 1969; **209**: 1889–1895.

13 Thompson JE, Austin DJ, Patman RD. Endarterectomy of the totally occluded carotid artery for stroke: results in 100 operations. *Archives of Surgery* 1967; **95**: 791–801.

14 Mead GE, O'Neill PA, McCollum CN. Is there a role for carotid surgery in acute stroke? *European Journal of Vascular and Endovascular Surgery* 1997; **13**: 112–121.

15 Meyer FB, Sundt TM Jr, Piepgras DG et al. Emergency carotid endarterectomy for patients with acute carotid occlusion and profound neurological deficits. *Annals of Surgery* 1986; **5**: 82–89.

16 Goldstone J, Moore WS. A new look at emergency carotid artery operations for the treatment of cerebrovascular insufficiency. *Stroke* 1978; **9**: 599–602.

17 Piotrowski JJ, Bernhard VM, Rubin JR et al. Timing of carotid endarterectomy after acute stroke. *Journal of Vascular Surgery* 1990; **11**: 45–52.

18 Eckstein HH, Schumacher H, Ringleb P, Allenberg JR. Indications for surgery in neurologically unstable patients. In: Branchereau A, Jacobs M (eds). *European Vascular Course: New Trends and Developments in Carotid Artery Disease*, pp. 77–92. Armont: Futura, 1998.

19 Eckstein HH, Schumacher H, Lanbach H et al. Early carotid endarterectomy after non-disabling ischaemic stroke: adequate therapeutical option in selected patients. *European Journal of Vascular and Endovascular Surgery* 1998; **15**: 423–428.

4.2

When should I perform carotid endarterectomy after a completed stroke?

Mark W Sebastian (USA)
Anthony D Whittemore (USA)

INTRODUCTION

Acute stroke is a common condition. Each year more than 500 000 strokes and more than 150 000 stroke-related deaths occur in the US. Stroke is the third leading cause of death in the US and remains the leading cause of disability in our society. Atherothrombotic disease is responsible for a significant percentage of these strokes, and selected patients with atherothrombotic carotid lesions ipsilateral to their cerebral infarction may be candidates for CEA to prevent further strokes or even to minimize the sequelae from an acute stroke.

In the early 1960s acute anticoagulant therapy of carotid territory strokes was associated with clinical improvement in selected patients. These data were unfortunately confounded by the fact that delayed treatment of fixed strokes of greater than 24 h duration resulted in no symptomatic improvement or no clinical benefit. Antithrombotic therapy was furthermore felt to contribute to intracerebral bleeding as a result of reperfusion injury and extension of the infarction from bleeding within compromised but not infarcted tissue.[20] Anticoagulation for the treatment of acute stroke was, therefore, temporarily abandoned.

Likewise, the role of CEA in acute stroke patients was uncertain. CEA was initially performed on symptomatic patients to treat crescendo TIAs or completed stroke with carotid occlusion. Multiple early case reports revealed that only 7–10% of patients with completed stroke were improved after early operation, and that perioperative mortality was as high as 21%.[21–27] Wiley and coworkers in 1964 reported a series in which 5 of 9 patients undergoing endarterectomy for acute stroke died from intracranial hemorrhage.[28] Because of results like

these, CEA was deemed inappropriate in the setting of acute stroke. Wylie et al. suggested that 6 weeks after acute stroke, the blood–brain barrier stabilized and the risk of hemorrhagic conversion of the stroke lessened.[28] The 6-week waiting period after acute stroke was then generally accepted as the safest means for managing stroke patients.

The advent of CT scanning in the late 1970s provided the means to differentiate between hemorrhagic and ischemic infarction and to determine accurately the size and location of the infarction.[29,30] The advent of accurate brain imaging promised improved patient selection.

CURRENT PRACTICE

Despite the dismal early results of CEA for acute stroke, the rationale for early intervention remained clear and attractive. The basic concept underlying the treatment of acute stroke is twofold: first, to minimize extension of cerebral injury due to ongoing hypoperfusion or embolization, and second, to revive penumbral cerebral tissue that is injured, though not infarcted.

One major problem with the policy of routinely waiting 6 weeks prior to endarterectomy in acute stroke victims is the morbidity and frequency of recurrent stroke. Patients suffering an ischemic stroke who are treated non-operatively have an annual risk for recurrent stroke of 5–21%. Furthermore, approximately 30% of the recurrent cerebral ischemic episodes in these patients are fatal. Retrospective review of patients waiting 6 weeks after acute stroke for CEA demonstrated that approximately 20% suffered recurrent stroke during the waiting period.[31] Furthermore, prospective studies suggest that 10% of patients suffer CT-

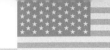

documented reinfarctions during the waiting period.[30] This high incidence of reinfarction has prompted reassessment of the 6-week period.

By the early 1980s, series began to appear reporting low morbidity and mortality with urgent CEA after limited acute stroke. Our group at Brigham and Women's Hospital initially reported a small series of 28 patients in 1984 and expanded the database to 44 patients by 1987.[21,32] These patients were operated on within 4 weeks of an acute stroke, with an operative mortality of 2.3% and no perioperative strokes. Sixty-two percent of patients had CT-documented evidence of infarction in the cerebral hemisphere ipsilateral to the significant carotid stenosis. One of the significant findings in this series was the frequent requirement for intraoperative shunting based on electroencephalographic criteria, a requirement approximately fourfold greater in acute stroke patients than in elective patients. Other retrospective series subsequently reported no significant difference in morbidity between groups of patients who had surgery for ipsilateral carotid stenosis after a stroke at 1–2 weeks, 3–4 weeks, and 5–6 weeks. By the mid 1980s the dogma requiring 4–6 weeks delay after acute stroke had been abandoned. Most recently, analysis of the NASCET data demonstrated no benefit derived from waiting the classical 4–6 weeks following stroke.[33]

Current management of patients presenting with an acute stroke should include three initial steps. First, the patient's baseline neurologic deficit must be precisely defined and neurologic status closely monitored. Second, during this period of initial evaluation and stabilization, the patient must undergo CT scan or magnetic resonance imaging to rule out hemorrhage or mass lesion and document the size of the infarct. Third, a duplex scan of the extracranial carotid arteries must be obtained to identify any potentially correctable carotid lesion. Following this evaluation, the role of thrombolytic therapy should be considered by both surgical and neurologic teams. The patient's level of consciousness is closely monitored, prognosis is determined, and neurologic exam frequently repeated until the patient has stabilized. The patient's comorbid conditions are assessed and managed as well as possible during this period of neurologic assessment. When the patient's neurologic status has stabilized, urgent CEA is considered if the infarct is localized and significant viable hemispheric territory remains at risk.

Contraindications to early surgery after acute stroke include inability to control hypertension, alteration in mental status, severe headache, a fixed neurologic deficit of such magnitude that the prognosis for meaningful recovery is poor even with revascularization, a large-volume infarct on CT scan, significant cerebral edema, and, of course, intracranial hemorrhage. In these patients subsequent neurologic recovery may permit delayed endarterectomy to prevent later recurrent stroke.

Thus, the timing of surgery after acute stroke is individualized, based on the patient's clinical status, the findings on brain imaging studies, and the severity of the carotid lesion. Appropriate individualization of therapy for these patients requires the efforts of stroke neurologists and cerebrovascular surgeons working as a team.

REFERENCES

20 Genton E, Barnett HJM, Fields WS, Gent M, Hoak JC. XIV. Cerebral ischemia: the role of thrombosis and of antithrombotic therapy. Joint Committee for Stroke Resources. Stroke 1977; 8: 150–174.

21 Whittemore AD, Ruby ST, Couch NP, Mannick JA. Early carotid endarterectomy in patients with small, fixed neurologic deficits. Journal of Vascular Surgery 1984; 15: 795–698.

22 Giordano JM, Trout III HH, Kozloff L, DePalma RG. Timing of carotid endarterectomy after stroke. Journal of Vascular Surgery 1985; 2: 250–254.

23 Goldstone JR, Moore WS. A new look at emergency carotid artery operations for the treatment of cerebrovascular insufficiency. Stroke 1978; 9: 599–602.

24 Meyer FB, Sundt TM, Peipgras DG, Sandok BA, Forbest G. Emergency carotid endarterectomy for patients with acute carotid occlusion and profound neurologic deficits. Annals of Surgery 1986; 203: 82–87.

25 Goldstone J, Moore WS. Emergency carotid artery surgery in neurologically unstable patients. Archives of Surgery 1976; 111: 1284–1291.

26 Goldstone J, Effeney DJ. The role of carotid

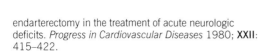
endarterectomy in the treatment of acute neurologic deficits. *Progress in Cardiovascular Diseases* 1980; **XXII**: 415–422.

27 Mentzer RM Jr, Finkelmeier BA, Crosby IK, Wellons HA Jr. Emergency carotid endarterectomy for fluctuating neurologic deficits. *Surgery* 1981; **89**: 60–66.

28 Wylie EF, Hein MF, Adams JE. Intracranial hemorrhage following surgical revascularization for treatment of acute strokes. *Journal of Neurosurgery* 1964; **21**: 212–218.

29 Haykal HA, Rumbaugh CL. Cerebrovascular accident: angiography/radionuclide brain scan/CT. *Postgraduate Radiology* 1984; **4**: 181–202.

30 Dosick SM, Whalen RC, Gale SS, Brown OW. Carotid endarterectomy in the stroke patient: computerized axial tomography to determine timing. *Journal of Vascular Surgery* 1986; **2**: 214–219.

31 Piotrowski J, Bernhard V, Rubin J *et al.* Timing of carotid endarterectomy after acute stroke. *Journal of Vascular Surgery* 1990; **2**: 45–52.

32 Whittemore AD, Mannick JA. Surgical treatment of carotid disease in patients with neurologic deficits. *Journal of Vascular Surgery* 1987; **5**: 910–916.

33 Gasecki AP, Ferguson GG, Eliasziw M *et al.* Early endarterectomy for severe carotid artery stenosis after a nondisabling stroke: results from the North American Symptomatic Carotid Endarterectomy Trial. *Journal of Vascular Surgery* 1994; **20**: 288–295.

4.3   Editorial Comment

1   Evidence from several series and analysis of the NASCET data debunk the previously held dogma that a 6-week waiting period between stroke and CEA is mandatory.
2   A 6-week or greater waiting period still seems most prudent in patients with more severe neurologic deficits, large-volume infarcts on CT/MRI, and significant comorbidity such as poorly controlled hypertension.
3   Expedited surgery is appropriate in those with stable neurologic deficits, minimal CT findings and critical carotid lesions (preocclusive stenosis, free-floating thrombus, etc.) deemed at high risk for early recurrent stroke.
4   Other patients with a stable neurologic deficit and a severe but not critical responsible carotid lesion may be operated on electively within 6 weeks of their stroke without adversely affecting outcome.
5   Certain stroke patients will never be candidates for endarterectomy despite compelling carotid lesions. Such patients include those moribund from massive hemispheric stroke, those with severe multi-infarct dementia, those with massive hemispheric defects on CT/MRI, and those with middle cerebral artery occlusion without recanalization.

The traditional decision to defer CEA for 6 weeks after a completed stroke is based on data derived from 1964 which suggested a high risk of hemorrhagic transformation of the infarction with early operation. With improvements in brain imaging, blood pressure management, and perioperative care, it now seems possible to select those patients at higher risk for early recurrent stroke than for hemorrhagic transformation. The timing of surgery can now be based on criteria other than the fear of intracranial hemorrhage. The nature of the carotid lesion and the patient's overall neurologic status, correlated with brain imaging data, are now the principal criteria determining the timing of CEA in stroke patients.

5.1

In patients with combined carotid and coronary artery disease, should I perform a staged or synchronous procedure?
Peter RF Bell (Europe)

INTRODUCTION

Atherosclerosis is a generalized disease and patients presenting with one aspect of this condition have a significant chance of having similar pathology in other vascular beds. What then are the chances of a patient with coronary artery disease also having a severe carotid artery stenosis? Opinions vary but recent studies using duplex ultrasound suggest that haemodynamically significant carotid lesions occur in 10–18% of patients.[1] The converse is also true, in that patients with significant carotid artery disease also have an increased risk of coronary artery disease. As a result, these patients have an increased risk of perioperative myocardial infarction, which is one of the important causes of morbidity and mortality following carotid surgery. Moreover, as the age of patients undergoing cardiac procedures increases, so too will the number of patients with coexistent carotid artery disease.[2]

PREDICTING RISK

Before embarking on a discussion as to when an operation should be performed, one should first ask the question: Does the presence of severe carotid stenosis increase the risk of stroke in patients undergoing either cardiac valve replacement or coronary artery bypass graft (CABG)? The presence of severe symptomatic carotid artery disease is generally accepted to be a marker of higher perioperative risk.[3] However, the risk attached to asymptomatic carotid stenosis is more difficult to define. For those patients undergoing CABG with coexistent severe, asymptomatic carotid artery disease, the risk of operative stroke is 6–14% as compared to < 2% in those with no evidence of carotid artery disease.[4,5] For those aged less than

45 years, the risk of perioperative stroke is 0.2% as compared with 1% for those aged under 65 years.[6,7] However, once a patient's age exceeds 65 years, the overall risk may increase to 9%.[6,7] The combination of age > 60 years together with a carotid stenosis > 75% increases the operative stroke risk to 15% as compared to 0.6% in similar patients with no carotid stenosis.[1]

Thus, despite the lack of controlled, randomized trials, it seems intuitive that having a severe carotid artery stenosis (whether asymptomatic or symptomatic) does place the cardiac patient at increased risk of suffering a perioperative stroke. However, one should also remain aware that the increased risk may not be solely attributable to the presence of a carotid stenosis, as stroke could also be due to thromboembolic events from other sources such as the aortic arch. Before proceeding to bypass, aortic clamps are applied, which can dislodge emboli into the cerebral circulation. The presence of a carotid stenosis may, therefore, simply be a marker of that increased risk.

PATIENT SELECTION

There are two common scenarios that present to the vascular and cardiac surgeons. The first is the symptomatic carotid patient with coexistent ischaemic heart disease who usually presents to the vascular surgeon, while the second is the cardiac surgery patient who is found to have a coexistent severe carotid artery stenosis.

In the former, the priority is the prevention of stroke and I would prefer to undertake carotid endarterectomy (CEA) as a discrete procedure once it had been satisfied that there was no excessive cardiac risk. On occasions this can be difficult, but our policy would be to refer patients with cardiac failure and poor functional capacity, recent myocardial infarction, unstable angina, severe valvular heart disease and symptomatic arrhythmias for formal cardiological assessment. If the prevailing view was that the cardiac risk was acceptable, I would proceed with CEA without coronary revascularization. If, however, the converse were true, then the patient should proceed to urgent coronary angiography with a view to either coronary angioplasty or CABG (see later).

In the second group of patients, the immediate priority is the treatment of the underlying cardiac problem. The presence of coexistent severe carotid artery disease requires careful assessment in order to minimize the risks of perioperative stroke. In those situations where the carotid stenosis is also symptomatic, the overall decision is more straightforward, as the patient will require both CABG and CEA. The question of timing is discussed below.

The situation regarding patients with asymptomatic carotid disease is more complicated. The evidence above suggests that patients with coexistent asymptomatic carotid artery disease are at greater risk of stroke, not only in the natural history,[8] but particularly when undergoing cardiac surgery. As will be seen, my own personal preference is to perform a synchronous operation in carefully selected patients. These include patients with one carotid artery blocked and the other severely stenosed, as evidence suggests that these patients are at higher risk of stroke, even if they do not have a CABG.[9] Patients with bilateral severe carotid artery disease are a difficult group of patients upon whom to advise, but currently we recommend operating on the carotid artery supplying the dominant hemisphere. However, it is indeed the case that in the 150 patients in whom the Unit have performed a combined CEA and CABG, 3 patients with bilateral disease have suffered a stroke in the non-operated hemisphere, which raises the issue as to whether bilateral procedures should have been performed.

The most difficult subgroup of all are those patients with severe unilateral asymptomatic disease. We have tried to rationalize this problem by using transcranial Doppler (TCD) to evaluate flow patterns within the circle of Willis. If the scan shows good cross-over flow towards the hemisphere supplied by the stenosed artery, then it would seem reasonable not to operate upon these patients. Those with no evidence of recruitment of collateral flow via the anterior or posterior communicating arteries are considered for a synchronous procedure. A summary of our selection policy is presented in Figure 5.1.

STAGED OR SYNCHRONOUS?

Notwithstanding the lack of control data, if we assume that some form of treatment for both symptomatic and asymptomatic carotid disease might be necessary, the question arises as to how one should deal with this. Should the operation be done synchronously or as a staged event?

This debate has been going on for many years and does not end with the simple alternatives

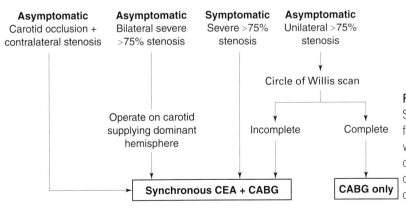

Fig. 5.1
Suggested investigative pathway for the management of patients with combined coronary and carotid artery disease. CEA, carotid endarterectomy; CABG, coronary artery bypass graft.

proposed in the title of this chapter. For example, the potential number of variables within each group are such that it would be difficult to design a randomized controlled study to answer the question. These variables include concurrent comorbidity, especially cardiac status, unilateral carotid disease, bilateral stenoses, unilateral stenosis and contralateral occlusion, symptomatic versus asymptomatic and vertebral artery problems. Moreover, should the carotid artery disease be dealt with before or after CABG, on bypass or off bypass? As a result, most surgeons have evolved views about what should or should not be done without any evidence upon which reliably to base their decisions.

Staged procedures

A number of series have been reported where CEA is performed before the cardiac procedure. The obvious disadvantages are the risks and costs associated with having to do two procedures. Mortality rates range between 0 and 7%[10,11] and stroke rates between 0 and 6%.[1,12] All of these series are, of course, blighted by the usual problems of historical controls and exclusions. One question – should the CEA be performed as a staged procedure after CABG – appears to have been answered by Hertzer's study, where CEA was performed after CABG but within 10 days. Here there was an unacceptably high rate of stroke after the initial cardiac procedure.[13]

In an overview of the published literature, the American Heart Association confirmed this finding (Table 5.1). As a rule, staged procedures with CEA performed first were predominantly complicated by myocardial infarction, while those where the CEA was performed after CABG tended to be complicated by stroke.[14] Therefore, if the staged procedure is to be opted for, it would seem logical to do this before the CABG.

A further modification of this approach would be to perform CEA under local anaesthetic prior to CABG.[15] There is, however, little evidence that operations performed under locoregional anaesthesia are less risky than those performed under general anaesthesia (especially in high-risk cardiac patients) because of the tendency towards elevated blood pressure and plasma noradrenaline levels.[16]

Table 5.1

Overview of operative risk associated with staged and synchronous procedures

Procedure	Stroke	Myocardial infarction	Death
Synchronous CEA + CABG	6.2%	4.7%	5.6%
CEA first, then staged CABG	5.3%	11.5%	9.4%
CABG first, then staged CEA	10%	2.7%	3.6%

CEA, carotid endarterectomy; CABG, coronary artery bypass graft
Derived from a meta-analysis of the published literature between 1970 and 1992.[14]

Synchronous procedures

The obvious advantage of this approach is that the patient only has to undergo one operation and one anaesthetic. The disadvantages are that if the CEA takes too long the patient may be exposed to excessive anaesthetic risks and may even die before going onto bypass.

The pros and cons of a synchronous procedure are confusing. While unacceptably high complication rates have been reported,[17] other studies have described excellent outcomes[18] and an overview confirms that the combined death/stroke/myocardial infarction risk is more evenly balanced.[14] In my own centre, the combined death/stroke and myocardial infarction rate at 30 days is about 6%, which includes the risk of stroke in the contralateral hemisphere.

One of the rationales underlying our preference for the synchronous procedure is that CEA should only be performed to lessen the risk of perioperative stroke in patients who otherwise have to undergo a cardiac procedure. Although the published data suggest that CEA could be performed as a staged procedure prior to CABG, if the patient were to develop on-table cardiac problems there is relatively little one can do. The advantage of the synchronous procedure is that,

Table 5.2
American Heart Association guidelines for synchronous carotid and cardiac surgery in patients with asymptomatic carotid artery disease

	Acceptable	Uncertain	Inappropriate
CEA risk < 3%* + life expectancy > 5 years	Unilateral > 60% stenosis Bilateral > 60% stenosis		
CEA risk 3–5%* + life expectancy > 5 years		Unilateral > 70% stenosis Bilateral > 70% stenosis	
CEA risk 5–10%* + life expectancy > 5 years		Bilateral > 70% stenosis	Unilateral > 70% stenosis

CEA, carotid endarterectomy
*CEA risk means 30-day death/any stroke rate in patients with an asymptomatic carotid stenosis. Adapted from Biller et al.[19]

should such an adverse event occur, the patient is already prepared to go on to bypass should the need arise.

Of course, the decision to proceed to synchronous (or even staged) procedures is dependent on a track record of low CEA risk. Because our current stroke and death rate following elective CEA is about 2%, we feel more comfortable about advocating a synchronous approach in this difficult situation. The American Heart Association have recently published new guidelines (Table 5.2) regarding the appropriateness of performing synchronous procedures[19] and this is primarily dependent on the operative risk during elective CEA in asymptomatic patients.

The technique of the synchronous procedure is important. Our own protocol requires the patients to be prepared in theatre for both operations from the outset. In very high risk patients, a balloon pump can be inserted via the groin into the aorta, or the chest opened in preparation for urgent bypass, but usually the cardiac team harvest the long saphenous vein while the vascular team perform the CEA. A segment of thigh vein is used for carotid patching and, usually, the CEA is completed at the same time that the vein harvesting is completed, thereby avoiding unnecessarily prolonging the procedure. A further important practical point is to ensure that the neck wound is not closed at the end of the CEA. We did this in our first two cases and had to reopen the neck because of haematoma formation. Although a small dose of heparin (5000 iu) is used during CEA, the larger doses employed during bypass inevitably mean that some bleeding will occur. Our usual practice is to close the neck loosely while the CABG proceeds with formal drainage and closure upon its completion.

CONCLUSIONS

No randomized trials have been performed to identify the relative merits of staged and synchronous procedures. Depending upon the staging, the risk of either myocardial infarction or stroke is increased. Synchronous procedures appear to be associated with a blend of the two. There is, however, compelling evidence that CEA after CABG is unwise.

Accordingly, the choice will remain up to individuals as the question as to whether or not an operation should be done and how it should be done remains unanswered. This dilemma may change in the future as more minimally invasive endovascular techniques emerge.

The course of action finally taken will depend on the results of individual centres. If the combined stroke/myocardial infarction/death rate using the synchronous technique is acceptable, it is clearly preferable to performing two separate operations. Patient preference certainly lies in this direction. In the long run, the best results will probably be obtained in centres where the results of CEA in patients without significant cardiac disease are lowest. Yet again, this is another example of the need for careful audit.

REFERENCES

1 Faggioli GL, Curl GR, Ricotta JJ. The role of carotid screening before coronary artery bypass. *Journal of Vascular Surgery* 1990; **12**: 724–729.

2 Jausseran JM, Bergeron P, Reggi M *et al.* Single stage carotid and coronary artery surgery: indications and results. *Journal of Cardiovascular Surgery* 1989; **30**: 407–413.

3 Ricotta JJ, Faggioli GL, Castilone A *et al.* Risk factors for stroke after open heart surgery. *Journal of Vascular Surgery* 1995; **21**: 359–364.

4 Ricotta JJ. The approach to patients with carotid bifurcation disease in need of coronary artery bypass grafting. *Seminars in Vascular Surgery* 1995; **8**: 62–69.

5 Brenner BJ, Brief DK, Alpert J *et al.* The risks of stroke in patients with asymptomatic stenosis undergoing cardiac surgery. *Journal of Vascular Surgery* 1987; **5**: 269–279.

6 Gardner TJ, Horneffer PJ, Manolio TA, Hoff SJ, Pearson TA. Major stroke after coronary bypass surgery: changing magnitude of the problem. *Journal of Vascular Surgery* 1986; **3**: 6844–6687.

7 Tuman KJ, McCarthy RJ, Najafi H, Ivankovich AD. Differential effects of advanced age on neurologic and cardiac risks of coronary artery operations. *Journal of Thoracic and Cardiovascular Surgery* 1992; **104**: 1510–1517.

8 Executive Committee for the Asymptomatic Carotid Atherosclerosis Study. Endarterectomy for asymptomatic carotid artery stenosis. *Journal of the American Medical Association* 1995; **273**: 1421–1428.

9 Bock RW, Grag-weal C, Mock PA *et al.* The natural history of asymptomatic carotid artery disease. *Journal of Vascular Surgery* 1993; **17**: 160–171.

10 Pillai L, Guttierez I, Curl GR *et al.* Evaluation and treatment of carotid stenosis in open heart surgery patients. *Journal of Surgical Research* 1994; **57**: 212–215.

11 Rosenthal D, Caudill DR, Lamis PA. Carotid and coronary artery disease: a rational approach. *American Journal of Surgery* 1984; **52**: 332–335.

12 Bernhard VM, Johnson WD, Petersen JJ. Carotid artery stenosis: association with surgery for coronary artery disease. *Archives of Surgery* 1972; **105**: 837–840.

13 Hertzer NR, Loop FD, Beven EG. Surgical staging for simultaneous coronary and carotid disease: a study including prospective randomisation. *Journal of Vascular Surgery* 1989; **9**: 455–463.

14 Moore WS, Barnett HJM, Beebe HG *et al.* Guidelines for carotid endarterectomy. *Circulation* 1995; **91**: 566–579.

15 Fiorani P, Starigin E, Speziale F *et al.* General anaesthesia versus cervical block and perioperative complications in carotid artery surgery. *European Journal of Vascular and Endovascular Surgery* 1997; **13**: 37–42.

16 Forsell C, Takolander R, Bergqvist D, Johannsson A. Local versus general anaesthesia in carotid surgery: a prospective randomised trial. *European Journal of Vascular Surgery* 1989; **3**: 503–509.

17 Bass A, Krupski WC, Dilli R *et al.* Combined carotid endarterectomy and coronary artery revascularisation: a sobering review. *Israeli Journal of Medical Science* 1992; **28**: 27–32.

18 Halpin DB, Riggins S, Carmichael JD *et al.* Management of carotid and coronary artery disease. *Southern Medical Journal* 1994; **87**: 187–189.

19 Biller J, Feinberg WM, Castaldo JE *et al* Guidelines for carotid endarterectomy: a statement for healthcare professionals from a special writing group of the Stroke Council, American Heart Association. *Stroke* 1998; **29**: 554–562.

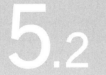

5.2 In patients with combined carotid and coronary artery disease, should I perform a staged or synchronous procedure?

William C Mackey (USA)

BACKGROUND

When screened with duplex ultrasound, up to 22% of coronary bypass patients are found to have 50% or greater carotid stenosis, and up to 12% to have 80% or greater carotid stenosis.[20–22] The presence of carotid disease in coronary bypass patients is clearly associated with perioperative stroke. In a retrospective study of 1179 cardiac surgery patients, > 50% carotid stenosis was associated with a sixfold increase in stroke risk, but the anatomic distribution of the strokes did not correlate with the side of the carotid lesion.[20]

In addition, more than 50% of patients presenting for CEA have clinically apparent coronary disease (angina, prior infarction, or ischemic electrocardiogram abnormalities), and approximately 50% of patients with symptomatic or asymptomatic carotid disease will have abnormal nuclear angiocardiograms.[23,24] Myocardial infarction is by far the leading cause of perioperative and late death following carotid surgery.[23]

Approximately 309 000 patients underwent coronary bypass in the US in 1992 (American Heart Association, 1995 Statistical Supplement). As above, up to 12% (or over 36 000) would be predicted to have 80% or greater carotid stenosis. Since the benefit of CEA in both symptomatic and asymptomatic patients with 80% or greater carotid stenosis has been clearly demonstrated, a policy of ignoring carotid disease in coronary bypass patients is not tenable. The incidence and clinical significance of carotid lesions in coronary bypass patients amply demonstrate the need for a well-defined management algorithm for patients presenting with surgically significant coronary and carotid disease.

One significant problem in analyzing outcome by choice of treatment in patients presenting with both coronary and carotid disease is the multiple potential causes of stroke in coronary bypass patients. While the presence of carotid disease appears to represent a significant marker for perioperative stroke risk, the carotid lesion itself may not be responsible for each stroke. The carotid lesion may simply be a marker for severe atherosclerosis. While Ricotta et al.[20] found a sixfold increase in stroke risk in coronary bypass patients presenting with carotid disease, the location of the strokes did not correlate with the side for the carotid lesion.

Embolization from aortic atheroma at the time of cross-clamping is probably the most frequent cause of stroke in coronary bypass patients. In their study published in the New England Journal of Medicine, Roach et al.[25] found proximal aortic atherosclerosis to be the most significant predictor of postoperative neurologic events (odds ratio 4.52), followed by history of neurologic disease (3.19), use of intra-aortic balloon pump (2.60), diabetes (2.59), and hypertension (2.31). Aortic atheromata, pump-related air or thromboembolism, cardiogenic embolism, hypoperfusion related to carotid or intracranial occlusive disease and low cardiac output, and intracranial hemorrhage are all potential sources for stroke in coronary bypass patients. Carotid endarterectomy cannot, therefore, prevent all strokes in coronary bypass patients.

CURRENT TREATMENT OPTIONS

The options for management of coexisting carotid and coronary disease include CEA followed by coronary bypass (staged approach), coronary bypass followed by CEA (reversed staged approach), and simultaneous CEA and coronary bypass (synchronous approach). A meta-analysis of the outcomes of these management strategies based on 56 English-language reports between 1970 and 1992 failed to reveal a distinct outcome advantage for any of the three.[26] In Table 5.3, the results of this meta-analysis are summarized. These results are consistent with an intuitive understanding of the issues involved. Performing the carotid endarterectomy first yields the lowest stroke risk but results in higher myocardial infarction ($P = 0.01$) and mortality ($P = 0.02$) risks. Performing the coronary bypass first yields the lowest mortality risk but a significantly higher stroke risk ($P < 0.05$).[26] The simultaneous CABG–CEA strategy resulted in intermediate stroke, myocardial infarction, and death rates.[26] The authors concluded: 'The optimal strategy for management of patients with combined coronary and carotid disease will be established only by a well-designed prospective randomized trial'.[26]

Table 5.3
Probability of adverse outcome by management strategy

	Stroke	MI	Death
Simultaneous	0.062	0.047	0.056
Staged (CEA, CABG)	0.053	0.115	0.094
Reversed staged (CABG, CEA)	0.100	0.027	0.036

MI, myocardial infarction; CEA, carotid endarterectomy; CABG, coronary artery bypass graft.
Reproduced from Moore et al.[26] with permission.

Unfortunately, no large-scale randomized trial has yet been conducted. Hertzer et al. evaluated these three strategies in a study which included randomization for some patients.[27] In this study, 129 patients with unilateral asymptomatic lesions were eligible for randomization to simultaneous versus reversed staged strategies, but because of cardiac risk were not eligible for randomization to the staged strategy. Mortality (4.2% vs 5.3%) and stroke morbidity (2.8% vs 14%) were lower in the simultaneous than in the reversed-staged group ($P = 0.042$ for stroke morbidity).[27] Only 24 patients with very stable cardiac status were eligible for a staged strategy, which was associated with stroke and death rates of 4.2%.[27]

In the study of Hertzer et al. patients with more critical coronary and carotid disease were managed on a case-by-case basis, with 99 undergoing simultaneous treatment (6.1% mortality and 7.1% stroke) and 23 undergoing coronary bypass followed by carotid endarterectomy (0% mortality but 16.1% stroke morbidity).[27]

In the absence of a large-scale prospective randomized trial, clinical practice must be guided by the available literature, which consists mostly of reports of the experience of individual institutions with their chosen management protocol. A review of this literature is confusing. Contemporary series of patients managed with simultaneous CABG–CEA include mortality rates ranging from 2% to 12% and stroke morbidity rates ranging from 1% to 15%.[28–30] Review of these contemporary series suggests that this wide variability in outcome is due to significant variations in patient selection for simultaneous procedures. Those centers which aggressively screen coronary bypass patients for carotid lesions and offer synchronous operations to those with unilateral asymptomatic carotid lesions report the lowest stroke morbidity and mortality rates. Hertzer et al. reported a 4.2% mortality rate and a 2.8% stroke rate in 71 patients with unilateral asymptomatic carotid lesions.[27] Chang et al. reported on 189 patients who underwent synchronous procedures with a mortality rate of 2% and a stroke rate of 1%.[28] Contralateral occlusion was present in only 13 (6.9%) and severe bilateral stenoses in only 6 (3.2%) of these patients.[28]

On the other hand, those centers restricting synchronous procedures to higher-risk patients with carotid symptoms, with critical bilateral stenoses, or with unilateral critical stenosis and contralateral occlusion report less favorable results. In the past our approach was to restrict the synchronous approach to those patients with symptoms of severe bilateral disease, and our stroke morbidity and mortality rates were 9% and 8% respectively.[31]

Similarly, Curl et al.[29] reported stroke and mortality rates of 6.3% and 11.7% respectively in 34 high-risk patients, and Coyle et al.[30] found perioperative stroke and death rates of 15.4% and 10.8% respectively. Those patients who would appear most likely to benefit from synchronous carotid endarterectomy and coronary bypass suffer the highest morbidity and mortality with this approach.

Curl and colleagues[29] advocate the staged approach based on their finding that 65% of patients with surgical carotid and coronary disease can safely undergo pre-bypass carotid endarterectomy with excellent stroke (3.1%) and mortality (3.1%) rates. Hertzer et al. however, found that fewer than one-third of coronary bypass patients at the Cleveland Clinic were eligible for this approach because of the perceived cardiac risk associated with the endarterectomy.[27]

Similarly, the reversed staged approach, while associated with the lowest mortality and myocardial infarction rates, may be associated with an unacceptable stroke rate – 14% in Hertzer's randomized series and 16% in his non-randomized group.[27]

While all authorities agree that a large-scale prospective randomized trial is necessary to define the optimal management strategy for patients with both carotid and coronary disease, the logistical and ethical considerations involved in the planning of such a trial are formidable. Based on the above-cited meta-analysis, it may not be justifiable simply to assign patients randomly to one of the three strategies. Patients with unstable cardiac disease and/or very ominous coronary anatomy should not be eligible for randomization to the staged approach. Patients with particularly ominous carotid anatomy and/or active cerbrovascular symptoms should not be eligible for randomization to the reversed staged approach. If a strict three-way randomization protocol is attempted in such a trial, patient accrual may be very slow, since the management strategies may not be seen as equally acceptable for all patients. On the other hand, if a variety of randomization protocols are offered based on the severity of the coronary and carotid disease, the statistical power of the study will be significantly diluted and very large numbers of patients will have

to be randomized to reach scientifically valid conclusions.

Recently a proposal for a large-scale randomized prospective trial was submitted to the National Institutes of Health. This protocol included two separate randomization schemes based on cardiac risk. Patients deemed at high cardiac risk would be randomly assigned to simultaneous or reversed staged management strategies, while those deemed to be at lower coronary risk would be randomly assigned to staged or simultaneous strategies. This study has not been funded.

SYNCHRONOUS, STAGED, OR REVERSED STAGED?

In the absence of persuasive data, it is impossible to articulate one correct management protocol. Management of patients presenting with surgical disease in both the coronary and carotid arteries must be based on common sense and a knowledge of the existing literature, confusing and flawed as it may be. A logical approach to these patients is outlined in Table 5.4.

Table 5.4
Suggested management algorithm for simultaneous carotid and coronary disease

	Carotids		
	Critical	Severe	Elective
Coronaries			
Critical	Synchronous	Synchronous	Reversed?
Severe	Synchronous	Synchronous	Synchronous
Elective	Staged	Staged	Staged

For definitions see text.

In Table 5.4, critical coronary disease is defined as severe left main stenosis, severe left main equivalent or triple-vessel disease, unstable (requiring intravenous nitrates, etc.) or post-infarction angina, or severely depressed left ventricular function. Severe coronary disease is defined as multivessel coronary disease with limiting but stable angina and moderately depressed

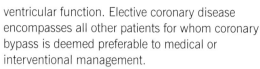

ventricular function. Elective coronary disease encompasses all other patients for whom coronary bypass is deemed preferable to medical or interventional management.

Critical carotid disease is defined as active carotid territory transient ischemic attacks or recent stroke related to a 70–99% carotid stenosis or a 70–99% asymptomatic carotid stenosis opposite an occluded carotid. Severe carotid disease is defined as bilateral asymptomatic 70–99% stenoses. Elective carotid disease is defined as a unilateral asymptomatic 70–99% stenosis.

With the recommended management algorithm, patients with critical carotid and coronary disease would undergo a synchronous coronary bypass–CEA, because there is no rational alternative. Operative risk in these patients is increased (5–10% mortality and stroke rates) because of their severe systemic atherosclerosis, but the staged or reversed staged approaches would probably be associated with even higher mortality or stroke rates. This group is very likely to have severe arch atherosclerosis and a high risk of stroke on this basis. Epiaortic ultrasound imaging and the use of surgical techniques designed to minimize aortic manipulation may be useful in this group in the prevention of perioperative strokes.

Patients with critical coronary and severe carotid disease are probably also best served by the synchronous approach. Staging in these patients is unacceptable, and reversed staging may be associated with a very high stroke risk based on their bilateral high-grade stenoses. Although a few surgeons would advocate synchronous bilateral endarterectomies and coronary bypass in these patients, most would correct the more critical or, if equal, the dominant hemisphere lesion with the coronary bypass and leave the opposite side for later.

The reversed staged strategy seems only applicable in patients with critical coronary disease and elective carotid disease. Prolongation of the coronary bypass by the addition of CEA in these patients may be difficult to justify. If, however, the

unilateral carotid lesion is preocclusive, reversed staging may not be appropriate.

Patients with elective coronary disease and carotid disease in any of the above categories are probably best served by staged procedures (endarterectomy followed by coronary bypass). With modern anesthetic and surgical techniques, the cardiac risk of endarterectomy in these patients is very low. The coronary bypass can be carried out within 72 h of the endarterectomy in almost all cases. Patients with bilateral critical carotid lesions and elective coronary disease are probably best managed by first performing CEA on the more severe of the carotid lesions (or, if the lesions are of equal severity, on the dominant hemisphere lesion), and then performing a synchronous coronary bypass and contralateral CEA.

An alternative to the management algorithm shown in Table 5.4 is to recommend synchronous procedures for all patients presenting with surgical disease in the carotid and coronary circulations. Recently, some authors have advocated routine synchronous procedures based on excellent results at their institutions.[32,33] When associated with acceptable morbidity rates, this approach undoubtedly results in less resource utilization and shorter inpatient stay than the more individualized management plan outlined above. While routine use of synchronous endarterectomy and coronary bypass is certainly the simplest approach to these difficult patients, it may not be the safest approach for all patients in all settings.

The choice of optimal therapy for patients with significant coronary and carotid disease becomes even more complex when the various endovascular options for treating these lesions are considered. As these treatment modalities – especially carotid angioplasty/stenting – mature, they may provide safer alternatives to traditional surgical therapy in this very high risk population. All reasonable management strategies for coexistent carotid and coronary disease must be evaluated in scientifically valid comparative studies.

REFERENCES

20 Ricotta JJ, Faggioli GJ, Castilone A, Hassett JM. Risk factors for stroke after cardiac surgery. *Journal of Vascular Surgery* 1995; **21**: 359–364.

21 Schwartz LB, Bridgman AH, Kieffer RW *et al*. Asymptomatic carotid artery stenosis and stroke in patients undergoing cardiopulmonary bypass. *Journal of Vascular Surgery* 1195; **21**: 146–153.

22 Gerraty RP, Gates PC, Doyle JC. Carotid stenosis and perioperative stroke risk in symptomatic and asymptomatic patients undergoing vascular or coronary surgery. *Stroke* 1993; **24**: 1115–1118.

23 Mackey WC, O'Donnell TF, Callow AD. Cardiac risk in patients undergoing carotid endarterectomy: impact on perioperative and long-term mortality. *Journal of Vascular Surgery* 1990; **11**: 226–234.

24 Love BB, Grover-McKay M, Biller J *et al*. Coronary artery disease and cardiac events with asymptomatic and symptomatic cerebrovascular disease. *Stroke* 1992; **23**: 939–945.

25 Roach GW, Kanchuger M, Mangano CM *et al*. Adverse cerebral outcomes after coronary bypass surgery. *New England Journal of Medicine* 1996; **335**: 1857–1863.

26 Moore WS, Barnett HJM, Beebe HG *et al*. Guidelines for carotid endarterectomy: a multidisciplinary consensus statement from the ad hoc committee, American Heart Association. *Stroke* 1995; **26**: 188–201.

27 Hertzer NR, Loop FD, Beven EG *et al*. Surgical staging for simultaneous coronary and carotid disease: a study including prospective randomization. *Journal of Vascular Surgery* 1989; **9**: 455–463.

28 Chang BB, Darling C, Shah DM *et al*. Carotid endarterectomy can be safely performed with acceptable mortality and morbidity in patients requiring coronary artery bypass grafts. *American Journal of Surgery* 1994; **168**: 94–97.

29 Curl GR, Pillai L, Raza ST *et al*. Staged vs combined carotid endarterectomy in coronary bypass patients. Abstract presented at Ninth Eastern Vascular Society Meeting, Buffalo, 5/5/1995.

30 Coyle KA, Gray BC, Smith RB *et al*. Morbidity and mortality associated with carotid endarterectomy; effect of adjunctive coronary revascularization. *Annals of Vascular Surgery* 1995; **9**: 21–27.

31 Mackey WC, Khabbaz K, Bojar R, O'Donnell TF. Simultaneous carotid endarterectomy and coronary bypass: perioperative risk and long-term survival. *Journal of Vascular Surgery* 1996; **24**: 58–64.

32 Akins CW, Moncure AC, Daggett WM *et al*. Safety and efficacy of concomitant carotid and coronary operations. *Annals of Thoracic Surgery* 1995; **60**: 311–318.

33 Takach TJ, Reul GJ, Cooley DA *et al*. Is an integrated approach warranted for concomitant carotid and coronary artery disease? *Annals of Thoracic Surgery* 1997; **64**: 16–22.

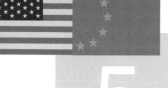

5.3 Editorial Comment

KEY POINTS

1   There is no evidence from randomized trials to support the preferential use of staged as opposed to synchronous procedures.
2   In patients presenting with symptomatic carotid disease, the priority is stroke prevention. Only those patients with evidence for high-risk coronary artery disease which cannot be corrected by prior medical or endovascular means should be considered for staged or synchronous procedures.
3   In patients presenting with coronary disease, the priority is prevention of myocardial infarction. Only those patients considered at high risk for perioperative stroke should be considered for staged or synchronous procedures.
4   If the stroke/death rate for CEA for asymptomatic disease is > 5%, according to American Heart Association guidelines, the role of prophylactic endarterectomy prior to CABG is uncertain.

The authors agree that the presence of significant carotid disease in CABG patients substantially increases the risk of perioperative stroke, and that the carotid disease may not be the causative agent of the strokes but rather only a marker for the severity of generalized atherosclerosis in the aortic arch and elsewhere.

In patients presenting with carotid disease who are found to have coronary disease, the priority is stroke prevention. The ends of stroke prevention can be served only if the endarterectomy can be performed safely. With expert anesthetic management most patients with coronary disease can undergo endarterectomy without preceding coronary revascularization. Coronary disease will adversely affect longevity and should be evaluated and treated aggressively as part of the patient's ongoing medical care. CEA patients with unstable coronary disease will require pre-endarterectomy coronary angiography and subsequent coronary angioplasty followed by CEA or combined CEA-CABG.

In patients presenting with coronary disease primarily (the most common situation), the priority is prevention of myocardial infarction and death. The safety of CABG in patients with severe carotid disease is compromised both by the carotid lesions and by the severity of the patient's systemic atherosclerosis. In selected patients, such as those with concomitant carotid symptoms or compelling carotid anatomy, the safety of the procedure may be enhanced by treating the carotid lesion either before or at the same time as the CABG. These are high-risk patients. With any treatment algorithm, strokes will occur as a result of arch lesion embolization, intracranial occlusive disease, poor cardiac function with hypotension, vertebrobasilar disease, pump-related air or particulate embolization, or contralateral carotid lesions. It is indeed difficult to prove the benefit of CEA in this patient population.

While randomized trials could be designed to define better the management of patients with both coronary and carotid disease, the logistical issues involved in the design of such a trial seem daunting. For now, each institution must carefully design and evaluate its management of these patients, with an eye toward minimizing short-term morbidity and mortality and optimizing long-term quality survival.

6.1 Is there a role for carotid surgery in patients with non-hemispheric or vertebrobasilar symptoms?

Roger M Greenhalgh (Europe)

INDICATIONS: SYMPTOMS OR ANATOMY?

There are locations in the world where vertebral artery surgery is relatively frequently performed. It seems rather strange that some centres perform very much more vertebral artery surgery than others implying that more patients are referred to them and that therefore they see more of the patients requiring the operation. Certainly, vertebral artery surgery is rarely performed in most tertiary vascular centres and only one or two centres in the world stand out as performing larger numbers of vertebral operations than others. Some specialize in proximal vertebral reimplantation and others in an operation on the distal vertebral artery. It is a matter of great interest why patients are referred to these centres because anatomical abnormalities are found by chance during angiography to determine whether the patients have true vertebrobasilar symptoms. Working as I do in a regional vascular service alongside a regional neurovascular service for the whole of the west of London, I find that confirmation of the presenting symptom of vertebrobasilar insufficiency is made with extreme caution by even the most experienced neurologist. In my experience, symptoms of vertebrobasilar insufficiency can just as easily be associated with severe bilateral carotid artery disease which is otherwise relatively easily corrected.

PATIENT PRESENTATION AND THE IMPORTANCE OF THE CIRCLE OF WILLIS

An experienced neurologist will occasionally diagnose so-called misery perfusion in patients with symptoms which they attribute to vertebrobasilar insufficiency. These symptoms usually include double vision and a sense of instability or unsteadiness on the feet and dizziness. These symptoms are thought by the neurologist to relate to poor hind brain perfusion. Neurologists also describe a particular visual symptom in these patients in which vision is affected when the patient enters a bright room. The neurologists are then able to examine the eyes and, by gentle orbital pressure, which distorts blood flow to the retina, diagnose misery perfusion clinically; in these patients, the vertebrobasilar nature of the symptoms is more certain. Every neurologist is very cautious about making this diagnosis but, in my experience, when they do, the patients almost always have bilateral severe carotid artery stenoses.

Because of the finding of severe bilateral carotid artery stenoses in these patients, one assumes that the input of arterial pressure to the circle of Willis from each carotid artery has led in some way to poor perfusion to the posterior cerebral circulation. This implies that the vertebral and basilar arteries are not providing enough perfusion. Sometimes angiography can demonstrate a reason for this but there can sometimes be no anatomical explanation on angiography and thus no vertebral artery surgery comes into question. If posterior cerebral perfusion is reduced, then perfusion to the front of the brain is also likely if the carotid arteries are the reason for this.

Function of the brain supplied by the anterior cerebral artery seems much more difficult to assess even than vertebrobasilar insufficiency! It usually requires psychological assessment, but sometimes patients can be so drowsy and have obvious personality change that they and their relatives know they are different from earlier years. Anecdotally, there are a number of patients who have had carotid surgery performed in our regional centre to increase

57

circle of Willis perfusion. In these there has been a correction of personality with a return to the type of person the patient was decades before. One such was a senior lecturer in the preclinical department in the medical school where I work. He was a docile gentleman with a passive accepting smile and his lectures had become uninteresting and without zip and zest. His wife knew that he was not the man of his youth. He had symptoms of double vision and dizziness and was found to have a total occlusion of one carotid artery and a 99% stenosis of the other and no vertebral or basilar disease. A neurological colleague recommended carotid surgery, which was performed with correction of double vision, dizziness, unsteadiness of gait and with an unexpected and dramatic personality change. His wife found again 'the man I married' and the lectures suddenly regained their liveliness.

Others will not place great store on my personal observation but seeing is believing and this triggered a thought process that the improvement in this patient must have been through increased flow to the anterior portion of the brain and to the posterior portion of the brain through improved perfusion in each direction through the circle of Willis, which was complete in this case. Following this experience, we have recently sought to document patients thought to have posterior circulation symptoms of vertebrobasilar insufficiency who have undergone carotid endarterectomy.

CAROTID ENDARTERECTOMY FOR VERTEBROBASILAR INSUFFICIENCY

The consecutive series described above is unpublished and consists of 19 patients, in which there are complete data on 18. (The 19th patient died.) In these 18 patients, a consultant neurologist diagnosed vertebrobasilar insufficiency on the basis of double vision and dizziness with confirmatory suggestive signs of misery perfusion. The patients underwent the same preoperative investigation and operative treatment as described in my chapter on emergency surgery (Chapter 3). All patients were treated with Javid intraluminal shunts, as it was felt that, in every case, the 'master artery' was being operated upon and the

flow of blood to the brain was already restrictive and dependent upon that carotid vessel. In most patients, the contralateral carotid artery was occluded and the operated vessel had severe stenosis of certainly greater than 70% and usually greater than 90%. It is not always easy to be certain which carotid artery should be operated upon, but if any lateralization was suggested from the symptoms, then the appropriate symptomatic side was operated upon in the first instance. The surgeon must be prepared to operate on the second side if symptoms do not subside following the first operation. This was performed once in this series. Dexamethasone was used with the premedication and for 2 days thereafter because of the expected increase in blood flow using the procedure designed for that purpose.

In the 2-year period since we have been alerted to this problem, all 18 patients have had their presenting symptoms corrected by carotid surgery – unilateral in 17 and bilateral in the 18th patient.

DISCUSSION

These data amount to no more than pilot information upon which a future study can be based. Neurologists are extremely reluctant to accept that symptoms of vertebrobasilar insufficiency can be corrected by operation on the anterior circulation when they have attributed the symptoms to a paucity of posterior cerebral circulation. Conventional neurological wisdom is that surgery to the anterior circulation cannot be expected to benefit posterior circulation symptoms. However, if the circle of Willis is complete, allowing increased carotid perfusion flow to benefit the posterior circulation, then such symptoms might be expected to be corrected. My own observation is that carotid surgery has relieved symptoms of vertebrobasilar insufficiency in those patients in whom we demonstrated no restriction to blood flow in the vertebral or basilar arteries. We have taken to performing magnetic resonance angiography to image the circle of Willis in all such patients before carotid surgery and to be certain that the circle of Willis is complete. In addition, transcranial imaging by duplex ultrasound of the circle of Willis is now becoming possible and this is a helpful preoperative assessment. To clinch this suspicion, it will be necessary to use functional magnetic resonance imaging of the brain to show a change in perfusion to the front and back of the brain caused by carotid surgery; this change should be associated with improved vertebrobasilar symptoms (posterior circulation) and psychological assessments (anterior circulation).

CONCLUSIONS

For the moment, my personal view is that there is a limited role for carotid surgery in patients with vertebrobasilar insufficiency but that this role is far from proven at the present time. I have great scepticism about the value of vertebral artery surgery and little experience of vertebrobasilar insufficiency being relieved by surgery to the vertebral artery.

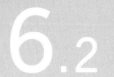

6.2

Is there a role for carotid surgery in patients with non-hemispheric or vertebrobasilar symptoms?

John Ricotta (USA)

Kara Kvilekval (USA)

The indications for carotid endarterectomy have become increasingly well defined since the Asymptomatic Carotid and Atherosclerosis Study (ACAS) and North American Symptomatic Carotid Endarterectomy Trial (NASCET) studies. The primary mechanism of stroke in the anterior circulation is generally accepted to be embolic, originating from a stenosis in the internal carotid artery or occasionally from a more proximal lesion; hypoperfusion is of secondary importance as the result of collateral flow and cerebral autoregulation. In contradistinction, although emboli from the vertebral or subclavian arteries may occasionally cause ischemia in the vertebrobasilar circulation,[1] hypoperfusion is presumed to be the main etiology of vertebrobasilar symptoms. Carotid endarterectomy has become the treatment of choice for those patients with hemispheric symptoms and a high-grade stenosis of the carotid artery. There is no consensus, however, about the efficacy of carotid endarterectomy in patients with non-hemispheric symptoms.

The difficulty arises in part from the array of symptomatology that can be ascribed to ischemia in the vertebrobasilar system, and the multiple potential etiologies of these symptoms. As a result, these patients often present a diagnostic challenge. Patients with non-hemispheric symptoms may complain of dizziness (or light-heartedness), vertigo, diploplia, ataxia, dysarthria, drop attacks, paresthesias, headaches, bilateral or alternating limb weakness, visual blurring, and syncope. Differential diagnosis includes cardiac dysrhythmia, autonomic dysfunction, microangiopathy, migraine, middle- or inner-ear disease and non-organic syndromes. The diagnostic work-up is tailored to the history and physical and may include Holter monitoring,

echocardiography, tilt-table studies, auditory and vestibular testing, medication history, and brain imaging or electroencephalogram, in addition to evaluation of vertebrobasilar insufficiency from a stenotic, embolic, or compressive source.

In patients whose symptoms are thought to be vertebrobasilar in origin, and who have a concurrent high-grade carotid stenosis, carotid endarterectomy may have a beneficial effect if collateral pathways to the posterior circulation and brainstem are intact. In these patients, non-hemispheric or vertebrobasilar symptoms may be relieved if improvement in flow in the posterior circulation can be established from the anterior circulation through an intact circle of Willis or other collateral pathways. However, as we will note, demonstration of intact collateral circulation is not always practical.

HISTORICAL STUDIES

Studies have suggested conflicting results for the relief of non-hemispheric symptoms by carotid endarterectomy. Humphries et al.[2] found that carotid endarterectomy relieved the complaints of vertigo in all patients with associated significant carotid stenosis. Fields et al.[3] found no outcome difference of medical versus surgical treatment of non-hemispheric symptoms. McNamara et al.[4] found that 44% of patients treated with carotid endarterectomy continued to experience their preoperative symptoms, in contrast to only 15% of those patients who had hemispheric signs preoperatively. Ford et al.[5] reported that in those patients complaining of non-hemispheric symptoms, the majority benefited from carotid endarterectomy. The benefit was maximal in patients without stenosis in the subclavian or

vertebral system (71%), although even those patients with stenosis did benefit in the majority of cases (61%).

Rosenthal et al.[6] retrospectively reviewed 114 patients complaining of vertebrobasilar insufficiency either alone or in conjunction with anterior circulation signs who underwent angiography and carotid endarterectomy. They found improvement in 80% of the patients postoperatively and, of those alive in the 10-year follow-up period, 88% remained asymptomatic. Patients who did not have relief of symptoms in this study ultimately were found to have a variety of disorders: cardiac arrhythmia, seizure disorders, diabetic or hypertensive retinopathy, idiopathic hypertrophic subaortic stenosis and labyrinthitis. In this series, a subset of patients had the gradients measured across the bifurcation at the time of surgery. Fifty-nine of the 80 patients who improved after endarterectomy in this subset had minimal gradients across the carotid bifurcation found at surgery, leading these authors to conclude that an embolic etiology was more important than hypoperfusion. Others, however, have found that a hemodynamically significant stenosis in the carotid artery is an important predictor of success.

Ouriel et al.[7] studied 107 patients undergoing carotid endarterectomy for non-hemispheric symptoms. They divided these patients into those with classic vertebrobasilar ischemia and those not meeting classic criteria. Classic symptoms consisted of a non-hemispheric motor deficit, a non-hemispheric sensory deficit, a visual loss in both homonymous fields, ataxia or vertigo, plus diplopia, or dysarthria in combination with one of the other symptoms but not alone. Non-classic symptoms were vertigo, syncope, confusion, seizures, dysarthria, and diploplia. They found that, in those patients with classic vertebrobasilar symptoms, 73% became asymptomatic postoperatively, whereas only 43% became asymptomatic in the group with non-classic symptoms. Carotid stump pressures were measured in this study and found to have no correlation with results. Carotid stenosis of greater than 60% was, however, significantly related to results. In those patients with vertebrobasilar symptoms and a carotid stenosis >60%, 77%

became asymptomatic after carotid endarterectomy; when the stenosis was < 60%, only 36% became asymptomatic.

In a subsequent study, Ouriel et al.[8] found that patients with an abnormal OPG were much more likely to be asymptomatic than those with a normal OPG (72% vs 36%). This study also showed better results in those patients with classic non-hemispheric symptoms. These studies suggest that an increase in perfusion in the anterior system improved that of the posterior system. Ricotta et al.[9] reviewed their long-term follow-up of 61 patients undergoing carotid endarterectomy for non-hemispheric symptoms. They only operated on patients with > 60% carotid stenosis. In this study, mean follow-up was 42.3 months. Symptoms recurred in 11 patients (18%): (3/11 patients did not have initial relief of symptoms, while the other 8 patients were symptom-free for 23–111 months). In contradistinction to earlier studies, symptomatic recurrence was not more frequent in patients with non-classic vertebrobasilar symptoms.

Overall, these studies suggest that carotid endarterectomy can relieve vertebrobasilar symptoms by augmenting flow to the brainstem or posterior circulation. This can be important when normal extracranial flow is compromised intracranially by disease or developmental anomalies or when vertebral flow is compromised by extracranial obstruction or hypoplasia of the subclavian or vertebral arteries.

RELATION BETWEEN ANTERIOR AND POSTERIOR CIRCULATIONS

Support for a functional interrelationship between the anterior and posterior circulations comes from several studies. Bogusslavsky and Regil[10] examined patients with non-hemispheric signs with high-grade carotid stenosis who had no evidence of significant vertebrobasilar or subclavian stenosis and compared them to patients with stenosis in both anterior and posterior circulations. They found that patients without angiographic evidence of vertebral, subclavian, or posterior circulation stenosis more often demonstrated improvement in symptoms following correction of their carotid lesion than those patients who had stenosis in both, and postulated a steal effect. They also found that patients with disease in both circulations were at a higher risk of significant stroke, stressing the interdependence of the two circulations.

Harward et al.[11] studied patients with vertebrobasilar symptoms in whom a posterior communicating artery (PCA) was angiographically visualized. In those patients in whom the PCA was visualized, 71% became asymptomatic and 21% had improvement of their symptoms after ipsilateral carotid endarterectomy, whereas in those without a PCA visualized, only 37% became asymptomatic and 30% showed improvement. Interestingly, there was no difference in carotid stump pressures measured at surgery; however, this likely reflected the contribution of the contralateral carotid rather than the vertebrobasilar system.

Yonas et al.[12] were able to study 9 patients with internal carotid artery stenosis and vertebrobasilar symptoms using pre- and postoperative cerebral blood flow studies with xenon enhanced computed tomography scans. They found that global cerebral perfusion and posterior cerebral perfusion increased after carotid endarterectomy. Archie[13] examined improvement in anterior hemodynamics by improving posterior circulation. He studied 12 patients with vertebrobasilar symptoms and unreconstructable carotid arteries who underwent posterior circulation reconstruction (both anatomic and extra-anatomic) by measuring carotid back-pressures with the reconstruction open and closed. In these patients there was significant improvement in intraoperative carotid stump pressure when the reconstruction was open compared to the pressure with temporary occlusion.

Others have not found a correlation between preoperative functional studies and outcome. Baker and Barnes[14] studied patients with and without reversal of flow in the frontal artery (a branch of the ophthalmic artery) and found no correlation between preoperative Doppler findings and the likelihood of alleviation of non-hemispheric symptoms by carotid endarterectomy, although symptoms were relieved in 67% and improved in 28%. It appears that the concept of augmenting cerebral flow by relieving significant carotid stenosis is a sound one; however, these studies also demonstrate the difficulties of quantifying collateral flow both before and after surgery.

In most studies, relief of non-hemispheric symptoms by carotid endarterectomy is not as predictable as relief of anterior circulation symptomatology. Patient selection may be a critical issue. Reliable preoperative quantification of collateral circulation between the anterior and posterior vasculature should greatly improve patient selection.

The vertebral arteries arise from the subclavian arteries, join to form the basilar artery, and then join the circle of Willis. This vertebrobasilar system and its branches supplies the medulla, pons, midbrain, and superior and inferior cerebellum.[15] The posterior circulation and the anterior circulation communicate through the circle of Willis. Anatomic studies have shown that a normal circle of Willis is present in 52% of normal brains, with abnormalities of the posterior communicating artery (string-like or absent) being the most common anomaly. Additionally, the posterior cerebral arises from the ipsilateral internal carotid artery (embryonic derivation) in 15–30% of cases.[16,17]

With the advent of non-invasive testing, functional assessment of the collateral circulation has been theoretically possible. Use of both the duplex scan and the transcranial Doppler to assess the anterior, posterior, and intracerebral vessels has been studied. Bendick and Jackson found that the duplex scanner could be used to distinguish normal from abnormal vertebral flow, and reversal of flow in the vertebral arteries. They found that vertebral artery flow could be quantified in 96% of patients. Bendick and Glover[19] further tried to define the threshold for vertebral flow in those patients with carotid artery stenosis and vertebrobasilar symptoms.[19,20] They found that, using a calculated value of net vertebral flow (obtained by adding the two velocities), 60% of patients with high vertebral net flows (>200 ml/min) were found to have a significant carotid lesion. However, those patients with vertebrobasilar symptoms were less likely to have high net flows than those with hemispheric signs (52% vs 65%).

Transcranial Doppler (TCD) and duplex have allowed the evaluation of intracerebral vessels.[21–24]

This technique is limited by the temporal bony window and is highly technician-dependent. The study of the PCA is more difficult than that of the anterior cerebral or anterior communicating arteries. Detection of the PCA was possible in just over 60% of patients studied.[25,26] If the PCA was able to be visualized, results were as reliable as those of angiography.

Several pitfalls still exist in the use of TCD for evaluation of collaterals:

1 misinterpretation of hyperdynamic collaterals as stenosis;
2 displacement of arteries by space-occupying lesions;
3 misinterpretation of physiologic changes within the circle of Willis;
4 inability to distinguish vasospasm and stenosis;
5 inability to distinguish reactive hyperemia and stenosis in those patients undergoing evocative studies.[27]

Thus, TCD, although promising in the anterior and vertebral circulation, does not seem to be a reliable method of assessing the collateral circulation to the posterior cerebral arteries.

Magnetic resonance angiography (MRA) may be more promising. MRA has been shown to be able to image accurately the direction of blood flowing through the cerebral arteries and the presence or absence of collateral flow in the circle of Willis.[28] There are potential advantages of MRA over TCD: MRA creates images with high spatial resolution and can demonstrate vascular lesions; it provides an unrestricted field of view; and furthermore, posterior circulation collaterals and fetal circulation can be visualized. Computed tomographic (CT) angiography may also be useful in the future in defining the anatomy of the circle of Willis, as well as that of carotid stenosis.[29] Collateral circulation can be measured non-invasively using single-photon emission computed tomography (SPECT), xenon CT, or positron emission tomography (PET).[30,31] SPECT and xenon CT measure regional cerebral blood flow, while PET measures regional cerebral metabolism. While discussion of these techniques is beyond the scope of this chapter, each can be used to identify marginally perfused areas of the brain. If these can be correlated with symptoms, then it may be possible to identify subgroups of patients who can be improved by repair of hemodynamically significant stenosis.

CONCLUSIONS

The exact role of carotid surgery in the treatment of vertebrobasilar insufficiency remains undefined. The data on asymptomatic stenosis have made this question moot to a degree, since at present the indications for surgery for patients who are asymptomatic are quite similar to those for patients with vertebrobasilar insufficiency (a hemodynamically significant stenosis). We believe that the presence of vertebrobasilar insufficiency provides additional impetus to perform carotid endarterectomy, since not only is the risk of late stroke reduced but more than two-thirds to three-quarters of patients experience long-term relief of symptoms.

Available data suggest that patients with vertebrobasilar insufficiency and isolated carotid stenosis fare better than those with carotid and vertebral/subclavian lesions in whom only the carotid lesion is repaired. Our current practice is to perform the carotid endarterectomy first and defer vertebrobasilar reconstruction until a later time, and then only in patients with persistent symptoms. An alternative may be to combine carotid endarterectomy with carotid subclavian bypass or vertebral artery transposition into the common carotid artery. While this may further improve the efficacy of surgery, we have insufficient clinical experience with this approach to determine whether or not it is justified on a routine basis.

REFERENCES

1 Ricotta JJ, Ouriel K, Green RM, DeWeese JA. Embolic lesions from the subclavian artery causing transient vertebrobasilar insufficiency. *Journal of Vascular Surgery* 1986; 4: 372–375.

2 Humphries AW, Young JR, Beven EG, LeFevre FA, DeWolfe VG. Relief of vertebrobasilar symptoms by carotid endarterectomy. *Surgery* 1965; 57: 48–52.

3 Fields WS, Maslenikov V, Meyer JS, Hass VK,

Remington RD, Macdonald M. Joint study of extracranial arterial occlusion. *Journal of the American Medical Association* 1970; **211**: 1993–2003.

4 McNamara JO, Heyman A, Silver D, Mandel ME. The value of carotid endarterectomy in treating transient cerebral ischemia of the posterior circulation. *Neurology* 1977; **27**: 282–284.

5 Ford JJ, Baker VY'H, Ehrenhaft JL. Carotid endarterectomy for nonhemispheric transient ischemic attacks. *Archives of Surgery* 1975; **110**: 1314–1317.

6 Rosenthal D, Cossman D, Ledig B, Callow AD. Results of carotid endarterectomy for vertebrobasilar insufficiency. *Archives of Surgery* 1978; **113**: 1361–1364.

7 Ouriel K, May AG, Ricotta JJ, DeWeese JA, Green RM. Carotid endarterectomy for nonhemispheric symptoms: predictors of success. *Journal of Vascular Surgery* 1984; **1**: 339–345.

8 Ouriel K, Ricotta JJ, Green RM, DeWeese JA. Carotid endarterectomy for nonhemispheric cerebral symptoms – patient selection with ocular pneumoplethysmography. *Journal of Vascular Surgery* 1986; **4**: 115–118.

9 Ricotta JJ, O'Brien MS, DeWeese JA. Carotid endarterectomy for non-hemispheric ischemia: long-term follow-up. *Cardiovascular Surgery* 1994; **2**: 561–566.

10 Bogusslavsky J, Regil F. Vertebrobasilar transient ischemic attacks in internal carotid artery occlusion or tight stenosis. *Archives of Neurology* 1985; **42**: 64–68.

11 Harward TRS, Wickborn IG, Otis SM, Bernstein EF, Dilley RB. Posterior communicating artery visualization in predicting results of carotid endarterectomy for vertebrobasilar insufficiency. *American Journal of Surgery* 1984; **148**: 43–50.

12 Yonas H, Steed DL, Latchaw RE, Gur D, Peltzman AB, Webster MW. Relief of nonhemispheric symptoms in low flow states by anterior circulation revascularization. A physiologic approach. *Journal of Vascular Surgery* 1987; **5**: 289–297.

13 Archie JP. Improved carotid hemodynarnics with vertebral reconstruction. *Annals of Vascular Surgery* 1992; **6**: 138–141.

14 Baker WH, Barnes RW. The cerebrovascular Doppler examination in patients with nonhemispheric symptoms. *Annals of Surgery* 1977; **186**: 190–192.

15 Johnson NM, Christman CW. Posterior circulation infarction: anatomy, pathophysiology, and clinical correlation. *Seminars in Ultrasound, CT and MRI* 1995; **16**: 237–252.

16 Alpers BJ, Berry RG, Paddison RM. Anatomical studies of the circle of Willis in normal brain. *AMA Archives of Neurology and Psychiatry* 1959; **81**: 409–418.

17 Alpers BJ, Berry RG. Circle of Willis in cerebral vascular disorders. *Archives of Neurology* 1963; **8**: 398–402.

18 Bendick PJ, Jackson VP. Evaluation of the vertebral arteries with duplex sonography. *Journal of Vascular Surgery* 1986; **3**: 523–530.

19 Bendick PJ, Glover JL. Vertebrobasilar insufficiency: evaluation by quantitative duplex flow measurements. *Journal of Vascular Surgery* 1987; **5**: 594–600.

20 Bendick PH, Glover JL. Hemodynarnic evaluation of vertebral arteries by duplex ultrasound. Noninvasive diagnosis of vascular diseases. *Surgical Clinics of North America* 1990; **70**: 235–244.

21 Ringelstein EB, Zeumer H, Poeck K. Non-invasive diagnosis of intracranial lesions in the vertebrobasilar system. A comparison of Doppler sonographic and angiographic findings. *Stroke* 1985; **16**: 848–855.

22 Grolimund P, Seiler RW, Aaslid R, Huber P, Zurbruegg H. Evaluation of cerebrovascular disease by combined extracranial and transcranial Doppler sonography. *Stroke* 1987; **18**: 1018–1024.

23 Schneider PA, Rossman ME, Totem S, Otis SM, Dilley RB, Bernstein EG. Transcranial Doppler in the management of extracranial cerebrovascular disease: implications in diagnosis and monitoring. *Journal of Vascular Surgery* 1988; **7**: 223–231.

24 Chimowitz NU, Furlan AJ, Jones SC *et al.* Transcranial Doppler assessment of cerebral perfusion reserve in patients with carotid occlusive disease and no evidence of cerebral infarction. *Neurology* 1993; **43**: 353–357.

25 Schneider PA, Ringelstein EB, Rossman ME *et al.* Importance of cerebral collateral pathways during the carotid endarterectomy. *Stroke* 1988; **19**: 1328–1334.

26 Baumgartner RW, Baumgartner I, Mattle HP, Schroth G. Transcranial color-coded duplex sonography in the evaluation of collateral flow through the circle of Willis. *American Journal of Neuroradiology* 1997; **18**: 127–133.

27 Bernstein EG. Role of transcranial Doppler in carotid surgery. Noninvasive diagnosis of vascular diseases. *Surgical Clinics of North America* 1990; **70**: 225–234.

28 Edelman RR, Mattle HP, O'Reilly GV, Wentz KU, Liu C, Zhao B. Magnetic resonance imaging of flow dynamics in the circle of Willis. *Stroke* 1990; **21**: 56–65.

29 Wilting JE, Zonneveld FW. Computed tomographic angiography. In: Lanzer P, Lipton M (eds) *Diagnostics of Vascular Diseases*, pp. 114–134. London: Springer-Verlag, 1997.

30 Vlasenko A, Petit-Toboue MC, Bouvard G, Morello R, Derlon JM. Comparative quantitation of cerebral blood volume: SPECT versus PET. *Journal of Nuclear Medicine* 1997; **38**: 919–924.

31 Ekholm S, Forsell-Aronsson E, Starck G *et al.* Phosphorus-31 NM spectroscopy in the preoperative evaluation of symptomatic-unilateral carotid artery stenosis. *Acta Radiologica* 1996; **37**: 288–291.

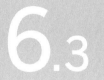

6.3 Editorial Comment

KEY POINTS

1 The significance, natural history, and pathogenesis of many non-hemispheric and vertebrobasilar symptoms are not well defined.

2 Non-hemispheric or vertebrobasilar symptoms may be relieved by carotid endarterectomy (CEA), though no clear patient selection criteria exist. Current imaging and physiologic studies cannot predict which patient's symptoms will be effectively treated by CEA.

3 Patients with non-hemispheric or vertebrobasilar symptoms and critical carotid disease, especially bilateral high-grade stenoses or unilateral occlusion and contralateral high-grade stenosis, are most likely to derive symptomatic relief from CEA, especially if there are no obvious intracranial or vertebrobasilar lesions to explain the symptoms.

4 The role of direct vertebral reconstruction, alone or in concert with CEA, remains ill-defined.

5 Neurologic assessment and thorough preoperative evaluation are essential in dealing with these patients.

As Drs Ricotta and Kvilekval point out, the question of the appropriateness of CEA for high-grade carotid stenosis with vertebrobasilar or non-hemispheric symptoms is to some extent made moot by the ACAS study. Since, in selected patients, high-grade asymptomatic carotid lesions are appropriate for endarterectomy, the presence of symptoms possibly related to hemodynamic insufficiency may not be a critical factor in deciding for or against surgical intervention. Certainly, the observation that most of these patients will be relieved of their symptoms after CEA is reassuring. Still, given the current state of our knowledge in this area, it would be difficult to recommend CEA for non-hemispheric or vertebrobasilar symptoms in a high-risk patient who would not otherwise be a candidate for CEA for asymptomatic disease.

Several difficult questions remain to be answered before clear treatment guidelines can be formulated for these patients. When, if ever, is direct vertebral reconstruction indicated? When should vertebral reconstruction be combined with CEA? What preoperative imaging, hemodynamic, or physiologic data are relevant to the decision-making process?

7.1 Should cost-effectiveness influence patient selection for carotid surgery?
A Ross Naylor (Europe)
Peter Rothwell (Europe)

INTRODUCTION

Until recently, cost-effectiveness was a relatively alien concept to most clinicians who had otherwise tended to justify clinical practice on the basis of training, personal experience and the results of familiar trials. For some, the concept may even be construed as a threat to clinical independence. Part of the problem is the way in which cost-effectiveness analysis is performed because, for the majority of clinicians, the mode in which it is presented seems unintelligible, and barely applicable to clinical decision-making. Moreover, there is a prevailing view that it often fails to reflect the conscience of society.[1]

COST-EFFECTIVENESS ANALYSIS

The principle upon which cost-effectiveness analysis is based is the recognition that most treatment strategies lie somewhere between the extremes of those which provide benefit without cost (highly desirable) and those highly undesirable ones which confer no benefit while incurring cost.[1]

Cost-effectiveness analysis requires the net costs of an intervention to be balanced against the health effects. The former is calculated from medical and non-medical outgoings but, by tradition, indirect costs such as loss of tax revenue or salary from the patient and/or spouse carer are not included.[2] Quantifying health effect is difficult and has led to the evolution of quality-adjusted life years (QALYs). By dividing the net costs by the net effects, one arrives at an estimate of the cost-effectiveness ratio (CR), which is the incremental cost per QALY saved. For example, the CR for coronary artery bypass surgery versus medical therapy in patients with severe angina and left mainstem disease is $3800 per QALY saved.[3]

The QALY encompasses both quantity and quality of life.[2] The QALY is calculated by multiplying the projected life expectancy of the patient by a quality adjustment. The quality adjustment (termed the quality of life weight) for a given condition ranges between 0 (death) and 1 (perfect health). In studies on cerebrovascular disease, the quality adjustment for stroke is 0.39, a value derived from the literature.[4] Thus, if the predicted life expectancy of a patient suffering a stroke was 8.2 years, the QALY would be 3.20.

In order to apply this concept to clinical practice, one must apply the analysis to populations as a whole. Because the numbers required are unlikely to be encountered in clinical practice, most authors use a decision analysis model which computes all the possible scenarios and outcomes for a large, hypothetical population of individuals. In that way, one can determine a CR which can then be remodelled by altering one or more of the parameters (e.g. not doing angiography, increased operative risk, etc.).

However, one or two lingering doubts remain. First, having calculated the CR, how does one really know if it is cost-effective? Second, how can one be sure that the use of hypothetical, statistical patients reflects true clinical practice? Determining the threshold for cost-effectiveness is arbitrary but, as a rule, treatments that cost < $50 000 per QALY saved are considered cost-effective while those in excess of $50 000 are not.[1] The second issue remains the biggest cause for concern because, depending upon the risks and costs used in the model, one could probably produce almost any CR you wanted. Thus, as will be shown, one must carefully review all the available information before comparing two apparently similar studies.

CLINICAL EFFECTIVENESS AND COST-EFFECTIVENESS

Screening for carotid artery disease

The Asymptomatic Carotid Atherosclerosis Study (ACAS) showed that carotid endarterectomy (CEA) conferred a 54% relative reduction in the risk of stroke over best medical therapy alone[5] and focused attention on whether a screening programme (usually duplex ultrasound) could be both clinically effective and cost-effective in selecting patients for CEA.

However, although one study has suggested that in patients with a 20% prevalence of detecting a stenosis > 60%, screening might be cost-effective with a CR of $35 130 per QALY,[6] the results overall are contradictory. Yin and Carpenter[7] have suggested that screening might be cost-effective ($39 495 per QALY), but only if certain criteria were met. These included a disease prevalence of > 4.5%, a duplex specificity of 91%, that the stroke risk of medically treated patients exceeded 3.3% per annum, that the relative risk reduction conferred by surgery was > 37% and that the operative risk was 160% less than that reported in NASCET and ACAS.[7] In contrast, Lee et al. found that screening followed by selective angiography incurred an incremental cost of $120 000 per QALY which only fell below $50 000 under conditions the authors considered to be implausible. These included provision of free duplex machines, perfect test characteristics and a 40% prevalence of detecting a stenosis > 60%.[8] On a more practical note, for any screening programme to prevent more strokes than it causes (including those strokes caused by angiography or following surgery in false-positive patients), evidence suggests that clinicians would first have to identify a population with a predicted prevalence of 20% for detecting a stenosis > 60%. Assuming that this were possible, such a programme would only prevent about 100 strokes per 10 000 patients screened.[9] Thus, for now, there seems to be little evidence to suggest that screening for asymptomatic carotid artery disease is cost-effective.

Reducing the costs associated with carotid endarterectomy

There have been numerous attempts to rationalize the use of angiography, computed tomographic (CT) scanning, general anaesthesia, intensive care, postoperative surveillance and reducing overall hospital stay. Given that CEA costs the US health care system > $1.2 billion per annum, this seems a not unreasonable approach.[10]

Angiography has always been viewed as the 'gold standard' for selecting patients for CEA. However, with the advances in colour duplex technology and magnetic resonance angiography (MRA) few of these absolute indications probably now apply. Only 1% of lesions are currently outwith the scanning range of modern duplex machines,[11] routine angiography alters decision-making in < 2% of patients[12] and reliance on Duplex does not compromise the surgeon's ability to complete the procedure.[13] In addition, even when one includes the fact that a very small number of strokes might occur in patients with either a false-positive or negative duplex diagnosis of a 70–99% stenosis, continued reliance on contrast angiography increases the CR to $99 200 per QALY as compared with duplex alone.[14]

There is also increasing evidence that preoperative CT scans are neither clinically effective nor cost-effective. Commonly quoted reasons for performing a CT scan include the need to document cerebral infarcts, unexpected pathology such as tumour and also to aid in the prediction of operative risk. In fact, there is increasing evidence to suggest that CT scans do not influence operative decision-making, they do not exclude patients from angiography or surgery, they do not reliably predict those at risk of perioperative stroke but that they do add significantly to the overall cost.[15] Apart from the evaluation of patients with asymptomatic disease, surely the time to do a CT scan is in the acute phase of stroke when the differentiation between infarction and haemorrhage is vital.

Discharge within 24 h of surgery is now increasingly the norm in the US, where it has largely been driven by changes in health care reimbursement. In the UK, resistance to implementing such a strategy is probably conceptual as opposed to being based upon evidence which otherwise suggests that the average $5000 savings per case and increased efficiency are not offset by an increased surgical risk.[16,17]

A further controversial subject is serial postoperative surveillance. Clinical and non-invasive imaging follow-up has been advocated on the grounds that it can prevent late stroke through the early detection of recurrent stenoses or disease progression in the non-operated artery. In fact, the overall incidence of recurrent stenosis after CEA is 1–2% per annum,[18,19] the incidence of significant disease progression in the non-operated artery about 1% per annum[20] and the incremental cost per stroke prevented by surveillance about $126 950 per QALY saved.[21] Moreover, the ACAS study showed that only 0.15% of surgical patients developed a symptomatic, recurrent stenosis requiring reoperation and that there was no correlation between late stroke and recurrent stenosis.[22] Can anyone demonstrate a valid clinical or cost-effective reason for continuing with serial postoperative surveillance?

Surgery for symptomatic disease

Trials have clearly shown that CEA is not only clinically effective,[23,24] but that it is also cost-effective, with a CR of $4000 to $39 000 per QALY saved.[2,25] However, CEA will only remain cost-effective provided that the relative risk reduction exceeds 30%, the operation remains durable beyond 5 years, the stroke risk for medically treated patients exceeds 4.6% per annum and the operative stroke risk does not increase significantly.[2] Thus, it remains implicit that patients selected for carotid surgery should be at high risk of stroke and that the operative risk is kept to the minimum.

The most important variable is therefore the initial operative risk but virtually every study on cost-effectiveness has used the NASCET and ACAS risks in the decision-making model. In a recent systematic review of the literature, the spread of published operative risk ranged from 0 to >20%.[26] Accordingly, it remains difficult for individual surgeons to envisage how their own operative risk subsequently influences the long-term benefit of the procedure and also the relative cost implications.

Table 7.1

The effect of the initial operative risk on prevention of major stroke in patients with an 80–99% symptomatic stenosis

Risk of operative CVA/death	Surgery: risk of any CVA/death at 3 years	Medical: risk of any CVA/death at 3 years	Absolute risk reduction	Relative risk reduction	CVA/death prevented/ 1000 CEAs	No. of CEAs to prevent 1 CVA/death
0%	3.7%	22.4%	18.7%	83.5%	187	5.3
1%	4.7%	22.4%	17.7%	79.0%	177	5.6
2%	5.7%	22.4%	16.7%	74.6%	167	6.0
3%	6.7%	22.4%	15.7%	70.1%	157	6.4
4%	7.7%	22.4%	14.7%	65.6%	147	6.8
5%	8.7%	22.4%	13.7%	61.2%	137	7.3
6%	9.7%	22.4%	12.7%	56.7%	127	7.9
7%	10.7%	22.4%	11.7%	52.2%	117	8.5
8%	11.7%	22.4%	10.7%	47.8%	107	9.3
9%	12.7%	22.4%	9.7%	43.3%	97	10.3
10%	13.7%	22.4%	8.7%	38.8%	87	11.5

CVA, cerebrovascular accident; CEA, carotid endarterectomy. Data reanalysed from the European Carotid Surgery Trial.[23]

Table 7.1 presents a simple reanalysis of the European Carotid Surgery Trial (ECST) data with regard to the prevention of major stroke or operative death at 3 years using the newly recommended threshold of 80–99% stenosis.[23] The ECST 80% stenosis threshold is equivalent to a 60% stenosis using the North American Symptomatic Carotid Endarterectomy Trial (NASCET) criteria.[27] As can be seen, the clinical effectiveness of CEA rapidly diminishes as the initial operative risk increases. For example, in a unit with a 30-day operative risk of 2%, CEA will prevent 167 strokes per 1000 CEAs, which equates to six CEAs being necessary to prevent one stroke. If, however, the initial risk were 10% (as was recently reported in the Carotid and Vertebral Artery Transluminal Angioplasty Study[28], the relative risk reduction falls from 75% to 39% and CEA will only prevent 87 strokes per 1000 CEAs. Table 7.2 presents a simplified overview of the impact of the initial operative risk on the overall cost of performing CEA, assuming that CEA costs £2500 ($4000) and that the average cost of treating

and rehabilitating an acute stroke patient is £25000 ($40000). As can be seen, once the 30-day operative risk exceeds 8%, the costs of rehabilitation exceed the potential savings on strokes prevented.

Surgery for asymptomatic disease

Following the ACAS alert, there was a 64% increase in the number of CEAs performed annually in Florida, with the largest single increase being observed in patients aged over 84 years. The result was a $56 million increase in the annual costs for CEA.[29] However, while the data supporting the clinical effectiveness and cost-effectiveness of operating on symptomatic patients are compelling, the same cannot easily be said about operating on asymptomatic patients.

The problem remains that, while CEA reduces the risk of late stroke, the actual risk reduction is only about 1% per annum. Moreover, CEA does not seem to prevent disabling stroke, it has little effect in women and there is no demonstrable correlation

Table 7.2
Effect of the initial operative risk on the cost of preventing major stroke or surgical death in 100 patients with a symptomatic 80–99% carotid stenosis

Operative risk (%)	Cost of 100 CEAs (£1000)	Cost of operation-related strokes (£1000)	Cost of treating late strokes after CEA (£1000)	Cost of stroke in medical patients (£1000)	Net cost (£1000)
0	250	0	92.5	560	+217.5
1	250	25	92.5	560	+192.5
2	250	50	92.5	560	+167.5
3	250	75	92.5	560	+142.5
4	250	100	92.5	560	+117.5
5	250	125	92.5	560	+92.5
6	250	150	92.5	560	+67.5
7	250	175	92.5	560	+42.5
8	250	200	92.5	560	+17.5
9	250	225	92.5	560	−7.5
10	250	250	92.5	560	−32.5

CEA, carotid endarterectomy. Data derived from risks reported in the final results of the European Carotid Surgery Trialists' Collaborative Group[23] and based on the assumption that CEA costs £2500 and acute and rehabilitation costs for stroke average £25000.

Table 7.3
The effect of the initial operative risk on prevention of major stroke in patients with a 60–99% asymptomatic carotid stenosis

Risk of operative CVA/death	Surgery: risk of any CVA/death at 3 years	Medical: risk of any CVA/death at 3 years	Absolute risk reduction	Relative risk reduction	CVA/death prevented/ 1000 CEAs	No. of CEAs to prevent 1 CVA/death
0.0%	2.8%	11.0%	8.2%	74.5%	82	12.2
1.0%	3.8%	11.0%	7.2%	65.5%	72	13.9
2.0%	4.8%	11.0%	6.2%	56.4%	62	16.1
3.0%	5.8%	11.0%	5.2%	47.3%	52	19.2
4.0%	6.8%	11.0%	4.2%	38.2%	42	23.8
5.0%	7.8%	11.0%	3.2%	29.1%	32	31.3

CVA, cerebrovascular accident; CEA, carotid endarterectomy. Data recalculated from Asymptomatic Carotid Atherosclerosis Study.[5]

Table 7.4
Effect of the initial operative risk on the cost of preventing major stroke or surgical death in 100 patients with an asymptomatic 60–99% carotid stenosis

Operative risk (%)	Cost of 100 CEAs (£1000)	Cost of operation-related strokes (£1000)	Cost of treating late strokes after CEA (£1000)	Cost of stroke in medical patients (£1000)	Net cost (£1000)
0	250	0	70	275	−45
1	250	25	70	275	−70
2	250	50	70	275	−95
3	250	75	70	275	−120
4	250	100	70	275	−145
5	250	125	70	275	−175

CEA, carotid endarterectomy. Data derived from risks reported in the final results of the Asymptomatic Carotid Atherosclerosis Study[5] and based on the assumption that CEA costs £2500 and acute and rehabilitation costs for stroke average £25 000.

between the degree of stenosis and stroke risk.[5] Although the 30-day risk in ACAS was 2.3% (including the angiographic risk), the worry remains that these results will not be translated into routine clinical practice. Accordingly, the overall clinical benefit may be much less. Table 7.3 summarizes the effect of CEA on overall stroke prevention in asymptomatic individuals relative to the initial operative risk. As with symptomatic patients (Table 7.1), the overall benefit of CEA is inextricably linked to the initial operative risk. Similarly, uncritical generalization of the ACAS findings is unlikely to generate any savings regarding costs of strokes prevented versus costs of rehabilitation (Table 7.4).

A number of studies have addressed the issue of whether operating on asymptomatic patients is cost-effective and, at first sight, the results appear contradictory. Cronenwett et al. employed the ACAS data and concluded that CEA was cost-effective with an incremental CR of only $8000 per QALY saved. However, operating upon patients aged over 80 years of age was never cost-effective.[30] Kuntz and Kent[25] also used the ACAS data in their model but did not include the angiographic stroke rate within the 30-day risk. In their study, CEA now had a CR of $52 700 per QALY, which increased to $100 900 per QALY if the operative risk increased to 4% and fell to $13 500 per QALY saved if the cost of CEA was halved. Finally, Matchar et al.[2] included asymptomatic patients with a bruit in their model. They found that the CR was $247 500 per QALY and concluded that it would never be cost-effective to perform CEA in all patients with an asymptomatic stenosis > 60%. However, their model included the duplex screening costs, all angiographic strokes, an allowance for the 90% sensitivity and specificity of duplex (including operative strokes in false-positive patients), an operative mortality rate of 1.5% and, perhaps most controversially, a 30-day stroke rate of 5%. These results therefore appear to confirm the surgeon's worst fears that any CR value can be achieved if one really wants.

REFERENCES

1 Finlayson SRG, Birkmeyer JD. Cost-effectiveness analysis in surgery. Surgery 1998; 123: 151–156.
2 Matchar DB, Pauk J, Lipscomb J. A health policy perspective on carotid endarterectomy: cost, effectiveness and cost-effectiveness. In: Moore WS (ed.) Diagnostic Endocrinology, pp 650–689 New York: Harcourt.
3 Weinstein MC, Stason WB. Cost-effectiveness of coronary artery bypass surgery. Circulation 1982; 66 (Suppl): III56–III66.
4 Gage BF, Cardinalli AB, Albers GW, Owens DK. Cost-effectiveness of warfarin and aspirin for prophylaxis of stroke in patients with non-valvular atrial fibrillation. Journal of the American Medical Association 1995; 274: 1839–1845.
5 Executive Committee for the Asymptomatic Carotid Atherosclerosis Study. Endarterectomy for asymptomatic carotid artery stenosis. Journal of the American Medical Association 1995; 273: 1421–1461.
6 Derdeyn CP, Powers WJ. Cost-effectiveness of screening for asymptomatic carotid atherosclerotic disease. Stroke 1996; 27: 1944–1950.
7 Yin D, Carpenter JP. Cost-effectiveness of screening for asymptomatic carotid stenosis. Journal of Vascular Surgery 1998; 27: 245–255.
8 Lee TT, Solomon NA, Heidenreich PA, Oehlert J, Garber AM. Cost-effectiveness of screening for carotid stenosis in asymptomatic persons. Annals of Internal Medicine 1997; 126: 337–346.
9 Whitty CJM, Sudlow CLM, Warlow CP. Investigating individual subjects and screening populations for asymptomatic carotid stenosis can be harmful. Journal of Neurology, Neurosurgery and Psychiatry 1998; 64: 619–623.
10 Luna G, Adye B. Cost-effective carotid endarterectomy. American Journal of Surgery 1995; 169: 516–518.
11 Renton S, Crofton M, Nicolaides A. Impact of duplex scanning on vascular surgical practice. British Journal of Surgery 1991; 78: 1203–1207.
12 Ballard JL, Deiparine MK, Bergan JJ, Bunt TJ, Killeen JD, Smith LL. Cost-effective evaluation and treatment for carotid disease. Archives of Surgery 1997; 132: 268–271.
13 Loftus IM, McCarthy MJ, Pau H et al. Carotid endarterectomy without angiography does not compromise operative outcome. European Journal of Vascular and Endovascular Surgery 1998; 16: 489–493.
14 Kent KC, Kuntz KM, Patel MR et al. Peri-operative imaging strategies for carotid endarterectomy: an analysis of morbidity and cost-effectiveness in symptomatic patients. Journal of the American Medical Association 1995; 274: 888–893.
15 Martin JD, Valentine RJ, Myers SI, Rossi MB, Patterson CB, Clagett GP. Is routine scanning necessary in the pre-operative evaluation of patients undergoing carotid endarterectomy? Journal of Vascular Surgery 1991; 14: 267–270.
16 Musser DJ, Calligaro KD, Dougherty MJ, Raviola CA, DeLaurentis DA. Safety and cost-efficiency of 24-hour hospitalization for carotid endarterectomy. Annals of Vascular Surgery 1996; 10: 143–146.
17 Ammar AD. Cost-efficient carotid surgery: a comprehensive evaluation. Journal of Vascular Surgery 1996; 24: 1050–1056.
18 Frericks H, Kievit J, van Baalan JM, van Bockel JH. Carotid recurrent stenosis and risk of ipsilateral stroke: a systematic review of the literature. Stroke 1998; 29: 244–250.
19 Naylor AR, John T, Howlett J, Gillespie I, Allan P, Ruckley CV. Serial surveillance imaging does not alter clinical outcome following carotid endarterectomy. British Journal of Surgery 1996; 83: 522–526.
20 Naylor AR, John T, Howlett J, Gillespie I, Allan P, Ruckley CV. Fate of the non-operated carotid artery after contralateral endarterectomy. British Journal of Surgery 1995; 83: 44–48.
21 Patel ST, Kuntz KM, Kent KC. Is routine duplex ultrasound surveillance after carotid endarterectomy cost-effective? Surgery 1998; 124: 343–351.

22 Moore WS, Kempczinski RF, Nelson JJ, Toole JF. Recurrent carotid stenosis: results of the Asymptomatic Carotid Atherosclerosis Study. *Stroke* 1998; **29**: 2018–2025.

23 European Carotid Surgery Trialists' Collaborative Group. Randomised trial of endarterectomy for recently symptomatic carotid stenosis: final results of the MRC European Carotid Surgery Trial (ECST). *Lancet* 1998; **351**: 1379–1387.

24 Barnett HJM, Taylor DW, Eliasziw M *et al.* Benefit of carotid endarterectomy in patients with symptomatic moderate or severe stenosis. *New England Journal of Medicine* 1998; **339**: 1415–1425.

25 Kuntz KM, Kent KC. Is carotid endarterectomy cost-effective? An analysis of symptomatic and asymptomatic patients. *Circulation* 1996; **94** (Suppl 1): II194–II198.

26 Rothwell PM, Slattery J, Warlow CP. A systematic review of the risks of stroke and death due to endarterectomy for symptomatic carotid stenosis. *Stroke* 1996; **27**: 260–265.

27 Donnan GA, Davis SM, Chambers BR, Gates PC. Surgery for prevention of stroke. *Lancet* 1998; **351**: 1372–1373.

28 CAVATAS Investigators. Results of the Carotid and Vertebral Artery Transluminal Angioplasty Study (CAVATAS). Proceedings of the Annual Vascular Society Meeting of Great Britain and Ireland (Hull, November 1998).

29 Huber TS, Wheeler KG, Cuddeback JK, Dame DA, Flynn TC, Seeger JM. Effect of the Asymptomatic Carotid Atherosclerosis Study on carotid endarterectomy in Florida. *Stroke* 1998; **29**: 1099–1105.

30 Cronenwett JL, Birkmeyer JD, Nackman GB *et al.* Cost-effectiveness of carotid endarterectomy in asymptomatic patients. *Journal of Vascular Surgery* 1997; **25**: 298–309.

7.2

Should cost-effectiveness influence patient selection for carotid surgery?

Jack L Cronenwett (USA)

John D Birkmeyer (USA)

IS COST-EFFECTIVENESS RELEVANT?

The idea that cost considerations should influence the care of individual patients is foreign to many physicians who were taught to select the best management independent of cost. Rapidly rising health care expenditures, however, have forced society in general, and physicians in particular, to examine their practice in terms of cost-effectiveness. In fact, many physicians have unconsciously made patient management decisions based on cost-effectiveness in the presence of scarce resources. A common example involves the choice to limit preoperative cardiac assessment with sophisticated but expensive testing, even though it might be 'safer' to obtain all studies in all patients. Thus, in many ways, physicians have already assumed a role as cost managers, and their decisions concerning individual patients are influenced by cost considerations.[31]

Furthermore, physicians are increasingly involved in policy-making decisions for larger patient groups that might involve the development of clinical pathways for a local hospital, reimbursement policy for an HMO, or statewide guidelines for health care resource allocation. In all of these cases it is important not only to weigh the risks and benefits of a given procedure, but also to determine whether the expected benefits justify the health care resources consumed.[32] To assist in this decision-making, it is possible to perform formal economic analyses to compare alternative treatment strategies with respect to their resource usage and their expected outcome.[33]

ASSESSING COST-EFFECTIVENESS

The cost-effectiveness of a given procedure is defined as its cost divided by its benefit. Typically,

marginal cost-effectiveness is calculated, where the costs and benefits of two alternative strategies are compared. Thus, the C/E (cost-effectiveness ratio) of strategy A versus strategy B is defined as [cost A – cost B]/[benefit A – benefit B].

It is important for costs and benefits to be analyzed from the same perspective, which could reflect the viewpoint of the patient, the hospital, the third-party payer, or society at large.[34] Although each perspective may be relevant depending on the specific question being asked, the societal perspective is usually most relevant. For example, a study performed from a hospital perspective might determine that early discharge of patients following vascular surgery to a rehabilitation center was very cost-effective because of reduced length of stay. However, this perspective ignores the cost of the rehabilitation, which might invalidate its conclusion from a broader, societal perspective.

It is also important to recognize that charges for health care do not reflect actual costs. Charges are determined by the marketplace, and by a variety of accounting practices which may shift cost responsibilities within an institution. Costs are calculated by determining the actual value of supplies, wages, utilities, etc. that are required for a specific treatment. Some analyses also include indirect costs, such as lost wages by the patient or relatives who provide home care. Because of difficulties in estimating such indirect costs, however, most analyses include only direct costs. Unfortunately, the literature is replete with reports in which charges are used as a surrogate for costs, often in a misleading and inaccurate manner.

Measuring the benefits of health care is equally complicated, because different interventions result in diverse outcomes that are difficult to compare. For example, one intervention might improve survival, while another might relieve suffering or improve well-being. The most commonly used metric to compare these different outcomes is quality-adjusted life expectancy, measured in QALYs. This summary measurement captures the effect of an intervention on both the quantity and quality of life. To adjust absolute life expectancy for quality of life, time spent in imperfect health is multiplied by a fraction between 0 (death) and 1 (perfect health), which is determined by individuals or society to be the relative value of that health state. For example, based on interviews with patients following major stroke, it was determined that their quality of life was 40% of perfect health. Thus, if a patient lived 10 years following a myocardial infaction or stroke, the quality-adjusted survival would be 0.40×10, or 4 QALYS. When comparing the cost-effectiveness of two alternative procedures, it is necessary to compare their costs, measured in dollars, and their benefits, measured in QUALYs. Thus, a C/E is defined in terms of dollars/QALYs. Since most people value current benefits more than remote future benefits, it is customary to discount future benefits (and costs) by approximately 5% per year.[34]

For a rigorous cost-effectiveness analysis, it is necessary to know or estimate the exact outcome of the treatment strategies being compared. Since this differs among individual patients, and is defined by probabilities rather than precision, a decision analysis model is used to protect all of the possible treatment outcomes, their probabilities, and their associated costs. One such model, a Markov analysis, projects the outcome of a hypothetical cohort of patients from their initial health state until their death, based on the probabilities for different events as derived from the medical literature.[35] For example, a 65-year-old man with an asymptomatic carotid stenosis might live normally for 5 years, then experience a major stroke, and die 5 years later. The Markov analysis would calculate quality-adjusted survival for this patient based on the number of years in each health state, reducing the value of life after stroke, as noted above. A similar patient might live 20 years with no stroke. Based on the probabilities for all of these events, the Markov

analysis calculates the average quality-adjusted life expectancy for each cohort of patients with certain baseline characteristics. It also assigns a cost to each outcome, and calculates the ultimate cost per QALY. Finally, this analysis compares the C/E for two different strategies. The strategy that improves quality-adjusted life expectancy is preferred, and the C/E determines the incremental cost for achieving that incremental benefit. Although there is no rigid definition for cost-effective therapy, it is generally agreed that procedures with an incremental CR < $20000/QALY are very cost-effective, while procedures with an incremental CR > $100000 are not cost-effective.[36] In the intermediate range, many procedures are considered

Table 7.5
Cost-effectiveness of selected medical practices

Medical practice	Cost/QALY
Treatment of mild–moderate hypertension compared with no treatment	
Propranolol	$13000
Captopril	$87000
Hemodialysis for end-stage renal disease	$53000
Total hip replacement for severe osteoarthritis	$4600
Coronary artery bypass compared to medical treatment of severe angina	
Left main disease	$7000
Single-vessel disease	$51000
Transplantation compared with medical treatment	
Heart	$33000
Kidney	$20000
Treatment of hyperlipidemia with cholestyramine	$189000
Universal precautions for HIV prevention in health care workers	$770000

QALY, quality-adjusted life years; HIV, human immunodeficiency virus.

cost-effective, depending on a variety of factors that influence public opinion (Table 7.5).

An important benefit of decision analysis modeling is the ability to vary the baseline assumptions about patient characteristics, outcome probabilities, or costs, in order to determine whether the choice of optimal therapy is sensitive to these variables (sensitivity analysis). Thus, in formulating a decision model, the plausible range for key variables and costs is studied, which allows one to ask questions such as: what if the cost of surgery were lower? Or, what if the patients were older? This then identifies the key variables that will change the correct treatment choice, which helps physicians focus on the relevant issues for individual patients.[37]

COST-EFFECTIVENESS OF CAROTID ENDARTERECTOMY IN ASYMPTOMATIC PATIENTS

Natural history studies have demonstrated a 2–5% annual ipsilateral stroke risk for patients with internal carotid artery (ICA) stenoses > 50% diameter reduction, increasing with stenosis severity.[38–42] Based on reduced stroke rates reported after CEA, prophylactic surgery has been recommended to prevent future stroke in asymptomatic patients with severe carotid stenosis.[43] This concept was tested in the ACAS, which compared aggressive medical management with CEA for patients with asymptomatic 60–99% ICA stenoses.[38] This randomized, prospective, multicenter trial demonstrated that the annual ipsilateral stroke rate was reduced from 2.3% per year under medical management to 1% per year by endarterectomy (P = 0.004). Although the relative reduction in stroke risk of 54% by endarterectomy was significant, the absolute 5-year stroke reduction from 11% to 5.1% seemed less substantial. In fact, the ACAS authors noted that 19 endarterectomies would need to be performed to prevent one stroke in 5 years[38] and it was suggested that this would not be cost-effective because of the expense associated with carotid surgery.[44] In order to answer this question, however, formal decision analysis is required, because the cost of stroke is also high, and asymptomatic patients might develop transient ischemic attacks (TIAs) or minor stroke, and undergo the cost of

endarterectomy anyway. For this reason, we performed a cost-effectiveness analysis to determine whether patients with characteristics similar to average patients in ACAS should undergo CEA based on cost-effectiveness guidelines.[45]

In our decision analysis model, we examined the outcome of hypothetical cohorts of asymptomatic patients with 60–99% ICA stenoses who were initially selected for best medical management or surgical treatment (medical management plus endarterectomy).[45] We assumed that patients undergoing medical management would receive aspirin therapy and risk factor reduction as in ACAS, but would not undergo endarterectomy as long as they remained asymptomatic. Unlike ACAS, but to reflect more accurately current clinical practice, we assumed that patients in the medical group would undergo endarterectomy if they experienced a TIA or minor stroke. For a base-case analysis, we used average demographic data from ACAS (age = 67 years, 66% men).[38] We assumed a 2.3% annual ipsilateral stroke rate (50% major stroke) and a postoperative 30-day stroke and death rate of 2.3% based on ACAS, which included the risk of arteriography. For patients in the medical group who developed TIAs or minor strokes and then underwent endarterectomy, we used outcome probabilities from the NASCET.[46] We calculated expected long-term survival based on ACAS results that included an excess mortality from generalized atherosclerosis, in addition to specific cerebrovascular events. We estimated the quality of life after stroke based on a published assessment in elderly patients (0.39 after first major stroke),[47] and assumed that patients with minor stroke had complete resolution by 3 months. We calculated the cost of CEA at $8500 and arteriography at $1600 based on a cost-accounting system in which both fixed hospital overhead costs and variable costs specifically related to this diagnosis were derived from our institution.[45] This calculation included an estimate of physician costs, based on current Medicare reimbursement. We estimated the cost of major stroke at $34000 during the first year followed by $18000 annually, based on population-based reports.[48,49] We applied a discount rate of 5% to adjust future costs and health benefits to their present value.

For the average patient in the ACAS study, our calculations indicated that quality-adjusted life expectancy for patients in the medical group was 7.87 QALYs versus 8.12 QALYs for patients in the surgical group – a difference of 0.25 QALYs (3 months) in favor of surgical treatment.[45] The predicted lifetime cost was $12 407 for medical treatment and $14 448 for surgical treatment – a difference of $2041 in favor of medical treatment. Thus, the incremental C/E for surgical treatment was $2041/0.25 QALYS, or $8000 per QALY compared with medical treatment. Thus, for the average patient in the ACAS study, endarterectomy was clearly cost-effective when compared with other commonly accepted medical practices (Table 7.5).

A detailed analysis indicated that the majority of costs in the medical group were associated with stroke, while most costs in the surgical group were associated with endarterectomy (Fig. 7.1). It is noteworthy that 26% of medically managed patients experienced TIAs or minor stroke during follow-up which led to CEA (TIAs at 2.1% per year and minor stroke at 1.1% per year based on ACAS). Not surprisingly, the proportion of patients who experience such symptoms is substantially increased for younger patients with longer life expectancy (32% for 60-year-old patients versus only 14% for 80-year-old patients). Our model predicted that this would occur at a median time of 5.5 years following initial evaluation. The cost of stroke was substantial in our model, with a projected lifetime cost of $192 000 following a major stroke.

IMPACT OF KEY VARIABLES ON COST-EFFECTIVENESS

Sensitivity analysis indicated that life expectancy had the most significant influence on cost-effectiveness.[45] Although age is only a proxy for life expectancy, it is the most accurate predictor in large population-based models. For individual patients, many other variables can be used to predict life expectancy more accurately. However, in decision analysis models, age is a useful surrogate for life expectancy, and its impact on the cost-effectiveness of carotid endarterectomy for asymptomatic > 60% ICA stenosis is shown in Figure 7.2. This demonstrates that, for patients younger than 70 years, the incremental cost of surgical treatment was < $20 000/QALY and clearly cost-effective. It also demonstrates that, for patients younger than 60 years, surgery was dominant (both more effective and less expensive). Above age 70, the cost of surgical treatment increased exponentially and exceeded $100 000/QALY by age 79. This exponential increase in the C/E with increasing age is an important concept that can be attributed to decreased life expectancy in older patients, with reduced opportunity to experience

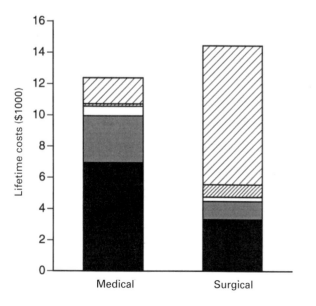

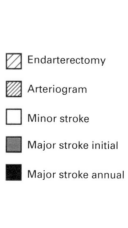

Fig. 7.1
Lifetime cost estimates (discounted at 5%) for medical and surgical treatment of 67-year-old patients with > 60% asymptomatic carotid stenosis. Medical patients experienced total costs that were $2000 less than for surgical patients, heavily allocated to care after major stroke. Costs for surgical patients were predominantly influenced by initial procedural costs.[45]

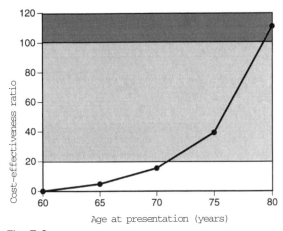

Fig. 7.2
Cost-effectiveness of surgical treatment compared with medical management as a function of age in the base-case analysis of patients with > 60% asymptomatic carotid stenosis.[45] Shading indicates three categories of cost-effectiveness: < $20 000 per quality-adjusted life year, clearly cost-effective; $20 000–100 000, intermediate cost-effectiveness; > $100 000, not cost-effective. By these definitions, surgical treatment is cost-effective until at least age 72, and perhaps age 79.

the benefit of prophylactic endarterectomy after incurring the initial cost.

The second variable with a major influence on cost-effectiveness is the ipsilateral stroke rate observed during medical management (Fig. 7.3). It is difficult to predict the precise stroke risk for a given patient. The estimate of 2.3% per year from ACAS is very similar to the rate of 2.4% per year for male patients in the Veterans' Administration Cooperative Study with 50–99% ICA stenoses.[40] This is also similar to the annual ipsilateral stroke rate of 2.3% observed during follow-up of asymptomatic patients with 50–79% ICA stenoses by Mansour et al.[41] However, individual patient factors undoubtedly influence this result. For example, there is convincing evidence that progression of ICA stenoses during follow-up substantially increases stroke risk. In the asymptomatic patients with 50–79%, ICA stenosis followed by Mansour et al., the stroke rate was only 0.23% per year if the stenosis remained stable, but fully 6.8% per year if the stenosis progressed to > 80%[41] This detrimental effect of ICA stenosis progression has been noted by others.[50] Carotid

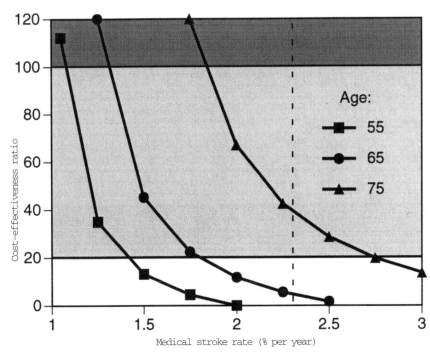

Fig. 7.3
Cost-effectiveness of surgical treatment for > 60% asymptomatic carotid stenosis as a function of ipsilateral stroke rate during medical management for three different age groups.[45] For young patients (age 55), surgery is cost-effective even at low annual stroke risk (1.5% per year). For older patients (age 75), surgery is cost-effective only if medical stroke risk is high (> 2.5% per year). The broken line at 2.3% annual stroke risk indicates the base-case assumption based on the Asymptomatic Carotid Atherosclerosis Study.

ulceration and low plaque density also appear to increase stroke risk during medical management.[43,51] Thus, as shown in Fig. 7.3, prophylactic endarterectomy is probably not cost-effective for stable, non-progressive ICA stenoses, but is cost-effective, even for elderly patients, with significant stenosis progression when stroke rate during medical management likely exceeds 3% per year.

The final important variable that determines cost-effectiveness of endarterectomy is the risk of perioperative stroke or death.[45] This emphasizes the importance of evaluating surgeon-specific outcomes when considering a recommendation for prophylactic carotid endarterectomy. Published guidelines suggest that endarterectomy for asymptomatic patients should only be offered when the perioperative stroke death rate is < 3%,[43] which would clearly be cost-effective according to our analysis (Fig. 7.4). Unfortunately, population-based studies suggest that these results are often not achieved, especially in hospitals that perform a low volume of carotid surgery.[52]

WHEN IS CAROTID SURGERY COST-EFFECTIVE?

Our analysis indicates that life expectancy is the most important factor for selecting patients for cost-effective carotid surgery.[45] Older patients have less opportunity to enjoy the benefit of carotid surgery, even though this is known to reduce stroke risk. For asymptomatic patients, our analysis suggests that endarterectomy is cost-effective until about age 75, assuming an average life expectancy for this group of patients. For patients who are 75–80 years of age, the cost of endarterectomy increases to the upper limit of the acceptable range, so that only patients with particularly good life expectancy would be optimal candidates for surgery. For asymptomatic patients over 80, it is unlikely that endarterectomy will be cost-effective, unless the expected stroke risk during medical management is much higher than normal, such as with documented progression from < 80% to > 80% ICA stenosis. These conclusions assume a low perioperative risk.

For symptomatic patients with carotid stenosis, the same key variables apply, but the threshold for each is lower, since the stroke risk is higher and the benefit of surgery is greater in absolute terms. In fact, for most patients with symptomatic carotid disease, surgery is not only more effective, but is also less expensive. However, for patients with a very short life expectancy of only several years, even surgery for carotid symptoms might not prove cost-

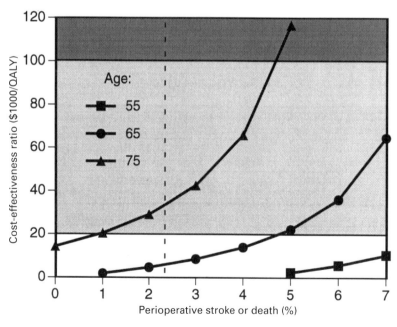

Fig. 7.4
Cost-effectiveness of surgical treatment for > 60% asymptomatic carotid stenosis as a function of perioperative stroke or death rate for three different age groups.[45] For young patients, surgery is cost-effective even at higher operative event rates. For older patients, however, the perioperative event rate must be much lower for surgical treatment to be cost-effective. The broken line at 2.3% indicates the base-case assumption for perioperative event rate based on the Asymptomatic Carotid Atherosclerosis Study.

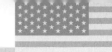

effective. The impact of age on decision-making is important because carotid atherosclerosis increases with age, so that most carotid stenoses are found in the very group of patients who are least likely to benefit from surgical treatment, underscoring the importance of careful patient selection.

Cost-effectiveness analysis should not substitute for clinical judgment when recommending appropriate treatment for individual patients. However, this technique identifies the important variables, such as age and stroke risk, which should influence decision-making. Overall, our

results indicate that carotid endarterectomy is cost-effective in asymptomatic patients < 75 years of age with > 60% ICA stenosis when compared with other commonly accepted medical practices.[45] Application of this conclusion requires excellent surgical results and at least average life expectancy. Future efforts directed toward better prediction of stroke risk in individual patients would increase the accuracy of these prediction models. Even at present, we believe that cost-effectiveness analysis facilitates the selection of appropriate patients for carotid surgery.

REFERENCES

31 Finlayson SR, Birkmeyer JD. Cost-effectiveness analysis in surgery. *Surgery* 1998; **123**: 151–156.
32 Russell LB, Gold MR, Siegel JE, Daniels N, Weinstein MC. The role of cost-effectiveness analysis in health and medicine. Panel on Cost-effectiveness in Health and Medicine. *Journal of the American Medical Association* 1996; **276**: 1172–1177.
33 Weinstein MC, Siegel JE, Gold MR, Kamlet MS, Russell LB. Recommendations of the Panel on Cost-effectiveness in Health and Medicine. *Journal of the American Medical Association* 1996; **276**: 1253–1258.
34 Drumond MF, Richardson WS, O'Brien BJ, Levine M, Heyland D. Users' guides to the medical literature. XIII. How to use an article on economic analysis of clinical practice. A. Are the results of the study valid? Evidence-based Medicine Working Group. *Journal of the American Medical Association* 1997; **277**: 1552–1557.
35 Beck JR, Pauker SG. The Markov process in medical prognosis. *Medical Decision Making* 1983; **3**: 419–458.
36 Laupacis A, Feeny D, Detsky AS, Tugwell PX. How attractive does a new technology have to be to warrant adoption and utilization? Tentative guidelines for using clinical and economic evaluations. *Canadian Medical Association Journal* 1992; **146**: 473–481.
37 O'Brien BJ, Heyland D, Richardson WS, Levine M, Drummond MF. Users' guides to the medical literature. XIII. How to use an article on economic analysis of clinical practice. B. What are the results and will they help me in caring for my patients? Evidence-based Medicine Working Group. *Journal of the American Medical Association* 1997; **277**: 1802–1806.
38 Asymptomatic Carotid Atherosclerosis Study Group. Endarterectomy for asymptomatic carotid artery stenosis. *Journal of the American Medical Association* 1995; **273**: 1421–1428.
39 European Carotid Surgery Trialists Group. European carotid surgery trial: interim results for symptomatic patients with severe (70–99%) or with mild (0–29%) carotid stenosis. *Lancet* 1991; **337**: 1235–1243.
40 Hobson RW, Weiss DG, Fields WS *et al.* Efficacy of carotid endarterectomy for asymptomatic carotid stenosis. The

Veterans Affairs Cooperative Study Group. *New England Journal of Medicine* 1993; **328**: 221–227.
41 Mansour MA, Mattos MA, Faught WE *et al.* The natural history of moderate (50% to 79%) internal carotid artery stenosis in symptomatic, nonhemispheric, and asymptomatic patients. *Journal of Vascular Surgery* 1995; **21**: 346–357.
42 Norris JW, Zhu CZ, Bornstein NM, Chambers BR. Vascular risks of asymptomatic carotid stenosis. *Stroke* 1991; **22**: 1485–1490.
43 Moore WS, Barnett HJ, Beebe HG *et al.* Guidelines for carotid endarterectomy. A multidisciplinary consensus statement from the ad hoc Committee, American Heart Association. *Stroke* 1995; **26**: 188–201.
44 Mayberg MR, Winn HR. Endarterectomy for asymptomatic carotid artery stenosis. Resolving the controversy. *Journal of the American Medical Association* 1995; **273**: 1459–1461.
45 Cronenwett JL, Birkmeyer JD, Nackman GB *et al.* Cost-effectiveness of carotid endarterectomy in asymptomatic patients. *Journal of Vascular Surgery* 1997; **25**: 298–309; discussion 10–11.
46 North American Symptomatic Carotid Endarterectomy Trialists. Beneficial effect of carotid endarterectomy in symptomatic patients with high-grade carotid stenosis. *New England Journal of Medicine* 1991; **325**: 445–453.
47 Gage BF, Cardinalli AB, Albers GW, Owens DK. Cost-effectiveness of warfarin and aspirin for prophylaxis of stroke in patients with nonvalvular atrial fibrillation. *Journal of the American Medical Association* 1995; **274**: 1839–1845.
48 Thorngren M, Westling B. Utilization of health care resources after stroke. A population-based study of 258 hospitalized cases followed during the first year. *Acta Neurologica Scandinavica* 1991; **84**: 303–310.
49 Terent A, Marke LA, Asplund K *et al* Costs of stroke in Sweden. A national perspective. *Stroke* 1994; **25**: 2363–2369.
50 Roederer GO, Langlois YE, Jager KA *et al.* The natural history of carotid arterial disease in asymptomatic patients with cervical bruits. *Stroke* 1984; **15**: 605–613.

51 Geroulakos G, Domjan J, Nicolaides A *et al.* Ultrasonic carotid artery plaque structure and the risk of cerebral infarction on computed tomography. *Journal of Vascular Surgery* 1994; **20**: 263–266.

52 Fisher ES, Malenka DJ, Solomon NA *et al.* Risk of carotid endarterectomy in the elderly. *American Journal of Public Health* 1989; **79**: 1617–1620.

7.3 Editorial Comment

KEY POINTS

1 While advocacy for our individual patients is paramount, surgeons also have a duty to promote optimal resource utilization.
2 Decision analysis modeling enables clinicians to compare the cost-effectiveness of different management strategies in a standardized format.
3 Limiting preoperative studies and postoperative length of stay could potentially reduce overall costs without compromising safety, thereby favorably altering the CEA cost–benefit ratio.
4 Major determinants of the cost-effectiveness of CEA are patient age (expected longevity), symptom status, and perioperative mortality/stroke morbidity.
5 CEA for symptomatic patients is cost-effective under virtually all realistic modeling parameters.
6 The cost-effectiveness of CEA for asymptomatic patients remains controversial and highly dependent on modeling parameters such as age and perioperative risk.

It is now possible for surgeons to understand more fully the benefits and costs associated with CEA under specific conditions in their individual hands. For example, using Naylor and Rothwell's method of analysis, a surgeon with a 3% perioperative stroke morbidity/mortality rate for CEA in symptomatic patients with an 80–99% stenosis will prevent 157 strokes for every 1000 endarterectomies performed. However, under the same conditions, a surgeon whose operative risk is 9% will prevent only 97 strokes per 1000 CEAs, such that all savings associated with stroke prevention are lost. Similarly, in Cronenwett and Burkmeyer's analysis, a surgeon who operates for an asymptomatic critical stenosis in a 65-year-old male with a 3% perioperative risk achieves a cost–benefit ratio of approximately $10 000/QALY (a highly cost-effective result). However, if the surgeon's perioperative risk is 7%, the C/E is approximately $65 000/QALY (a dubiously cost-effective result). In asymptomatic 75-year-olds, even with a 4% perioperative risk, the cost–benefit ratio is again approximately $65 000/QALY (and again dubious).

In the era of managed care, this type of analysis is critical to demonstrate the comparative value of CEA. This is especially important since CEA will soon be compared with interventional treatments for stroke prevention. In addition, such analyses provide a method with which to compare the performance of individual surgeons or vascular centers against the standards set in the randomized trials. It is important to keep in mind that the cost components of these calculations are variable and easily altered by reducing expenditure for preoperative evaluation and postoperative care, but that injudicious expenditure reduction could also result in adverse effects on benefit.

Finally, as both authors have commented, the utility of cost-effectiveness analysis is entirely dependent on the quality of the baseline assumptions used for the calculations. Readers of this literature are cautioned to check carefully underlying assumptions when attempting to interpret conclusions based on decision analyses.

Part Two   Evaluation and Preoperative Management

8.1 Is duplex ultrasound alone sufficient for preoperative imaging?
Peter R Taylor (Europe)

INTRODUCTION

For most patients undergoing carotid endarterectomy (CEA), the answer to the question posed in the title of this chapter is a qualified yes. This is not a new subject: references relating to this subject have been available for more than 15 years,[1-3] but it still continues to arouse much debate.[4-6] However, a recent audit of CEA practice in the UK and Ireland has shown that preoperative assessment by duplex was performed in 96% of cases, an angiogram in 55%, a computed tomographic (CT) scan in 38% and magnetic resonance imaging in 14%, suggesting that clinical practice is changing towards a policy of non-invasive assessment.[7]

However, reliance upon duplex requires the surgeon to put considerable faith in the technologist and there are a number of questions that must be asked in each institution before duplex can replace angiography as the principal imaging modality to select patients for carotid surgery. The major issues that must be addressed are the accuracy of duplex in grading the severity of the stenosis; the scanning limits of duplex ultrasound and whether reliance on duplex leads to an increased risk of the surgeon encountering unexpected findings at operation which may compromise the safety of the operation.

ACCURATE MEASUREMENT OF CAROTID STENOSIS?

Two international studies have unequivocally shown that CEA confers a six- to 10-fold reduction in the long-term risk of stroke in symptomatic patients with a severe ipsilateral carotid stenosis in excess of 70% as compared with best medical therapy alone.[8,9] The measurement of the degree of stenosis in the two studies was based on the percentage reduction in luminal diameter on angiography. In the European trial, however, the denominator was the diameter of the carotid bulb. In the North American trial, the denominator was the diameter of the distal internal carotid artery (ICA) at the point where the arterial walls became parallel. More recently, a third method of quantifying the degree of stenosis has been proposed and termed the carotid stenosis index. Here the denominator is the diameter of the disease-free common carotid artery below the bifurcation.[10]

How accurate is angiography and what is the interobserver and intraobserver error? The difficulties involved in objectively measuring, as opposed to subjectively 'eyeballing' an angiogram, were highlighted in a recent study which showed that, even when using a high-resolution work station with computerized calipers, the degree of agreement was no better than a radiologist simply eyeballing the angiogram.[11] This study also showed that, in expert hands, duplex scanning was as good as, if not better than, computation of the degree of stenosis on angiography. The main proviso was the experience and expertise of the duplex operator, together with a high-resolution scanning machine. Evidence suggests that, under these circumstances, duplex has a sensitivity and specificity of > 90% in detecting a stenosis in excess of 70%.[12-14]

There are, however, two specific problems associated with reliance on duplex. These include the identification of occlusion (as opposed to trickle flow) and the fact that severe calcification can prevent ultrasound interrogation of the stenosis. The advent of colour flow and 'power' duplex has, however, increased the accuracy of the ultrasound diagnosis of occlusion[15] and magnetic resonance angiography (MRA) may have a complementary role in confirming the diagnosis of a thrombosed carotid artery in difficult cases. However, at present, due to limitations in software, expense and availability, MRA is usually used in a secondary role to duplex.

Calcification will always be a problem with ultrasound-based methods, but it should be borne in mind that severe calcification can also reduce the diagnostic accuracy of digital subtraction angiography, CT angiography and MRA. The overall problem with calcification reduces as the experience of the operator increases and can be partly circumvented by sampling the velocity immediately proximal and distal to the calcified plaque. In practical terms, plaque calcification sufficient to render reliable interpretation of the carotid plaque unsafe by ultrasound occurs in < 5% of patients, who should undergo investigation by other means.

EXTENT OF DISEASE?

To date, angiography has been the gold standard against which all other imaging modalities are compared. Its use has been recommended in order to visualize the upper limits of the carotid plaque, inflow disease, syphon disease and intracranial disease. However, there is now increasing evidence that many of these important characteristics can be evaluated by both extra- and transcranial duplex and transcranial Doppler technology.

Distal limits of the plaque

Duplex reports should include whether it is possible to visualize a disease-free ICA above the plaque. If this is the case, then the surgeon should not encounter any unexpected problems at operation. If the distal end of the plaque is not seen clearly, then it is essential that either intra-arterial digital subtraction angiography or MRA be performed. However, these secondary investigations rarely alter the decision as to whether the patient should have surgery, as this is primarily based upon clinical findings and the degree of stenosis. It does, however, make the surgeon aware that the operation may be potentially difficult and that the higher reaches of the ICA may need to be exposed. Paradoxically, the most commonly encountered feature that can make the operation more challenging is the finding of a

posterior tongue of plaque which extends above the main stenosis. This does not tend to impinge on the arterial lumen and, as a rule, is difficult to detect with duplex and almost impossible with angiography.

Is there proximal disease?

Duplex performed by an experienced operator can detect haemodynamically significant lesions proximal to the carotid bifurcation. Some can be imaged directly by angling the duplex probe down into the thorax behind the sternum. Any haemodynamically significant inflow stenoses which cannot be directly imaged will, however, affect the waveform in the proximal common carotid artery. Spectral broadening with a damped low-velocity flow is thus highly suggestive of inflow disease provided the contralateral common carotid artery is normal. This again is an indication for referring patients for angiography or MRA.

However, in reality, significant intrathoracic disease is extremely rare and in a review of 1000 arch angiograms this was only identified in 1.8%.[16] Clinically significant proximal lesions can be treated synchronously at operation with retrograde balloon angioplasty performed via the arteriotomy used for CEA. If this is done, the ICA should be temporarily clamped to prevent distal embolization.

Is there syphon disease?

Tandem lesions were previously considered to be a relative contraindication to CEA. However, while some would consider that the presence of significant disease at both the carotid bifurcation and the carotid syphon does not confer tandem risk,[17] a recent overview of the available literature suggests that coexistent syphon disease may slightly increase the excess risk of perioperative stroke.[18] Accordingly, any patient with duplex evidence of a high-resistant or reverberant distal ICA signal should undergo angiography in order to exclude a severe syphon stenosis. The presence of a lesser degree of syphon disease should not serve as a contraindication to surgery as CEA will increase the perfusion pressure proximal to the syphon disease, thus reducing the risk of distal thrombosis, whilst removing a potential proximal embolic source.

Is there intracranial occlusive or aneurysmal disease?

It has also been suggested that angiography is the only method for reliably assessing intracranial occlusive and aneurysmal disease. However, the addition of transcranial colour duplex ultrasound to conventional pulsed-wave transcranial Doppler (TCD) has largely rendered angiography redundant in this respect. Although TCD can readily diagnose significant intracranial stenoses through the detection of high-velocity jets,[19] there is no evidence that the presence of intracranial stenotic disease adversely affects operative risk. The only situation where it may influence decision-making with regard to patient selection for CEA is the presence of middle cerebral artery (MCA) mainstem occlusion. The latter is, however, extremely rare as patients with stroke secondary to MCA occlusion without recanalization rarely improve sufficiently to be considered for surgery.

The diagnosis of intracranial aneurysm has similarly been used by some authorities as justification for performing routine angiography in all patients being assessed for CEA. However, the pick-up rate for significant intracranial aneurysm is low – 4.5% in one series comprising 576 patients.[20] Of these, only 7 subsequently underwent surgery for the intracranial problem, 6 of which were after CEA. In our experience, only 1 patient in 300 (0.3%) was found to have an intracerebral aneurysm that was large enough to cause postponement of surgery. However, it is possible (but unproven) that undiagnosed aneurysms may predispose towards an increased risk of intracerebral haemorrhage within 30 days of surgery.

ADDITIONAL BENEFITS FROM ULTRASOUND

Plaque characterization?

High-resolution duplex scanning has the added advantage that, in addition to evaluating the degree of stenosis, plaque morphology can also be characterized. In this respect, angiography is unreliable in predicting plaque morphology and the presence of luminal thrombus. Steffen *et al.* have proposed four duplex-derived subtypes based on the degree of echogenicity of the plaque,[21] and this has been shown to correlate with the number of cerebral infarcts detected by CT scan.[22] Although this may be important in the future selection of asymptomatic patients who might benefit from CEA, it currently does not help in the selection of symptomatic patients and is the subject of ongoing research.

Is there recruitment of the collateral circulation?

Advocates of angiography have suggested that selective digital subtraction angiography of each carotid artery is the best method to determine whether there is recruitment of collateral flow within the circle of Willis. In practical terms this usually means reversed flow in the anterior cerebral artery ipsilateral to the stenosed ICA but it can also mean enhanced flow through the posterior communicating arteries.

However, evidence suggests that angiography is a relatively poor means of evaluating the state of the collateral circulation.[23] TCD is currently the optimal method for evaluating collateral flow patterns within the brain; this can also be augmented, if necessary, by compression of the common carotid artery in the root of the neck as a way of simulating the effects of carotid clamping or occlusion.[24]

IS IT SAFE TO OPERATE WITHOUT DUPLEX?

What is the safety of the investigation?

Duplex is a very safe, non-invasive examination which in experienced hands and with state-of-the-art equipment gives accurate information regarding the degree of stenosis, the length of the lesion and the characteristics of the plaque. It is repeatable and relatively inexpensive and can detect stenoses proximal and distal to the carotid bifurcation.

Intravenous digital subtraction angiography is also safe, but often gives poor-quality images and has largely been abandoned by most UK institutions. It is contraindicated in patients with poor left ventricular function and in those with borderline cardiac failure in whom the larger volume of contrast may cause problems.

Intra-arterial digital subtraction angiography carries a 1–2% risk of major neurological complications, which are increased if selective carotid angiograms are performed as opposed to arch studies.[25,26] Angiography is associated with some discomfort in accessing the intravascular space and also involves ionizing radiation. It is expensive compared to duplex and does not give any useful information about plaque characteristics. Occasionally, angiography will show the surface characteristics of the plaque but the sensitivity is low. MRA is non-invasive but very expensive and not freely available. Moreover, unlike duplex, it cannot readily be performed in the outpatient clinic. In a recent prospective study, MRA did not alter the management of any patient with carotid stenosis.[27] Development of the software, a decrease in cost and an increase in availability are therefore essential before this technique will find a routine place in the investigation of patients with carotid occlusive disease.

Operative risk

Surgeons may also be worried that reliance upon duplex will increase the risk of unexpected findings at operation and so potentially increase the risks of the procedure. In practice, however, it is usually the case that before a surgeon stops requesting routine angiograms, he or she will have developed a standardized protocol within their duplex department, which should be based on a comparative series of duplex and angiographic findings. With experience, simple criteria such as an inability to image above the plaque, high-resistance signals suggestive of syphon disease or spectral broadening and damped inflow signals will warn of the need for referring patients for selective angiography or MRA. By adopting such a protocol, it is possible to reduce the rate of angiograms to < 5% and evidence suggests that this is not associated with unexpected findings at operation, or an increase in the operative risk.[28]

How can standards be maintained?

All patients should be discussed at regular neurovascular meetings with a neurologist, vascular technologist, neuroradiologist and vascular surgeon. The results of carotid interventions should be regularly audited at this meeting. The introduction of new personnel into the non-invasive vascular laboratory should be carefully monitored with initial checking of every carotid duplex scan by an experienced operator. Subsequently cross-checks between different duplex operators should be carried out at random and for difficult cases. Comparison of duplex with angiography or MRA should be done whenever these are performed.

In summary, in experienced hands, duplex has a sensitivity and specificity of > 90% in diagnosing a > 70% carotid stenosis and, provided careful criteria are employed, it should be possible to identify the small subgroup who will require corroborative angiography or MRA. High-resistance, reverberant signals in the distal ICA suggest stenotic or occlusive disease in the carotid syphon and are an indication for selective angiography. Spectral broadening and a damped inflow signal suggest inflow disease and are an indication for angiography. If the duplex technologist can image normal artery above the stenosis, the surgeon should be able to complete the operation. The presence of intracranial stenotic, occlusive or aneurysmal disease rarely alters management decisions. Reliance on a protocol of duplex plus selective angiography does not compromise patient safety or operability. Duplex scanning is very operator-dependent. For those centres with inexperienced technologists, routine angiography should continue to be performed until reliable correlation has been achieved.

REFERENCES

1 Blackshear WM Jr, Connar RG. Carotid endarterectomy without angiography. *Journal of Cardiovascular Surgery* 1982; **23**: 477–482.
2 Ricotta JJ, Holen J, Schenk E *et al*. Is routine angiography necessary prior to carotid endarterectomy? *Journal of Vascular Surgery* 1984; **1**: 96–102.
3 Crew JR, Dean M, Johnson JM. Carotid surgery without angiography. *American Journal of Surgery* 1984; **148**: 217–220.
4 Shifrin EG, Bornstein NM, Kantarovsky A *et al*. Carotid endarterectomy without angiography. *British Journal of Surgery* 1996; **83**: 1107–1109.
5 Chen JC, Salvian AJ, Taylor DC, Teal PA, Marotta TR, Hsiang YN. Can duplex ultrasonography select appropriate

patients for carotid endarterectomy? *European Journal of Vascular and Endovascular Surgery* 1997; **14**: 451–456.

6 Khaw K-T. Does carotid duplex imaging render angiography redundant before carotid endarterectomy? *British Journal of Radiology* 1997; **70**: 235–238.

7 McCollum PT, da Silva A, Ridler DM, de Cossart L and the Audit Committee for the Vascular Surgical Society Carotid endarterectomy in the UK and Ireland: audit of 30-day outcome. *European Journal of Vascular and Endovascular Surgery* 1997; **14**: 386–391.

8 North American Symptomatic Carotid Endarterectomy Trial Collaborators. Beneficial effect of carotid endarterectomy in symptomatic patients with high-grade stenosis. *New England Journal of Medicine* 1991; **325**: 445–453.

9 European Carotid Surgery Triallists Collaborative Group. MRC European Carotid Surgery Trial: interim results for symptomatic patients with severe (70–99%) or with mild (0–19%) carotid stenosis. *Lancet* 1991; **337**: 1235–1243.

10 Bladin CF, Alexandrov AV, Murphy J, Maggisano R, Norris JW. Carotid stenosis index. A new method of measuring internal carotid artery stenosis. *Stroke* 1995; **26**: 230–234.

11 Padayachee TS, Cox TCS, Modaresi KB, Colchester ACF, Taylor PR. The measurement of internal carotid artery stenosis: comparison of duplex with digital subtraction angiography. *European Journal of Vascular and Endovascular Surgery* 1997; **13**: 180–185.

12 Faught WE, Mattos MA, van Bemmelen PS *et al*. Colour flow Duplex scanning of carotid arteries: new velocity criteria based on receiver operator characteristic analysis for threshold velocities used in the symptomatic and asymptomatic carotid trials. *Journal of Vascular Surgery* 1994; **19**: 818–828.

13 Moneta GL, Edwards M, Chitwood RW *et al*. Correlation of North American Symptomatic Carotid Endarterectomy Trial (NASCET) angiographic definition of 70–99% stenosis with Duplex scanning. *Journal of Vascular Surgery* 1993; **17**: 152–159.

14 Neale ML, Chambers JL, Kelly AT Reappraisal of duplex criteria to assess significant carotid stenosis with special reference to reports from NASCET and ECST. *Journal of Vascular Surgery* 1994; **20**: 642–649.

15 Lee DH, Gao FQ, Rankin RN, Pelz DM, Fox AJ. Duplex and color Doppler flow sonography of occlusion and near occlusion of the carotid artery. *American Journal of Neuroradiology* 1996; **17**: 1267–1274.

16 Akers DL, Markowitz IA, Kerstein MD. The value of aortic arch study in the evaluation of cerebrovascular insufficiency. *American Journal of Surgery* 1987; **154**: 230–232.

17 Mackey WC, O'Donnell TF, Callow AD. Carotid endarterectomy in patients with intracranial vascular disease: short-term risk and long-term outcome. *Journal of Vascular Surgery* 1989; **1**: 432–438.

18 Rothwell PM, Slattery J, Warlow CP. A systematic review of clinical and angiographic predictors of stroke and death due to carotid endarterectomy. *British Medical Journal* 1997; **315**: 1571–1577.

19 Delcker A, Turowski B. Diagnostic value of three-dimensional transcranial contrast duplex sonography. *Journal of Neuroimaging* 1997; **7**: 139–144.

20 Pansegrau T, Robicsek F. The clinical value and cost effectiveness of intracranial angiography in the management of carotid bifurcation disease; is it necessary? *Cardiovascular Surgery* 1997; **5** (Suppl. 1): 38–39.

21 Steffen CM, Gray-Weale AC, Byrne KE *et al*. Carotid atheroma: ultrasound appearance in symptomatic and asymptomatic patients. *Australia and New Zealand Journal of Surgery* 1989; **59**: 529–534.

22 Geroulakos G, Domjan J, Nicolaides A *et al*. Ultrasonic carotid plaque characterisation and the risk of cerebral infarction on computed tomography. *Journal of Vascular Surgery* 1994; **20**: 263–266.

23 AbuRahma AF, Robinson PA, Short Y, Lucente FC, Boland JP. Cross-filling of circle of Willis and carotid stenosis by angiography, duplex ultrasound and oculopneumoplethysmography. *American Journal of Surgery* 1995; **169**: 308–312.

24 Giller CA, Mathews D, Walker B, Purdy P, Roseland AM. Prediction of tolerance to carotid artery occlusion using transcranial Doppler ultrasound. *Journal of Neurosurgery* 1994; **81**: 15–19.

25 Hankey GJ, Warlow CP, Sellar RJ. Cerebral angiographic risk in mild cerebrovascular disease. *Stroke* 1990; **21**: 209–222.

26 Heiserman JE, Dean BL, Hodak JA *et al*. Neurologic complications of cerebral angiography. *American Journal of Neuroradiology* 1994; **15**: 1401–1407.

27 Erdoes LS, Marek JM, Berman SS *et al*. The relative contributions of carotid duplex scanning, magnetic resonance angiography and cerebral angiography to clinical decision making: a prospective study in patients with carotid occlusive disease. *Journal of Vascular Surgery* 1996; **23**: 950–956.

28 Loftus IM, McCarthy MJ, Pau H *et al*. Carotid endarterectomy without angiography does not compromise operative outcome. *European Journal of Vascular and Endovascular Surgery* 1998; **16**: 489–493.

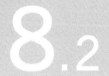

8.2

Is duplex ultrasound alone sufficient for preoperative imaging?

Andrew H Schulick (USA)
Richard P Cambria (USA)

INTRODUCTION

Recent randomized trials have demonstrated the efficacy of CEA in preventing ischemic stroke in both symptomatic[29,30] and asymptomatic patients.[31] Atherosclerotic stenosis of the carotid bifurcation can be detected and quantified by several different techniques. From the perspectives of patient safety, cost containment, and physician satisfaction, the optimal test or tests prior to CEA remains controversial. Since local resources, precision in non-invasive diagnosis, and CEA case volume may vary considerably, the appropriate diagnostic algorithm prior to CEA should not necessarily be considered uniform over different practice environments.

Angiography has remained the gold standard for classifying the severity of carotid bifurcation disease. It provides information relative to arch vessel disease, the degree and extent of bifurcation and ICA disease, the status of at least the anterior circle of Willis, and an accurate localization of the carotid bifurcation, all in a format that is readily interpretable by surgeons. All recently completed large randomized trials of CEA (North American Symptomatic Carotid Endarterectomy Trial (NASCET), Asymptomatic Carotid Atherosclerosis Study (ACAS), European Carotid Surgery Trial (ECST)) stratify patients based on the degree of carotid artery stenosis as defined by angiographic criteria.[29-31] Routine angiography, however, significantly adds to the morbidity (stroke, contrast reaction, puncture site problems) and cost of surgical treatment. Decision analysis based on ACAS data suggests that routine use of preoperative cerebral angiography, despite the diagnostic advantages, results in an increased 5-year stroke risk.[32] Had all

patients been subjected to cerebral angiography, fully 40% of the estimated 30-day stroke morbidity and mortality of ACAS patients would have been directly attributable to arteriography itself (1.2% stroke rate of angiography; 2.7% total risk of stroke in surgical arm, including strokes due to angiography).[31] The complications associated with cerebral angiography have stimulated the quest to perform CEA based solely on non-invasive testing. In the last decade, duplex scanning has emerged as the non-invasive test of choice. Compared to angiography, duplex scanning is less expensive and is essentially risk-free to the patient. In addition, duplex scanning can provide information on plaque composition, which may potentially have prognostic implications with respect to the natural history of specific lesions.[33]

With regard to stratification of the severity of carotid artery stenosis, data obtained by angiography and duplex scanning are not interchangeable.[34,35] Strict adherence to results of randomized trials dictates that duplex data alone are insufficient as a basis to perform CEA, and prominent voices in the neurologic literature have called for routine angiography prior to CEA.[36] In our view, this posture is unreasonable and indeed wasteful in environments where quality control documentation of the accuracy of duplex scanning has been demonstrated. In this chapter, we seek to define first, those conditions in which duplex scanning is adequate as a sole examination prior to CEA and second, the appropriate role for the selective application of angiography.

DUPLEX SCANNING

Duplex scanning combines B-mode ultrasound imaging with pulsed Doppler flow detection. In

contemporary practice, B-mode imaging is used to locate the carotid bifurcation, identify anatomic characteristics of the artery wall and plaque, and define the point of maximum stenosis for Doppler insonation; pulsed Doppler spectral waveform analysis allow interrogation of a defined sample volume on the B-mode image, and is used to assess the severity of arterial stenosis. The Doppler-shifted frequency is directly proportional to red blood cell velocity, and the magnitude of the shift is governed by the equation:

$$f_s = 2\,Vf_0\cos 2/C$$

where f_s is the frequency shift, V the velocity, f_0, the transmitted frequency, 2 the angle of insonation, and C the speed of sound in tissue (1540 m/s).

The Doppler-generated data are processed using fast Fourier transform spectral analysis. The resulting sonogram is displayed with frequency (velocity) on the ordinate and time on the abscissa. The degree of arterial stenosis is determined by flow velocity criteria generated by pulsed Doppler. In an idealized system, the relationship between red blood cell velocity and lumen size is expressed as:

$$r_1^2V_1 = r_2^2V_2$$

where r is the radius of the tube and v is velocity.

Another commonly used parameter to gauge the degree of arterial stenosis is spectral broadening. In a laminar flow system, red blood cells have near uniform velocity. In areas of vessel stenosis, where turbulence occurs, red blood cell velocity becomes heterogeneous and is recorded as broadening of pulsed Doppler waveforms. Color flow Doppler imaging is a newer technique wherein color assignments are based on flow direction and a single mean frequency estimate made for each site in the B-mode image. While spectral waveform analysis actually gives more detailed information on flow at each individual site, color Doppler allows flow information for the entire B-mode image to be displayed simultaneously. Quantitative and qualitative spectral waveform criteria for classifying the severity of carotid artery stenosis such as peak systolic velocity, ICA to common carotid artery (CCA)

velocity ratio, end diastolic velocity, and the presence and degree of spectral broadening have been validated to a high degree of correlation with independently interpreted contrast angiograms. Several groups have defined various values for these criteria and have demonstrated a high degree of internal accuracy and consistency within their respective laboratories in detecting significant arterial stenoses.[37-44] The lack of standardization between vascular laboratories is multifactorial and includes differences in ultrasound equipment, scanning technique, angle of insonation, and technologist experience.[45-47]

The degree of ICA stenosis is stratified in many vascular laboratories according to criteria developed at the University of Washington[37]:

1 no stenosis;
2 1–15% diameter stenosis;
3 16–49%;
4 50–79%;
5 80–99%;
6 occluded;
   the degree of stenosis in this system is defined as the ratio of the residual luminal diameter of the ICA to the diameter of the normal carotid bulb.

Unfortunately, this stratification scheme does not meld easily with data from either the ACAS or NASCET studies in which CEA is recommended for angiographic stenoses greater than or equal to 60% and 50%, respectively. Moreover, in these two studies, stenosis is defined as the ratio of residual luminal diameter of the ICA to the diameter in the normal distal ICA. Newer studies have proposed to redefine duplex criteria in a manner more consistent with that used in ACAS and NASCET;[38-44] the confusion, however, has made appropriate patient selection for CEA somewhat unclear.

In our own vascular laboratory we have developed duplex criteria directly correlated with the actual residual luminal diameter of surgical pathologic specimens obtained en bloc from CEA, rather than the percent stenosis determined angiographically.[48] Information obtained from TCD suggests that significant hemodynamic changes (alterations of flow in the ophthalmic artery, carotid siphon, and

Table 8.1
Various Doppler criteria to determine residual lumen ≤1.5 mm and their sensitivities, positive predictive value, negative predictive value, and accuracies

	Sensitivity	Specificity	PPV	NPV	Accuracy
PSV > 220	99	26	82	86	82
PSV > 360	85	78	93	62	82
PSV > 440	58	100	100	42	68
EDV > 115	82	70	90	53	79
EDV > 155	63	100	100	45	72
Carotid index > 3.5	99	35	83	89	84
Carotid index > 5.5	80	78	94	53	80
Carotid index > 10	30	100	100	30	46
PSV > 440 or EDV > 130 or carotid index > 9	82	87	95	59	83
Highly specific criteria: PSV > 440 or EDV > 155 or carotid index > 10	72	100	100	52	79
Highly sensitive criteria: PSV > 200 (and EDV > 140 or carotid index > 4.5)	96	61	89	82	88

PPV, positive predictive value; NPV, negative predictive value. PSV and EDV values are centimeters per second.
Reproduced from Suwanwela et al.[48] with permission.

intracranial circulation) due to carotid arterial stenosis occur when the residual luminal diameter of the ICA is ≤1.5 mm;[49] such indirect studies can occasionally add useful confirmatory information on the hemodynamic significance of a lesion identified by duplex scanning. We have therefore defined a significant stenosis of the ICA as ≤1.5 mm, and have developed appropriate carotid duplex criteria. The results can achieve 100% specificity or high sensitivity (96%) by adjusting the velocity criteria (Table 8.1). Defining severe stenosis as a residual lumen of 1.5 mm appears justified as this degree of narrowing corresponds roughly to a 60–75% stenosis by ACAS and NASCET criteria. In addition, this method obviates the need to obtain angiography for correlation, and accumulating evidence suggests that pathologic validation of duplex criteria is more accurate than angiographic correlation in quantifying the severity of a stenotic lesion.

CAROTID ENDARTERECTOMY WITHOUT ANGIOGRAPHY

Since the vast majority of cases of carotid disease consist of bifurcation atherosclerosis, and once the degree of stenosis is established the angiographic anatomy has little influence on the technical components of CEA, the need for angiography has been questioned. A variety of studies have found that angiography changes few operative plans,[50-55] but poses a significant risk of complications.[56] In terms of cost, cerebral angiography for carotid stenosis is upwards of 10 times as expensive as duplex scanning. In one study, preoperative angiography increased total charges by 43% per patient.[57]

The most important considerations regarding the decision to perform CEA based on the results of duplex scanning alone are the quality control issues and validated accuracy of the vascular laboratory. Indeed, in an active referral practice of vascular surgery, a common observation is the wide spectrum of expertise with which carotid non-invasive testing is performed. Typically, the direction of error is in the overestimation of the degree of stenosis. Validation of any laboratory must be obtained through a consistent history of correlation between duplex scanning and angiographic or pathologic data. In addition, each vascular laboratory should be monitored periodically by a sanctioned quality control commission. The results of duplex must be considered in the context of the clinical presentation of the patient, e.g., the management of apparent total carotid occlusion on duplex will be determined by clinical, not anatomic, variables. The surgeon performing CEA without angiography should, ideally, be experienced in vascular duplex scanning and should be present at the time of the studies or review videotapes of the studies with the responsible technologist. This will aid in assessing the technical components of the study, such as adequacy of arterial visualization, and the presence of topographic characteristics of the ICA, such as coiling, which might adversely affect the accuracy of the study yet not be readily appreciated on analysis of flow velocity data alone.

Proponents of angiography cite certain limitations of duplex scanning as reasons to obtain preoperative angiography in all potential surgical patients. Careful review of these objections, however, fails to provide sufficiently compelling arguments to encourage other than the selective use of angiography. First: duplex scanning cannot reliably image aortic arch and intracranial disease. Significant proximal stenosis is often associated with innominate or subclavian disease which can be identified on physical examination. Severe proximal CCA stenosis occurs infrequently and can generally be identified as a diminished or non-palpable carotid pulse or on duplex scan as turbulent flow and spectral broadening in the more distal CCA.[58] In the authors' opinion, arch-level CCA stenosis which does not produce palpable diminution of the CCA pulse can be safely ignored in the absence of symptoms. When indicated, proximal lesions may be further assessed by MRA as an alternative to contrast angiography. The presence of intracranial cerebrovascular pathology such as siphon stenosis and berry

aneurysms, in general, have no bearing on the decision to perform carotid endarterectomy. Most experienced surgeons recommend correcting significant carotid bifurcation disease even in the presence of these lesions.[59–61]

Second: duplex scans are dependent on flow and may be less accurate in the presence of severe contralateral ICA disease. Although determination of ICA stenosis in the presence of contralateral occlusion or severe stenosis may be subject to error because of altered flow dynamics, several groups have defined modified duplex criteria which have demonstrated a high degree of correlation with independently interpreted angiograms.[62,63] It should be possible for other experienced vascular laboratories to accumulate their own criteria in a similar fashion. Alternatively, MRA may serve as a confirmatory study in this situation.

Third: duplex scanning cannot reliably distinguish between high-grade stenosis and ICA occlusion. Duplex scanning can, however, suggest the need for further evaluation; this is especially important in the clinical circumstance where hemispheric symptoms are referable to the side ipsilateral to the purported occlusion; this situation suggests that the ICA may not be occluded, or is in the process of occluding, and demands further investigation. MRA has proven very reliable in making the distinction between high-grade arterial stenosis and occlusion, with virtually 100% accuracy in most series;[64–66] routine angiography in this circumstance, although still currently indicated, may eventually prove unnecessary.

Since Blackshear and Connar's sentinel report in 1982,[67] many groups have reported series of CEA performed without utilizing preoperative angiography; the results of major series are summarized in Table 8.2. The decision to operate was based largely on data from duplex scanning, although other non-invasive tests were occasionally obtained. Overall, the degree of stenosis determined by duplex scanning was found to correlate closely to surgical pathologic findings. The reported combined perioperative stroke morbidity and mortality rate is low, confirming CEA without angiography as a safe approach. Whether CEA without angiography improves on currently achieved stroke morbidity and

Table 8.2
Early results reported in major large series of carotid endarterectomy performed without preoperative angiography

Author	Year	Cases	Stroke	TIA	Death
Sandmann et al.[68]	1983	91	0 (0%)	0 (0%)	0 (0%)
Crew et al.[69]	1984	65	1 (1.5%)	1 (1.5%)	0 (0%)
Hill et al.[70]	1990	101	1 (1%)	2 (2%)	0 (0%)
Wagner et al.[71]	1991	255	5 (2%)	1 (0.4%)	0 (0%)
Cartier et al.[72]	1993	130	2 (1.5%)	2 (1.5%)	2 (1.5%)
Shifrin et al.[73]	1996	109	2 (1.8%)	0 (0%)	2 (1.8%)
Campron et al.[74]	1998	75	0 (0%)	1 (1.3%)	1 (1.3%)
Total		826	11 (1.3%)	7 (0.9%)	5 (0.6%)

TIA, transient ischemic attack.

mortality statistics has not been studied. Certainly, omission of angiography defrays the additional costs associated with the study, and avoids the small but definite morbidity of angiography.

Duplex ultrasound is highly reliable in detecting severe carotid stenosis except under certain specific circumstances; in these situations, cerebral angiography is required for clarification. The indications for angiography prior to CEA are as follows (Table 8.3):

1   inadequate or incomplete duplex scan;
2   hemispheric symptoms in the presence of a lesion of 50% or less (i.e., non-stenotic), as determined by duplex scanning;
3   vertebrobasilar symptoms, or non-hemispheric symptoms in which further brain imaging has ruled out lesions such as tumor and chronic subdural, arteriovenous malformations;
4   abnormal flow patterns in the common carotid artery, as determined by duplex scanning, unequal upper-extremity pressures, or other signs of aortic arch disease;
5   suggestion by duplex scanning that the ICA may be occluded in an actively symptomatic patient;
6   significant discrepancy between history, physical, duplex scanning, and other imaging studies;
7   recurrent carotid artery stenosis – our experience has indicated that duplex scanning in this

Table 8.3
Indications from preoperative cerebral angiography prior to carotid endarterectomy

Inadequate or incomplete duplex scan

Hemispheric symptoms in the presence of non-stenotic lesion by duplex

Atypical/non-hemispheric symptoms

Signs of proximal disease by duplex or physical examination

Occluded internal carotid artery by duplex (dependent on clinical presentation)

Discrepancy between duplex and clinical evaluation

Recurrent carotid artery stenosis

situation is less accurate than in primary stenosis.

As suggested earlier, forthcoming studies and refinements of MRA may narrow this list of indications for preoperative angiography even

further. On the other hand, should carotid stenting emerge as a viable therapeutic alternative for the treatment of carotid artery stenosis, a resurgence in angiography may result.

AUTHORS' PERSPECTIVE

A technically acceptable duplex scan of the carotid artery performed in a vascular laboratory with validated accuracy is a safe, cost-effective alternative to angiography prior to CEA. This determination has led us to pursue a policy of selective preoperative angiography only for the indications listed in Table 8.3. In the senior author's experience (RPC), the utilization of preoperative angiography has progressively declined over the past 5 years. In 1991, virtually all patients were studied with angiography and, by 1994, the figure was 50%. In contemporary practice, less than 20% of patients are evaluated with angiography. The combined perioperative stroke and death rates have remained unchanged, in the 1% range.

CEA performed on the basis of results from duplex scanning alone is an appropriate strategy in environments with documented duplex scan accuracy and sufficient surgical volume, and can be applied to all but a select group of patients.[75] Those who do require preoperative angiography are readily identified by a combination of duplex scanning, history, and physical examination, making routine diagnostic angiography unnecessary. This perspective is not borne of concern over the potential major morbidity of carotid angiography. In his personal experience with nearly 800 CEAs over a span of 12 years, the senior author has had but a single case in which major stroke complicated carotid angiography performed at the Massachusetts General Hospital. Rather, since diagnostic precision is not sacrificed by the highly selective use of angiography in our practice environment, such practice is both logical and cost-effective.

REFERENCES

29 North American Symptomatic Carotid Endarterectomy Trial Collaborators. Beneficial effect of carotid endarterectomy in symptomatic patients with high-grade carotid stenosis. *New England Journal of Medicine* 1991; **325**: 445–453.

30 European Carotid Surgery Trialists' Collaborative Group. MRC European surgery trial: interim results for symptomatic patients with severe (70–99%) carotid stenosis. *Lancet* 1991; **337**: 1235–1243.

31 Executive Committee for the Asymptomatic Carotid Atherosclerosis Study. Endarterectomy for asymptomatic carotid artery stenosis. *Journal of the American Medical Association* 1995; **273**: 1421–1428.

32 Kuntz KM, Kent KC, Whittemore AD, Skillman JJ. Carotid endarterectomy in asymptomatic patients – is contrast angiography necessary? A morbidity analysis. *Journal of Vascular Surgery* 1995; **22**: 706–714.

33 Reilly LM. Importance of carotid plaque morphology. In: Bernstein EF (ed.) *Vascular Diagnosis*, p. 333. St Louis: Mosby-Year Book, 1993.

34 Ricci MA. The changing role of duplex scan in the management of carotid bifurcation disease and endarterectomy. *Seminars in Vascular Surgery* 1998; **11**: 3–11.

35 Moneta GL, Saxon RR, Taylor LM Jr, Porter JM. Carotid imaging before carotid endarterectomy. *Seminars in Vascular Surgery* 1995; **8**: 21–28.

36 Barnett HJM, Eliasziw M, Meldrum HE, Taylor DW. Do the facts and figures warrant a 10-fold increase in the performance of carotid endarterectomy on asymptomatic patients? *Neurology* 1996; **46**: 603–608.

37 Strandness DE Jr. Extracranial arterial disease. In: Strandness DE Jr (ed.) *Duplex Scanning in Vascular Disorders*, pp. 113–158. New York: Raven Press, 1993.

38 Moneta GL, Porter JM, Cummings CA et al. Correlation of North American Symptomatic Carotid Endarterectomy Trial (NASCET) angiographic definition of 70% to 99% internal carotid artery stenosis with duplex scanning. *Journal of Vascular Surgery* 1993; **17**: 152–157.

39 Mattos MA, Sumner DS, Ramsey DE et al. Carotid endarterectomy without angiography: is color-flow duplex scanning sufficient? *Surgery* 1994; **116**: 776–782.

40 Neale ML, Appleberg M, Roche J et al. Reappraisal of duplex criteria to assess significant carotid stenosis with special reference to reports from the North American Symptomatic Carotid Endarterectomy Trial and the European Carotid Surgery Trial. *Journal of Vascular Surgery* 1994; **20**: 642–649.

41 Moneta GL, Porter JM, Strandness DE Jr et al. Screening for asymptomatic internal carotid artery stenosis: duplex criteria for discriminating 60% to 99% stenosis. *Journal of Vascular Surgery* 1995; **21**: 989–994.

42 Carpenter JP, Davis JT, Lexa FJ. Determination of sixty percent or greater carotid artery stenosis by duplex Doppler ultrasonography. *Journal of Vascular Surgery* 1995; **22**: 697–703.

43 Hood DB, Sumner DS, Barkmeier LD et al. Prospective evaluation of new duplex criteria to identify 70% internal carotid artery stenosis. *Journal of Vascular Surgery* 1996; **23**: 254–261.

44 Alexandrov AV, Burns PN, Murphy J, Hamilton P,

Mclean A, Brodie DS. Correlation of peak systolic velocity and angiographic measurement of carotid stenosis revisited. *Stroke* 1997; **28**: 339–342.

45 Alexandrov AV, Grotta JC, Hamilton P, Brodie DS, Vital D. Grading carotid stenosis with ultrasound. An interlaboratory comparison. *Stroke* 1997; **28**: 1208–1210.

46 Kuntz KM, Kent KC, Skillman JJ, Whittemore AD. Duplex ultrasound criteria for the identification of carotid stenosis should be laboratory specific. *Stroke* 1997; **28**: 597–602.

47 Fillinger MF, Cronenwett JL, Walsh DB *et al*. Carotid duplex criteria for a 60% or greater angiographic stenosis: variation according to equipment. *Journal of Vascular Surgery* 1996; **24**: 856–864.

48 Suwanwela N, Can U, Furie KL *et al*. Carotid Doppler ultrasound criteria for internal carotid artery stenosis based on residual lumen diameter calculated from en bloc carotid endarterectomy specimens. *Stroke* 1996; **27**: 1965–1969.

49 Can U, Furie KL, Suwanwela N *et al*. Transcranial Doppler ultrasound criteria for hemodynamically significant internal carotid artery stenosis based on residual lumen diameter calculated from en bloc endarterectomy specimens. *Stroke* 1997; **28**: 1966–1971.

50 Ricotta JJ, Holen J, Schenk E *et al*. Is routine arteriography necessary prior to carotid endarterectomy? *Journal of Vascular Surgery* 1984; **1**: 96–102.

51 Walsh J, Markowitz I, Kerstein MD. Carotid endarterectomy for amaurosis fugax without angiography. *American Journal of Surgery* 1986; **152**: 172–174.

52 Goodson SF, Meyer JP, Kikta MJ, Schuler JJ, Bishara RA, Flanigan DP. Can carotid duplex scanning supplant arteriography in patients with focal carotid territory symptoms? *Journal of Vascular Surgery* 1987; **5**: 551–557.

53 Moore WS, Baker JD, Busuttil RW, Machleder HI, Quinones-Baldrich WJ, Ziomek S. Can clinical evaluation and noninvasive testing substitute for arteriography in the evaluation of carotid artery disease? *Annals of Surgery* 1988; **208**: 91–94.

54 Dawson DL, Zierler RE, Kohler TR. Role of arteriography in the preoperative evaluation of carotid artery disease. *American Journal of Surgery* 1991; **161**: 619–624.

55 Dawson DL, Kohler TR, Clowes AW, Strandness DE Jr, Zierler RE. The role of duplex scanning and arteriography before carotid endarterectomy: a prospective study. *Journal of Vascular Surgery* 1993; **18**: 673–680.

56 Hankey GJ, Warlow CP, Sellar RJ. Cerebral angiographic risk in mild cerebrovascular disease. *Stroke* 1990; **21**: 209–222.

57 Garrard CL, Money SR, Bowen JC *et al*. Cost savings associated with the nonroutine use of carotid angiography. *American Journal of Surgery* 1997; **174**: 650–653.

58 McLaren JT, Drezner AD, Donaghue CC. Accuracy of carotid duplex examination to predict proximal and intrathoracic lesions. *American Journal of Surgery* 1996; **172**: 149–150.

59 Moore WS. Does tandem lesion mean tandem risk in patients with carotid artery disease? *Journal of Vascular Surgery* 1988; **7**: 454–455.

60 Ladowski JS, Webster MW, Yonas HO, Steed DL. Carotid endarterectomy in patients with asymptomatic intracranial aneurysm. *Annals of Surgery* 1984; **200**: 70–73.

61 Orrechia PM, Clagett GP, Youkey JR *et al*. Management of patients with symptomatic extracranial carotid artery disease and incidental intracranial berry aneurysm. *Journal of Vascular Surgery* 1985; **2**: 158–164.

62 Fujitani RM, Taylor SM, Wang LM, Mills JL. The effect of unilateral internal carotid arterial occlusion upon contralateral duplex study: criteria for accurate interpretation. *Journal of Vascular Surgery* 1992; **16**: 459–467.

63 AbuRahma AF, Alberts S, Pollack JA, Khan S, Robinson PA, Richmond BK. Effect of contralateral severe stenosis or carotid occlusion on duplex criteria of ipsilateral stenosis: comparative study of various duplex parameters. *Journal of Vascular Surgery* 1995; **22**: 751–761.

64 Heiserman JE, Drayer BP, Fram EK *et al*. Carotid artery stenosis: clinical efficacy of two-dimensional time-of-flight MR angiography. *Radiology* 1992; **182**: 761–768.

65 Huston J 3rd, Lewis BD, Wiebers DO, Meyer FB, Riederer SJ, Weaver AL. Carotid artery: prospective blinded comparison of two-dimensional time-of-flight MR angiography with conventional angiography and duplex US. *Radiology* 1993; **186**: 339–344.

66 Mittl RL, Broderick M, Carpenter JP *et al*. Blinded-reader comparison of magnetic resonance angiography and duplex ultrasonography for carotid artery bifurcation stenosis. *Stroke* 1994; **25**: 4–10.

67 Blackshear WM, Connar RG. Carotid endarterectomy without angiography. *Journal of Cardiovascular Surgery* 1982; **23**: 477–482.

68 Sandmann W, Hennerici M, Nullen H *et al*. Carotid artery surgery without angiography; risk or progress? In Greenhalgh RM, Rose FC (eds) *Progress in Stroke Research II*, pp. 447–460. London: Pitman, 1983.

69 Crew JR, Dean M, Johnson JM *et al*. Carotid surgery without angiography. *American Journal of Surgery* 1984; **148**: 217–220.

70 Hill JC, Carbonneau K, Baliga PK, Akers DL, Bell WH 3rd, Kerstein MD. Safe extracranial vascular evaluation and surgery without preoperative arteriography. *Annals of Vascular Surgery* 1990; **4**: 34–38.

71 Wagner WH, Treiman RL, Cossman DV, Foran RF, Levin PM, Cohen JL. The diminishing role of diagnostic arteriography in cartotid artery disease: duplex scanning as definitive preoperative study. *Annals of Vascular Surgery* 1991; **5**: 105–110.

72 Cartier R, Cartier P, Fontaine AF. Carotid endarterectomy without angiography. The reliability of Doppler ultrasonography and duplex scanning in preoperative assessment. *Canadian Journal of Surgery* 1993; **36**: 411–416.

73 Shifrin EG, Aronovich B, Portnoi I *et al*. Carotid endarterectomy without angiography. *British Journal of Surgery* 1996; **83**: 1107–1109.

74 Campron H, Fontaine AF, Cartier R. Prophylactic carotid endarterectomy without arteriography in patients without hemispheric symptoms: surgical morbidity and mortality and long-term follow-up. *Annals of Vascular Surgery* 1998; **12**: 10–16.

75 Dawson DL, Fujitani RM, Roseberry CA: Preoperative testing before carotid endarterectomy: a survey of vascular surgeons' attitudes. *Annals of Vascular Surgery* 1997; **11**: 264–272.

8.3 Editorial Comment

KEY POINTS

1 Duplex ultrasound technology has supplanted angiography as the routine imaging study prior to CEA and has significantly refined the indications for angiography.
2 In experienced hands, duplex has a sensitivity and specificity of ≥90% for detecting a stenosis > 70%.
3 The presence of significant inflow disease is suggested by diminished carotid pulse and/or spectral broadening or a damped inflow signal and is an indication for angiography.
4 The presence of high resistance or reverberant signals in the distal ICA suggests significant stenotic or occlusive disease in the carotid siphon and is an indication for angiography.
5 If the ultrasound technologist cannot image normal carotid artery above the plaque, an angiogram should be performed in order to identify patients with significant distal disease extension.
6 A caveat in the reliance on duplex prior to CEA is the absolute dependence on the experience of the operator. Before abandoning a policy of routine angiography, each vascular laboratory must perform comparative studies and maintain a protocol of quality control checks thereafter.

There is increasing consensus that, in experienced hands, duplex ultrasound is a reliable method of grading stenosis and can refine the indications for contrast angiography. In addition, unexpected operative findings which might compromise operability or patient safety. Thus, for those institutions where the surgeon has confidence in the duplex findings and clearly defined criteria for grading stenosis, angiography may be necessary in fewer than 10% of patients. This is obviously advantageous because angiography is associated with significant risk and cost and a duplex scan can be performed in a single-visit vascular clinic.

While there will be some variability among individuals with respect to the duplex criteria for a surgically significant lesion, each laboratory should also compare its criteria with standards such as the Strandness criteria. In this respect, the method based on detecting a residual luminal diameter ≤1.5 mm proposed by Drs Schulick and Cambria represents a modification of the Strandness criteria and requires further evaluation in larger comparative studies. Any method which will enable surgeons and vascular technologists to ensure greater accuracy is to be welcomed, although the Schulick–Cambria method is ultimately dependent on the diameter of the normal ICA. For example, a 1.5 mm residual lumen in a 3 mm artery will be a 50% stenosis while a similar lumen in a 5 mm artery will represent a 70% stenosis. To our knowledge, there is no evidence that residual luminal diameter has a better correlation with stroke risk than the percent diameter stenosis.

The areas of ongoing controversy relate to first, the effect of acoustic shadowing on interpretation of the waveform, second, the differentiation between subocclusion and total occlusion and third, the fact that incorrect clinical decisions may be made in the small number of patients with false-positive or negative duplex findings. Plaque calcification causing acoustic shadowing has always been a potential problem, but most experienced technologists can usually interrogate the waveform at some point in the plaque by adjusting the angle and plane of insonation. If, however, there is evidence of circumferential calcification which totally impedes access, an angiogram is necessary. Similarly, the differentiation between occlusion and subocclusion is very much dependent upon operator experience. For those less experienced centers this probably means that a number of patients will require confirmatory angiography. Finally, it is conceivable that a small number of strokes might occur in

patients with either a false-positive or negative duplex diagnosis of a 70–99% stenosis. However, the available evidence suggests that any potential benefit derived from a policy of routine angiography would be negated by the stroke risk associated with angiography.

In practice, therefore, for those centers with highly experienced duplex services, patients will rarely require angiography and probably very few will need adjunctive MRA studies. For those centers with less experienced duplex services, there may be a need for increased reliance on MRA as a means of selecting patients for angiography whilst their vascular laboratory gains more experience.

9.1

Is there a role for preoperative magnetic resonance angiography?
Peter RD Humphrey (Europe)

INTRODUCTION

The author must first declare a major bias in favour of a policy of non-invasive work-up for the detection of carotid stenosis. Our own unit largely relies upon duplex ultrasound and magnetic resonance angiography (MRA) and only occasionally do we now perform intra-arterial digital subtraction angiography (DSA). However, despite recent advances in technology, it is important to balance the potential advantages of MRA against its current limitations. At present, about 80% of MRA studies are of good or excellent quality, 15% are of reduced quality but still diagnostic, whilst about 5% are of sufficiently poor quality to preclude reliable interpretation.[1–3]

TECHNICAL CONSIDERATIONS

The generation of an MRA scan requires the patient to be surrounded by a magnetic field which causes individual protons in the water molecules in the field of view to become aligned with their axis to the magnetic field. A radiofrequency pulse is then emitted which excites the protons and causes them to rotate. Following this, the protons realign themselves within the magnetic field and thereafter emit energy, which is received by a coil adjacent to the patient's head.

The time-of-flight MRA technique uses rapid radiofrequency pulses, during which time stationary tissues are unable to emit strong enough signals to the receiving coil and, as a result, generate a black or grey colour on the ensuing image (Fig. 9.1A). In contrast, flowing blood is not influenced by previous radiofrequency pulses and is able to emit a stronger signal, which is displayed as white on the final MRA scan (Fig. 9.1A).

To obtain the best images, it is important to have short repetition times, a fast gradient echo and relatively low flip angles. This will create many slices of baseline data in which the vessels stand out and the background stationary tissue is basically lost (Fig. 9.1A).

With two-dimensional MRA (2D MRA), multiple thin (2–3mm) slices are imaged in sequence and then reconstructed to give a 12cm field of view. In three dimensional MRA (3D MRA), a block of tissue (up to 8cm) is imaged at one time and then divided up into tomographic slices. The principal advantage of 2D MRA is that very low flow states can be imaged (Fig. 9.1E), whilst with 3D MRA there is a higher spatial resolution overall, but trickle flow may be missed (Fig. 9.1C). In practice, most current MRA scanners provide both 2D and 3D MRA images. When hard copies of the MRA are taken, it is best to keep both the baseline and the angiographic data as it is sometimes useful to consult the former if the angiographic data are difficult to interpret (Fig. 9.1A–F). Once the final image has been generated, it can be evaluated in much the same way as a conventional angiogram with regard to the calculation of stenosis (Figs 9.2 and 9.3).

DISADVANTAGES OF MRA

MRA requires up to 30min to acquire the data and the quality of the image is compromised by any motion artefact induced by patient swallowing or movement. During this time, the patient may also have trouble with claustrophobia. Clinicians should note that the level of the carotid bifurcation (usually between the third and sixth cervical vertebra) can vary and, unless a number of preliminary sagittal localizing studies are performed, it may be difficult to

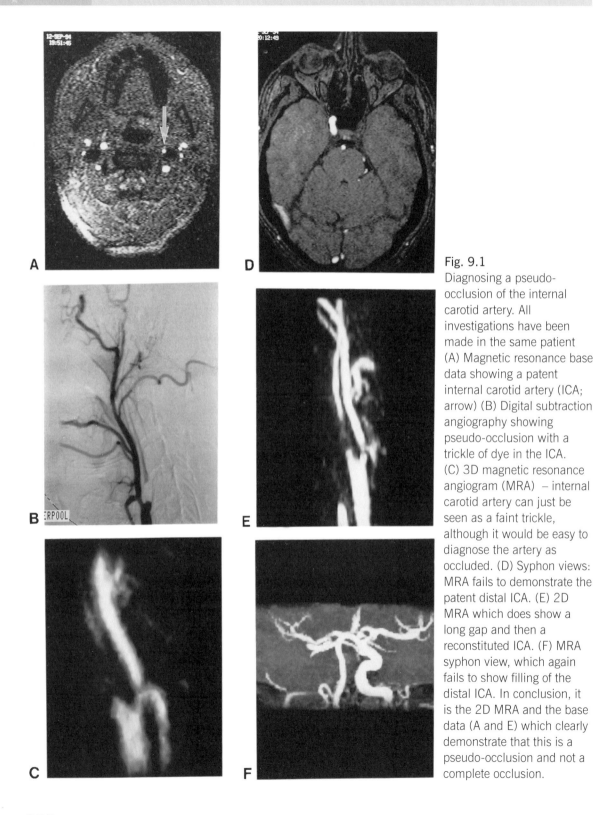

Fig. 9.1
Diagnosing a pseudo-occlusion of the internal carotid artery. All investigations have been made in the same patient (A) Magnetic resonance base data showing a patent internal carotid artery (ICA; arrow) (B) Digital subtraction angiography showing pseudo-occlusion with a trickle of dye in the ICA. (C) 3D magnetic resonance angiogram (MRA) – internal carotid artery can just be seen as a faint trickle, although it would be easy to diagnose the artery as occluded. (D) Syphon views: MRA fails to demonstrate the patent distal ICA. (E) 2D MRA which does show a long gap and then a reconstituted ICA. (F) MRA syphon view, which again fails to show filling of the distal ICA. In conclusion, it is the 2D MRA and the base data (A and E) which clearly demonstrate that this is a pseudo-occlusion and not a complete occlusion.

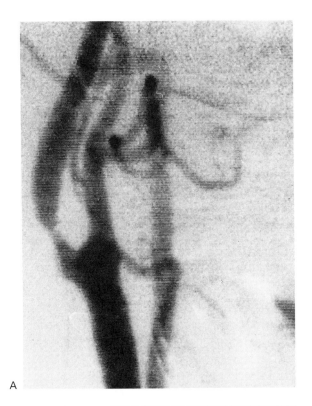

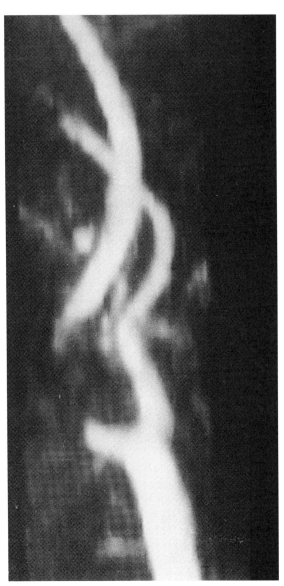

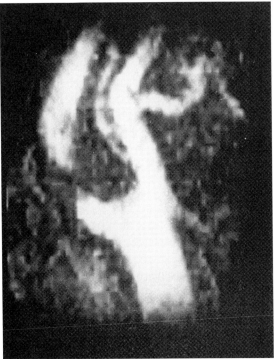

Fig. 9.2
(A) Intra-arterial digital subtraction angiogram showing a severe stenosis of the internal carotid artery. The same stenosis is examined using (B) 2D and (C) 3D magnetic resonance angiogram (MRA). Note that the 3D MRA provides a clearer image of the stenosis than 2D MRA. The 2D MRA image is associated with a larger signal gap. Reproduced with permission from the Young et al.[4]

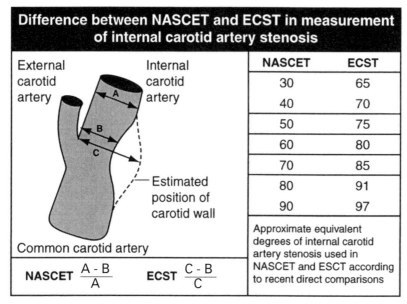

Difference between NASCET and ECST in measurement of internal carotid artery stenosis

External carotid artery

Internal carotid artery

— Estimated position of carotid wall

Common carotid artery

$$\text{NASCET}\ \frac{A - B}{A} \qquad \text{ECST}\ \frac{C - B}{C}$$

NASCET	ECST
30	65
40	70
50	75
60	80
70	85
80	91
90	97

Approximate equivalent degrees of internal carotid artery stenosis used in NASCET and ESCT according to recent direct comparisons

Fig. 9.3
Methods of measuring the degree of carotid stenosis. Measurement B, the original internal carotid lumen, is made at the point of maximal stenosis (i.e. not necessarily the carotid bulb). Reproduced with permission from Donnan et al.[16]

ensure that the bifurcation lies in the centre of the field of view. On rare occasions, the patient may be too large to enter the tunnel of the scanner and MRA is absolutely contraindicated in patients with a pacemaker.[4]

In 2D MRA images, turbulent, non-laminar flow patterns within the stenosed artery can cause local loss of signal which may lead to a systematic overestimation of the degree of stenosis. On occasions there can even be a complete loss of the signal which might then be misinterpreted as a complete occlusion. As will be seen, complete flow voids with distal refilling with 3D MRA are virtually diagnostic of a stenosis > 70% (Fig. 9.2C). However, for those who rely on 2D images alone, up to 15% of flow voids may be encountered in patients with a stenosis < 70%.[2] Similarly, current MRA methods are unable reliably to interpret plaque morphology, largely because of the variable degree of signal loss within the stenosed artery.[5]

3D MRA scans have a relatively small field of view (< 8cm) and are poor at differentiating a subtotal occlusion from complete occlusion (Fig. 9.1C). Moreover, clinicians should be aware that low flow in a carotid dissection will give the same appearance as trickle flow through a subocclusion. Similarly, patients with looped carotid arteries can pose a problem if 2D MRA is used because the scan will misinterpret the apparent flow reversal within one of the components of the loop and lend to the conclusion that there is an underlying occlusion. In practice, this is rarely a problem if both 2D and 3D MRA are employed.

ADVANTAGES OF MRA
MRA is non-invasive, can be performed as an outpatient examination and does not require the use of contrast agents. However, the use of gadolinium to enhance difficult images may be of benefit in selected patients in the future. There is also the advantage that an MRA scan can be combined with an MR imaging study, which will identify any organic pathology at the same sitting. In contrast to 2D MRA, the presence of a flow void on 3D MRA is almost invariably indicative of a severe carotid stenosis (Fig. 9.4). In contrast, 2D MRA is especially good at identifying trickle flow through a pseudo-occlusion (Fig. 9.1E).

The principal advantage of MRA over duplex is the ability to image the arch vessels, carotid syphon and intracranial circulation, although this does require several studies. As will be seen, however, current MRA technology does have problems with regard to the accurate diagnosis of intracranial

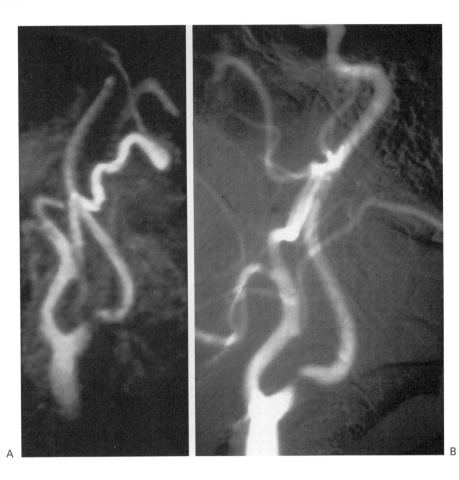

Fig. 9.4
(A) Magnetic resonance angiogram (MRA) and (B) contrast arteriogram. MRA can provide a precise anatomic depiction of carotid bifurcation disease.

A

B

disease and, although MRA can image the carotid syphon, there may be problems with interpretation because of low flow above a critical inflow stenosis (Fig. 9.1D and 9.1F), the tortuosity of the distal ICA and artefacts due to air in the adjacent sinuses.[3]

INTER- AND INTRAOBSERVER VARIABILITY

A number of studies have compared the different methods of measuring stenosis and the associated inter- and intraobserver variability for DSA.[6–9] Relatively few, however, have evaluated observer variability in DSA and MRA using the same cohort of patients.

In a recent study, we compared observer variability for four different methods of measuring carotid stenosis using a population of patients who underwent MRA and DSA.[1] Patients who had evidence of a flow void on 3D MRA were excluded because it has been shown that this correlates closely with a 70–99% stenosis and precise measurements are not possible with a gap. Instead, our aim was to focus attention on observer variability in the interpretation of stenoses not associated with a flow void which, in clinical practice at least, should be the most difficult subgroup in which to categorize disease severity. The four methods of measuring stenosis were:

1 the European Carotid Surgery Trial (ECST) method;
2 the North American Symptomatic Carotid Endarterectomy Trial (NASCET) method;
3 the common carotid method;
4 the 'eyeballing method' (Fig. 9.3).

Two independent observers graded the DSA and 2D

Table 9.1
Intraobserver variability for DSA and MRA in 73 carotid arteries

	Median absolute differences (95% CI)		95% limits of agreement (95% CI)	
	DSA	MRA	DSA	MRA
Intraobserver 1 agreement				
Common carotid method	2% (2–4)	6% (5–8)	−11 to +11	−22 to +27
ECST method	4% (3–6)	5% (3–7)	−16 to +17	−20 to +26
NASCET method	4% (3–5)	6% (4–8)	−10 to +14	−16 to +24
Eyeballing method	4% (0–5)	5% (4–9)	−15 to +17	−22 to +15
Intraobserver 2 agreement				
Common carotid method	4% (3–5)	3% (2–5)	−16 to +16	−23 to +21
ECST method	5% (3–8)	6% (4–9)	−18 to +19	−23 to +23
NASCET method	4% (3–6)	5% (3–6)	−16 to +15	−24 to +22
Eyeballing method	4% (0–5)	4% (0–9)	−14 to +14	−20 to +23

DSA, digital subtraction angiography; MRA, magnetic resonance angiography; ECST, European Carotid Surgery Trial; NASCET, North American Symptomatic Carotid Endarterectomy Trial; CI, confidence interval. (Adapted from Young et al.[1] with permission.

and 3D MRA images on two occasions 3 months apart.

Table 9.1 summarizes the intraobserver variability associated with the four different methods of measuring stenosis. The median value for the absolute difference between measurement 1 and measurement 2 for each of the scrutineers was 4–5% for DSA and 3–6% for MRA.[1] Overall, this equates to a typical measurement error of ±4% for DSA and ±5% for MRA. However, as can be seen, the 95% limits of agreement (which represent the range of values within which 95% of the results of a second reading would be expected to lie) are wider but better for DSA than for MRA.[1]

Table 9.2 summarizes the interobserver agreement for DSA and MRA. As can be seen, the interobserver variability in measuring the degree of stenosis using DSA was 5–8% and, for MRA, 5–13%. Interestingly, the lowest variability was noted in the eyeballing method of determining stenosis.[1]

A measure of interobserver variability is important as it tells us how stenosis measurements might be interpreted in clinical practice as no two observers will diagnose the same value for stenosis. In our study, we observed that one observer systematically reported tighter degrees of stenosis than the other. Although this systematic difference could be overcome by a numerical correction for bias, it does reinforce the point that multiple observers in numerous institutions using different DSA and MRA machines and different calipers will incur considerable variability for any given stenosis.[1] This could lead to some patients with a true severe stenosis being denied surgery, whilst some patients with less severe disease might undergo an inappropriate operation.

COMPARISON BETWEEN MRA, DSA AND DUPLEX

Following the development of 3D MRA, a number of publications have compared MRA with DSA but few have used the same patient cohort to provide comparable data for MRA, DSA and duplex ultrasound. Table 9.3 presents sensitivity and specificity analyses for MRA versus DSA and duplex

Table 9.2
Interobserver variability for DSA and MRA in 73 carotid arteries

	Median absolute differences (95% CI)		95% limits of agreement (95% CI)	
	DSA	MRA	DSA	MRA
Interobserver agreement				
Common carotid method	7% (6–10)	13% (7–16)	−12 to +24	−19 to +41
ECST method	7% (6–10)	12% (10–16)	−13 to +26	−13 to +37
NASCET method	8% (5–9)	8% (6–12)	−12 to +24	−18 to +32
Eyeballing method	5% (4–9)	5% (4–9)	−20 to +20	−23 to +20

DSA, digital subtraction angiography; MRA, magnetic resonance angiography; ECST, European Carotid Surgery Trial; NASCET, North American Symptomatic Carotid Endarterectomy Trial; CI, confidence interval. Adapted from Young et al.[1] with permission.

Table 9.3
Sensitivity and specificity of magnetic resonance angiography and duplex ultrasound in the diagnosis of a carotid stenosis or occlusion using contrast angiography as the gold standard

Reference	Stenosis	Magnetic resonance angiography			Duplex	
		sensitivity	specificity	2D/3D	Sensitivity	Specificity
Young et al.[1]	30–99%	89%	82%	2D+3D	93%	82%
Young et al.[1]	70–99%	86%	93%	2D+3D	89%	93%
Patel et al.[2]	70–99%	84%	75%	2D	94%	83%
Patel et al.[2]	70–99%	94%	85%	3D	94%	83%
Turnipseed et al.[12]	70–99%	100%	93%	2D	93%	93%
Mittl et al.[13]	70–99%	92%	75%	2D	81%	82%
Jackson et al.[14]	60–100%	86%	70%	2D+3D	89%	93%
Young et al.[1]	70–100%	90%	95%	2D+3D	93%	92%
Patel et al.[2]	Occlusion	100%	100%	2D+3D	88%	94%
Currie et al.[15]	Occlusion	100%	100%	3D	95%	100%
Young et al.[1]	Occlusion	80%	99%	2D+3D	93%	99%

versus DSA where the same patient population was used. Even allowing for the fact that the surgical plaque is the true gold standard and that DSA is subject to variability of its own, MRA and duplex compare very well with DSA. One of the problems with performing comparative analyses is that one has to select a gold standard. In this situation, it is invariably angiography, and thus duplex and MRA can only ever come second best – it will never be possible for duplex or MRA to be equivalent to IADSA as the maximum level of agreement cannot exceed the intraobserver variability for IADSA.

Overall, MRA and duplex findings correlate in about 90% of patients. Each technique, however, has advantages that can be employed selectively or in combination to ensure accurate management planning for individual patients. For example, MRA is unable reliably to interpret plaque morphology (for which duplex is the current imaging gold standard) but, as very few surgeons currently base their decision to operate upon the presence or absence of ulceration, this is therefore largely irrelevant. 2D MRA is the method of choice for differentiating between an occlusion and subocclusion and MRA has a sensitivity and specificity approaching 100% in this situation (Table 9.3). Accurate diagnosis of occlusion remains a problem for duplex ultrasound (especially with less experienced operators) and, in this situation, MRA is a useful corroborative investigation and may replace DSA in this role.

ASSESSMENT OF INTRACRANIAL DISEASE USING MRA

One of the quoted benefits of MRA is that it can image disease outwith the scanning range of duplex ultrasound. Although in theory this is true, there is relatively little in the way of validation and evidence suggests that MRA imaging of the syphon and intracranial circulation is not without problems.

Anzola et al. found that MRA tended to overestimate the degree of stenosis within the middle cerebral artery (MCA) mainstem and two-thirds of MCA stenoses were misdiagnosed as occlusions.[10] Similarly, Patel et al. concluded that MRA may be a relatively unreliable method for identifying intracranial stenoses, as many lesions identified on MRA were not evident during contrast angiography.[2] Imaging the carotid syphon can also be difficult because of its tortuosity and because of artefacts caused by air in the adjacent sinuses.[3] A particular problem with distal ICA lesions is the loss of signal associated with severe inflow ICA stenoses.[2]

Cine-phase contrast MRA has demonstrated that MRA is able to identify patterns of collateral recruitment within the brain,[11] but MRA is generally poorer than transcranial Doppler (TCD) at identifying reversed flow in the ipsilateral ophthalmic artery.[10] Comparative studies with TCD and angiography suggest that TCD is more sensitive at demonstrating the anatomical patterns of collateral recruitment, i.e. flow reversal in the ophthalmic artery, flow reversal in the anterior cerebral artery and recruitment of flow from the posterior cerebral arteries, but that MRA is perhaps better at identifying which collateral source has the greatest functional importance.[10] Thus, the

precise role for MRA in evaluating intracranial disease and patterns of collateral flow remains to be established.

HOW MIGHT MRA BE USED IN CLINICAL PRACTICE?

There is now increasing evidence that MRA and/or duplex can safely and reliably replace routine DSA in the selection of patients for carotid surgery. It is imperative, however, that any unit planning to establish a non-invasive procedure should validate their results in a reasonably sized study against DSA (at least 50 patients/100 arteries) before starting to issue independent reports. If severe stenoses are missed it may be some time before this comes to light as the natural history for carotid stenosis is otherwise relatively good.

MRA complements Doppler/duplex ultrasound and gives the surgeons hard angiographic films to examine when operating. Combining both Doppler/duplex and MRA helps to ensure a measure of quality control for both ultrasound and MRA and keeps the risks of investigation to a minimum. In those centres with limited access to duplex or less experienced technicians, MRA may be the logical alternative to routine DSA. For units that continue to perform conventional DSA, it is clearly important that the local risk of angiography is quoted before the test proceeds. My own personal viewpoint is that patients do not need to be exposed to angiographic risk provided there is agreement between Doppler/duplex ultrasound and MRA.

Our usual policy is therefore to perform Doppler/duplex ultrasound as the initial assessment in any patient who describes carotid territory symptoms. If > 50% stenosis is diagnosed by ultrasound and the patient is prepared to consider carotid endarterectomy (CEA), we would then proceed to MRA. A final decision is made regarding the appropriateness of surgery once the MRA data are available.

In practice, this means that all patients with a 70–99% stenosis on both ultrasound and MRA are then referred for CEA. In fewer than 5% of cases we would now perform conventional angiography and this is currently reserved for those patients in whom MRA and duplex disagree significantly.

ACKNOWLEDGEMENTS

It is a pleasure to acknowledge my colleague, Dr Gavin Young, who was instrumental in much of the work in comparing DSA, MRA and ultrasound and in the interobserver and intraobserver studies.

REFERENCES

1 Young GR, Humphrey PRD, Nixon TE, Smith ETSS. Variability in measurement of extracranial internal carotid artery stenosis as displayed by both digital subtraction and magnetic resonance angiography: an assessment of three caliper techniques and visual impression of stenosis. *Stroke* 1996; **27**: 467–473.

2 Patel MR, Kuntz KM, Klufas RA *et al.* Pre-operative assessment of the carotid bifurcation: can magnetic resonance angiography and Duplex ultrasonography replace contrast angiography? *Stroke* 1995; **26**: 1753–1758.

3 Saouaf R, Grassi CJ, Hartnell GG, Wheeler H, Suojanen JN. Complete MR angiography and Doppler ultrasound as the sole imaging modalities prior to carotid endarterectomy. *Clinical Radiology* 1998; **53**: 579–586.

4 Young GR, Humphrey PRD, Shaw MDM, Nixon TE, Smith ETSS. Comparison of magnetic resonance angiography, duplex ultrasound and digital subtraction angiography in assessment of extracranial internal carotid artery stenosis. *Journal of Neurology, Neurosurgery and Psychiatry* 1994; **57**: 1466–1478.

5 Spartera C, Morettini G, Marino G *et al.* Detection of internal carotid artery stenosis: comparison of 2D-MR angiography, duplex scanning and arteriography. *Journal of Cardiovascular Surgery (Torino)* 1993; **34**: 209–213.

6 Rothwell PM, Gibson RJ, Slattery J, Sellar RJ, Warlow CP for the European Carotid Surgery Trialists' Collaborative Group. Equivalence of measurements of carotid stenosis. A comparison of three methods on 1001 angiograms. *Stroke* 1991; **25**: 2435–2439.

7 Rothwell PM, Gibson RJ, Slattery J, Warlow CP for the European Carotid Surgery Trialists' Collaborative Group. Prognostic value and reproducibility of measurements of carotid stenosis. A comparison of three methods on 1001 angiograms. *Stroke* 1994; **25**: 2440–2444.

8 Eliasziw M, Smith RF, Holdsworth DW, Fox AJ, Barnett HJM for NASCET Group. Further comments on the measurement of carotid stenosis from angiograms. *Stroke* 1994; **25**: 2445–2449.

9 Young GR, Sandcock PAG, Slattery J, Humphrey PRD, Smith ETSS, Brock L. Observer variation in the interpretation of intra-arterial angiograms and the risk of inappropriate decisions about carotid endarterectomy. *Journal of Neurology, Neurosurgery and Psychiatry* 1996; **60**: 152–157.

10 Anzola GP, Gasparotti R, Magoni M, Prandini F. Transcranial Doppler sonography and magnetic resonance angiography in the assessment of collateral hemispheric flow in patients with carotid artery disease. *Stroke* 1995; **26**: 214–217.

11 Miralles M, Dolz JL, Cotillas J *et al.* The role of the circle of Willis in carotid occlusion: assessment with phase contrast MR angiography and transcranial duplex. *European Journal of Vascular and Endovascular Surgery* 1995; **10**: 424–430.

12 Turnipseed WD, Kennell TW, Turski PA, Acher CW, Hoch JR. Magnetic resonance angiography and duplex scanning: non-invasive tests for selecting symptomatic carotid endarterectomy candidates. *Surgery* 1993; **114**: 643–648.

13 Mittl RL, Broderick M, Carpenter JP *et al.* Blinded-reader comparison of magnetic resonance angiography and duplex ultrasonography for carotid bifurcation stenosis. *Stroke* 1994; **25**: 4–10.

14 Jackson MR, Chang AS, Robles HA *et al.* Determination of 60% or greater carotid stenosis: a prospective comparison of magnetic resonance angiography and duplex ultrasound with conventional angiography. *Annals of Vascular Surgery* 1998; **12**: 236–243.

15 Currie IC, Murphy KP, Jones AJ *et al.* Magnetic resonance angiography or IADSA for diagnosis of carotid pseudo-occlusion. *European Journal of Vascular Surgery* 1994; **8**: 562–566.

16 Donnan GA, Davis SM, Chambers BR, Gates PC. Surgery for prevention of stroke. *Lancet* 1998; **351**: 1372–1373.

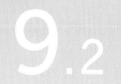

9.2

Is there a role for preoperative magnetic resonance angiography?

Sheela T Patel (USA)

K Craig Kent (USA)

INTRODUCTION

Contrast arteriography (CA) is the traditional method for evaluating the carotid bifurcation prior to CEA. However, the incidence of stroke associated with CA is not insignificant and this morbidity must be included when calculating the overall risk of intervention for carotid artery disease. In the Asymptomatic Carotid Atherosclerosis Study (ACAS), the combined perioperative stroke and death rate associated with CEA was 2.7%. However, almost 50% of this neurologic morbidity was related to CA (1.2%).[17] CA is also associated with insertion site complications, renal dysfunction, and contrast reactions, as well as ionizing radiation. Furthermore, the cost of CA is significant. The cost (not charge or reimbursement) of CA can range from $1500 to $2500 and is much greater than that of other less invasive modalities such as duplex ultrasound or MRA. Because of its invasive nature and the associated inconvenience and discomfort, patient acceptance of CA is poor.

All of these issues have led to an increasing interest in the use of non-invasive modalities for the preoperative imaging of carotid artery disease. MRA and duplex ultrasonography (DU) are the two non-invasive methods that have received the greatest attention, although spiral CT angiography is currently being evaluated in a number of institutions. Each of these techniques has inherent advantages and disadvantages. Although all three modalities have been used for preoperative imaging, this chapter will focus on the technique of MRA.

MRA is a variant of magnetic resonance imaging that has been used increasingly in the evaluation of patients with cerebrovascular occlusive disease. The carotid bifurcation, because of its straight-line configuration and the rapid velocity of blood flow, is especially well suited for evaluation by MRA. MRA is virtually free of immediate complications provided that patients are accurately screened for metallic implants. The cost of MRA is a fraction of that of CA. An appealing advantage of MRA over DU is that it anatomically displays the intracranial and extracranial circulation in a format strikingly similar to that of a conventional arteriogram, even though fundamentally different properties of blood vessels are depicted (Fig. 9.4). Moreover, MRA can be performed in conjunction with magnetic resonance imaging of the brain with only a small increase in examination time and therefore cost.

In this section the theory behind MRA will be outlined as well as the clinical role of this test in the preoperative evaluation of patients with carotid artery stenosis. A preoperative imaging algorithm which includes a combination of DU and MRA will be proposed.

BASIC PRINCIPLES AND THEORY

A basic understanding of the physics of magnetic resonance imaging is important for a full appreciation of its role in clinical imaging. The hydrogen ion (proton) when placed in a magnetic field and pulsed with radiofrequency waves becomes excited and absorbs energy. When these particles 'relax', they re-emit this energy, which can then be detected as a signal. To create arteriograms the magnetic resonance magnet creates a condition in which protons in flowing blood produce stronger signals than the protons in stationary tissue. The resultant variation in signal production allows flowing blood to be differentiated from adjacent tissue. Thus, while CA depends on the opacification

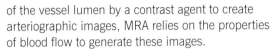

9.2 Is there a role for preoperative magnetic resonance angiography?

of the vessel lumen by a contrast agent to create arteriographic images, MRA relies on the properties of blood flow to generate these images.

The MRA technique most often used for evaluation of the carotid bifurcation is referred to as time-of-flight (TOF). The TOF sequence can be acquired in either a 2D or 3D mode. With the 2D TOF sequence, excitation occurs sequentially in slices perpendicular to the blood vessel. This process continues until a stack of slices encompassing the full length of the blood vessel to be imaged is accumulated. In the 3D TOF sequence, the entire vessel is excited at once and then subdivided into small sequential partitions for later reconstruction. These slices or partitions constitute the source data. A reconstructed image resembling that of a conventional angiogram can be produced by compiling the source data. A special post-processing computer algorithm (called the maximum-intensity projection or MIP) is employed to create this image.

2D and 3D TOF sequences have different properties and strengths, which act in complementary ways to enhance the reliability of information obtained from MRA (Table 9.4). In the 2D TOF technique, there is minimal signal loss since each slice is excited individually. This technique is particularly valuable in conditions in which there is slow blood flow, such as might occur with a preocclusive lesion. As such, 2D TOF allows MRA reliably to differentiate between a high-grade stenosis and a carotid artery occlusion. There is less likelihood of image degradation secondary to motion artefacts with 2D TOF since patients can move slightly between successive slice excitations without significant consequence.

The length of artery that can be imaged with 2D is also greater than with 3D TOF, allowing better visualization of the proximal common and distal internal carotid arteries. In 3D TOF, the patient must remain immobile throughout the entire imaging sequence since there is only one period of excitation. The partitions of 3D TOF are thinner than the slices of 2D TOF. This provides higher spatial resolution, allowing a more accurate estimation of the degree of stenosis compared to 2D TOF, albeit the imaging time requirements being greater. Because the imaging volume is excited simultaneously and not in the form

Table 9.4

Comparison of two-dimensional (2D) and three-dimensional (3D) train-of-flight magnetic resonance angiography

	2D	3D
Estimate degree of stenosis	Poor	Excellent
Differentiate occlusion from stenosis	Excellent	Good
Image tortuous, kinked, coiled vessels	Poor	Excellent
Imaging time	Shorter	Longer
Susceptibility to motion artifact	Less	More

of perpendicular slices, a vessel may be oriented in any direction in 3D TOF. Thus, 3D TOF is better for imaging tortuous vessels and areas of turbulent flow. Because of their individual inherent and complementary advantages, both techniques should be routinely performed when MRA is used to evaluate the carotid bifurcation.

MRA IN THE EVALUATION OF CAROTID ARTERY DISEASE

Understanding the precise degree of stenosis is critically important in selecting candidates for carotid endarterectomy. Table 9.5 summarizes modern series examining the sensitivity and specificity of MRA for detection of stenosis and occlusion and including more than 100 carotid bifurcation examinations. MRA is extremely sensitive in the detection of carotid stenosis, to the extent that a normal or near-normal MRA can effectively exclude the presence of a hemodynamically significant lesion. The specificity of MRA for the detection of carotid artery stenosis has been less consistent. This is related to the potential for MRA to overgrade the degree of stenosis. The explanation for this tendency is as follows. Turbulence is found distal to a high-grade stenosis. Because turbulent blood swirls and the flow is no longer perpendicular to the imaging plane, no signal is generated. An area of turbulence

Table 9.5
Sensitivity and specificity of magnetic resonance angiography for stenosis and occlusion in selected series

	Technique	Stenosis		Occlusion	
		Sensitivity (%)	Specificity (%)	Sensitivity (%)	Specificity (%)
Patel et al.[18]	3D	94	85	100	100
Anderson et al.[19]	2D and 3D	96	78	93	–
White et al.[20]	2D	85	86	80	100
Young et al.[21]	2D and 3D	86	93	80	99
Chiesa et al.[22]	3D	84	87	86	97
Laster et al.[23]	2D	93	97	100	99
Spartera et al.[24]	2D	89	84	82	99

appears dark on the processed image, implying the presence of a larger plaque or stenosis than actually exists. With a high-grade stenosis there may be complete loss of signal. This latter finding is called a signal void.

Signal voids are particularly common when 2D TOF techniques are employed. Riles et al.[25] observed for 2D TOF MRA a sensitivity of 100% and a specificity of 60% for detecting stenoses of 50–99%. Litt et al.[26] similarly used 2D TOF and observed a 96% specificity and 53% specificity. Overestimation with 2D TOF MRA more frequently occurs when a moderate carotid artery stenosis is present. Heiserman et al.[27] found that 2D TOF MRA overestimated the grade of stenosis in only 12% of arteries overall. However, stenosis was overestimated in 48% of the carotid arteries with moderate (50–75%) stenosis, as shown by CA. This tendency is particularly undesirable since the differentiation between a moderate and high-grade stenosis is often a critical part of the decision of whether or not to proceed with CEA. When optimum MRA techniques are used (3D TOF or multiple overlapping then slab acquisition (MOTSA)), we and others have found that a signal void, with rare exceptions, correlates with a 70–99% stenosis. When 2D TOF techniques are used, a signal void may result from a lesser degree of stenosis or just a tortuous artery.

In MRA studies where low specificities are reported, the technique that has been invariably used is 2D TOF. Over the past several years, it has become increasingly clear that 3D TOF is significantly more accurate than 2D MRA techniques for determining the degree of stenosis. The use of 3D TOF with its greater spatial resolution helps to eliminate the problem of signal void. In our own study, we found a sensitivity and specificity of 92% and 83% for 3D TOF versus 83% and 75% when images were created using 2D techniques.[18] Similar findings have been reported by others.[28,29] The data are so convincing that 3D TOF has become the gold standard for MRA in determining the degree of carotid stenosis.

Reviewing source or axial images is another way of increasing the accuracy of MRA. When axial images are post-processed to create a reconstructed image of the entire carotid artery, inevitably some of the data is lost. Thus, vascular stenoses can be exaggerated in reconstructed images. The evaluation of individual source images, particularly at the level of the greatest stenosis, can avoid such errors or overgrading. Anderson et al.,[29] in a study of 3D TOF MRA, observed that use of source rather than reconstructed images significantly increased specificity by reducing this tendency for overestimation.

MOTSA is a newly introduced MRA technique for the evaluation of carotid artery stenosis. This technique theoretically combines the best features of 2D and 3D TOF sequences, resulting in high resolution as well as sensitivity to slow flow. Blatter et al.[30] found that stenoses were less likely to be overestimated with MOTSA than with 2D TOF.

However, a comparison of MOTSA and 3D TOF has not been made. Moreover, several post-processing problems with the MOTSA sequence have been identified and the technique in general requires further investigation.

It is important to note that the accuracy of non-invasive techniques, including MRA, is most often judged by comparing these techniques to CA. However, CA may occasionally under- or overestimate the degree of stenosis. In our own studies with MRA, we have identified a number of instances where MRA was more accurate than CA in depicting the degree of stenosis.[18] This is often related to the fact that CA provides only a 2D image. Despite the routine use of both anteroposterior and lateral views, there are circumstances where a web or a small focal stenosis can be missed or underestimated by CA. Intuitively, a more accurate determination of stenosis might be expected from MRA, related to its ability to image the carotid artery in a 3D format. Pan et al.[31] prospectively studied lesion size with DU, MRA, and CA in 28 patients who underwent 31 carotid endarterectomies, and compared the percent of carotid stenosis as determined by these imaging techniques to the histologic findings of the resected carotid atheroma. These authors found that MRA more accurately depicted the histologic stenosis than did CA. Studies such as this are difficult to interpret because of the inability accurately to measure the degree of stenosis in excised plaque. However, there are clearly circumstances where MRA, because of its capability of imaging a vessel in three dimensions, may more accurately depict a stenotic lesion than a conventional arteriogram.

The ability of a non-invasive test to differentiate between a high-grade carotid stenosis and an occlusion is critically important to the surgeon performing CEA. An attempted endarterectomy on a patient with a carotid occlusion results in wasted resources and unwanted morbidity. Of equal concern is the danger of not treating a threatening high-grade carotid stenosis that is misinterpreted by a non-invasive study as an occlusion. One of the important advantages of 2D TOF MRA is its ability to differentiate a carotid artery occlusion from a high-grade > 90% stenosis (Fig. 9.5). Our own data demonstrate that the accuracy of MRA in differentiating a carotid stenosis from an occlusion is 100%.[18] The sensitivity and specificity of MRA in diagnosing occlusion are shown in Table 9.5. The inexperienced MRA interpreter may mistake a collateral or a branch of the external carotid artery (e.g., the ascending pharyngeal artery) as the internal carotid artery. This error can be avoided by evaluating both 2D and 3D images since the latter provides a more accurate representation of the external carotid artery. Source images from both studies are also helpful in making this differentiation.

The characteristics of carotid plaque are potentially important in identifying patients at high risk for stroke (Fig. 9.6). The relationship between the surface features of plaque (smooth, rough, ulcerated) as well as its internal composition (intraplaque hemorrhage, lipids, cholesterol, calcium, etc.) and the potential for subsequent stroke have been studied extensively. Using data from NASCET, Eliasziw et al.[32] found a strong correlation between ulceration and stroke. Unoperated patients having a greater than 70% carotid stenosis and plaque ulceration as demonstrated on preoperative arteriogram had up to a three-fold increased risk of stroke over 2 years compared to patients without ulceration. Park et al.[33] prospectively recorded the plaque characteristics of 1008 endarterectomy specimens over a 14-year period and demonstrated that the presence of intraplaque hemorrhage was associated with more advanced stenosis. Unfortunately, with current techniques, MRA is inaccurate in the detection of ulceration. This inaccuracy is related to diminished and turbulent flow of blood within the crater of the ulcer leading to signal loss. Thus, flowing blood within the ulcer is not imaged and thus the ulcer is obscured. In our studies we found MRA to be an extremely poor predictor of ulceration.[18] 3D TOF MRA yielded a sensitivity of 22% compared to CA for the detection of ulceration. Others have reported similar findings.[34,35] Even CA is inconsistent in its ability to identify plaque ulceration. Chiesa et al.[22] used surgical specimens to compare the efficacy of both CA and MRA in detecting plaque ulceration. Large ulcerations in the

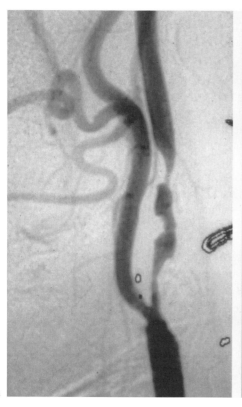

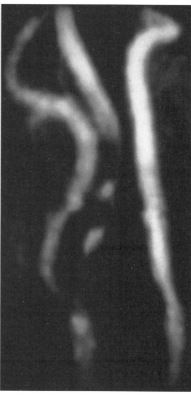

A   B

Fig. 9.5
(A) Contrast arteriogram demonstrating a long-segment irregular high-grade stenosis of the internal carotid artery. (B) The accuracy of magnetic resonance angiography in differentiating high-grade stenosis from occlusion is excellent.

surgical specimen were detected by CA and MRA in only 67% and 33% of cases, respectively.

Experimental MRA techniques may prove useful for delineating plaque composition. Using high-resolution imaging of endarterectomy specimens, different constituents of plaque, including calcium, hemorrhage, fat, and fibrosis, can be identified. Extremely small slices and a very fine matrix are needed for these studies. Unfortunately, these techniques are not yet available for clinical use.

Intracranial disease has been reported in 20–50% of patients undergoing CA. Pathologic entities include intracranial aneurysms and tandem atherosclerotic stenoses. Intracranial aneurysms were identified in 39 of 1500 CAs obtained as part of NASCET, yet only 6 (0.4%) were deemed clinically important. In general, asymptomatic intracranial aneurysms do not pose an increased risk of rupture when a patient undergoes CEA.[36] Hemodynamically significant stenosis of the intracranial internal carotid artery is also unusual,

occurring in less than 5% of patients with extracranial carotid stenosis.[37]

Several studies suggest that the presence of intracranial disease does not impact on perioperative mortality and morbidity or the long-term stroke rate after CEA. Roederer et al.[38] observed carotid siphon abnormalities in 84% of 282 carotid arteries. Neither the existence nor the severity of these siphon lesions was associated with an increased risk of a subsequent neurological event. Mackey et al.[39] compared the short- and long-term outcome after CEA of 134 patients with significant intracranial disease to that of 463 patients with no intracranial disease. They found that the perioperative stroke and mortality rate as well as the late incidence of stroke was nearly identical in these two groups. Although the data are convincing that mild to moderate intracranial lesions do not predispose to stroke following CEA, detection of a severe tandem siphon stenosis might lead to abandonment of plans for endarterectomy, particularly in patients with

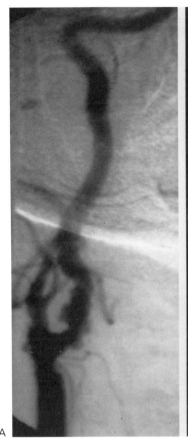
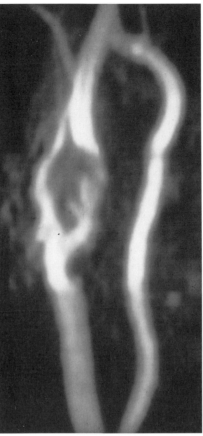

Fig. 9.6
(A) Contrast arteriogram revealing type C ulceration at the origin of the internal carotid artery. Because of three-dimensional imaging, magnetic resonance angiography (MRA) in this circumstance provides a more accurate depiction of this ulcer. However, in general, MRA is less accurate than contrast arteriography in defining ulceration.

A   B

asymptomatic carotid disease. MRA can accurately identify these intracranial lesions. Because of their small size and tortuosity, delineation of intracranial vasculature requires high-resolution imaging with 3D TOF. We found that 3D TOF MRA had a sensitivity of 82% and specificity of 95% for the presence of a 50–99% stenosis of the intracranial internal carotid artery.[18] MRA is also useful in detecting intracranial aneurysms.[40] The ability of MRA to detect intracranial disease is an important advantage over duplex ultrasound in some clinical settings.

As with intracranial disease, the clinical importance of detecting intrathoracic disease is unclear. Intrathoracic disease is less common than intracranial disease. Akers *et al.*[41] observed intrathoracic abnormalities in only 1.8% of 1000 cerebral angiograms. Two-thirds of these abnormalities were suspected prior to angiography

because of the finding of unequal brachial artery blood pressures on clinical examination. Despite the rarity of proximal disease, many surgeons continue to require preoperative contrast arch aortograms. MRA has the ability to image the arch and the proximal great vessels, although a separate examination focusing on the chest rather than the neck is required. Respiratory motion, cardiac pulsations, and turbulent flow, coupled with the large field of view needed to accommodate the relevant anatomy make intrathoracic imaging particularly troublesome. The coils used to image the carotid bifurcation and the intracranial vessels do not cover the aortic arch. Only a body coil, which has less signal sensitivity, is able to image the entire aortic arch and the origins of the great vessels. Despite these inherent complexities, several authors have observed good correlation between MRA and

CA in detecting disease in the aorta and great vessels.[42,43] The preferred method for imaging the arch is 3D TOF with injection of the intravascular contrast, gadolinium. Gadolinium has no nephrotoxicity and a low incidence of allergic reaction.[42,43]

There are situations where MRA cannot be used. Patients requiring invasive monitoring or mechanical respiration as well as patients with metallic surgical clips or cardiac pacemakers are unable to be studied with MRA because of interactions between metallic objects and the magnetic field. Because patients must remain immobile for a prolonged period of time in a cylindrical chamber, claustrophobia is another contraindication to MRA, although careful use of sedation can often overcome this problem. Patients must also be able to follow instructions (i.e, hold their breath, not swallow) in order to produce an image that is free of motion artifacts. Since MRA is based on blood flow, poor-quality images may be generated in patients with marginal cardiac output.

SUGGESTED CAROTID IMAGING ALGORITHM

At many centers, surgeons are proceeding with carotid endarterectomy on the basis of DU alone. This practice is analyzed in detail in Chapter 8. However, a discussion of the relative efficacy of DU versus MRA in the preoperative evaluation of carotid stenosis is warranted. The accuracy of DU relies heavily on the experience, skill, and dedication of the technologist and interpreter of this study. Although interpretation of MRA also requires training and expertise, the performance of MRA is simple once correct protocols are established. Moreover, if an inadequate MRA is obtained, the poor quality of the images is readily apparent to both radiologists and surgeons alike. This same ability to monitor the quality of studies is not available to the surgeon who does not perform DU.

DU is also unable to define accurately the anatomy of the intracranial and intrathoracic circulation. The presence of disease in both circulations can be inferred from DU; however, the overall sensitivity for detecting disease in these locations is poor. Differentiation between a high-grade stenosis and arterial occlusion with DU may be problematic. The false diagnosis of an occlusion can be made if the internal carotid artery courses medially or an occlusion can be missed if a branch of the external carotid artery is mistaken for the internal carotid artery. Artifacts originating from calcified plaque, or acoustic shadows, can compromise the quality of DU. DU is difficult in patients with short, broad necks or tortuous arteries. Because DU is based on flow velocities for the determination of lesion severity, hyperdynamic states caused by sepsis, inotropic agents, anemia, or contralateral carotid occlusion can lead to an overestimation of the degree of stenosis. The use of DU for the detection of carotid stenosis in the subset of patients who have contralateral carotid occlusion is particularly problematic. Falsely elevated velocities in the patent carotid artery can lead to inappropriate carotid endarterectomy in this high-risk patient subset. Surgeons' hesitation to proceed with endarterectomy on the basis of duplex alone may result in overutilization of CA. A recent survey indicated that, although 73% of respondents agreed that CEA based on DU alone was acceptable if appropriate indications were present, 79% still routinely performed CA.[44]

DU and MRA can be complementary techniques for evaluating carotid artery disease; the benefit of combining the results of these two techniques has become increasingly apparent. MRA can provide both proximal and distal anatomic information that is unavailable through DU. Moreover, MRA has a greater ability to differentiate high-grade stenosis and occlusion. Although calcification and adipose tissue can compromise the quality of DU imaging, these do not interfere with MRA. Conversely, DU can provide information on plaque composition or ulceration that is not available through MRA. Our studies have shown that, in terms of accuracy, DU and MRA are complementary. In our study, the accuracy of DU and MRA (86% and 88%, respectively) increased to 94% when the results of these two tests were combined.[18] Fortunately, the deficiencies of MRA are often different from those of DU.

It is also important to consider cost when choosing non-invasive strategies. Using decision-analytic techniques, we found that the combination of DU and MRA was a more cost-effective method of

preoperative evaluation for CEA when compared to DU, MRA, or CA alone.[45] The advantage of the combination of MRA and DU over DU alone was related to the increase in accuracy that this combination affords.

Preoperative CA contributes significantly to the total cost and risk of CEA. Utilizing MRA and DU without CA will reduce the cost and risk of surgery without compromising patient selection. This is particularly important in the subset of patients with asymptomatic carotid stenosis in whom the cost-effectiveness and risk–benefit ratio of CEA are open to question. With the advent of carotid stenting, reducing the cost and improving the safety of CEA becomes an even more important consideration. Although its current accuracy is sufficient to allow its widespread use for carotid imaging, technical improvements and increasing experience with MRA will certainly further enhance the quality of the images in years to come.

REFERENCES

17 Executive Committee for the Asymptomatic Carotid Atherosclerosis Study. Endarterectomy for asymptomatic carotid artery stenosis. *Journal of the American Medical Association* 1995; **273**: 1421–1428.

18 Patel MR, Kuntz KM, Klufas RA *et al*. Preoperative assessment of the carotid bifurcation: can magnetic resonance angiography and duplex ultrasonography replace contrast arteriography? *Stroke* 1995; **26**: 1753–1758.

19 Anderson CM, Lee RE, Levin DL *et al*. Measurement of internal carotid artery stenosis from source MR angiograms. *Radiology* 1994; **193**: 219–226.

20 White JE, Russell WL, Greer MS *et al*. Efficacy of screening MR angiography and Doppler ultrasonography in the evaluation of carotid artery stenosis. *American Surgery* 1994; **60**: 340–348.

21 Young GR, Humphrey PRD, Shaw MDM *et al*. Comparison of magnetic resonance angiography, duplex ultrasound, and digital subtraction angiography in assessment of extracranial internal carotid artery stenosis. *Journal of Neurology, Neurosurgery and Psychiatry* 1994; **57**: 1466–1478.

22 Chiesa R, Melissano G, Castellano R *et al*. Three dimensional time-of-flight magnetic resonance angiography in carotid artery surgery: a comparison with digital subtraction angiography. *European Journal of Vascular Surgery* 1993; **7**: 171–176.

23 Laster RE, Acker JD, Halford HH *et al*. Assessment of MR angiography versus arteriography for evaluation of cervical carotid bifurcation disease. *American Journal of Neuroradiology* 1993; **14**: 681–688.

24 Spartera C, Morettini G, Marino G *et al*. Detection of internal carotid artery stenosis: comparison of 2D-MR angiography, duplex scanning, and arteriography. *Journal of Cardiovascular Surgery* 1993; **34**: 209–213.

25 Riles TS, Eidelman EM, Litt AW *et al*. Comparison of magnetic resonance angiography, conventional angiography, and duplex scanning. *Stroke* 1992; **23**: 341–346.

26 Litt AW, Eidelman EM, Pinto RS *et al*. Diagnosis of carotid artery stenosis: comparison of 2DFT time-of-flight MR angiography with contrast angiography in 50 patients. *American Journal of Neuroradiology* 1991; **12**: 149–154.

27 Heiserman JE, Drayer BP, Fram EK *et al*. Carotid artery stenosis: clinical efficacy of two-dimensional time-of-flight MR angiography. *Radiology* 1992; **182**: 761–768.

28 Huston J, Nichols DA, Luetmer PH *et al*. MR angiographic and sonographic indications for endarterectomy. *American Journal of Neuroradiology* 1998; **19**: 309–315.

29 Anderson CM, Saloner D, Lee RE *et al*. Assessment of carotid artery stenosis by MR angiography: comparison with X-ray angiography and color coded Doppler ultrasound. *American Journal of Neuroradiology* 1992; **13**: 989–1003.

30 Blatter DD, Bahr AL, Parker DL *et al*. Cervical carotid MR angiography with multiple overlapping thin-slab acquisition: comparison with conventional angiography. *American Journal of Radiology* 1993; **161**: 1269–1277.

31 Pan XM, Saloner D, Reilly LM *et al*. Assessment of carotid artery stenosis by ultrasonography, conventional angiography, and magnetic resonance angiography: correlation with ex vivo measurement of plaque stenosis. *Journal of Vascular Surgery* 1995; **21**: 82–89.

32 Eliasziw M, Streifler JY, Fox AJ *et al*. Significance of plaque ulceration in symptomatic patients with high-grade carotid stenosis. *Stroke* 1994; **25**: 304–308.

33 Park AE, McCarthy WJ, Pearce WH *et al*. Carotid plaque morphology correlates with presenting symptomatology. *Journal of Vascular Surgery* 1998; **27**: 872–879.

34 Huston J, Lewis BD, Wiebers DO *et al*. Carotid artery: prospective blinded comparison of two-dimensional time of flight MR angiography with conventional angiography and duplex ultrasound. *Radiology* 1993; **186**: 339–344.

35 Wilkerson DK, Keller I, Mezrich R *et al*. The comparative evaluation of three dimensional magnetic resonance for carotid artery disease. *Journal of Vascular Surgery* 1991; **14**: 803–811.

36 Ladowski JS, Webster MW, Yonas HO *et al*. Carotid endarterectomy in patients with asymptomatic intracranial aneurysm. *Annals of Surgery* 1984; **200**: 70–73.

37 Mattos MA, van Bemmelen PS, Hodgson KJ *et al*. The influence of carotid siphon stenosis on short- and long-term outcome after carotid endarterectomy. *Journal of Vascular Surgery* 1993; **17**: 902–911.

38 Roederer GO, Langlois YE, Chan ARW *et al*. Is siphon disease important in predicting outcome of carotid endarterectomy? *Archives of Surgery* 1983; **118**: 1177–1181.

39 Mackey WC, O'Donnell TF, Callow AD. Carotid

endartectomy in patients with intracranial vascular disease: short-term risk and long-term outcome. *Journal of Vascular Surgery* 1989; **10**: 432–438.

40 Ross JS, Masaryk TJ, Modic MT *et al*. Intracranial aneurysms: evaluation by MR angiography. *American Journal of Radiology* 1990; **155**: 159–165.

41 Akers DL, Markowitz IA, Kerstein MD. The value of aortic arch study in the evaluation of cerebrovascular insufficiency. *American Journal of Surgery* 1987; **154**: 230–232.

42 Carpenter JP, Holland GA, Golden MA *et al*. Magnetic resonance angiography of the aortic arch. *Journal of Vascular Surgery* 1997; **25**: 145–151.

43 Prince MR. Gadolinium-enhanced MR aortography. *Radiology* 1994; **191**: 155–164.

44 Dawson DL, Roseberry CA, Fujitani RM. Preoperative testing before carotid endarterectomy: a survey of vascular surgeons' attitudues. *Annals of Vascular Surgery* 1997; **11**: 264–272.

45 Kent KC, Kuntz KM, Patel MR *et al*. Perioperative imaging strategies for carotid endarterectomy: an analysis of morbidity and cost-effectiveness in symptomatic patients. *Journal of the American Medical Association* 1995; **274**: 888–893.

9.3 Editorial Comment

It seems ironic that, 5 years ago, the presence of a flow void was viewed as the major limitation of MRA because of its tendency to overestimate the severity of a carotid stenosis. The subsequent advent of 3D TOF suggests that a flow void is now highly predictive of a severe stenosis! Accordingly, MRA is increasingly being viewed as an alternative or at least an adjunct to duplex ultrasound in the selection of patients for angiography, not least because of its capability to image both the intra- and extracranial circulation. In practice, however, unless the surgeon has rapid access to both 2D and 3D images, MRA will be limited in its overall application because duplex has the unique advantage of being able to be performed in the outpatient clinic. Moreover, there is no evidence that the ability to diagnose intracranial vascular lesions by MRA alters outcome, nor that MRA is any better than duplex in predicting the likelihood of inflow disease. In addition, MRA is not able to provide any reliable data on plaque morphology, which may assume increasing clinical importance in the future. If, however, you are a firm believer in the concept that knowledge of the intracranial circulation prior to CEA is mandatory, then MRA will fulfill that role. Moreover, the ability to combine MRA with magnetic resonance imaging could be a trump card for the future if one believes that the exclusion of extremely rare occult structural lesions is critical prior to CEA.

In practice, those centers with access to experienced vascular laboratories will probably conclude that MRA provides little in the way of additional data. However, for those with no access to a vascular laboratory or inexperienced duplex technologists, MRA is the preferred option with regard to selecting patients for angiography. As with duplex, however, it is essential that MRA is compared with angiography and that regular quality control checks are made thereafter.

10.1

Which patients should undergo contrast angiography?

Torben V Schroeder (Europe)

Niels Levi (Europe)

Henrik H Sillesen (Europe)

INTRODUCTION

In the past, contrast angiography was viewed as the gold standard for selecting patients for carotid endarterectomy (CEA). Its use was justified on the basis that:

1 it was the only accurate method for grading stenosis;
2 it was essential for excluding proximal aortic arch, carotid syphon and intracranial disease;
3 it was essential for differentiating subtotal from total carotid occlusion;
4 important features might be missed that would otherwise compromise the surgeon's ability to complete the operation.

However, with the recent advances in colour duplex technology and the evolution of magnetic resonance angiography (MRA), few of these absolute indications probably now apply. In particular, the ability to quantify obstructive lesions at the carotid bifurcation is at least as good as that of angiography.[1-5]

Duplex ultrasound has become the routine screening method for the identification of carotid artery disease due to its non-invasiveness and widespread availability. In an increasing number of institutions, duplex scanning has also been adopted as the only imaging technique prior to CEA with selected cases undergoing angiography. This concept is compelling, because carotid arteriography is unpleasant, expensive, and carries a small but important risk of stroke. On the other hand, some clinicians continue to feel that knowledge about the status of the proximal inflow vessels as well as the carotid syphon and intracranial is of equal importance in order to plan appropriate treatment.

In 1994, we undertook a review of 50 consecutive CEAs where all patients had undergone preoperative duplex scans and carotid arteriograms. The results indicated that in 47 patients (94%) the angiogram would not have altered the management strategy had only the duplex findings been available.[6] However, surgery was subsequently abandoned in three cases despite having the benefit of preoperative angiography: in one case, a lesion extended to the base of the skull, while in two patients 30–50% stenoses were encountered. Ironically, the duplex studies in the latter patients had correctly predicted that the stenoses were of the order of 50–60%. Based on this pilot study experience, we decided to proceed to a policy of CEA without angiography provided that duplex indicated the presence of a severe stenosis with a clearly visible distal limit to the plaque. From a mere 56% of CEAs based on duplex alone in 1995, more than 90% are currently based solely on duplex examination.[7]

ACCURATE MEASUREMENT OF CAROTID STENOSIS

CEA is only beneficial if applied correctly, i.e. in patients with a severe internal carotid artery (ICA) stenosis with or without symptoms.[8-10] It is therefore crucial that the severity of the stenosis is categorized correctly, otherwise the results of the randomized studies are no longer applicable. Arteriography has long been considered the gold standard and the technique is well established in all vascular surgical units. However, serious drawbacks, in terms of morbidity and cost,[11] subsequently led to increasing debate as to whether less invasive imaging techniques would be safer but equally as effective.[12]

Doppler ultrasound and duplex scanning have, for many years, been accepted as being of sufficient accuracy to identify correctly patients who should undergo angiography prior to surgery, i.e. using duplex as a screening procedure.[13] After the first report in 1979 by von Reutern,[14] an increasing number of publications have indicated that carotid surgery can be performed safely on the basis of ultrasound alone.[5,7,11,15–18] Only Geuder et al.[19] recommended continued routine use of arteriography based on the observation that angiography altered the management strategy in 8% of patients in their series. However, Chervu and Moore[20] reanalysed this data and subsequently concluded that arteriography would only have changed the management in a few cases had standard indications and patient handling been applied.

In a later prospective series, Erdoes et al.[21] concluded that angiography was useful in clarifying decision-making in 30% of patients who were otherwise considered candidates for carotid surgery. However, most situations in which the management was altered were patients with moderate stenoses (50–70%) and atypical symptoms. These situations should not be encountered if only those patients as defined in the symptomatic multicentre studies are considered for surgery.[8,9]

However, the principal catalyst for change has remained the indisputable fact that angiography remains associated with a not insubstantial risk of neurological events.[10] A 1–2% risk may not seem to be too much, but when taken in the context of a 30-day operative risk of 5%, arteriography may thus increase the overall risk by 20–30%.

IS DUPLEX ULTRASOUND RELIABLE?

While the benefits of avoiding arteriography are obvious, the most important question remains as to whether duplex is accurate and reliable and whether the limited ability to identify concomitant proximal or distal lesions in the vascular tree has any impact. A large number of publications suggest that duplex scanning does provide accurate information regarding the degree of carotid stenosis.[1–3,5,22] By adding B-mode plaque assessment, duplex may

even provide more clinically useful information than angiography.[23,24]

However, duplex studies are ultimately operator-dependent. As with the institution that performs the surgical procedure, each vascular laboratory should also have a track record of duplex findings agreeing with angiographic results. It is not sufficient simply to depend on criteria described in other centres. It is therefore necessary that the criteria for determining a particular degree of stenosis be individualized for each laboratory by basing them on its own data.[25,26] These guiding principles are emphasized by the Intersocietal Commission for the Accreditation of Vascular Laboratories.[27] Individual validation also circumvents those problems relating to the fact that the standard ultrasound classification of high-grade stenosis, i.e. 50–79% and 80–99%, do not coincide with the stenosis thresholds developed in the international trials, i.e. 50–69% and 70–99%.[2,28–30]

WHEN SHOULD ANGIOGRAPHY BE CONSIDERED?

A number of specific indications have been identified in which duplex examination may be less reliable, e.g. in the presence of a contralateral severe stenosis or occlusion[31,32] and ipsilateral occlusion/pseudo-occlusion.[1,33] Arteriography is also occasionally mandated in the patient in whom the bifurcation is not easily visualized or where the distal limit of the disease cannot be seen.

Patients with a narrow distal ICA (the ubiquitous 'string sign') warrant special mention. The appearance of the string sign may reflect underfilling because of an extremely low distal perfusion pressure, but it may also be due to hypoplasia of the carotid artery, which is less amenable to a successful endarterectomy.[34] In either event, these patients should be identified and undergo arteriography before the final decision is made.

Another potential limitation is the failure of duplex to identify lesions of the arch and intracranial vessels. Significant arch lesions are probably encountered in fewer than 1% of patients.[35] Unequal arm blood pressures and abnormal flow signals (spectral broadening, damped low-velocity waveforms in the common carotid artery) may suggest this and should prompt the surgeon to proceed to arteriography. Similarly, severe distal disease may be inferred from an unexpectedly high-resistance waveform, i.e. a steep systolic acceleration and low diastolic flow velocity. This again is an indication for formal angiography.

Significant intracranial lesions are also rare and seldom alter the outcome of carotid surgery.[36,37] Published data suggest that transcranial Doppler (TCD) may reliably identify severe carotid arterial disease with a high sensitivity, but low specificity.[38] This should not be surprising because TCD evaluates the haemodynamic effect of the carotid stenosis on distal outflow while also taking into account the contribution of the intracranial collateral circulation.

Publications that have addressed the potential value of MRA suggest that its accuracy may be similar to that of duplex regarding the identification of a high-grade ICA stenosis. Perhaps more importantly, the overall accuracy may be improved if duplex and MRA are combined.[39,40] To date, however, prospective decision-making analyses have found that MRA is unlikely to influence management decisions when the duplex study is unequivocal.[21]

In conclusion, angiography is an effective means of visualizing anatomic abnormalities within the extracranial and intracranial circulation but carries a 1–2% risk of procedural stroke. CEA can be performed safely without arteriography in most patients and reliance upon duplex does not compromise patient safety or operability. Preoperative arteriography is, however, recommended in the following situations:

1   if there is uncertainty about the reliability of the vascular laboratory performing the duplex scanning;
2   if the examination is less than perfect;
3   if the distal limitation of the atherosclerotic lesion cannot be visualized.

REFERENCES

1   Ricotta JJ, Bryan FA, Bond MG et al. Multicenter validation study of real time (B-mode) ultrasound, arteriography and pathological examination. Journal of Vascular Surgery 1987; 6: 512–520.
2   Neale ML, Chambers JL, Kelly AT et al. Reappraisal of duplex criteria to assess significant carotid stenosis with special reference to reports from the North American Symptomatic Carotid Endarterectomy Trial and the European Carotid Surgery Trial. Journal of Vascular Surgery 1994; 20: 642–649.
3   Moneta GL, Edwards JE, Papanicolaou G et al. Screening for asymptomatic internal carotid artery stenosis: duplex criteria for discriminating 60% and 99% stenosis. Journal of Vascular Surgery 1995; 21: 989–994.
4   Pan XM, Saloner D, Reilly LM et al. Assessment of carotid artery stenosis by ultrasonography, conventional angiography, and magnetic resonance angiography: correlation with ex vivo measurement of plaque stenosis. Journal of Vascular Surgery 1995; 21: 82–89.
5   Colledge J, Wright R, Pugh N, Lane IF. Colour-coded duplex assessment alone before carotid endarterectomy. British Journal of Surgery 1996; 83: 1234–1237.
6   Sillesen H, Henriksen B, Schroeder TV. Er arteriografi nødvendig ved udredning og behandling af patienter med carotis stenose. [Carotid stenosis: is arteriography necessary?] Ugeskr. Læger 1996; 158: 6617–6619.
7   Schroeder TV, Grønholdt MLM, Sillesen HH. Carotid endarterectomy without angiography. Journal of Vascular Investigation 1998; 4: 5–9.
8   European Carotid Surgery Trialists' Collaborative Group. MRC European Carotid Surgery Trial: interim results for symptomatic patients with severe (70–99%) or with mild (0–29%) carotid stenosis. Lancet 1991; 337: 1235–1243.
9   North American Symptomatic Carotid Endarterectomy Trial Collaborators. Beneficial effect of carotid endarterectomy in symptomatic patients with highgrade carotid stenosis. New England Journal of Medicine 1991; 325: 445–453.
10 Executive Committee for the Asymptomatic Carotid Atherosclerosis Study. Endarterectomy for asymptomatic carotid artery stenosis. Journal of the American Medical Association 1995; 273: 1421–1428.
11 Faught E, Trader SD, Hanna GR. Cerebral complications of angiography for transient ischaemia and stroke: prediction of risk. Neurology 1979; 29: 4–15.
12 Dawson DL, Zierlev E. Strandness DE, Clowes AW, Kohler TR. The role of duplex scanning and arteriography before carotid endarterectomy: a prospective study. Journal of Vascular Surgery 1993; 18: 673–683.
13 Sumner DS, Russell JB, Miles RD. Are noninvasive tests sufficiently accurate to identify patients in need of carotid arteriography? Surgery 1982; 91: 700–706.
14 Von Reutern GM, Ortega-Schurkamp E, Spillner S. Is noninvasive Doppler sonography alone sufficient to indicate carotid surgery? In: Meyer JS, Lechner M, Reivich M (eds) Cerebral Vascular Disease II. International Congress Service, pp. 46–49. New York: Elsevier, 1979.
15 Ricotta JJ, Holen J, Schenk E et al. Is routine angiography necessary prior to carotid endarterectomy? Journal of Vascular Surgery 1984; 1: 96–102.
16 Ranabaldo C, Davies J, Chant A. Duplex scanning alone before carotid endarterectomy: a 5-year experience.

European Journal of Vascular Surgery 1991; **5**: 415–419.

17 Colgan MP, Grouden M, Moore DJ, Shanik GD. Carotid endarterectomy without preoperative angiography. In: Greenhalgh RM (ed.) *Vascular Imaging for Surgerons*, pp. 121–127. WB Saunders: London, 1995.

18 Shifrin EG, Bornstein N, Kantarovsky A *et al*. Carotid endarterectomy without angiography. *British Journal of Surgery* 1996; **83**: 1107–1109.

19 Geuder JW, Lamparello PJ, Riles TS, Giangola G, Imperato AM. Is duplex scanning sufficient evaluation before carotid endarterectomy? *Journal of Vascular Surgery* 1989; **9**: 193–201.

20 Chervu A, Moore WS. Carotid endarterectomy without arteriography. *Annals of Vascular Surgery* 1994; **8**: 296–302.

21 Erdoes LS, Marek JM, Mills JL *et al*. The relative contributions of carotid duplex scanning, magnetic resonance angiography, and cerebral arteriography to clinical decisionmaking: a prospective study in patients with carotid occlusive disease. *Journal of Vascular Surgery* 1996; **23**: 950–956.

22 Sillesen H, Just S, Hansen L, Schroeder T. Ultralyd farve-Doppler undersøgelse af arteria carotis. Prospektiv sammenligning med arteriografi. *Ugeskr Laeger* 1994; **156**: 7035–7038.

23 European carotid plaque study group. Carotid artery plaque composition – relationship to clinical presentation and ultrasound B-mode imaging. *European Journal of Vascular and Endovascular Surgery* 1995; **10**: 23–30.

24 El-Barghouty NM, Nicolaides A, Bahal V, Geroulakos G, Androulakis A. The identification of the high risk carotid plaque. *European Journal of Vascular and Endovascular Surgery* 1996; **11**: 470–478.

25 Chang Y-J, Golby AJ, Albers GW. Detection of carotid stenosis. From NASCET results to clinical practice. *Stroke* 1995; **26**: 1325–1328.

26 Howard G, Baker WH, Chambless LE *et al*. An approach for the use of Doppler ultrasound as a screening tool for hemodynamically significant stenosis (despite heterogeneity of Doppler performance). A multicenter experience. *Stroke* 1996; **27**: 1951–1957.

27 The Intersocietal Commission for the Accreditation of Vascular Laboratories. Essentials and standards for accreditation in noninvasive vascular testing. Part II. *Vascular Laboratory operations. Extracranial cerebrovascular testing*. IACVL, 1995.

28 Faught WE, Mattos MA, van Bemmelen *et al*. Color flow duplex scanning of carotid arteries: new velocity criteria based on receiver operator characteristic analysis for threshold stenoses used in the symptomatic and asymptomatic carotid trials. *Journal of Vascular Surgery* 1994; **19**: 818–828.

29 Hood DB, Mattos MA, Mansour A *et al*. Prospective evaluation of new duplex criteria to identify 70% internal carotid artery stenosis. *Journal of Vascular Surgery* 1996; **23**: 254–262.

30 Moneta GL, Edwards JM, Chitwood RW *et al*. Correlation of North American Symptomatic Carotid Endarterectomy Trial (NASCET) angiographic definition of 70–99% internal carotid artery stenosis with duplex scanning. *Journal of Vascular Surgery* 1993; **17**: 152–159.

31 Spadone DP, Barkmeier LD, Hodgson KJ *et al*. Contralateral internal carotid artery stenosis or occlusion: pit fall of correct ipsilateral classification – a study performed with color-flow imaging. *Journal of Vascular Surgery* 1990; **70**: 201–211.

32 AbuRahma AF, Richmond BK, Robinson PA, Khan S, Pollack JA, Alberts S. Effect of contralateral severe stenosis or carotid occlusion on duplex criteria of ipsilateral stenoses: comparative study of various duplex parameters. *Journal of Vascular Surgery* 1995; **22**: 751–762.

33 Berman SS, Devine JJ, Erdoes LS, Hunter GC. Distinguishing carotid artery pseudo-occlusion with color flow doppler. *Stroke* 1995; **26**: 434–438.

34 Archie JP. Carotid endarterectomy when the distal internal carotid artery is small or poorly visualized. *Journal of Vascular Surgery* 1994; **19**: 23–31.

35 Akers DI, Markowitz IA, Kerstein MD. The value of aortic arch study in the evaluation of cerebrovascular insufficiency. *American Journal of Surgery* 1987; **154**: 220–223.

36 Roederer GO, Langlois YE, Chan ARW, Chikos PM, Thiele BL, Strandness DE. Is siphon disease important in predicting outcome of carotid endarterectomy? *Archives of Surgery* 1983; **118**: 1177–1181.

37 Akers DL, Bell WH, Kerstein MD. Does intracranial duplex study contribute to evaluation of carotid artery disease? *American Journal of Surgery* 1985; **156**: 87–90.

38 Wilterdink JL, Feldmann E, Furie KL *et al*. Transcranial Doppler ultrasound reliably identifies severe internal carotid artery stenosis. *Stroke* 1997; **28**: 133–136.

39 Patel MR, Kuntz KM, Klufas RA *et al*. Preoperative assessment of the carotid bifurcation. Can magnetic resonance angiography and duplex ultrasonography replace contrast angiography? *Stroke* 1995; **26**: 1753–1758.

40 Kent KC, Kuntz KM, Patel D *et al*. Perioperative imaging strategies for carotid endarterectomy. An analysis of morbidity and cost-effectiveness in symptomatic patients. *Journal of the American Medical Association* 1995; **274**: 888–893.

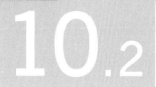

10.2 Which patients should undergo contrast angiography?
Patrick J Lamparello (USA)

INTRODUCTION

CEA has been proven effective in reducing the risk of ischemic stroke in patients with carotid artery stenosis in several studies, including the North American Symptomatic Carotid Endarterectomy Trial (NASCET) and the Asymptomatic Carotid Atherosclerosis Study (ACAS).[41,42] Currently, the focus has shifted to making the evaluation and treatment of these patients safer and more cost-effective. The approach to the investigation and management of extracranial cerebral vascular disease has changed significantly since the early 1980s, largely as a result of the dramatic advances in imaging technology. Computed tomography (CT) and magnetic resonance imaging (MRI) have virtually replaced angiography as a primary diagnostic modality. Non-invasive duplex Doppler screening evaluations of the cervical carotid circulation can now be performed effectively and inexpensively using a combination of high-resolution ultrasound imaging to delineate anatomic detail and Doppler ultrasound scanning to determine the hemodynamic significance of lesions identified by anatomic imaging. Supraorbital and TCD ultrasound examinations provide information about the state of the intracranial portions of the carotid circulation. These examinations have a steep learning curve and are more operator-dependent. Although they are still used in many non-invasive laboratories, they are not nearly as well accepted as duplex scanning. Similarly, oculoplethysmography, once a common examination, is rarely used and has been largely replaced by duplex scanning.

Historically, angiography was the method of choice for definitive evaluation of vascular lesions of both the extracranial and intracranial circulation because of the complex three-dimensional nature of the vascular system and the need for very high resolution images. Currently, both magnetic resonance angiography (MRA) and computed tomographic angiography (CTA), are supplanting conventional angiography for this definitive evaluation. CTA has the disadvantage of requiring potentially nephrotoxic contrast administration. Conventional catheter-directed angiography is no longer the gold-standard diagnostic modality. The utility of angiography now lies primarily in its use in guiding and monitoring catheter-directed treatments. These treatments include thrombolytic infusion, balloon angioplasty, stent placement, and transcatheter embolization.

Traditionally, potential candidates for CEA were evaluated initially with duplex. If significant disease was noted on duplex, the patient was subjected to contrast angiography for confirmation and for surgical planning. Although increasing numbers of surgeons are comfortable performing carotid artery surgery based solely on duplex findings, the majority still use angiography in most cases.[43] The duplex scan occasionally can be in error, does not yield readily interpretable anatomic images for surgeons, and is technician-dependent. Many surgeons will use the duplex scan as the sole imaging study only when the risks of angiography are excessive, such as in the patient with renal insufficiency or documented contrast allergy. The role of duplex ultrasonography in the evaluation of endarterectomy patients is covered in detail in Chapter 8.

Because conventional catheter cerebral angiography is invasive, with potential complications, the use of magnetic resonance imaging in replacing angiography has been

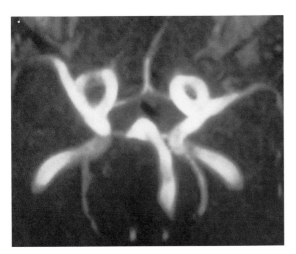

Fig. 10.1
NIRA demonstrating intracranial circulation and the circle of Willis.

Table 10.1
Comparison of recent correlative studies on duplex scanning, magnetic resonance angiography (MRA), and conventional catheter-directed angiography (CCA) of patients with suspected carotid artery stenosis

Authors	Sensitivity compared to CCA		
	Duplex	MRA	Combination
White et al.[45]	88%	84%	
Buijs et al.[46]	77%	81%	
Huston et al.[47]			85%
Polak et al.[48]			96%
Pan et al.[49]		95%	
Mattle et al.[50]	86%	100%	100%
Kido et al.[51]	86%	100%	

proposed. The advantages of MRA over conventional contrast angiography are clear. The ability to assess with increasing accuracy normal as well as diseased cervical and intracranial vessels allows us to obtain the necessary information without the risks of catheterization, contrast injection, and radiation (Fig. 10.1). To date, clinical correlation studies using MRA have established its role. MRA has come to replace conventional contrast angiography in most carotid disease patients. MRA is discussed in detail in Chapter 9.

Recently, the non-invasive combination of duplex and MRA has been compared with angiography and validated as accurate. Our group studied a total of 75 carotid arteries with MRA, conventional angiography, and duplex scanning.[44] The residual lumen at the carotid plaque was measured on conventional angiography and used as a basis for evaluating the nuclear medicine angiographic readings and duplex scan interpretations. Our findings were similar to those of others. When the duplex scan and MRA were in agreement, correlation with cerebral angiography, was 100%. Another important observation was that two patients in this study sustained strokes while undergoing conventional cerebral angiography.

Table 10.1 lists the results of recent studies and investigations found in the literature on MRA and carotid artery disease. It should be emphasized, however, that if the magnetic resonance angiographic image is of suboptimal quality or if it differs from the duplex scan, it may be necessary to obtain further diagnostic information with a cerebral angiogram.

WHEN IS CONTRAST ANGIOGRAPHY NECESSARY?

As morbidity and mortality rates for CEA continue to improve, the risks of stroke from conventional angiography receive more attention. Depending upon the patient being studied, the risks of conventional carotid angiography have been reported to be between 0.5% and 4%.[52] Therefore, the risks of angiography and its attendant catheter manipulation are not trivial. Most recently, the angiographic stroke risk in the ACAS study (1.2%) was noted to be very close to the stroke risk associated with surgery (1.5%).[42] Even if the risk of carotid angiography approached zero, the cost would still exceed that of MRA, thereby making the latter more attractive for the evaluation of surgical candidates for CEA. Currently, many institutions are using duplex scanning and MRA as the sole tests in assessing the carotid bifurcation before surgery. This is done only when the two tests are in agreement and the quality of the images are satisfactory to the vascular surgeon.

While MRA and/or duplex ultrasound have displaced conventional catheter angiography as the imaging studies of choice prior to carotid surgery, there are still situations when a cerebral angiogram is warranted:

1   Some patients may not tolerate the close surroundings of a magnetic resonance scanner. As the technology changes, this should be less of a problem. Duplex alone, CTA, or conventional angiography may be used in this situation.

2   Some patients may not lie still enough for a satisfactory magnetic resonance image to be obtained. Oftentimes, mild sedation will overcome this problem. As scanning times decrease, this should be less frequently a problem.

3   Patients who have pacemakers and implanted defibrillators cannot undergo MRA. The magnetic field strength and radio-wave energy will cause the electronic device to malfunction. Implanted electronic devices are now undergoing investigation for shielding of electromagnetic radiation. Those devices that are shielded may not be adversely affected by MR scanning in the future. At our institution, we would proceed with carotid surgery based upon an adequate duplex scan that was reviewed firsthand by the surgeon. If the surgeon is uncomfortable with surgery on the basis of duplex scanning alone, then a CT can be obtained. If this is inadequate, then the surgeon may obtain a cerebral angiogram.

4   Most of the information presented in this article has been limited to patients with atherosclerosis of the carotid bifurcation. Obviously, other disease entities may cause the need for carotid artery surgery. Among these are fibromuscular dysplasia, carotid artery dissection, and carotid artery aneurysms. Surgery for these disorders is usually complex and requires significant planning. Detailed information, such as the extent of the disease process, is required. Sometimes this information may only be obtained with a contrast angiogram. At our

institution, the patients would undergo MRA first. When other pathological entities, such as those listed above, are suspected, the surgeon would consider whether there is satisfactory information to plan further therapeutic interventions or whether a cerebral angiogram is required.

5   Contrast angiography is currently required for the conduct of interventional procedures such as angioplasty, stenting, or stent graft placement. In addition, occasionally, preoperative test occlusion of the carotid is required to determine the adequacy of collateral flow in the event that the carotid must be ligated. This information may be useful in patients who have undergone previous surgery and/or radiation to the neck for such problems as head and neck carcinoma.[53] Balloon test occlusion currently requires contrast angiography. As the technology of MRA evolves,

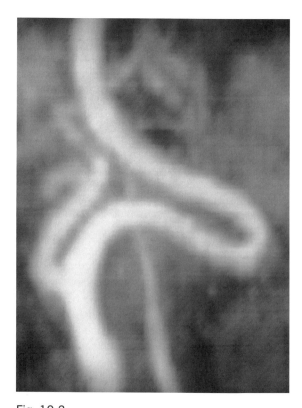

Fig. 10.2
Magnetic resonance angiogram image of extremely tortuous internal carotid artery.

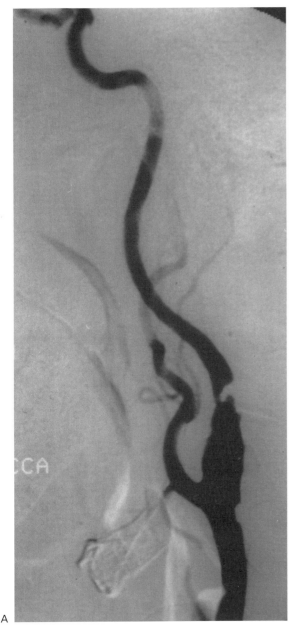
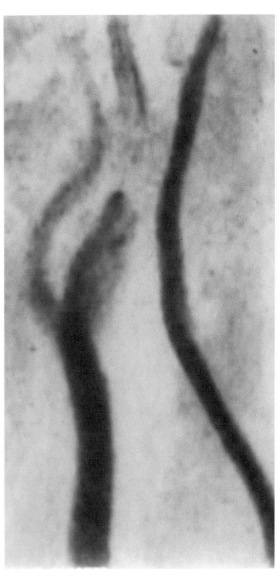

Fig. 10.3
Comparison of conventional contrast angiogram of a patient with recurrent carotid artery stenosis (A) with magnetic resonance angiogram (B).

many interventional procedures may be able to be performed using open magnetic resonance scanners rather than conventional angiography.

6   Vascular surgeons will occasionally encounter unusual carotid artery anatomy. Redundancy or excessive tortuosity may result in a suboptimal magnetic resonance image. Magnetic resonance angiography has the advantage of allowing the

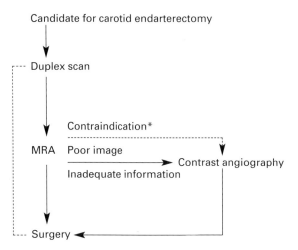

Fig. 10.4

Algorithm for evaluation of patients for carotid endarterectomy. *If patient has contraindication to MRA, such as a pacemaker.

surgeon to review the hard copy. If this image is not satisfactory, then it is important for the surgeon to evaluate the patient further. This evaluation may require conventional cerebral angiography. As the images produced by magnetic resonance scanning have improved (Fig. 10.2), excessive tortuosity or redundancy of a carotid artery may be adequately evaluated by MRA.

7   With the increasing frequency of the performance of carotid artery endarterectomies, and a recurrence rate of approximately 1%, many vascular surgeons are finding it necessary to perform re-do carotid surgery.[54] Previously, it was necessary to perform a cerebral angiogram on

these patients. The information gained from angiography, including the nuances of anatomy, that formerly was not apparent on MRA, may be helpful to the surgeon at the time of the re-do surgery. As magnetic resonance images have improved, the information that was thought only able to be obtained on cerebral angiography may be available on MRA (Fig. 10.3). This is another situation where the surgeon has to evaluate the magnetic resonance angiogram, and if the information seen on the image is adequate for the planned re-do carotid surgery, no further evaluation will be required. If it is not adequate, then cerebral angiography is indicated.

CONCLUSIONS

- Almost all patients undergo carotid surgery based on a duplex scan and/or MRA.
- Contrast angiography is indicated for patients who are unable to undergo or who have inadequate information obtained from MRA and duplex.
- As technology advances, cerebral angiograms will rarely be performed for diagnosis but will continue to have a role in association with interventional procedures.

Given the rapid development of MRA technology over the past few years, it is certain that many more advance in technology will occur in the future. Experience with magnetic resonance and duplex imaging will improve. The algorithm shown in Fig. 10.4 summarizes the points in this chapter. Although it is applicable to today's practice, it is certain to change in the future.

REFERENCES

41 North American Symptomatic Carotid Endarterectomy Trial Collaborators. Beneficial effect of carotid endarterectomy in symptomatic patients with high grade carotid stenosis. *New England Journal of Medicine* 1991; **325**: 445–453.

42 Executive Committee for the Asymptomatic Carotid Atherosclerosis Study. Endarterectomy for asymptomatic carotid atherosclerosis. *Journal of the American Medical Association* 1995; **273**: 1421–1426.

43 Ricotta JJ, Holen J, Schenk E et al. Is routine angiography necessary prior to carotid artery endarterectomy? *Journal of Vascular Surgery* 1984; **1**: 96–102.

44 Riles TS, Eidelman EM, Litt EW et al. Comparison of magnetic resonance angiography, conventional angiography, and duplex scanning. *Stroke* 1992; **23**: 341–346.

45 White JE, Russell WL, Greer MS et al. Efficacy of screening NM angiography and Doppler ultrasonography in the evaluation of carotid artery stenosis. *American Surgeon* 1994; **60**: 340–348.

46 Buijs PC, Klop RB, Eikelboom BC et al. Carotid bifurcation imaging: magnetic resonance angiography compared to conventional angiography and Doppler ultrasound.

European Journal of Vascular Surgery 1993; **7**: 245–251.

47 Huston J, Lewis ED, Wiebers DO *et al*. Can duplex scanning supplant arteriography in patients with focal carotid territory symptoms? *Journal of Vascular Surgery* 1987; **5**: 551–557.

48 Polak JF, Kalina B, Donaldson MC *et al*. Carotid endarterectomy: preoperative evaluation of candidates with combined Doppler sonography and MR angiography. *Radiology* 1993; **186**: 333–338.

49 Pan XM, Anderson CM, Reilly LM *et al*. Magnetic resonance angiography of the carotid artery combining two and three dimensional acquisitions. *Journal of Vascular Surgery* 1992; **16**: 609–615.

50 Mattle BP, Kent KC, Edelman RR *et al*. Evaluation of the extracranial carotid arteries: correlation of magnetic resonance angiography, duplex ultrasonography, and conventional angiography. *Journal of Vascular Surgery* 1991; **13**: 838–845.

51 Kido DK, Panzer RJ, Szumowski J *et al*. Clinical evaluation of stenosis of the carotid bifurcation with magnetic resonance angiographic techniques. *Archives of Neurology* 1991; **48**: 484.

52 Mani R, Eisenberg R, McDonald E *et al*. Complications of catheter cerebral arteriography: analysis of 5000 procedures. *American Journal of Roentgenology* 1978; **131**: 861–865.

53 Rockman CB, Riles TS, Fisher F *et al*. The surgical management of carotid artery stenosis in patients with previous neck irradiation. *American Journal of Surgery* 1996; **172**: 191–195.

54 Gagne PJ, Riles TS, Lamparello PJ. Long-term follow-up of patients undergoing reoperation for recurrent carotid artery disease. *Journal of Vascular Surgery* 1993; **18**: 991–1001.

KEY POINTS

1 Routine angiography was previously advocated because it was:
   • the imaging method used in the randomized trials;
   • the only method of grading stenosis;
   • the only reliable method for excluding inflow or intracranial disease;
   • essential in preventing unexpected findings at operation.
2 The fundamental disadvantages of angiography are the risk of stroke, significant cost, and the risks of contrast- or puncture-related complications.
3 Advances in duplex and MRA have now limited the indications for angiography.

If it were not for the invasive nature of angiography and the risk of procedural stroke, many of the debates about angiography, duplex, and MRA would be academic. Unfortunately, the risk of angiographic stroke is a very real phenomenon. In the ACAS study, angiographic stroke was responsible for almost 50% of the overall perioperative risk.

Angiography has always been perceived to be the gold standard with regard to determining the severity of carotid disease when, in reality, direct plaque examination should assume this role. Moreover, whilst angiography provides anatomic data (provided at least two planar images are available), it provides no hemodynamic information and little reliable information on plaque morphology. Accordingly, even with angiography, mistakes can occur with regard to interpretation of the degree of any stenosis. Evidence now clearly shows that provided certain criteria are met, reliance on duplex and/or MRA does not compromise the safety of surgery and little in the way of unexpected findings is encountered. It should be borne in mind that the factor most likely to render CEA more difficult is the failure to identify the posterior tongue of plaque preoperatively. Because this usually causes little in the way of luminal stenosis, angiography, MRA and duplex are not reliable predictors of its presence. MRA is probably just as effective as angiography in evaluating intracranial disease but, to date, there is no conclusive evidence that either is superior in terms of outcome.

Thus, while the indications for carotid angiography are increasingly limited, it is not an obsolete or discredited procedure. Patients who would still qualify for angiographic assessment include those in whom:

1 there is no access to either duplex or MRA;
2 duplex suggests inflow or distal ICA disease;
3 duplex cannot image the upper or lower limits of the plaque;
4 duplex interpretation is confounded by extensive acoustic shadowing;
5 carotid subocclusion has to be excluded;
6 the findings of MRA and duplex are either difficult to interpret or discordant;
7 there is an inability to undergo MRA because of claustrophobia or the presence of metallic objects and a reliable vascular laboratory is unavailable.

Finally, for medicolegal reasons it is essential that all surgeons who continue to advocate routine angiography prior to CEA include the additional 1–2% risk of angiographic stroke when discussing the general risks of the operation with the patient. It is unacceptable simply to quote the overall operative risk in this situation.

11.1

Does routine preoperative CT scanning alter patient management?
Dafydd Thomas (Europe)

INTRODUCTION

In order to achieve the maximum clinical benefit from carotid endarterectomy (CEA), a perioperative morbidity and mortality rate of less than 5% is required. To achieve this in otherwise high-risk individuals with generalized arterial disease is not easy. Evidence suggests that the international trial results are not instantly generalizable to routine clinical practice and that, following the publication of these trials, the combined death and any-stroke rate may be higher than was anticipated.[1]

Thus, for many surgeons, good outcome statistics are likely to be threatened by including patients who have complicating or even conflicting intracranial conditions. CEA would be, for example, contraindicated in a patient with intracranial aneurysm, where carotid ligation might be a more appropriate operation to prevent haemorrhage.

UNEXPECTED PATHOLOGY ON CT SCAN?

However, the chances of encountering unexpected or unusual pathology on computed tomographic (CT) scan in a patient presenting with a transient ischaemic attack (TIA) in association with a carotid stenosis in excess of 70% is < 2% (St Mary's experience; unpublished). The implication, therefore, is that since only a small percentage of CT brain scans will show an unexpected lesion, e.g. tumour, arteriovenous malformation, hydrocephalus, intracranial aneurysm, or haemorrhage sufficient to contraindicate surgical treatment, why bother to arrange a CT scan in the first place, particularly when this might cause delay in the surgical treatment and involve unnecessary expense?

It is this author's view that much useful information can be obtained from brain imaging and simply to exclude it from an investigative protocol on the basis that the pick-up rate of unexpected findings is low is misguided and could leave one vulnerable to medicolegal action.

CEREBRAL ISCHAEMIC INJURY?

Patients who present with purely ocular ischaemic symptoms with absolutely classical altitudinous disturbances with or without emboli on retinoscopy are the least likely to have coexistent cerebral hemispheric pathology as compared with patients who present with hemisensory/motor signs. Thus, if a policy of selective CT or MRI had to be implemented on the grounds of availability or expense, then this would be the only group of patients in whom I would feel that preoperative brain imaging was unnecessary. But even in this group the presence of coincidental intracranial problems, including silent infarcts, needs to be considered.

A CT brain scan is adequate in most instances for excluding cerebral tumours and intracranial haemorrhage. The CT scan is, however, poor at demonstrating small ischaemic lesions. An important minority of otherwise uncomplicated TIA patients will have evidence of established ischaemic lesions in the cerebral hemispheres. In particular, the CT scan is very poor at demonstrating vascular lesions within the brainstem and cerebellum.

CT scans do show carotid territory infarcts in 20% of patients presenting with a hemispheric TIA and in approximately 66% of patients who present with a clinical stroke. The presence of such a lesion on CT scan may increase the perioperative risk of stroke at the time of CEA,[2] and this may be one of several important factors to include when planning the care of individual patients and in discussing the risks/benefits of surgery with the patient and relatives.

The situation becomes even more complex when discussing the management of patients with asymptomatic disease. Because a significant part of our lives is spent asleep and because only 20% of the brain is clinically evocative, many patients may actually have suffered a TIA or minor stroke which is not clinically apparent. If the patient is then found to have a severe carotid stenosis, is this patient now considered symptomatic or asymptomatic? Should carotid surgery be offered or withheld? In the future, the presence of silent infarcts on CT scan or MRI might tip the balance towards advising surgical intervention.

LARGE- OR SMALL-VESSEL DISEASE?

In the author's experience, magnetic resonance is definitely the preferred method for imaging the brain[3] in order to appreciate fully the extent of any cerebral ischaemic lesions. Not only does it show infarcts more reliably, but it is very much better at showing smaller ischaemic lesions and more diffuse vascular changes. It is not uncommon to see multiple small infarcts in patients who present with one clinical TIA or retinal ischaemic event. Approximately 80% of the brain is clinically silent and sometimes moderate or even large asymptomatic infarcts are discovered in the frontal or non-dominant temporal lobes.

The presence of multiple (usually bilateral) small ischaemic lesions in the white matter suggests that the patient has significant small-vessel intracranial disease as opposed to thromboembolic disease. This small-vessel disease is more commonly associated with hypertension, diabetes and, possibly, hyperlipidaemia. The significance of differentiating between large- and small-vessel disease with regard to the role of CEA is unknown because none of the trials to date have addressed this particular question. One might argue that patients with diffuse small-vessel changes within the deeper structures of the brain are more at risk from perioperative neurological complications as a result of blood pressure fluctuations than are patients without such changes. Alternatively, this subgroup of patients might derive greater benefit by improving the overall inflow to the diseased lenticulostriate arteries. Certainly, blood pressure control and antiangina therapy has to be

implemented more cautiously in this group of patients because they seem more vulnerable to poor cerebral perfusion pressure.

These diffuse ischaemic changes on MRI, visualized less efficiently on CT (where they are termed leucoareosis), are also an adverse risk factor when considering the possibility of anticoagulant treatment. Such patients are much more likely to bleed and some neurologists now regard the presence of such changes as a relative contraindication to anticoagulant therapy.

NON-INVASIVE ANGIOGRAPHY

With increasing reliance on preoperative carotid duplex, we could be denied important information about the state of the intracranial vessels. However, with good-quality CT and/or magnetic resonance scanning it is now possible to produce adequate intracranial angiographic pictures, which can only improve preoperative assessment in complicated cases. Conventional angiography is likely to be phased out of routine carotid investigative practice in the near future because of the 1–2% risk of procedural stroke.[4]

CONCLUSIONS

The simple answer to the question posed in the chapter title is no! However, in the author's view, preoperative brain imaging is an important component of the protocol for investigating patients prior to CEA. Wherever possible, patients should undergo a magnetic resonance imaging brain scan and preferably a magnetic resonance angiogram. A CT is acceptable when magnetic resonance imaging is unavailable. Patients who present with amaurosis fugax in the absence of hemispheric symptoms are the only subgroup where elective brain imaging may be unnecessary. The relatively low cost, as compared with the total package of endarterectomy, is justified. With the increasing emphasis on appropriateness of CEA in various situations, the extra information available for scanning should improve informed decision-making. Finally, there are potential medicolegal consequences for not having performed a preoperative scan of the brain, as this might be interpreted as having constituted suboptimal preoperative assessment and would make any defence of a postoperative complication more difficult.

REFERENCES

1 Hsai DC, Krushat WM, Moscoe LM. Epidemiology of carotid endarterectomy among Medicare beneficiaries: 1985–1996 update. *Stroke* 1998; **29**: 346–350.

2 Rothwell PM, Slattery J, Warlow CP. A symptomatic comparison of the risks of stroke and death due to carotid endarterectomy for symptomatic and asymptomatic stenosis. *Stroke* 1996; **27**: 266–269.

3 Bryan RN, Levy LM, Whitlow D *et al.* Diagnosis of acute cerebral infarction. Comparison of CT and MR imaging. *American Journal of Neuroradiology* 1991; **12**: 611–620.

4 Whitty CJM, Sudlow CLM, Warlow CP. Investigating individual subjects and screening populations for asymptomatic carotid stenosis can be harmful. *Journal of Neurology, Neurosurgery and Psychiatry* 1998; **64**: 619–623.

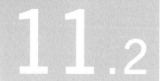

11.2

Does routine preoperative CT scanning alter patient management?
Magruder C Donaldson (USA)

INTRODUCTION

Development of safe, rapid, and accurate tools to image the brain has had a revolutionary impact on our understanding of the pathophysiology and natural history of diseases which affect the brain, among which is atherosclerosis of the extracranial carotid arteries.[5] CT and magnetic resonance imaging are widely available and can provide anatomic information to help refine the indications, timing, and impact of CEA. With the advent of magnetic resonance and CT (spiral) angiography, safe and minimally invasive imaging of the branches of the cerebrovascular tree is possible. The place of such angiographic techniques in patients with carotid disease is the subject of another section of this book. This chapter will focus on the impact of preoperative non-vascular brain imaging on management of patients who appear to be candidates for CEA.

DIAGNOSTIC VALUE OF BRAIN SCANS

Brain scans have revealed valuable information concerning the pathophysiology and natural history of extracranial carotid occlusive disease. Most notable have been studies indicating a high incidence of occult stroke among patients with carotid disease.[6–9] For example, even among patients with no discernible history of symptoms, scan defects on the side ipsilateral to disease in the carotid artery was found in 16% of patients.[6] With a history of TIA, the incidence of positive ipsilateral scans increased to 35%. There is also evidence that the prevalence of anatomic brain abnormality varies with the character of the plaque: heterogeneous and complex plaques detected by duplex ultrasound are associated with more CT scan lesions.[8,10] Taken together, this accumulated evidence strongly supports the importance of an atheroembolic pathophysiology for stroke related to extracranial carotid occlusive disease. In addition, these findings have made it clear that a history of symptoms is not a precise determinant of disease severity, since so many patients have been found with stroke and no history.

Equally startling has been the lack of anatomic CT findings among patients who present after a clinical stroke. For example, 24% of such patients had no evidence of infarct in one series[6] and fully 38% of stroke victims had normal scans in another study.[11] This lack of diagnostic sensitivity for correlates of clinical events is testimony to the fact that anatomy-based brain scans such as CT can only partially illuminate complex intracranial events.

Nonetheless, modern brain scanning has been critically important in understanding anatomic events following stroke. Most particularly, scans help make the crucial differentiation between strokes resulting from end-artery occlusion and those caused by hemorrhage. This has allowed increased precision in making a timely choice between use of anticoagulant or thrombolytic therapy for thromboembolic occlusive stroke and avoidance of anticoagulants after hemorrhagic stroke. In addition to findings of stroke, imaging has allowed identification of other intracranial pathology such as benign or malignant tumors, diffuse small-vessel infarctions (lacunes[12]), other forms of vascular disease such as berry aneurysm and arteriovenous malformation, brain atrophy, and post-traumatic lesions such as subdural hematoma.

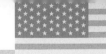

ROLE OF SCANS BEFORE CAROTID ENDARTERECTOMY

At present, CEA is performed for patients with high-grade extracranial carotid occlusive disease associated with no symptoms, TIA (including crescendo symptoms and amaurosis fugax), or completed stroke. Patients with a recent stroke are in many instances good candidates for a surgical approach relatively earlier in their course than had been previously felt to be safe.[13] Patients with acute fluctuating neurologic deficits (stroke in evolution) remain a challenging and controversial subset of stroke patients. The role of CT or magnetic resonance imaging is distinct in each of these categories of patients.[11,14-16]

Asymptomatic Patients

Data accumulated over the last 20 years has made it clear that patients with no history of neurologic event frequently harbor regions of damage in their brains.[6-8] Though impressive, the clinical relevance of this phenomenon remains unclear. Some researchers have found an increase in perioperative neurologic morbidity associated with silent infarcts[15,17,18] and have recommended routine CT scanning prior to CEA. Others, including the current author, have found no such predictive value.[11,14] Certainly, in most large series of patients undergoing CEA, the perioperative stroke rate is so low that adding a routine preoperative CT to all patients to help eliminate the 1–2% morbidity rate appears to be rather cost-ineffective. Furthermore, there are no data supporting the efficacy of CEA among patients with mild or moderate carotid disease and a silent ipsilateral brain infarct which might be revealed by a policy of routine scanning. Therefore, routine preoperative scans among truly asymptomatic patients do not appear to be justified at this time.

Transient Ischemic Attack Patients

Patients who have experienced intermittent transient neurologic symptoms may benefit from scanning in selected instances but not on a routine basis. A careful history remains the most important means of connecting extracranial carotid disease with neurologic symptoms and differentiating among syndromes which might mimic cerebrovascular TIA (Table 11.1). A classic pattern of transient monocular blindness or cortical motor or sensory events with an ipsilateral plaque detected by duplex ultrasound has a high level of specificity and confirmatory routine scans are extremely unlikely to yield further useful information.[6,11] Any peculiar feature of the symptoms (Table 11.2), however, should prompt wider consideration of other potential diagnoses. For example, headache, atypical patterns which do not fit known extracranial disease location or bilateral visual, motor, or sensory symptoms may be associated with other entities such as migraine, vertebrobasilar insufficiency or intracranial malignancy. Among other diagnostic studies, contrast arteriography, magnetic resonance angiography, or brain scan should be selectively pursued among these patients with a non-classical history to avoid misdiagnosis and consequent inappropriate therapy.

Table 11.1
Differential diagnosis of transient ischemic attack
Stokes–Adams attack
Seizure
Tumor
Subdural hematoma
Migraine
Cerebrovascular occlusive disease

Table 11.2
Atypical symptoms
Symptoms anatomically inappropriate to known extracranial carotid disease
Bilateral visual, motor, or sensory symptoms
Headache, either recurrent or severe
Unexplained vertigo and ataxia
Auditory symptoms
Seizures

Completed-Stroke Patients

Patients who present with a completed stroke generally have a scan shortly after the neurologic event to document the nature and extent of the brain

133

lesion, usually before carotid disease is causally implicated. Since scan infarcts are so common among patients with extracranial carotid disease who have not suffered clinical strokes, and since some patients with strokes have normal scans, a rigorous policy of routine preoperative scan among patients with completed stroke who are candidates for CEA is not justifiable. Some have argued that lacunar strokes are not related to carotid disease and therefore, if confirmed on scan, would exclude some stroke patients from surgical therapy designed to prevent another stroke.[12] On the other hand, others have argued that lacunes may indeed be caused by thromboembolism, making preoperative differentiation between lacunar and cortical stroke less relevant.[19]

Among patients who present acutely with a stable completed stroke it is advisable to delay intervention until it is clear that:

1   the stroke is not hemorrhagic;
2   circumstances point to an operable cause at the carotid bifurcation;
3   the stroke remains limited without clinical deterioration due to reactive edema or hemorrhage
4   the patient is otherwise a good surgical candidate.

All such patients may benefit from early scanning to exclude hemorrhage, and those in whom scans remain normal within the first several days of the event and whose clinical course remains stable may undergo CEA with expectation of minimal morbidity.[14,16,20,21] Increasing experience has indicated that many patients with scans showing a small thromboembolic stroke may also undergo CEA safely.[14,20,21] Thus, in part guided by preoperative scans, many patients with stroke can undergo early surgery within 2 weeks without waiting the traditional 4–6 weeks advised after the experience of the 1960s[13] and, more recently by others,[22] provided the above criteria have been satisfied (Fig. 11.1).

Stroke-in-Evolution Patients
Patients with acute fluctuating neurologic deficits which do not clear are a rare and difficult subgroup.

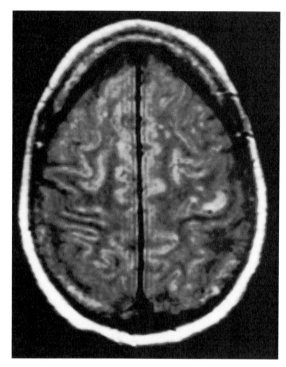

Fig. 11.1
Magnetic resonance image demonstrating small ischemic stroke in left middle cerebral artery distribution several days after onset of right-arm weakness. This image allowed differentiation from hemorrhagic event and correlation with high-grade left carotid stenosis, facilitating selection of this patient as a candidate for early carotid endarterectomy.

There is evidence that some patients with stroke in evolution may benefit from urgent CEA directed at removal of an ongoing cause of repeated or persistent ischemic insults and restoration of optimal flow to a region of brain ischemia which is presumed to be reversible.[23–25] These patients are usually easy to distinguish on clinical grounds from patients with crescendo TIA who return to a normal baseline between episodes and who should be treated like any patient with TIA, albeit more expeditiously. More difficult may be distinction from patients with acute completed stroke and minimal or no fluctuation who have established and irreversible infarction which will be presumably unresponsive to urgent surgery.

Optimal selection of potential candidates for CEA requires prompt characterization of the pathophysiology behind the neurologic presentation, including rapid confirmation of the presence of extracranial carotid disease and exclusion of a complicated or hemorrhagic intracranial process. Surgery may improve the chance of eventual recovery to normal in highly selected circumstances when:

1   there is compelling evidence of very recent carotid bifurcation occlusion or repeated atheroembolism from a high-grade carotid bifurcation plaque;
2   early brain scans show no hemorrhage and no infarction;
3   the patient is otherwise a good candidate for CEA.

Incidental Intracranial Disease

Intracranial aneurysms are present in about 2% of patients who present with significant extracranial carotid artery occlusive disease.[26] The great majority of these aneurysms are small. The risk of rupture of such aneurysms is related to their size; a threshold of 7–10 mm diameter is the usual indication for elective neurosurgical intervention. Though in theory anticoagulation and perioperative hypertension may contribute to rupture in association with CEA, no increased risk has been demonstrable by limited experience reported in the literature.[26–28] For this reason, when indications for clipping a large asymptomatic berry aneurysm and for CEA coexist, it is usually best to proceed with CEA and stage the clipping later. The only rationale for brain scanning before CEA with respect to berry aneurysms is thus to find the rare asymptomatic aneurysm which is large enough to be visualized and which might therefore best be treated later. This rationale is not sufficiently fruitful to support routine scans for this purpose.

Up to 15% of patients with significant extracranial carotid disease harbor tandem stenosis in the siphon portion of the intracranial carotid artery.[26,29,30]

Definitive diagnosis of such lesions requires preoperative contrast arteriography using either a selective or intra-arterial digital technique. Magnetic resonance angiography has also been useful, though somewhat fraught with artifactual false-positives. Fortunately, clinical experience supports the safety of CEA in patients with known siphon disease, particularly with < 80% stenosis.[26,31,32] Though not entirely resolved, this issue is not a compelling reason to perform routine preoperative intracranial arterial imaging, nor would it be a reason to pursue preoperative brain scanning to detect the small percentage of patients with siphon disease who might harbor calcifications evident on such scans.

Patients with known non-vascular intracranial disease may develop extracranial carotid artery disease which, taken by itself, may meet the indications for CEA. A recent scan should be available preoperatively in order to be certain that the intracranial status is clear and that a baseline is established.

An argument has been made that routine preoperative scanning should be done as a baseline for comparison should there be complications postoperatively. This approach is highly questionable from a cost–benefit standpoint, given the very low incidence of postoperative neurologic complications associated with CEA. Nonetheless, the medicolegal implications of such a baseline study may be a consideration in unusual circumstances.

Table 11.3
Indications for selective preoperative brain imaging

Strong
Unstable neurologic deficit
History of acute stroke

Moderate
Atypical transient symptoms
History of recent intracranial disease or trauma

Marginal
History of remote stroke
Medicolegal baseline

CONCLUSIONS

This analysis, supported by experience and the evidence in the literature, strongly supports a policy of CEA without routine preoperative brain scan. In a series testing such a policy, Martin et al.[11] performed routine CT scans on 469 patients. Scans were abnormal in 62% of patients with a history of stroke and in 14% of patients without a history of stroke. No tumors, aneurysms, arteriovenous malformations, or other unusual intracranial lesions were identified. Surgical judgment regarding selection of patients for CEA was not influenced by the preoperative scan.

Three postoperative strokes occurred among the 230 CEAs performed, none of which correlated with information derived from the preoperative CT.

A policy of selective preoperative scanning (Table 11.3) is clearly appropriate to help establish the diagnosis in patients with unusual symptoms and to help refine sophisticated management of the relatively rare patient who presents with small acute strokes or fluctuating stroke in evolution.

REFERENCES

5 Davis K, Taveras J, New P, Schnur J, Roberson G. Cerebral infarction diagnosis by computerized tomography analysis and evaluation of findings. Stroke 1975; 124: 643–664.
6 Street D, O'Brien M, Ricofta J et al. Observations on cerebral computed tomography in patients having carotid endarterectomy. Journal of Vascular Surgery 1988; 7: 798–801.
7 Grigg M, Papadakis K, Nicolaides A et al. The significance of cerebral infarction and atrophy in patients with amaurosis fugax and transient ischemic attacks in relation to internal carotid artery stenosis: a preliminary report. Journal of Vascular Surgery 1988; 7: 215–222.
8 Zukowski A, Nicolaides A, Lewis R et al. The correlation between carotid plaque ulceration and cerebral infarction seen on CT scan. Journal of Vascular Surgery 1984; 1: 782–786.
9 Calandre L, Gomara S, Beimejo F, Millan J, DelPozo G. Clinical CT correlations in TIA, RIND, and strokes with minimal residuum. Stroke 1984; 15: 663–666.
10 Geroulakos G, Domjan J, Nicolaides A et al. Ultrasonic carotid artery plaque structure and the risk of cerebral infarction on computed tomography. Journal of Vascular Surgery 1994; 20: 263–266.
11 Martin J, Valentine R, Myers S et al. Is routine CT scanning necessary in the preoperative evaluation of patients undergoing carotid endarterectomy? Journal of Vascular Surgery 1991; 14: 267–270.
12 Weisberg L. Diagnostic classification of stroke, especially lacunes. Stroke 1988; 19: 1071–1082.
13 Wylie E, Hein M, Adams J. Intracranial hemorrhage following revascularization for treatment of acute stroke. Journal of Neurosurgery 1964; 21: 212.
14 Ricotta J, Ouriel K, Green R, DeWeese J. Use of computerized cerebral tomography in selection of patients for elective and urgent carotid endarterectomy. Annals of Surgery 1985; 202: 783–787.
15 Graber J, Voliman R, Levine H, Scott R, Nabseth D. Stroke following carotid endarterectomy: risk predicted by preoperative CT scan. American Journal of Surgery 1984; 147: 492–497.
16 Dosick S, Whalen R, Gale S, Brown O. Carotid endarterectomy in the stroke patient: computerized axial tomography to determine timing. Journal of Vascular Surgery 1985; 2: 214.
17 Vollman R, Eldrup-Jorgensen J, Hoffman M. The role of cranial computed tomography in carotid surgery. Surgical Clinics of North America 1986; 66: 255–268.
18 Sise M, Sedwitz M, Rowley W, Shackford S. Prospective analysis of carotid endarterectomy and select cerebral infarction in 97 patients. Stroke 1989; 20: 329–332.
19 Milliken C, Futrell N. The fallacy of the lacune hypothesis. Stroke 1990; 21: 1251–1258.
20 Piotrowski J, Bernhard V, Rubin J et al. Timing of carotid endarterectomy after acute stroke. Journal of Vascular Surgery 1990; 11: 45–52.
21 Whittemore A, Mannick J. Surgical treatment of carotid disease in patients with neurologic deficits. Journal of Vascular Surgery 1987; 5: 910–916.
22 Giordano J, Trout H, Kozloff L, DePalma R. Timing of carotid artery endarterectomy after stroke. Journal of Vascular Surgery 1985; 2: 250–254.
23 Mentzer R, Finkelmeier B, Crosby I, Wellons H. Emergency carotid endarterectomy for fluctuating neurologic deficits. Surgery 1981; 89: 60–66.
24 Donaldson MC, Drezner AD. Surgery for acute carotid occlusion. Therapy in search of predictability. Archives of Surgery 1983; 118: 1266–1268.
25 Gertler J, Blankensteijn J, Brewster D et al. Carotid endarterectomy for unstable and compelling neurologic conditions: do results justify an aggressive approach? Journal of Vascular Surgery 1994; 19: 32–42.
26 Lord R, Raj T, Graham A. Carotid endarterectomy, siphon stenosis, collateral hemispheric pressure, and perioperative cerebral infarction. Journal of Vascular Surgery 1987; 6: 391–397.
27 Orecchia P, Clagett G, Youkey J et al. Management of patients with symptomatic extracranial carotid artery disease and incidental intracranial berry aneurysm. Journal of Vascular Surgery 1985; 2: 158–164.
28 Stern J. Management of extracranial carotid stenosis and intracranial aneurysms. Journal of Neurosurgery 1979; 51: 147–153.
29 Borozan P, Schuler J, LaRosa M et al. The natural history of isolated carotid siphon stenosis. Journal of Vascular Surgery 1984; 1: 744–749.
30 Craig D, Megurok K, Watridge C et al. Intracranial internal carotid artery stenosis. Stroke 1982; 13: 825–828.
31 Roederer G, Langlois Y, Chan A et al. Is siphon disease important in predicting outcome of carotid endarterectomy? Archives of Surgery 1983; 116: 1177–1181.
32 Schuler J, Flanigan D, Lim L et al. The effect of carotid siphon stenosis on stroke rate, death, and relief of symptoms following elective carotid endarterectomy. Surgery 1982; 92: 1058–1067.

11.3 Editorial Comment

KEY POINTS

1 Routine preoperative brain imaging is not cost-effective.
2 The significance of silent areas of infarction in otherwise asymptomatic patients is controversial.
3 Preoperative brain imaging is indicated in:
 • patients in the acute phase of stroke to exclude hemorrhage;
 • any patient under consideration for urgent or emergency CEA;
 • any patient with atypical symptoms or examination findings.

Both authors suggest that routine preoperative CT scanning is unnecessary, but there are subtle differences in emphasis that reflect the overall uncertainty regarding the role of preoperative imaging. It is also becoming increasingly clear that, were imaging to be indicated, magnetic resonance would be a better alternative to CT scan, although that will invariably depend on geographic factors.

The only indication for performing brain imaging in asymptomatic patients is if it is likely to alter decision-making in the future. The two authors disagree on the role of imaging in this situation, but this is more likely to reflect transatlantic attitudes towards surgery for asymptomatic disease. If you perform CEA routinely for severe asymptomatic disease, then no preoperative imaging seems necessary. If, however, the presence of silent areas of infarction might otherwise militate towards

operation, then either magnetic resonance or CT is indicated in asymptomatic patients.

It is our impression that the chances of encountering an intracranial hemorrhage with resolution of neurologic symptoms within 24 h is remote. Thus, most TIA patients will present electively and the rationale underlying the use of routine preoperative brain scans becomes less clear. The principal worry is that important intracranial pathology (especially a brain tumor) will be missed and that this will delay appropriate treatment and predispose to medicolegal action. Evidence suggests, however, that the chance of encountering a brain tumor in the setting of classical carotid territory symptoms plus a severe carotid stenosis is remote. The other argument supporting the use of routine preoperative scanning is that the presence of cortical infarcts increases the operative risk. This was probably true about 10 years ago and the inference was that these patients had less reserve for dealing with hypoperfusion or embolization. However, with increasing awareness of this possibility, thresholds for shunting have probably decreased, supplemented by the increasing use of monitoring and quality control methods. Currently, there is no clear-cut evidence that the presence of cerebral infarction is synonymous with a predictable increase in operative risk.

It would seem, therefore, that there is little in the way of compelling evidence to support routine preoperative brain imaging in TIA patients unless there is anything unusual in the clinical history. In that situation, referral to a neurologist is mandatory and he or she can decide what form of imaging is appropriate.

The rationale regarding the role of brain imaging in stroke patients is perhaps clearer. Surely the time to do this is within the first 2 weeks of the event. In that way, patients with intracranial hemorrhage are excluded from surgery. There is absolutely no point in delaying the scan as any evidence of hemorrhage will by then have disappeared. If there were any question of urgent or emergency surgery, preoperative CT or magnetic resonance imaging is obligatory. One residual dilemma is whether it is necessary to differentiate between lacunar and cortical infarcts. The editors currently conclude that there is no evidence that patients with carotid territory symptoms, a severe carotid stenosis, and a lacunar infarction should be denied surgery.

In conclusion, routine preoperative brain imaging is not cost-effective because the yield of unexpected findings which influence decision-making is low. For those who rely predominantly on preoperative duplex prior to surgery, the indications for brain imaging will be highly selected. However, for those using magnetic resonance angiography, it may seem appropriate to perform a magnetic resonance imaging study at the same time.

12.1 Which patients require preoperative assessment by a neurologist?

Dafydd Thomas (Europe)

In an ideal world, the simple answer to the question posed in this chapter title is everyone. Symptom analysis may, on occasions, be extremely difficult and neurological examination unrevealing. By involving a neurologist, overall patient selection should be improved and perioperative problems reduced.

INTRODUCTION

Carotid endarterectomy (CEA) is an operation which always needs to be treated with the utmost respect. If it goes wrong the patient, perceived by the family to have had relatively trivial preoperative symptoms, is rendered hemiplegic, dysphasic or dead. So although it may seem attractive to streamline the management of a patient presenting with 'straightforward' amaurosis fugax or hemiphenomena to duplex ultrasound and CEA, this approach may result in an increase in perioperative morbidity and mortality largely as a result of suboptimal patient selection.

A transient retinal or cerebral ischaemic attack associated with an ipsilateral carotid stenosis should be viewed as the tip of the vascular iceberg. The patient usually has widespread arterial disease, not only in the contralateral carotid, the intracranial vessels, the vertebrals and subclavian arteries, but also in the aortic arch, the heart and abdominal and leg vessels. To indulge in a quick 'smash-and-grab' procedure on just one aspect of a complicated case may not be doing the best for the patient in the long term. Rather, the transient ischaemic attack (TIA) might be regarded as a 'golden moment' for a proper assessment of the patient and all the other vascular problems.

In an ideal world, all patients presenting with neurological symptoms should be seen and assessed by a neurologist. In fact, only a relative minority of patients suffering the very important symptoms of a TIA find their way to an interested clinician of any specialty! The reason for this is largely educational and relates to both the patient and the primary-care physician. The former may have no idea of the importance of the transient symptoms and the latter may, in many cases, simply dismiss them and prescribe just a small dose of aspirin as appropriate therapy, despite its rather feeble protective effect.

THE ENDARTERECTOMY TRIALS

The design of the international trials, which have shown a benefit for CEA in selected patients[1,2] has been best medical treatment versus best medical treatment plus surgery. Virtually all patients included in these trials have been seen and assessed by a neurologist or similarly interested physician. Therefore, if surgery is to be contemplated without such a physician's involvement, the preconditions of the trials are not being satisfied and the trial results may become inapplicable. It is likely that the physician has had involvement not only in symptom clarification but also in the patient's selection for surgery as well as the planning of appropriate pharmacotherapy before and after surgery.

In addition, it should be noted that, in the international trials, only about 25% of patients in the best medical therapy group suffered a late stroke – one could say therefore that over 75% of those undergoing surgery did not actually need it. Quite rightly, there is increasing emphasis on identifying the 25% subgroup who are especially at risk and thus on the appropriateness of CEA in individual instances. The message that patients with more than 70% stenosis should be operated on and those with less than 70%

should not is now appreciated to be too simplistic.[1,2] Further subgroup analyses of the data have shown, for example, that patients with irregular and possibly ulcerated plaques with approximately 60% stenosis may be at just as much risk as patients with a 90% stenosis but with a smooth plaque.

It is now also appreciated that patients with purely retinal ischaemic events are at approximately half the risk of an ipsilateral stroke compared with a patient with either a hemisphere TIA or a combination of hemisphere and retinal TIAs. So the purely ocular patient may need to be considered separately. However, many such ocular patients will have had unsuspected hemisphere events and show residual neurological signs and may have abnormal brain scans.

There is also increasing emphasis on the different risk profiles constructed from the risk factors and the clinical and investigational findings. Endarterectomy in women seems to be more dangerous. There is also increased risk in patients with contralateral occlusion, those with hypertension and those with peripheral vascular disease. Modelling strategies are now being developed to allow the development of risk profiles for individual patients to help identify those with both asymptomatic and symptomatic carotid stenosis who are at greatest risk from ipsilateral stroke if treated solely with medical therapy, as well as defining those most likely to benefit from surgical treatment.

As a consequence, far fewer patients would need to be operated on to save one stroke. This would have obvious economic attractions as well as medical ones. The involvement of a multidisciplinary team in this decision-making process seems desirable, as well as inevitable, and would prove economical by targeting CEA appropriately.

INTERPRETATION OF SYMPTOMS

The interpretation of neurological symptoms that might otherwise masquerade as a TIA can be extremely difficult. One is often dealing with complicated cases with bilateral disease, some of whom have vertebrobasilar as well as carotid territory symptomatology. The interpretation of migrainous phenomena in the absence of typical headache, nausea and vomiting is not an area for those inexperienced in neurological assessment. In contrast, patients developing a carotid occlusion may experience migraine-like headaches on which TIA symptoms are superimposed.

Focal epilepsy can be even more difficult to diagnose because many focal epileptic attacks do not result in complete loss of consciousness but just a hemiphenomenon with or without an accompanying 'strange experience'. Such epileptic attacks occur not only from tumours or scarring, but also after small cortical infarcts. Speech disturbances also require appropriate diagnostic experience. Most non-neurologists have difficulty distinguishing dysphasia and dysarthria and many will not even have heard of the epileptiform disturbance of speech arrest and thus would never recognize it.

Subtle but persisting abnormal neurological signs imply that the TIA was, in fact, a minor stroke. This may at first sight seem pedantic, but evidence suggests that the perioperative risk may be increased in these patients. Moreover, the discovery of these deficits for the first time in the postoperative period might even lead to an erroneous diagnosis of operation-related stroke.

There are certain other areas of symptomatology that have been underemphasized – in particular, patients with poor cognitive function who are in the early stages of dementia. The subtle signs of this condition may well be missed by a non-neurologist and, in such cases, a detailed neurological assessment is required to identify the cause of the cognitive difficulties. Vascular disease is likely to be the reason in only a minority of such patients. CEA in early Alzheimer's disease might not be considered appropriate management!

MEDICAL TREATMENT

Medical treatment of patients with neurological and circulatory symptoms needs to be optimized. It would be unfortunate for the beneficial effect of endarterectomy to be countered by inappropriate blood pressure control or failure to tend to blood lipids and antiplatelet medication.

MEDICOLEGAL ASPECTS

Perioperative or postoperative events may be more difficult to defend if patients have not been assessed by an independent neurologist preoperatively. There may be room for criticism over the exact identification of the symptoms preoperatively and the exact indications for surgery may be challenged. A problem that might have existed preoperatively, for example dementia, might be significantly aggravated by the operation and anaesthetic and a postoperative problem may be entirely attributed to the operation rather than just being an emphasis of a preoperative problem for which the surgery was indicated, for example multi-infarct dementia rather than Alzheimer's disease.

In summary, CEA should not be performed in isolation. It needs to be carried out in a climate encouraging optimal medical care from a multidisciplinary approach. In particular, a postoperative physician's assessment is required in order to achieve an independent and therefore believable morbidity and mortality rate. This may be required by clinical audit in future. The cross-fertilization that takes place between specialties is of great importance, not only for patient care, but also for medical and surgical development. Anybody who has already enjoyed such an environment would be reluctant to accept that patients should have a CEA without neurological involvement. In the author's view, endarterectomy should not be performed without it. The extra delay involved must be minimized because early surgery is likely to be more effective. The extra expense is justifiable on patient selection alone.

REFERENCES

1 European Carotid Surgery Trialists' Collaborative Group MRC European carotid surgery trial: interim results for symptomatic patients with severe (70–99%) or with mild (0–29%) carotid stenosis. *Lancet* 1991; **337**: 1235–1243.

2 North American Symptomatic Carotid Endarterectomy Trial Collaborators. Beneficial effect of carotid endarterectomy in symptomatic patients with high-grade stenosis. *New England Journal of Medicine* 1991; **325**: 445–453.

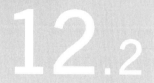

12.2

Which patients require preoperative assessment by a neurologist?
James M Estes (USA)

INTRODUCTION

There is considerable variability between vascular surgeons and neurologists in terms of the evaluation and management of patients with cerebrovascular disease. Many variables impact on this relationship, including the teaching status of the hospital (i.e., university-based or private), referral patterns, and characteristics of the individual staff members such as their experience and credentials. These relationships span the gamut. On one extreme is the practice where all candidates for CEA are evaluated and selected by neurologists who then refer to vascular specialists for surgery. In contrast to this is the setting where the vascular surgeon is referred patients from primary-care providers for evaluation of cerebrovascular disease. Depending on the clinical scenario, this surgeon may consider a secondary referral to a neurologist.

Practice patterns notwithstanding, most physicians are now under pressure to operate efficiently and minimize costs of patient care. Given the variability in practice patterns and increased cost-containment pressures, one must consider the appropriate role of a neurologist in the management of patients with cerebrovascular disease.

In general, patients presenting with critical carotid artery stenosis without symptoms do not need neurologic evaluation, as the decision to operate is based on the appropriate pathology and the absence of serious medical comorbidity. Cerebrovascular surgeons should also be able to manage patients with classic TIA and transient monocular blindness (TMB) symptoms without consultative assistance. However, patients presenting with atypical symptoms or acute stroke may benefit from an assessment by a neurologic specialist.

CONDITIONS WHEN NEUROLOGIC CONSULTATION IS NOT REQUIRED

Asymptomatic Carotid Stenosis

The decision to operate on asymptomatic patients with carotid stenosis is based on the vascular surgeon's assessment of the risks and benefits of surgery for the individual patient. The vascular surgeon should also have the expertise to request and properly interpret the appropriate carotid imaging studies. A neurologic consultation plays no role in the management of asymptomatic patients.

Classic Transient Ischemia and Monocular Blindness

Transient hemiparesis or monocular blindness in the setting of significant carotid stenosis mandates expeditious consideration of CEA due to the increased risk of stroke.[3] By definition, these patients have no new, persistent neurologic deficit and therefore neurologic consultation is unnecessary. When a significant carotid lesion on the appropriate side is identified in these patients, the decision to operate is usually straightforward.

This approach assumes that the responsible physician can discern symptoms of a TIA specifically associated with carotid stenosis. Dizziness, vertigo, syncope, and unexplained falls are atypical and non-specific symptoms frequently misdiagnosed as TIA by general practitioners and emergency room physicians.[4] Neurologic evaluation may be beneficial for such patients (see below).

CONDITIONS WHEN NEUROLOGIC CONSULTATION IS SUGGESTED

Acute Stroke

Detailed neurologic evaluation should be performed in all patients with fixed deficits. Ischemic insults to the brain can present as a myriad of clinical syndromes depending on the arterial branch affected (Table 12.1). Alterations in one or more aspects of motor function, sensory function, cognition, and personality may be seen. Some types of cerebral infarction may be subtle and only identifiable with specific testing. For example, occlusion of the posterior cerebral artery may cause contralateral homonymous hemianopia with macular sparing.[5] Patients with this disorder are often unaware of the peripheral blindness and thus careful visual field testing is required to elucidate it. Lacunar infarctions secondary to occlusion of small perforating vessels in the deep white-matter structures can produce lesions in the internal capsule that mimic classic hemiparesis and sensory loss from a middle cerebral artery territory stroke.[6]

The differential diagnosis of cerebral ischemia is extensive (Table 12.2). Therefore, in addition to a thorough history and physical examination, laboratory and radiologic testing is required to determine the cause when patients present with ischemic symptoms. A complete blood count, electrolyte and glucose determination, electrocardiogram, and computed tomographic (CT) scan of the brain comprise the basic diagnostic algorithm. History or electrocardiogram findings suggestive of myocardial infarction or atrial arrhythmia mandate echocardiography to assess for atrial or ventricular thrombi. Carotid duplex studies should be performed in patients over 50, younger patients at high risk for premature atherosclerosis, and those with suspected spontaneous or traumatic carotid dissection. Other tests are performed based on clinical necessity.

It is important to identify the affected area of cerebrum using clinical assessment and radiologic imaging, as this has important implications for treatment. The knowledgeable examiner can extract a great deal of useful information from a detailed history and physical examination. Brain imaging is required for patients with fixed deficits or in those with suspected intracranial bleeding (e.g. nuchal rigidity, severe headache, uncontrolled hypertension). Brain CT is the most useful initial imaging test as it is widely available and rapidly

Table 12.1
Clinical syndromes associated with major cerebrovascular occlusion

Vessel involved	Clinical syndrome
Anterior cerebral artery[9]	Motor and sensory loss in the contralateral foot and leg. May involve proximal arm Face spared
Bilateral anterior cerebral artery	Paraparesis, incontinence Akinetic mutism
Middle cerebral artery[10]	Contralateral hemiplegia, hemisensory loss, hemianopia May have depressed level of consciousness
Upper-division middle cerebral artery	Contralateral monoparesis of arm with facial involvement Motor aphasia (dominant side)
Lower-division middle cerebral artery	Contralateral visual field deficit Fluent aphasia (dominant side)
Unilateral posterior communicating artery[5]	Contralateral homonymous hemianopia with macular sparing
Bilateral posterior communicating artery	Cortical blindness
Basilar artery[5]	Quadriplegia, coma, 'locked-in' state
Lacunar infarction[6]	Pure motor or sensory deficit, ataxic hemiparesis Classic hemiplegia with sensory deficit

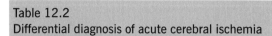

Table 12.2
Differential diagnosis of acute cerebral ischemia

Vascular causes
Inflammatory conditions
   Collagen vascular diseases
   Infectious agents (syphilis, tuberculosis, viral
     illness, ophthalmic herpes zoster)
   Arteritis (temporal arteritis, Takayasu's disease,
     polyarteritis nodosum)
   Granulomatoses (Wegener's granulomatosis,
     lymphatoid granulomatosis, granulomatosis
     angiitis)
Non-inflammatory conditions
   Carotid atherosclerosis
   Aortic arch atherosclerosis
   Arterial dissection (carotid, aorta)
   Fibromuscular hyperplasia
   Vasospasm (migraine, subarachnoid
     hemorrhage)
   Drug-induced (cocaine, amphetamine)

Hematologic causes
Polycythemia
Thrombophilic states
   Antithrombin III, protein C, protein S
     deficiencies
   Antiphospholipid antibodies
   Thrombocytosis
   Disseminated intravascular coagulopathy

Cardiac causes
Clot embolization
   Atrial fibrillation
   Recent myocardial infarction
   Ventricular aneurysm
   Paradoxical embolus
   Atrial myxoma

Other causes mimicking stroke
Brain neoplasm
Focal seizure
Hypoglycemic attack
Subdural hematoma
Cerebral contusion or hemorrhage

performed. CT is accurate in determining the presence of hemorrhage or mass lesions in the cerebrum. It is relatively insensitive in identifying acute cortical infarction, posterior fossa lesions, and lacunar infarction. Magnetic resonance imaging (MRI) is particularly sensitive to changes in water density (i.e. edema) and has greater accuracy than CT in identifying small acute infarctions and white-matter pathology. However, since ferromagnetic materials such as those found in monitoring equipment and intravenous pumps are not permitted in the MRI suite, it is not the ideal location for the acutely ill patient: brain CT is usually the initial test of choice.

Patients with significant carotid stenosis who present with acute stroke are optimally managed by collaboration between the vascular surgeon and neurologic specialist. The role of the neurologist is to characterize the deficit in detail and correlate these findings with the pathology identified by imaging studies. The vascular surgeon must choose the appropriate diagnostic test (e.g. duplex ultrasound, magnetic resonance angiography, contrast angiography) to assess the degree and nature of carotid atherosclerosis. This shared information, derived from the patient's symptoms, location of cerebral pathology, and carotid plaque morphology, is then used to determine whether the carotid lesion is the likely cause of the acute stroke.

The carotid plaque must be implicated as the source of cerebral infarction in order to justify early operative intervention. For example, a small parietal infarct ipsilateral to a critical carotid stenosis would justify an aggressive operative approach, whereas a critical carotid stenosis in the setting of multiple lacunar infarcts may not. Such a patient would benefit more initially from control of hypertension and supportive therapy.

The appropriateness and timing of CEA in the setting of acute stroke have been controversial and are beyond the scope of this discussion. The main justification for expeditious surgical intervention is prevention of recurrent ischemia from embolization or thrombosis of an unstable carotid plaque. It is the author's opinion that CEA should be performed without delay in alert patients with a stable, incomplete deficit, salvageable cerebral tissue, and acceptable medical risk.

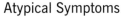

Atypical Symptoms

The evaluation and management of patients with extracranial carotid stenosis and atypical symptoms can be challenging. Presenting complaints in these patients include dizzy spells, syncope, vertigo, drop attacks, and global weakness. Blurred or double vision and other visual disturbances not consistent with TMB are also in this category. Many of these symptoms are non-specific and usually not due to carotid stenosis. These patients require a careful medical and neurologic evaluation to rule out conditions such as hypoglycemia, seizure disorder, intolerance to medications (particularly antihypertensives), labyrinthitis, cardiac conditions, and orthostatic hypotension.

Persistent unilateral visual symptoms in patients with a history of TMB warrant ophthalmologic evaluation. Carotid plaque embolization can lead to retinal artery thrombosis and retinal infarction that are evident on fundoscopic examination. Other retinal diseases such as hemorrhage or detachment may mimic retinal artery thrombosis and should be managed appropriately to avoid further visual compromise.

Syncope

Sudden loss of consciousness may be caused by acute cerebral hypoperfusion. Less severe reductions in blood flow may cause symptoms of dizziness or pre-syncope. Thorough neurologic evaluation is mandated in these patients to rule out seizure activity, metabolic conditions, and drug reactions, which may also cause these symptoms. Frequently a cardiac evaluation is required to assess for arrhythmias and aortic valvular stenosis (Stokes–Adams syndrome).

Duplex ultrasound assessment of the carotid and vertebral arteries should be routinely performed. If no obvious etiology for the symptoms is identified, then an assessment of the intracranial circulation is required using contrast angiography, magnetic resonance angiography, or transcranial Doppler.

Vertebrobasilar Symptoms

Symptoms of vertebrobasilar insufficiency (VBI) include many of those listed above as atypical symptoms for carotid atherosclerosis and may be due to embolic or hemodynamic causes. Hemodynamic lesions are typically transient and usually manifest in a predictable manner, i.e., after head turning, arm exercise, or decreased blood pressure. Embolic vertebrobasilar events occur unpredictably and often result in cumulative neurologic deficits.

Patients with suspected VBI are optimally managed by an initial medical and neurologic evaluation, discussed above. Imaging of the extra- and intracranial circulation is indicated if no other cardiac, neurologic, or metabolic cause is clearly identified.

Reinfarction After Previous Stroke

Patients with a stable pre-existing stroke who have recurrent infarction should be approached using the acute stroke algorithm outlined above. It is imperative to identify the new areas of damaged cerebrum and pursue an aggressive search for possible causes. Recurrent infarction, particularly when it occurs within several months of the initial stroke, is frequently caused by an ongoing source of embolization from the heart, although the aortic arch and carotid arteries may also serve as the embolic source.[7,8]

CONCLUSIONS

Cerebrovascular disease manifests in a broad spectrum of severity. Patients with carotid artery stenosis may be asymptomatic or present with fatal stroke. The trained vascular surgeon is uniquely capable of primarily managing patients with asymptomatic carotid disease or clear-cut transient monocular and hemispheric ischemia. However, patients with fixed neurologic deficits or atypical symptoms are optimally managed with the assistance of a neurologic specialist. The neurologist has the expertise to characterize neurologic deficits accurately, correlate physical findings with brain imaging abnormalities, and aid in the decision analysis regarding the appropriateness of CEA for acute stroke. In addition, the stroke neurologist possesses additional competency in differentiating vascular and non-vascular syndromes in patients with atypical symptoms.

The neurologist should play a primary role in the assessment and management of the acute stroke patient. However, optimal management of stroke, in a dedicated stroke center, requires a multidisciplinary group consisting of neurologists, vascular surgeons, neurosurgeons, and interventional radiologists. This group possesses the expertise to evaluate and treat the broad spectrum of diseases that cause acute brain ischemia.

REFERENCES

3 Beneficial effect of carotid endarterectomy in symptomatic patients with high-grade carotid stenosis. North American Symptomatic Carotid Endarterectomy Trial Collaborators. *New England Journal of Medicine* 1991; **325**: 445–453.

4 Ferro JM, Falcao I, Rodrigues G *et al*. Diagnosis of transient ischemic attack by the nonneurologist. A validation study. *Stroke* 1996; **27**: 2225–2229.

5 Caplan LR. Top of the basilar syndrome. *Neurology* 1980; **30**: 72.

6 Fisher CM. Lacunar strokes and infarcts: a review. *Neurology* 1982; **32**: 871.

7 Goldstein LB, Perry A. Early recurrent ischemic stroke. A case-control study. *Stroke* 1992; **23**: 1010–1013.

8 Broderick JP, Phillips SJ, O'Fallon WM, Frye RL, Whisnant JP. Relationship of cardiac disease to stroke occurrence, recurrence, and mortality. *Stroke* 1992; **23**: 1250–1256.

9 Bogousslavsky ECO, Regli F. Anterior cerebral artery territory infarction in the Lausanne stroke registry. *Archives of Neurology* 1990; **47**: 144.

10 Caplan L, Babikian V, Helgason C *et al*. Occlusive disease of the middle cerebral artery. *Neurology* 1985; **35**: 975–982.

Editorial Comment

KEY POINTS

1   In the ideal world, patient evaluation and care should be carried out by a multidisciplinary team of neurologists, surgeons and radiologists.
2   In the real world, the role of the neurologist inevitably reflects local referral patterns, staff interests and expertise, concerns over cost-effectiveness, and individualized institutional protocols.
3   Each institution must adopt protocols that promote patient safety and encourage a critical approach to patient selection and evaluation of surgical outcomes.
4   Irrespective of referral patterns, assessment by a stroke neurologist is mandatory for some patients. These include:
   • those with atypical symptoms or examination findings;
   • those being considered for surgery for vertebrobasilar or non-hemispheric symptoms;
   • any patient being considered for urgent or emergency surgery.
5   Assessment by a stroke neurologist is recommended in patients with prior stroke.

Certainly, a stroke neurologist should be involved in every case in which the role of cerebral vascular disease in the pathogenesis of the patient's presenting symptoms or signs is unclear. Likewise, the care of patients with acute stroke is sure to be improved by the careful, serial observations of a stroke neurologist.

The role of the stroke specialist in patients presenting with classical TIAs or amaurosis is less clear. In an ideal world, all patients should be reviewed by a stroke neurologist as part of the multidisciplinary team comprising neurologists, surgeons, neuroradiologists, and interventionists. However, in the real world this tends not to be possible. In the US cost containment enforced by managed care and in the UK the relative scarcity of stroke neurologists makes routine stroke specialist involvement impractical. Thus, in the real world, stroke specialists are not routinely involved in the care of patients with asymptomatic critical carotid disease or those who present with a classical carotid territory event and a critical carotid lesion. This position assumes, of course, that the vascular surgeon is capable of determining the absence of symptoms or the nature of any symptoms present. When there is any doubt over presentation, safety and medicolegal concerns mandate neurologic assessment. One basic rule at the New England Medical Center is that a stroke neurologist should see every patient who undergoes brain imaging studies.

One obvious reason for the discordant views on the role of the stroke neurologist expressed by our authors is that Dr Estes is a carotid surgeon, and Dr Thomas is a neurologist with a specialist interest in stroke. From the surgeon's point of view, involvement of the neurologist in the care of a straightforward patient referred in from a qualified ophthalmologist or experienced internist for carotid surgery would be superfluous, expensive, and potentially harmful to the referral relationship, especially in the US. It may be that the stroke neurologist perceives the surgeon to have a conflict of interest as the final arbiter of the appropriateness of surgery and the beneficiary of performance of the procedure. The stroke neurologist sees his or her role as that of gate-keeper and critical assessor of indications and outcomes. The importance of careful ongoing surgical audit of patient selection and outcomes, especially in centers without routine multidisciplinary input, is underscored in this debate.

13.1

Which non-cardiac medical conditions alter the operative risk?
Jonathan P Thompson (Europe)

INTRODUCTION

The individual assessment of perioperative risk is an important consideration when considering the pros and cons of carotid endarterectomy (CEA). In particular, it allows anaesthetists and surgeons to target preoperative investigations, perioperative monitoring and overall resources more effectively. CEA patients are usually elderly, with a high incidence of generalized vascular and coronary artery disease, hypertension, diabetes, cigarette smoking and related diseases.[1,2] Moreover, because CEA is essentially a prophylactic procedure, it must have well-defined selection criteria and minimum recommended standards for morbidity and mortality.[3-5]

Large, prospective studies have shown that most complications following CEA are related to preoperative risk factors and that the benefits of CEA will only be realized if the perioperative risk is low.[3-6] The role of cardiac risk factors in altering the outcome following carotid surgery has been detailed in another chapter. Information regarding how non-cardiac medical factors alter perioperative risk comes from a number of sources, including:

1   studies related to perioperative risk but not confined to vascular surgery;
2   studies confined to high-risk patients undergoing vascular surgery as a whole;
3   studies in patients undergoing CEA.

Although these apparently disparate sources will inevitably yield conflicting results, all contain useful information, and the reasons for the apparent discrepancies will be discussed.

OVERALL PERIOPERATIVE RISK

It is well established that medical fitness influences the incidence of perioperative complications. The (ASA) classification of physical status, which stratifies patients as being healthy, having mild, moderate or severe systemic disease or being moribund (grades 1–5 respectively), correlates with the *overall* risks of anaesthesia and surgery.[7] In a prospective randomized study of general anaesthesia in 17 201 patients undergoing a variety of surgical procedures, Forrest et al.[8] identified 20 significant predictors for adverse outcome. These included ASA physical status grade 3 or 4, a history of cardiac failure or myocardial infarction, age > 50 years and cardiovascular or neurological surgery. Specifically, a history of ventricular arrhythmia, hypertension, cardiac failure, myocardial ischaemia, myocardial infarction, smoking, ASA status and age were predictive of severe cardiovascular outcome. Similarly, a history of cardiac failure, myocardial ischaemia, chronic obstructive pulmonary disease, obesity, smoking, ASA status and male gender were predictive of severe respiratory outcome. In Forrest's study, diabetes mellitus and renal failure were not significant predictors of cardiovascular or respiratory risk, but these have been implicated in other studies[9-18] (Table 13.1).

Studies investigating perioperative morbidity have focused on cardiac risk.[9-11] These data are particularly relevant to patients undergoing CEA as both perioperative and longer-term morbidity/mortality are primarily related to stroke and cardiovascular morbidity.[2,19-21] Cardiac complications account for 37–50% and stroke for 15–18% of late mortality after CEA.[19-21] Indeed, the coexistence of old age, hypertension, diabetes, renal

Table 13.1
Factors affecting the overall perioperative risk of cardiovascular or respiratory morbidity or death in a variety of surgical patients

Factors affecting risk of cardiovascular or respiratory morbidity, or death	References
Ischaemic heart disease or previous myocardial infarct	Forrest,[8] Goldman,[9] Detsky,[10] Shah,[11] Eagle[12]
Cardiac failure	Forrest,[8] Goldman,[9] Detsky,[10] Eagle,[12] Ashton[13]
Age	Forrest,[8] Goldman,[9] Eagle,[12] Ashton,[13] Pedersen,[14] Browner[15]
ASA grade	Vacanti,[7] Forrest[8]
Hypertension	Forrest,[8] Eagle[12]
Diabetes	Eagle,[12] Foster[16]
Renal failure	Goldman,[9] Browner,[15] Pedersen[14]
Chronic obstructive pulmonary disease	Forrest,[8] Goldman,[9] Detsky,[10] Pedersen[14]
Arrhythmias	Forrest,[8] Goldman,[9] Detsky,[10] Eagle[12]
Obesity	Forrest[8]
Smoking	Forrest[8]
Poor exercise tolerance	Eagle,[12] McPhail[18]

impairment, chronic pulmonary disease, poor general condition, ischaemic heart disease, cardiac failure and cardiac arrhythmias has consistently been implicated as increasing cardiac risk as a whole.[12]

Table 13.2
Risk factors in vascular surgical or high-risk patients

Risk factors	
Ischaemic heart disease	Hertzer,[1] Eagle,[12] Raby,[26] Hollenberg,[27] Fleisher[24]
Diabetes mellitus	Hollenberg,[27] Eagle[45]
Hypertension	Browner,[15] Hollenberg[27]
Left ventricular hypertrophy	Hollenberg,[27] Eagle[45]
Renal impairment	Browner[15]
Age	Eagle[45]

PERIOPERATIVE RISK AND VASCULAR SURGERY

The second main source of data includes studies investigating perioperative risk in patients undergoing peripheral vascular surgery, i.e. not confined to CEA (Table 13.2). Since cardiovascular complications are more common in patients undergoing all types of vascular surgery,[13,22] investigators have again concentrated on perioperative cardiac risk, preoperative cardiac risk factors and methods of investigating or minimizing cardiac risk.[23] However, the existence of common risk factors in the same broad group of patients suggests that some useful information may be inferred from these studies.

Perioperative myocardial ischaemia has been associated with adverse cardiac outcome.[24,25] Raby et al.[26] have shown that silent perioperative myocardial ischaemia occurs in up to 30% of patients undergoing peripheral vascular surgery and was strongly associated with adverse postoperative events.[26] Hollenberg et al.[27] studied the incidence of postoperative myocardial ischaemia in 474 male veterans aged 38–89 undergoing major non-cardiac surgery under general anaesthesia. The patients either had clinical evidence of coronary artery disease or were considered at high risk for coronary artery disease (i.e. they were undergoing vascular surgery or had two of the following risk factors: age > 65 years, hypertension, smoking, hypercholesterolaemia, diabetes mellitus). In addition to proven coronary artery disease, hypertension, diabetes mellitus, left ventricular hypertrophy and digoxin therapy were found to be independent predictors of postoperative myocardial ischaemia. In-hospital mortality was 5%, and was significantly greater in those with preoperative hypertension, renal impairment or severe limitation of physical activity.[15]

PERIOPERATIVE RISK AND CAROTID ENDARTERECTOMY

The third group of data, and potentially the most relevant, would of course be prospective and specific to patients undergoing CEA (Table 13.3). However, most of the available data comes from small retrospective studies which have tended to concentrate on short-term cardiovascular complications or stroke. For example, a single hospital retrospective survey over 20 years following CEA in 279 patients highlighted age, non-insulin-dependent diabetes mellitus and hyperlipidaemia as predictors of early cerebral complications. Preoperative antiplatelet therapy (aspirin or dipyridamole) and a history of smoking were also associated with a decreased risk of complications.[28] Similarly, Assiddao and colleagues[29] found that postoperative hypertension was associated with a higher incidence of transient neurological deficit, and occurred more frequently in patients with preoperative hypertension, particularly if the hypertension was poorly controlled.

Similarly, preoperative cardiac dysrhythmias, renal insufficiency, systolic hypertension, intracranial carotid stenosis and progressive or recent (< 24h) neurological deficit were associated with postoperative hypertension[30] which in itself was associated with an increased risk of death, stroke and possibly cardiac complications.

In the largest single study, McCrory and colleagues[31] reported on 1160 records selected at random from patients who underwent CEA at 12 academic US medical centres between 1987 and 1990. The incidence of perioperative stroke or in-hospital death was 4.8%, while that of myocardial infarction was 2.1%. Adverse outcomes were significantly more common in patients with

ipsilateral hemispheric symptoms, hypertension (diastolic pressure > 110 mmHg), age > 75, a history of angina, internal carotid artery thrombus and a carotid syphon stenosis. The absolute risk was related to the number of risk factors present.

Significant medical risk (defined as the presence of angina, myocardial infarction within 6 months, cardiac failure, hypertension, chronic obstructive pulmonary disease, age > 70 or severe obesity) and neurological risk factors (recent or progressive neurological deficit, multiple transient ischaemic attacks (TIAs) or cerebral infarcts) were shown by Sundt et al. to be predictive of postoperative myocardial infarction or neurological deficit after CEA.[32] At long-term clinical and angiographic follow-up (mean 3.2 years) the authors found that late neurological complications correlated well with the same preoperative neurological risk factors.[33] These findings were confirmed in another retrospective study of 561 patients.[34] Late mortality and rate of myocardial infarction were more frequently encountered in patients with overt coronary artery disease at presentation or those with risk factors for coronary artery disease (diabetes, smoking or hyperlipidaemia).[35,36]

A meta-analysis of 36 studies published between 1980 and 1995 reporting perioperative (30-day) morbidity and mortality in patients undergoing CEA for symptomatic or asymptomatic carotid stenosis demonstrated five clinical characteristics associated with an increased risk of perioperative stroke or death.[37] These included:

1 surgery for cerebral compared to ocular symptoms at presentation;
2 female sex (odds ratio 1.44 (95% confidence interval (CI) 1.14–1.83));
3 age > 75 years (odds ratio 1.36 (95% CI 1.09–1.71));
4 systolic hypertension > 180 mmHg (odds ratio 1.82 (95% CI 1.37–2.41));
5 peripheral vascular disease (odds ratio 2.19 (95% CI 1.4–3.6)).

There was no association with diabetes, angina, recent myocardial infarction, cigarette smoking or presentation with cerebral TIA versus stroke.

Multiple regression analysis of data from the

Table 13.3
Studies of non-cardiac risk factors in carotid endarterectomy

Risk factor	Increased risk? Yes	Number of patients, study type	Increased risk? No	Number of patients, study type
Age	Rothwell[37]	Meta-analysis	Goldstein[46]	1160, retrospective
	ACAS[6]	659, prospective	Geary[47]	1572, retrospective
	Wong[39]	291, retrospective	Pinkerton[48]	607, retrospective
	McCrory[31]	1160, retrospective		
	Goldstein[46]	1160, retrospective		
	Salenius[28]	79, retrospective		
Female sex	Rothwell[37]	Meta-analysis	Geary[47]	1572, retrospective
Systolic hypertension	Rothwell[37]	Meta-analysis	Goldstein[46]	1160, retrospective
	Asiddao[29]	166, retrospective		
	McCrory[31]	1160, retrospective		
Peripheral vascular disease	Rothwell[37]	Meta-analysis		
Smoking	Mackey[35]	597, retrospective	Rothwell[37]	Meta-analysis
Diabetes	Mackey[35]	597, retrospective	Rothwell[37]	Meta-analysis
	Yeager[2]	224, retrospective		
Hyperlipidaemia	Mackey[35]	597, retrospective		
	Salenius[28]	279, retrospective		
Contralateral stenosis	Salenius[28]	279, retrospective	Goldstein[46]	1160, retrospective
	Rothwell[37]	Meta-analysis		
Recent or progressive neurological symptoms	McCrory[31]	1160, retrospective	Goldstein[46]	1160, retrospective
	Geary[47]	1572, retrospective		
	Sundt[32]	331, retrospective		
	Sieber[34]	561, retrospective		
Decreased risk				
Ocular symptoms only	Rothwell[37]	Meta-analysis		
Asymptomatic	Rothwell[38]	Meta-analysis		
Antiplatelet therapy	Wong[39]	91, retrospective		
	Salenius[28]	79, retrospective		

ACAS, Asymptomatic Carotid Atherosclerosis Study.

European Carotid Surgery Trial[38] confirmed that cerebral as opposed to ocular symptoms, female sex, systolic hypertension and peripheral vascular disease were independent risk factors for adverse outcome. The authors recognized the limitations of this type of review (variable quality of reports, possibility of publication bias in studies cited, effect of other confounding variables, demonstration of association rather than causality), but the results are nevertheless valuable. The association of peripheral vascular disease, presumably as a marker of generalized cardiovascular disease, and the lack of effect of other accepted risk factors such as recent myocardial infarction or angina (which may however increase the risk of non-fatal perioperative myocardial infarction) is interesting.

The importance of preoperative neurological status was confirmed in another meta-analysis using similar methods, where the overall rate of 30-day stroke or death was 5.18% in symptomatic patients compared with 3.35% in asymptomatic patients. This was attributable to the lower risk of non-fatal or fatal stroke in asymptomatic patients as the rates for non-stroke death were similar between the groups.[38] The protective effect of antiplatelet medication has been emphasized repeatedly.[28,39]

WHY ARE THERE DISCREPANCIES?

There are several reasons for the discrepancies between the various studies. Some factors which have been shown to predict increased risk elsewhere have not proved significant in patients undergoing CEA, e.g. diabetes, hyperlipidaemia and smoking. This may be because these risk factors are truly not clinically relevant, or because of limitations in study methodology, length of follow-up or definitions, or simply because the studies have used a few crude (i.e. retrospective) indices including death, myocardial infarction or stroke.[31] Similarly, improvements in medical therapy, e.g. thrombolysis and improved management of risk factors, may have changed the overall importance of certain risk factors.

Some studies have also included asymptomatic amongst symptomatic patients in their overall analyses, while surgical variables such as the presence of contralateral disease and surgical technique (use of shunts, anticoagulants or protamine) are rarely standardized. Moreover, the North American Symptomatic Carotid Endarterectomy Trial (NASCET) surgeons were pre-selected on the basis of a low perioperative stroke and death rate. Each of these factors will confound meaningful interpretation of risk factors unless controlled for from the outset.

The importance of chronological as well as physiological age is often ignored, and although the evidence is indirect,[9,10] poor general medical condition is an important individual consideration. It is intuitively obvious that patients with renal or respiratory impairment require increased perioperative monitoring and vigilance although, when specifically studied, these factors often have little effect on outcome. In fact, overall perioperative risk is increased in these patients, although the absolute effect is small in comparison with the risks from significant cardiovascular disease.[12,13]

CONCLUSIONS

Of those non-cardiac factors suspected to increase the perioperative risk in patients undergoing carotid endarterectomy, only female sex, age > 75 years, systolic hypertension and neurological status have consistently been associated with an adverse outcome. However, even systematic studies can only predict average group risk and may not necessarily predict subgroups or individuals at greater or lesser risk of morbidity and mortality. The effect of several coexistent factors may increase individual risk, even though they have no effect in isolation. Similarly, the possibility of end-organ damage should be considered if a condition such as hypertension or diabetes is present.

Since most perioperative medical morbidity is related to cardiac causes, non-cardiac risk factors for cardiovascular morbidity cannot be ignored in the individual patient. In addition to hypertension,[40] obesity, a history of chronic obstructive pulmonary disease, current smoking, diabetes mellitus and renal impairment increase the risk of myocardial ischaemia.[40–42] Similarly, patients with severe respiratory disease, current smoking or obesity are at greater risk of respiratory complications, and poor general medical condition or ASA status correlates broadly with adverse cardiovascular or respiratory outcome.

Of the proven risk factors, only hypertension is amenable to manipulation and, whilst the benefits of beta-blockade in decreasing myocardial ischaemia as well as long-term morbidity[43,44] are well established, the benefit of aggressive preoperative antihypertensive medication in patients with carotid stenosis is less certain.

Therefore, the overall morbidity and mortality associated with CEA may be decreased by thorough preoperative evaluation, identification of risk factors, perioperative medical therapy, optimal anaesthesia and monitoring, but patients are ultimately dependent on surgical expertise.

REFERENCES

1 Hertzer NR. Basic data concerning associated coronary disease in peripheral vascular patients. *Annals of Vascular Surgery* 1987; **1**: 616–620.

2 Yeager RA, Moneta GL, McConnell DB, Neuwelt EA, Taylor LM Jr, Porter JM. Analysis of risk factors for myocardial infarction following carotid endarterectomy. *Archives of Surgery* 1989; **124**: 1142–1149.

3 Moore WS, Barnett HJM, Beebe HG *et al*. Guidelines for carotid endarterectomy. *Circulation* 1995; **91**: 566–579.

4 European Carotid Surgery Trialists Collaborative Group. MRC European Carotid Surgery Trial: interim results for symptomatic patients with severe or with mild carotid stenosis. *Lancet* 1991; **337**: 1235–1243.

5 North American Symptomatic Carotid Endarterectomy Trial Collaborators. Beneficial effect of carotid endarterectomy in symptomatic patients with high-grade stenosis. *New England Journal of Medicine* 1991; **325**: 446–452.

6 Executive Committee for the Asymptomatic Carotid Atherosclerosis Study. Endarterectomy for asymptomatic carotid artery stenosis. *Journal of the American Medical Association* 1995; **273**: 1421–1428.

7 Vacanti CJ, Van Houten RJ, Hill RC. A statistical analysis of the relationship of physical status to postoperative mortality in 68 388 cases. *Anesthesia and Analgesia* 1970; **49**: 564–566.

8 Forrest JB, Rehder K, Cahalan MK, Goldsmith CH. Multicenter study of general anesthesia III. Predictors of severe perioperative adverse outcomes. *Anesthesiology* 1992; **6**: 3–15.

9 Goldman L, Caldera DL, Nussbaum SR. Multifactorial index of cardiac risk in noncardiac surgical procedures. *New England Journal of Medicine* 1977; **297**: 845–850.

10 Detsky AS, Abrams H, Forbath N, Scott JG, Hilliard JR. Cardiac assessment for patients undergoing noncardiac surgery: a multifactorial risk index. *Archives of Internal Medicine* 1986; **146**: 2131–2134.

11 Shah KB, Kleinman BS, Rao TLK, Jacobs HK, Mestan K, Schaafsma M. Angina and other risk factors in patients with cardiac diseases undergoing noncardiac operations. *Anesthesia and Analgesia* 1990; **70**: 240–247.

12 Eagle KA, Brundage BH, Chaitman BR *et al*. Guidelines for perioperative cardiovascular evaluation for noncardiac surgery. *Mayo Clinic Proceedings* 1997; **72**: 524–531.

13 Ashton CM, Petersen NJ, Wray NP *et al*. The incidence of perioperative myocardial infarction in men undergoing noncardiac surgery. *Annals of Internal Medicine* 1993; **118**: 504–510.

14 Pedersen T, Eliasen K, Henriksen E. A prospective study of risk factors and cardiopulmonary complications associated with anaesthesia and surgery: risk indicators of cardiopulmonary morbidity. *Acta Anaesthesiologica Scandinavica* 1990; **34**: 144–155.

15 Browner WS, Li J, Mangano DT. In-hospital and long-term mortality in male veterans following noncardiac surgery. *Journal of the American Medical Association* 1992; **268**: 228–232.

16 Foster ED, Davis KB, Carpenter JA, Abele S, Fray D. Risk of noncardiac operation in patients with defined coronary disease: the Coronary Artery Surgery Study (CASS) Registry experience. *Annals of Thoracic Surgery* 1986; **41**: 42–50.

17 Pedersen T, Eliasen K, Henriksen E. A prospective study of mortality associated with anaesthesia and surgery: risk indicators of mortality in hospital. *Acta Anaesthesiologica Scandinavica* 1990; **34**: 176–182.

18 McPhail N, Calvin JE, Shariatmadar A, Barber GG, Scobie TK. The use of preoperative exercise testing to predict cardiac complications following arterial reconstruction. *Journal of Vascular Surgery* 1988; **7**: 60–68.

19 Hertzer NR, Arison R. Cumulative stroke and survival 10 years after carotid endarterectomy. *Journal of Vascular Surgery* 1985; **2**: 661–668.

20 Mackey WC, O'Donnell TF Jr, Callow AD. Cardiac risk in patients undergoing carotid endarterectomy: impact on perioperative and long-term mortality. *Journal of Vascular Surgery* 1990; **11**: 226–234.

21 Easton JD, Wilterdink JL. Carotid endarterectomy: trials and tribulations. *Annals of Neurology* 1994; **35**: 5–17.

22 Gersh BJ, Rihal CS, Rooke TW, Ballard DJ. Evaluation and management of patients with both peripheral vascular and coronary artery disease. *Journal of the American College of Cardiology* 1991; **18**: 193–202.

23 Fleisher LA, Barash PG. Preoperative cardiac evaluation for non-cardiac surgery: a functional approach. *Anesthesia and Analgesia* 1992; **74**: 586–598.

24 Fleisher LA, Rosenbaum SH, Nelson AH, Barash PG. The predictive value of preoperative silent ischaemia for postoperative ischaemic cardiac events in vascular and nonvascular surgery patients. *American Heart Journal* 1991; **122**: 980–986.

25 Mangano DT, Browner WS, Hollenberg M, Li J, Tateo IM. Long-term cardiac prognosis following noncardiac surgery. *Journal of the American Medical Association* 1992; **268**: 233–239.

26 Raby KE, Barry J, Creager MA, Cook F, Weisberg MC, Goldman L. Detection and significance of intraoperative and postoperative myocardial ischaemia in peripheral vascular surgery. *Journal of the American Medical Association* 1992; **268**: 222–227.

27 Hollenberg M, Mangano DT, Browner WS, London MJ, Tubau JF, Tateo IM. Predictors of postoperative myocardial ischaemia in patients undergoing noncardiac surgery. *Journal of the American Medical Association* 1992; **268**: 205–209.

28 Salenius J-P, Harju E, Riekkinen H. Early cerebral complications in carotid endarterectomy: risk factors. *Journal of Cardiovascular Surgery* 1990; **31**: 162–167.

29 Asiddao CB, Donegan JH, Whitesell RC, Kalbfleisch JH. Factors associated with perioperative complications during carotid endarterectomy. *Anesthesia and Analgesia* 1982; **61**: 631–637.

30 Wong JH, Findlay JM, Suarez-Almazor ME. Hemodynamic instability after carotid endarterectomy: risk factors and associations with operative complications. *Neurosurgery* 1997; **41**: 35–40.

31 McCrory DC, Goldstein LB, Samsa GP *et al*. Predicting complications of carotid endarterectomy. *Stroke* 1993; **24**: 1285–1291.

32 Sundt TM, Sandok BA, Whisnant JP. Carotid endarterecotmy: complications and preoperative assessment of risk. *Mayo Clinic Proceedings* 1975; **50**: 301–306.

33 Sundt TM, Whisnant JP, Houser OW, Fode NC. Prospective study of the effectiveness and durability of carotid endarterectomy. *Mayo Clinic Proceedings* 1990; **65**: 625–635.

34 Sieber FE, Toung TJ, Diringer MN, Wang H, Long DM. Preoperative risks predict neurological outcome following carotid endarterectomy-related stroke. *Neurosurgery* 1992; **30**: 847–853.

35 Mackey WC, O'Donnell TF, Callow AD. Carotid endarterectomy in patients with intracranial vascular disease: short-term risk and long-term outcome. *Journal of Vascular Surgery* 1989; **10**: 432–438.

36 Hertzer NR. Clinical experience with preoperative coronary angiography. *Journal of Vascular Surgery* 1985; **2**: 510–515.

37 Rothwell PM, Slattery J, Warlow CP. Clinical and angiographic predictors of stroke and death from carotid endarterectomy: systematic review. *British Medical Journal* 1997; **315**: 1571–1577.

38 Rothwell PM, Slattery J, Warlow CP. A systematic comparison of the risks of stroke and death due to carotid endarterectomy for symptomatic and asymptomatic stenosis. *Stroke* 1996; **27**: 266–269.

39 Wong JH, Findlay JM, Suarez-Almazor ME. Regional performance of carotid endarterectomy. *Stroke* 1997; **28**: 891–898.

40 Allman KG, Muir A, Howell SJ, Hemming AE, Sear JW, Foex P. Resistant hypertension and preoperative silent myocardial ischaemia in surgical patients. *British Journal of Anaesthesia* 1994; **73**: 574–578.

41 Raby KE, Goldman L, Creager MA *et al*. Correlation between preoperative ischemia and major cardiac events after peripheral vascular surgery. *New England Journal of Medicine* 1989; **321**: 1296–1300.

42 Fleisher LA, Rosenbaum SH, Nelson AH, Barash PG. The predictive value of preoperative silent ischemia for postoperative ischemic cardiac events in vascular and nonvascular surgery patients. *American Heart Journal* 1991; **122**: 980–986.

43 Stone JG, Foex P, Sear JW, Johnson LL, Khambatta HJ, Triner L. Myocardial ischaemia in untreated hypertensive patients: effect of a single small oral dose of a beta-adrenergic blocking agent. *Anesthesiology* 1988; **68**: 495–500.

44 Mangano DT, Layug EL, Wallace A, Tateo I. Effect of atenolol on mortality and cardiovascular morbidity after noncardiac surgery. Multicenter study of perioperative ischaemia research group. *New England Journal of Medicine* 1996; **335**: 1713–1720.

45 Eagle KA, Coley CM, Newell JB *et al*. Combining clinical and thallium data optimizes preoperative assessment of cardiac risk before major vascular surgery. *Annals of Interna Medicine* 1989; **110**: 859–866.

46 Goldstein LB, McCrory DC, Landsman PB *et al*. Multicenter review of preoperative risk factors for carotid endarterectomy in patients with ipsilateral symptoms. *Stroke* 1994; **25**: 1116–1121.

47 Geary KJ, Ouriel K, Geary JE, Fiore WM, Green RM, DeWeese JA. Neurological events following carotid endarterectomy. *Annals of Vascular Surgery* 1993; **7**: 76–82.

48 Pinkerton JA Jr, Gholkar VR. Should patient age be a consideration in carotid endarterectomy? *Journal of Vascular Surgery* 1990; **11**: 650–658.

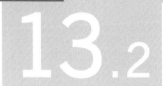

13.2 Which non-cardiac medical conditions alter the operative risk?

Allen D Hamdan (USA)

Frank B Pomposelli Jr (USA)

The major perioperative risks after CEA are neurological events, including TIAs and strokes, myocardial infarction, and death. Although cardiac risk factors play a major role in determining outcome, especially with regard to cardiac morbidity and mortality, several non-cardiac conditions may also have an impact.

DIABETES

Diabetes is a well-recognized risk factor for stroke and also increases the mortality and morbidity from any stroke. In addition, diabetics have a high incidence of pre-existing coronary artery disease which is often silent. Both factors may be responsible for the increased morbidity noted in previous reports on diabetics undergoing CEA.

An early study noted an increased number of strokes in diabetics with a rate of 20% versus 8.2% in non-diabetics. However, there were only 40 diabetics in this report and the overall stroke rate is higher than current standards.[49] A more recent series noted a 3.6% vs 2.2% stroke rate comparing diabetics to non-diabetics, respectively.[50] This relative equality of results was confirmed in a review of 9795 CEA procedures, including 2292 diabetics, which showed no statistically significant difference in stroke rate or mortality.[51]

We recently reported our experience comparing outcomes in 284 diabetics versus 448 non-diabetics undergoing CEA during the same 5-year period.[52] Diabetics undergoing CEA were younger and more likely to have pre-existing risk factors, including coronary artery disease (CAD) and congestive heart failure (CHF). They had a higher incidence of postoperative cardiac events (3.2% vs 1.1%) but on multiple logistic regression analysis neither diabetes

nor CAD proved to be risk factors for cardiac morbidity or mortality. The only clinical predictor was a history of CHF. In regard to postoperative stroke, diabetics and non-diabetics had similar rates (1.0% vs 1.1%). In conclusion, diabetics undergoing CEA need to be monitored closely for perioperative cardiac complications but should be expected to have similar rates of perioperative strokes as non-diabetics.

COAGULATION ABNORMALITIES

There are a number of well-recognized congenital coagulation abnormalities, including deficiencies of protein C, protein S, and antithrombin as well as the more recently described factor V Leiden. These conditions can be found in the general population as well as those undergoing CEA. Evidence that these conditions can adversely affect the results of peripheral vascular procedures has only recently been forthcoming. Moreover, the acquired coagulation abnormality, heparin-induced thrombocytopenia (HIT), may play a specific role in adverse outcomes in CEA.

The effect of protein C, protein S, and antithrombin deficiency as well as the presence of factor V Leiden (resistance to activated protein C (APC-R)) has not been specifically explored in regard to complications after CEA. It has been reported, however, that deficiency of protein C, protein S, or antithrombin can result in intracranial occlusive disease and infarction.[53] In a group of patients with all types of vascular disease, 14% of those undergoing infrainguinal artery reconstruction had APC-R, which is significantly higher than would be expected in a normal population. In addition, their graft patency rate was only 48% at 1 year compared with 88% in the controls. However, of the small group of patients

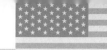

with carotid disease in this report, there was no increase in the percentage of patients with APC-R above what is seen in the general population. Unfortunately, data on the results of CEA in this cohort were not reported.[54] Taking into account these facts, in those undergoing CEA it would be reasonable to assume that patients with hypercoagulable states may have a higher risk of vessel thrombosis. These patients need to be treated with careful intraoperative anticoagulation and possibly prolonged postoperative warfarin. All patients prepared for CEA should be questioned by the surgeon for a history of hypercoagulability and routine screens should be employed in patients with a history of multiple episodes of venous thrombosis or multiple peripheral bypass failures within 30 days of the initial surgery.

HIT results when heparin, usually unfractionated, acts as an antigenic stimulus, probably with platelet factor 4, to form antibodies that lead to vessel wall damage, platelet deposition, and resultant thrombocytopenia. The concern is less for low platelet counts and bleeding diathesis than for thrombosis of vessels. The initial presentation requires about 4–5 days after heparin exposure to allow formation of immunoglobulin G antibodies and is independent of dose. The anamnestic response however can be very rapid. It is not uncommon for vascular patients to undergo multiple operations and thus be exposed to heparin on several occasions.

In a report looking at the cause of perioperative stroke, Riles et al. noted that a large percentage of cases were due to internal carotid artery thrombosis, which they ascribed to technical errors.[50] However, in a review of over 2000 patients at the Mayo Clinic Scottsdale, 6 of their 19 occlusions were considered to be associated with a heparin-induced coagulation disorder.[55] In addition, the Cleveland Clinic reported on 3 patients with suspected HIT who underwent successful CEA with the use of low-molecular-weight heparin (LMWH).[56] However, due to the possibility of cross-reactivity of LMWH, it should be used with caution in patients with HIT.[57] Our current practice is to use danaproid, an Xa inhibitor, and avoid any use of heparin.

Specific thrombin inhibitors may be the proper choice in the future. Since it is only possible to speculate on the true effect of HIT in post-CEA thrombosis, a good rule of thumb would be to check a platelet count on any patient who has been on heparin for 3 days or more and to have a low threshold to order the heparin antibody test.

RENAL FAILURE

It is well known that patients with chronic renal failure have a much higher incidence of death, usually from cardiovascular causes, than patients without renal failure. Specifically in peripheral vascular surgery, renal failure has been associated with increased risks of death and shorter long-term survival after aneurysm repair and lower-extremity vascular reconstruction. In one report, patients with renal insufficiency undergoing infrainguinal vascular reconstruction had a 5 times increase in mortality over patients with normal renal function, and 0 out of 11 patients on hemodialysis survived to 3 years.[58]

A review of 9795 CEA procedures found that dialysis-dependent renal failure produced a statistically significant increase in both mortality and stroke rate. The exact number of strokes and deaths was not reported.[51] In a review of 285 CEAs at the University of Mississippi, the investigators found an extremely high postoperative stroke rate (43%) in patients with creatinine > 2.9 mg/dl compared with a rate of 6% in patients without renal failure. In addition, it appeared that only 1 patient with severe renal insufficiency was alive and well 6 months after CEA. Although this is striking, only 7 patients fell into the category of severe renal insufficiency and their overall stroke rate appears to be higher than the average.[59] In our unpublished experience of 1001 CEAs over 7 years we had 73 patients who had creatinine greater than 1.5 mg/dl, including 3 patients on either hemo- or peritoneal dialysis. The stroke rate in the group with renal insufficiency was significantly higher than in the group with normal renal function (5.5% vs 1.08%).

Given the increased rate of stroke and mortality in patients with renal insufficiency undergoing CEA, recommendations for surgery in these patients should be based on careful evaluation. The surgeon needs to factor in the expected higher rates of complications in this group and should not anticipate the same low rates usually seen for carotid surgery. The American Heart Association consensus statement recommendations may underestimate the risks in renal failure patients.[60] Thus, a patient with CAD on long-standing hemodialysis may not be a good candidate for an incidentally discovered 80% internal carotid stenosis, but it may be reasonable to operate on the same patient with lateralizing TIAs and a high-grade stenosis.

GENDER

With increased rates of smoking in women and accelerated atherosclerosis after menopause, women are now comprising a higher percentage of patients with vascular disease. In relation to CAD there appears to be some treatment bias as well as different outcomes comparing women versus men.[61] With cerebrovascular disease, women have fewer strokes after TIAs and a lower mortality rate after strokes than men.[62]

A review from Northwestern Medical School compared results after CEA in women and men. At baseline, women tended to have less overt evidence of CAD. In comparing operative techniques, women had a higher rate of patch closure. The stroke rate was 3.2% in women and 1.5% in men but the difference was not statistically significant. There was no difference in perioperative cardiac events. However, using life-table analysis the estimated 5-year survival rates were significantly different: 95% in women and 85% in men.[63] Other reports have shown a higher restenosis rate in women compared to men. Two randomized trials identified that women have better results when patch angioplasty is employed.[64,65] In general, gender should not play a role in selecting patients for CEA at this time but most people agree that women (probably due to the smaller artery) will have a higher rate of restenosis if patch angioplasty is not employed.[66]

EXTREMES OF AGE

Most patients undergoing vascular procedures including CEA are over the age of 50. However, there are a small percentage of young patients who appear to have a premature and more aggressive form of atherosclerosis. In one study, young patients aged 25–40 with lower-extremity ischemia had

frequent failure of arterial reconstruction, greater need for repeated procedures, and a high amputation rate compared to an older cohort. Among a number of factors, hypercoaguability appeared to play a major role.[67] One report revealed that 45% of a cohort of patients under age 50 who were undergoing procedures for limb ischemia had some documented abnormality of the clotting/fibrinolytic system and this percentage increased to 100% of those patients who had graft thrombosis in less than 30 days.[68]

Another report, from the Cleveland Clinic, looked at CEA in patients under 50 and found that younger patients had a higher prevalence of smoking, lower high-density lipoprotein and, in women, a high rate of premature menopause. There was no increase in the perioperative stroke rate but there was a much higher percentage of recurrent carotid stenosis (32%) compared to a frequency-matched control of patients over age 60 (12%). Recurrence in the young-age group, however, was almost always asymptomatic.[69] Another report looking at CEA in patients younger than 45 revealed no real difference in perioperative complications but noted a much lower than expected long-term survival.[70]

At the other end of the spectrum is CEA in patients over age 75. This population may be extremely important to study since few patients in the NASCET or Asymptomatic Carotid Atherosclerosis Study (ACAS) were over 75 and no patients were more than 80 years old.[71,72] In addition, due to the increase in the total elderly population and the fact that an 80-year-old woman now has a life expectancy of 9 years and an 80-year-old man has a life expectancy of 7 years, it is likely that the number of very elderly patients requiring vascular procedures will increase.[73]

A number of reports have looked at the results of CEA in this patient population.[74–77] One study revealed no significant difference in stroke or death when comparing to a younger cohort but did find significant increase in mortality for other vascular procedures, such as abdominal aortic aneurysm repair and infrainguinal reconstruction.[77] The reported postoperative stroke and mortality rate in the elderly groups ranged from 2.3% to 6% in these series, which in some instances tended to be higher than the rates seen in younger patients, although these differences were not statistically significant. Of note, although the stroke rate itself was not prohibitive in one report, the mortality rate after stroke was 40%. There was also a fivefold increase in severe intracranial arterial disease (carotid siphon and circle of Willis) in older patients and it was postulated that this may account for the poor tolerance of strokes in this population. In addition, reports have noted a trend towards a longer length of stay in the elderly, especially with current practice trends of early postoperative discharge in patients undergoing CEA.[78]

In conclusion, age alone should not preclude a patient for CEA when the accepted indications are present. (See Chapter 7 for a discussion of the effect of age on the cost–benefit analysis of CEA.) A young patient undergoing CEA may prompt the surgeon to follow up for recurrent stenosis more closely, and possibly test for hypercoagulability. In addition it is reasonable to consider a cardiac evaluation in younger patients undergoing CEA due to the observed decrease in life expectancy, usually resulting from cardiac causes. In the patient older than 75, the surgeon must consider all risk factors in regard to expected survival of each patient, especially in the case of asymptomatic stenosis, where a statistical benefit in stroke reduction will not be realized unless patients live for at least 2 years.

PULMONARY DISEASE

Although pre-existing chronic obstructive pulmonary disease and cigarette use have been shown to increase postoperative respiratory complications after abdominal and thoracic surgery, several studies have not shown this to hold true after CEA.[79,80] Cervical incisions do not compromise respiratory function and most patients are eating and ambulatory by the next day. However, patients who continue to smoke cigarettes after CEA will have a higher rate of restenosis.[66]

SEVERE HYPERTENSION

Severe hypertension pre-, intra-, and postoperatively is common in patients undergoing CEA. In one series, 62% of patients undergoing CEA had a history of controlled hypertension and 58% manifested severe postoperative hypertension. Prior history of hypertension did not increase the risk of postoperative hypertension, while multivariate analysis revealed that diabetes was very closely associated with its development. Diabetics had a 93% incidence of postoperative hypertension versus 52% of non-diabetics.[81]

Reports have noted an increase in postoperative stroke and myocardial infarction in those patients with preoperative hypertension,[80,81] while others have noted an increase in neurologic complications in patients with postoperative hypertension s/pCEA.[81] Postoperative hypertension also appears to play a role in intracerebral hemorrhage, which is the most morbid form of postoperative stroke.[82] In addition, postoperative hypertension appears to be involved in the development of the hyperperfusion syndrome, whereby a loss of the brain's autoregulatory mechanism leads to a relative increase in local perfusion and edema, which is usually manifested by headaches and seizures 3–10 days after CEA.[83]

NEUROLOGIC STATUS

Numerous studies have looked at patients with contralateral carotid artery occlusions and have found no statistically significant difference in neurologic morbidity and mortality or long-term results. Very early studies revealed a combined stroke and death rate of 20–45% in this cohort but these operations were often performed in a setting of acute contralateral occlusion and stroke.[84] However, although the comparative rates did not reach statistical significance, the actual stroke rates in two larger series were 4.8–4.9% versus 2.5–2.6% for patients with contralateral occlusions and those without, respectively. It is unclear if a meta-analysis would uncover a true difference.[85,86] These patients are however at increased risk for postoperative intracerebral hemorrhage and hyperperfusion syndrome.[83]

Patients who have had recent strokes and then undergo CEA appear to be at higher risk for postoperative intracerebral bleeds, hyperperfusion syndrome, and another stroke.[83,87] The higher rate of perioperative strokes in patients who have had a prior stroke may be due to the inability of a zone of

Part Two: Evaluation and Preoperative Management

ischemic but viable tissue around a previous infarct (ischemic penumbra) to tolerate alterations in blood flow during clamping or due to hemodynamic instability.[88] Perioperative strokes are also more common in patients undergoing CEA for TIAs compared to asymptomatic patients (5.2% vs 3.35%).[89] The influence of prior stroke on the indications for CEA and resultant perioperative risks is discussed in Chapters 3 and 4.

There are few reports of patients with high-grade carotid stenosis and other intracranial pathology undergoing CEA. Intracerebral aneurysms can be seen on cerebral magnetic resonance angiography and angiograms in these patients. They are usually less than 10 mm in size and near the middle cerebral artery and intradural portion of the internal carotid artery. Due to size and location they are felt to be unlikely to rupture. Aneurysms that rupture are normally seen in the anterior and posterior communicating arteries. One series looked prospectively at 100 consecutive patients who had an angiogram for carotid stenosis and found 9

Table 13.4
Major non-cardiac conditions that a surgeon is likely to encounter

Risk factor	Increase in strokes	Increase in mortality	Comments
Diabetes	No	No	High silent CAD/monitor closely
Coagulation abnormalities	Unknown	Unknown	Question for HX/evaluate for HIT
Renal insufficiency	Yes	Yes	Carefully consider indications
Gender	No	No	Small arteries should be patched
Younger than 50	No	No	High rate of recurrent stenosis and limited life expectancy
Older than 75	No	No	Postoperative stroke has a high morbidity and mortality Carefully consider asymptomatic cases
Pulmonary disease	No	No	
Severe hypertension	Yes	No	May have a higher rate of HPS and intracerebral bleed
Pre-existing neurologic disease	Probably	No	Patients with co-existent intracranial disease may have higher risk

CAD, coronary artery disease; HIT, heparin-induced thrombocytopenia; HPS, hyperperfusion syndrome.

160

aneurysms, 2 arteriovenous malformations and 15 instances of severe intracranial atherosclerosis (siphon).[90] The reports of these patients with concurrent disease have described successful outcomes after CEA alone, clipping of the aneurysm alone, and performing both operations at the same time. The proper operation or sequence should be determined by the presenting symptoms, and the age and comorbidity of the patient.[91]

CONCLUSIONS

A number of potential risk factors need to be considered when evaluating a patient who has met the criteria for CEA. This chapter has attempted to review the major non-cardiac conditions that the surgeon is likely to encounter (Table 13.4). Diabetics can be expected to have the same stroke rates after CEA as non-diabetics but in general need closer postoperative monitoring and an awareness of the high possibility of silent CAD. Patients with known coagulation abnormalities must be treated with careful and continued postoperative anticoagulation. In addition, the general CEA population has to be routinely evaluated for coagulation problems, especially the patient on several days of intravenous

heparin who may develop HIT. Patients with renal failure are an especially challenging and difficult population and the risks of CEA may outweigh the benefits in some of these patients. Women and men should be treated identically since there appears to be no difference in results, although women and men with small arteries should be patched. Patients younger than 50 should be screened for CAD and hypercoagulable states and follow-up should be close, due to the high rate of restenosis. Patients older than 75 can safely undergo CEA, but in the case of asymptomatic disease an attempt should be made to estimate a specific patient's life expectancy before committing to CEA. Pre-existing pulmonary status probably has no effect on complications but may impact on the choice of regional versus general anesthesia. Severe hypertension should be controlled both pre- and postoperatively. It has been associated with increased stroke rates as well as intracerebral hemorrhage and the hyperperfusion syndrome. The impact of intracerebral pathology is unclear at this time and, although severe hypertension may present a challenging dilemma, the standard indications should apply.

REFERENCES

49 Salenius JP, Harju E, Riekkinen A. Early cerebral complications in carotid endarterectomy: risk factors. *Journal of Cardiovascular Surgery (Torino)* 1990; **31**: 162–167.

50 Riles TS, Imparato AM, Jacobowitz GR et al. The cause of perioperative stroke after carotid endarterectomy. *Journal of Vascular Surgery* 1994; **19**: 206–216.

51 Plecha EJ, King TA, Pitluk HC, Rubin JR. Risk assessment in patients undergoing carotid endarterectomy. *Cardiovascular Surgery* 1993; **1**: 30–32.

52 Akbari CM, Pomposelli FB Jr, Gibbons GW et al. Diabetes mellitus: a risk factor for carotid endarterectomy? *Journal of Vascular Surgery* 1997; **25**: 1070–1076.

53 Barinagarrementeria F, Brito CC, Izaguirre R, de la Pena A. Progressive intracranial occlusive disease associated with deficiency of protein S. *Stroke* 1993; **24**: 1752–1756.

54 Ouriel K, Green RM, DeWeese JA, Cimino C. Activated protein C resistance: prevalence and implications in peripheral vascular disease. *Journal of Vascular Surgery* 1996; **23**: 46–52.

55 Atkinson JL, Sundt TM, Kazmier FJ et al. Heparin-induced thrombocytopenia and thrombosis in ischemic stroke. *Mayo Clinic Proceedings* 1988; **63**: 353–361.

56 Gottlieb A, Tabares AH, Levy P et al. Use of low molecular weight heparin in patients with heparin-induced

thrombocytopenia undergoing carotid endarterectomy. *Anesthesiology* 1996; **85**: 678–681.

57 Warkentin TE, Levine MN, Hirsh J et al. Heparin-induced thrombocytopenia in patients treated with low-molecular-weight heparin or unfractionated heparin. *New England Journal of Medicine* 1995; **332**: 330–335.

58 Whittemore AD, Donaldson MC, Mannick JA. Infrainguinal reconstruction for patients with chronic renal insufficiency. *Journal of Vascular Surgery* 1993; **17**: 32–41.

59 Rigdon ER, Monajjem N, Rhodes RS. Is carotid endarterectomy justified in patients with severe chronic renal insufficiency? *Annals of Vascular Surgery* 1997; **11**: 115–119.

60 Moore WS, Barnett HJM, Beebe HG et al. Guidelines for carotid endarterectomy. *Stroke* 1995; **26**: 188–201.

61 Ayanian J, Epstein AM. Differences in the use of procedures between men and women hospitalized for coronary heart disease. *New England Journal of Medicine* 1991; **325**: 221–225.

62 Eager ED, Chesebro JH, Sacks FM et al. Cardiovascular disease in women. *Circulation* 1993; **88**: 1999–2009.

63 Schneider JR, Droste JS, Golan JF. Carotid endarterectomy in women versus men: patient characteristics and outcomes. *Journal of Vascular Surgery* 1997; **25**: 890–898.

64 Eikelboom BC, Ackerstaff RG, Hoeneveld H *et al*. Benefits of carotid patching: a randomized study. *Journal of Vascular Surgery* 1988; **7**: 240–247.

65 De Letter JAM, Moll FL, Welten RJT *et al*. Benefits of carotid patching: a prospective randomized study with long-term follow-up. *Annals of Vascular Surgery* 1993; **8**: 54–58.

66 Clagett GP, Rich NM, McDonald PT *et al*. Etiologic factors for recurrent carotid stenosis. *Surgery* 1983; **92**: 313–318.

67 Levy PJ, Hornung CA, Haynes JL, Rush DS. Lower extremity ischemia in adults younger than 40 years of age: a community-wide survey of premature arterial disease. *Journal of Vascular Surgery* 1994; **19**: 873–881.

68 Eldrup-Jorgensen J, Flanigan DP, Brace L *et al*. Hypercoaguable states and lower limb ischemia in young adults. *Journal of Vascular Surgery* 1989; **9**: 334–341.

69 Levy PJ, Olin JW, Piedmonte MR *et al*. Carotid endarterectomy in adults 50 years of age and younger: a retrospective comparative study. *Journal of Vascular Surgery* 1997; **25**: 326–331.

70 Mingoli A, Sapienza P, Feldhaus RJ *et al*. Carotid endarterectomy in young adults: is it a worthwhile procedure? *Journal of Vascular Surgery* 1997; **25**: 464–470.

71 Executive committee for the Asymptomatic Carotid Atherosclerosis Study. Endarterectomy for asymptomatic carotid artery stenosis. *Journal of the American Medical Association* 1995; **273**: 1421–1428.

72 North American Symptomatic Carotid Endarterectomy Trial Collaborators. Beneficial effect of carotid endarterectomy in symptomatic patients with high-grade stenosis. *New England Journal of Medicine* 1991; **325**: 445–453.

73 Manton KG, Vaupel JW. Survival after the age of 80 in the United States, Sweden, France, England and Japan. *New England Journal of Medicine* 1995; **333**: 1232–1235.

74 Roques XF, Baudet EM, Clerc F. Results of carotid endarterectomy in patients 75 years of age and older. *Journal of Cardiovascular Surgery* 1991; **32**: 726–731.

75 Perler BA, Williams GM. Carotid endarterectomy in the very elderly: is it worthwhile? *Surgery* 1994; **116**: 479–483.

76 Rosenthal D, Rudderman RH, Jones DH *et al*. Carotid endarterectomy in the octogenarian: is it appropriate? *Journal of Vascular Surgery* 1986; **3**: 782–787.

77 Plecha FR, Bertin VJ, Plecha EJ *et al*. The early results of vascular surgery in patients 75 years of age and older: an analysis of 3259 cases. *Journal of Vascular Surgery* 1985; **3**: 769–774.

78 Perler BA. The impact of advanced age on the results of carotid endarterectomy: an outcome analysis. *Journal of the American College of Surgeons* 1996; **183**: 559–564.

79 Goldstein LB, McCrory DC, Landsman PB *et al*. Multicenter review of preoperative risk factors for carotid endarterectomy in patients with ipsilateral symptoms. *Stroke* 1994; **25**: 1116–1121.

80 McCrory DC, Goldstein LB, Samsa GP *et al*. Predicting complications of carotid endarterectomy. *Stroke* 1993; **24**: 1285–1291.

81 Skydell JL, Machleder HI, Baker D *et al*. Incidence and mechanism of post-carotid endarterectomy hypertension. *Archives of Surgery* 1987; **122**: 1153–1155.

82 Pomposelli FB Jr, Lamparello PJ, Riles TS *et al*. Intracranial hemorrhage after carotid endarterectomy. *Journal of Vascular Surgery* 1988; **7**: 248–255.

83 Nielson TG, Sillesen H, Schroeder TV. Seizures following carotid endarterectomy in patients with severely compromised cerebral circulation. *European Journal of Vascular and Endovascular Surgery* 1995; **9**: 53–57.

84 Heyman A, Young WG Jr, Brown IW Jr. Long term results of endarterectomy of the internal carotid artery for cerebral ischemia and infarction. *Circulation* 1967; **36**: 156–168.

85 Mackey WC, O'Donnell TF, Callow AD. Carotid endarterectomy contralateral to an occluded carotid artery: perioperative risk and late results. *Journal of Vascular Surgery* 1990; **11**: 778–785.

86 McCarthy WJ, Wang R, Pearce WH *et al*. Carotid endarterectomy with an occluded contralateral carotid artery. *American Journal of Surgery* 1993; **166**: 168–172.

87 Mansoor GA, White WB, Grunnet M, Ruby ST. Intracerebral hemorrhage after carotid endarterectomy associated with ipsilateral fibrinoid necrosis: a consequence of the hyperperfusion syndrome? *Journal of Vascular Surgery* 1996; **23**: 147–151.

88 Green RM, Messick WJ, Ricotta JJ *et al*. Benefits, shortcomings and costs of EEG monitoring. *Annals of Surgery* 1985; **201**: 785–792.

89 Rothwell PM, Slattery J, Warlow CP. A systematic comparison of the risks of stroke and death due to carotid endarterectomy for symptomatic and asymptomatic stenosis *Stroke* 1996; **27**: 266–269.

90 Dippel DWJ, Vermeulen M, Braakman R, Habbema JDF. Transient ischemic attacks, carotid stenosis, and an incidental intracranial aneurysm. A decision analysis. *Neurosurgery* 1994; **34**: 449–458.

91 Griffiths PD, Worthy S, Gholkar A. Incidental intracranial vascular pathology in patients investigated for carotid stenosis. *Neuroradiology* 1996; **38**: 25–30.

13.3 Editorial Comment

KEY POINTS

1 Several non-cardiac risk factors influence the perioperative and late risk of stroke, myocardial infarction, and death.
2 Poorly controlled hypertension, chronic renal insufficiency, prior stroke, and severe peripheral vascular disease are associated with an increased risk of perioperative stroke.
3 Chronic renal failure and severe peripheral vascular disease are associated with increased perioperative mortality.
4 The effects of age, gender, diabetes, hyperlipidemia, and cigarette smoking on perioperative risk are unclear (and perhaps minimal once other confounding variables have been removed) but diabetes, hyperlipidemia, and smoking are associated with poorer long-term outcomes.

The respective authors stress that, while many non-cardiac conditions may adversely affect outcome following CEA, the precise impact of these conditions is difficult to assess because few studies have examined non-cardiac risk factors for CEA as apart from other vascular procedures, and the effect of individual non-cardiac risk factors may be difficult to analyze separately from cardiac risk factors, since most of the non-cardiac risk factors are also associated with increased cardiac risk. Despite these problems, it is apparent that several non-cardiac risk factors worsen outcome independently of their effects on cardiac risk. The most significant factors determining perioperative stroke risk (aside from technical error) include uncontrolled hypertension, chronic renal failure, prior stroke (especially recent stroke), and peripheral vascular disease. The most significant non-cardiac factors for perioperative death are chronic renal failure and severe peripheral vascular disease.

Age, as a continuous variable independent of other risk factors, has little influence on perioperative risk. As in most procedures, physiologic age is more important than chronologic age as a risk determinant. Age is, however, a major determinant of long-term survival and is therefore an important factor in risk–benefit analyses. The influence of gender on outcome remains controversial. In ACAS, females gained less benefit than men from surgery, with females suffering higher perioperative and angiographic risk. Other studies have not confirmed this difference. Smoking, diabetes, and hyperlipidemia appear to have a negligible effect on perioperative risk but a significant effect on long-term survival.

14.1

When is preoperative cardiac evaluation advisable?

Jonathan P Thompson (Europe)

INTRODUCTION

'This patient should be fit for carotid endarterectomy (CEA) provided that anaesthesia is stable and appropriate monitoring is used'. There is little benefit in this kind of opinion, sometimes offered by physicians, as this decision can *only* be made by the anaesthetist. However, not all patients can be referred for cardiological assessment before CEA, nor should they be. So, how can the surgeon and anaesthetist decide which patients would benefit most from cardiological referral?

Many patients undergoing CEA have coexistent coronary artery disease, which accounts for over 50% of early and late morbidity/mortality after CEA.[1–5] Data suggest that perioperative and long-term mortality following non-cardiac surgery in patients with documented coronary artery disease is reduced in those who undergo prior coronary revascularization.[1,6,7] For the individual patient, however, the risks of invasive cardiac testing and intervention must be considered and account taken of the potential to delay CEA. Moreover, the value of any cardiological referral depends on local expertise, the availability and quality of any subsequent investigations and the local results from cardiac interventions and carotid surgery.[8,9]

The rationale for requesting formal cardiological referral is:

1 to identify patients at highest risk of suffering perioperative myocardial ischaemia and infarction;
2 to optimize medical treatment of ischaemic heart disease, arrhythmias and ventricular failure;
3 to refer for coronary revascularization or other intervention where appropriate.

PREDICTING RISK?

A history of cardiac failure, valvular lesions (in particular aortic stenosis), arrhythmias, unstable angina and recent myocardial infarction predispose to increased perioperative cardiac morbidity and mortality.[1,4,10–16] The incidence of clinical cardiovascular complications after CEA may be lower than after other types of vascular surgery[11,15] but, all too frequently, perioperative myocardial infarctions are silent[16] and thereafter associated with a mortality of up to 50%. As a consequence, clinicians have attempted to predict overall risk by preoperative invasive and non-invasive testing, with conflicting results. Although a number of cardiac conditions increase the perioperative risk, invasive testing is pointless if it does not affect the overall treatment and outcome.[8,15]

If cardiological evaluation is sought to identify those who might benefit from coronary revascularization, it should also be noted that patients with carotid disease undergoing coronary artery bypass grafting (CABG) have an increased risk of stroke.[17] Patients with combined carotid and coronary artery disease therefore present a difficult clinical problem as they face a higher cardiac and neurological risk from either procedure (see Chapter 13).

CABG before CEA is only appropriate if associated with improved long-term survival[8,15] and is warranted by the patient's cardiac condition alone. CABG is rarely justified simply to 'get the patient through' a subsequent CEA.[11,15] Percutaneous transluminal coronary angioplasty (PTCA) or stenting may be useful alternatives to CABG, particularly in patients with single-vessel coronary artery disease.[18] Retrospective studies have shown that PTCA before non-cardiac surgery reduces the risks of perioperative cardiac death.[19–21] However, PTCA is not without risk, including the need for emergency CABG, and the overall risks are greater in patients with systemic vascular disease.[22] Unfortunately, in the absence of prospective data, the advantages of prior angioplasty or CABG in terms of morbidity and mortality in patients scheduled for CEA remain unproven.

HOW IS CARDIAC RISK CLASSIFIED?

Most of the information regarding preoperative cardiological evaluation comes from the US and, although there are some transatlantic differences,[23] it is generally applicable to European practice. Whilst the assessment of the very high or very low risk patient is relatively straightforward, there has been little consensus on developing a strategy for the patient of intermediate risk. In particular, how should one identify which patients with a history suggestive of ischaemic heart disease benefit from invasive preoperative assessment?

A number of authors have emphasized the importance of functional capacity as a marker of cardiac dysfunction and perioperative cardiac risk.[24–26] This has now been incorporated into the American College of Cardiology/American Heart Association (ACC/AHA) guidelines on perioperative cardiovascular evaluation.[15] In spite (or perhaps as a consequence) of the number of laboratory tests and invasive investigations available, these guidelines rely on a thorough history and clinical examination; the objective is to identify and assess potentially serious or correctable disorders.

Although most patients presenting for CEA can be expected to have significant coronary artery disease, which may be asymptomatic in up to 37%, the incidence of coronary stenosis is significantly higher in those with symptoms.[2,27] Furthermore, clinical suspicion of coronary artery disease is associated with a significant increase in perioperative cardiac morbidity[1] and a doubling in late mortality rates.[15,28] For example, angina associated with symptoms of left ventricular dysfunction (dyspnoea or syncope) may be particularly relevant as the patient may be at particular risk of perioperative hypotension or cardiac failure.[24]

The ACC/AHA guidelines (Table 14.1) define perioperative cardiac risk in terms of surgery-specific and patient-specific risk factors. CEA is classed as an intermediate-risk procedure and patients are allocated to one of three groups depending on the presence of major, intermediate or low predictors of clinical risk.

If the patient has undergone CABG within 5 years and is without current symptoms or signs, no further action is necessary. If, however, there is any evidence of recurrent symptoms, cardiology referral is recommended. Similarly, if the patient has not had a cardiological referral within 2 years and has major clinical predictors of perioperative cardiac risk (unstable coronary syndromes, decompensated congestive cardiac failure, symptomatic arrhythmias or severe valvular disease) coronary angiography or some other invasive assessment is indicated.

If patients are classified as having intermediate predictors of clinical risk using the ACC/AHA guidelines (mild angina, previous myocardial infarction, diabetes mellitus or compensated congestive cardiac failure), the decision to request formal cardiological assessment is based on an assessment of functional capacity. For example, the Duke Activity Status Index[29] grades physical activities according to the estimated oxygen requirements they impose. Basal oxygen requirements are rated as 1 metabolic equivalent (1 MET) and the aerobic demands of strenuous sports (e.g. swimming or football) exceeds 10 METs. Patients unable to sustain moderate physical activity as rated by 4 METs (e.g. walking on the flat at 4 mph, walking up a hill, climbing a flight of stairs, scrubbing floors or playing golf) require formal cardiological assessment.

The choice of first-line, non-invasive investigation depends upon local availability and symptom severity but may include exercise electrocardiogram (ECG), 24-h ECG, resting or stress echocardiography, radionuclide angiography or dipyridamole thallium scanning. No single preoperative test has proved superior for risk assessment[30] and local factors may dictate that cardiology referral is required before any of these non-invasive investigations can be performed.

Table 14.1
American College of Cardiology/American Heart Association guidelines as to clinical predictors of increased perioperative cardiovascular risk (myocardial infarction, congestive heart failure, death)

Major clinical predictors
Unstable coronary syndromes
- Recent* myocardial infarction with evidence of important ischaemic risk by clinical symptoms or non-invasive study
- Unstable or severe[†] angina (Canadian class III or IV; see Campeau[35])
- Decompensated congestive heart failure
- Significant arrhythmias:
  - High-grade atrioventricular block
  - Symptomatic ventricular arrhythmias in the presence of underlying heart disease
  - Supraventricular arrhythmias with uncontrolled ventricular rate
- Severe valvular disease

Intermediate clinical predictors
Mild angina pectoris (Canadian class I or II)
Prior myocardial infarction by history or pathological Q waves
Compensated or prior congestive heart failure
Diabetes mellitus

Minor clinical predictors
Advanced age
Abnormal electrocardiogram (left ventricular hypertrophy, left bundle-branch block, ST abnormalities)
Rhythm other than sinus (e.g. atrial fibrillation)
Low functional capacity (e.g. inability to climb one flight of stairs with a bag of groceries)
History of stroke
Uncontrolled systemic hypertension

---

*The American College of Cardiology National Database Library defines recent myocardial infarction as > 7 days but ″ 1 month (30 days).
[†]May include stable angina in patients who are unusually sedentary.
Reproduced with permission from Eagle *et al.*[15]

Depending on the results of non-invasive testing, further referral and investigation, e.g. coronary angiography, may be appropriate. Conversely, in patients with minor predictors of clinical risk (e.g. old age, isolated ECG abnormalities or atrial fibrillation with controlled ventricular rate, poor functional capacity *per se*, history of stroke or systemic hypertension), no specific tests are recommended.[15] Special precautions may, however, be required in some patients, such as control of hypertension without recourse to a cardiologist.

These guidelines were developed as a response to an increase in the volume of cardiological testing before non-cardiac surgery which had occurred despite a lack of adequately controlled data as to its effect on outcome. The American guidelines are universally applicable, though they assume the ready availability of both expert cardiologist and investigations. This situation may not always apply and therefore I would suggest a more pragmatic, practical approach which aims to target those at risk of perioperative myocardial ischaemia and infarction (Table 14.2).

166

Table 14.2
Specific indications for cardiology referral (see text for definitions)

Cardiac failure with poor functional capacity or poor results on non-invasive testing
Recent myocardial infarction (< 30 days) if surgery is urgent: otherwise delay surgery
Recent myocardial infarction (< 30 months) with poor functional capacity or limited physical activity
Severe or unstable angina, especially if associated with dyspnoea or syncope
Severe valvular disease
Symptomatic arrhythmias
Previous CABG or PTCA with recurrent symptoms, if not under cardiology review < 2 years

CABG, coronary artery bypass graft; PTCA, percutaneous transluminal coronary angioplasty.

WHICH CONDITIONS WARRANT REFERRAL TO A CARDIOLOGIST?

Congestive cardiac failure

Patients with untreated or severe symptoms or signs of cardiac failure should undergo a preliminary non-invasive assessment of cardiac function, e.g. echocardiography or multiple uptake gated acquisition (MUGA) scanning. Despite the limitations of extrapolating the results of resting echocardiography to the dynamic stresses of anaesthesia and surgery,[25] in view of the particular perioperative risks imposed by poor left ventricular function,[10–12] this should be optimized wherever possible. Patients with poor left ventricular function or significant aortic stenosis should thereafter be referred to a cardiologist.

Ischaemic heart angina

The presence of unstable or severe angina on minimal exercise (e.g. climbing a flight of stairs) is an indication for optimization of medical therapy and referral to a cardiologist. The ACC/AHA guidelines recommend coronary angiography as the initial investigation if revascularization is to be considered. Conversely, patients with stable cardiac symptoms

may undergo CEA with minimal extra risk. The risk of myocardial infarction in patients with stable coronary artery disease undergoing CEA is approximately 3.2%, compared with 0.8% in those without coronary artery disease.[4,17,31,32]

Our own approach is to assess whether a patient's coronary or carotid artery disease poses the greater risk on the basis of symptoms and functional capacity. In patients with symptomatic carotid artery disease but stable cardiac symptoms, I do not believe that the potential delays involved and the extra morbidity associated with coronary revascularization are justified. Patients with an asymptomatic carotid stenosis but severe or unstable angina are referred to a cardiologist with a view to coronary revascularization before CEA or as a combined procedure. If CABG were not considered necessary, we would attempt to optimize medical fitness and estimate perioperative cardiac and neurological risk. The increased risk is then discussed with the patient and, if accepted, we would proceed to CEA.

If patients have neurological symptoms and severe cardiac symptoms, similar considerations would apply, i.e. a cardiologist's opinion is sought, and combined or staged coronary and/or carotid surgery performed where appropriate. If coronary intervention is not considered necessary, CEA may be performed, taking all possible precautions in terms of anaesthesia and intra- and postoperative monitoring.

It should be stressed that this approach has been developed in a unit with low perioperative morbidity and mortality and may not be universally applicable.[33] Moreover, the optimal timing of CEA after CABG or PTCA is unknown. In the first few days, the coronary angioplasty site remains at risk of secondary thrombosis, whilst the risk of restenosis increases in the first few months. Although operation after 'at least several days' has been recommended,[15,23] in the absence of prospective controlled data a delay of 1 week after PTCA and 6 weeks after CABG seems reasonable.[18,23] Conversely, there are no data to show how long PTCA might protect against subsequent perioperative myocardial infarction, although restenosis is unlikely after 6 months. The ACC guidelines suggest that, if

167

at 6 months the patient is active and asymptomatic, it is reasonable to expect ongoing protection for up to 5 years.[15]

Peripheral vascular disease

Patients whose functional capacity or ability to exercise is limited by intermittent claudication present a particularly difficult problem with regard to the assessment of cardiological risk. These patients have a high prevalence of ischaemic heart disease and the ACC guidelines recommend alternative methods of functional assessment, such as dobutamine stress echocardiography or dipyridamole-thallium imaging.

These tests have a low positive predictive value for adverse cardiac outcomes, although adverse outcomes are rare if the test result is normal.[15] Our own experience suggests that, if a patient presenting for CEA has few symptoms of angina and no clinical or radiological evidence of cardiac failure, further investigation is unnecessary.

Arrhythmias

Patients with complete heart block, symptomatic ventricular arrhythmias or supraventricular arrhythmias with an uncontrolled ventricular rate (> 100 beats/min) should always be referred for formal cardiological assessment. This will allow optimization of medical therapy, including cardiac pacing if necessary, so as to enable CEA to be performed as soon as reasonably possible.

Previous myocardial infarction

Advances in cardiology over the last 15–20 years have gradually diminished the overall perioperative risk associated with recent myocardial infarction. For example, the widespread use of thrombolysis, percutaneous coronary angioplasty and secondary prevention after myocardial infarction have decreased the incidence of reinfarction within

6 months. The ACC has therefore abandoned the absolute time interval after infarction as an independent factor in perioperative cardiac risk,[15] although delaying elective surgery for 4–6 weeks is advised where possible. However, a recent myocardial infarction (within 7–30 days) remains a major predictor of perioperative cardiac risk.

Most patients who have suffered a myocardial infarction will already have been evaluated by a cardiologist and may have undergone exercise ECG testing during convalescence.[34] If not, the patient's current functional capacity should be assessed. Patients with good functional capacity and who have returned to full activity with no further cardiac symptoms require no further invasive testing. However, patients with either poor functional capacity or limited activity merit cardiology referral. In the absence of prospective data, we would currently prefer to delay CEA for 3 months after an acute myocardial infarction recognizing that this period is relatively arbitrary. If, however, the patient has unstable neurological symptoms, urgent cardiological assessment is essential.

CONCLUSIONS

Most patients presenting for CEA have underlying cardiac disease, but relatively few require formal cardiology referral. As a general rule, however, patients with the following should be referred for cardiological assessment:

1 cardiac failure with poor functional capacity;
2 recent myocardial infarction;
3 severe or unstable angina, especially if associated with dyspnoea or syncope;
4 severe valvular heart disease;
5 symptomatic arrhythmias;
6 previous CABG or PTCA in whom symptoms have recurred.

REFERENCES

1 Hertzer NR. Basic data concerning associated coronary disease in peripheral vascular patients. *Annals of Vascular Surgery* 1987; 1: 616–620.
2 Hertzer NR, Young JR, Beven EG. Coronary angiography in

506 patients with extracranial cerebrovascular disease. *Archives of Internal Medicine* 1985; 145: 849–852.
3 Hertzer NR, Arison R. Cumulative stroke and survival ten

years after carotid endarterectomy. *Journal of Vascular Surgery* 1985; **2**: 661–668.

4 Mackey WC, O'Donnell TF Jr, Callow AD. Cardiac risk in patients undergoing carotid endarterectomy: impact on perioperative and long-term mortality. *Journal of Vascular Surgery* 1990; **11**: 226–234.

5 Chimowitz MI, Weiss DG, Cohen SL et al. Cardiac prognosis of patients with carotid stenosis and no history of coronary-artery disease. *Stroke* 1994; **254**: 759–765.

6 Foster ED, Davis KB, Carpenter JA, Abele S, Fray D. Risk of noncardiac operation in patients with defined coronary disease: the Coronary Artery Surgery Study (CASS) registry experience. *Annals of Thoracic Surgery* 1986; **41**: 42–50.

7 Eagle KA, Rihal CS, Mickel MC et al. Cardiac risk of noncardiac surgery. Influence of coronary disease and type of surgery in 3368 operations. *Circulation* 1997; **96**: 1882–1887.

8 Fleisher LA, Eagle KA. Screening for cardiac disease in patients having noncardiac surgery. *Annals of Internal Medicine* 1996; **124**: 767–772.

9 Moore WS, Barnett HJM, Beebe HG et al. Guidelines for carotid endarterectomy. *Circulation* 1995; **91**: 566–579.

10 Detsky AS, Abrams H, Forbath N, Scott JG, Hilliard JR. Cardiac assessment for patients undergoing noncardiac surgery: a multifactorial risk index. *Archives of Internal Medicine* 1986; **146**: 2131–2134.

11 Gersh BJ, Rihal CS, Rooke TW, Ballard DJ. Evaluation and management of patients with both peripheral vascular and coronary artery disease. *Journal of the American College of Cardiologists* 1991; **18**: 193–202.

12 Mangano DT. Perioperative cardiac morbidity. *Anesthesiology* 1990; **72**: 153–184.

13 Mangano DT, Browner WS, Hollenberg M, London MJ, Tubau JF, Tateo IM. Association of perioperative myocardial ischaemia with cardiac morbidity and mortality in men undergoing noncardiac surgery: the study of the perioperative ischemia research group. *New England Journal of Medicine* 1990; **323**: 1781–1788.

14 Fleisher LA, Rosenbaum SH, Nelson AH, Barash PG. The predictive value of preoperative silent ischaemia for postoperative ischaemic cardiac events in vascular and nonvascular surgery patients. *American Heart Journal* 1991; **122**: 980–986.

15 Eagle KA, Brundage BH, Chaitman BR et al. Guidelines for perioperative cardiovascular evaluation for noncardiac surgery: report of the American College of Cardiology/American Heart Association task force on practice guidelines (committee on perioperative cardiovascular evaluation for noncardiac surgery). *Journal of the American College of Cardiologists* 1996; **27**: 910–948.

16 Charlson ME, Mackenzie CR, Ales K, Gold JP, Fairclough G, Shires GT. Surveillance for postoperative myocardial infarction after noncardiac operations. *Surgery, Gynaecology and Obstetrics* 1988; **167**: 407–414.

17 Wilke HJ, Ellis JE, McKinsey JF. Carotid endarterectomy: perioperative and anaesthetic considerations. *Journal of Cardiothoracic and Vascular Anesthesia* 1996; **10**: 928–949.

18 Rihal CS. The role of myocardial revascularisation preceding noncardiac surgery. *Progress in Cardiovascular Disease* 1998; **40**: 383–404.

19 Elmore JR, Hallett JW, Gibbons RJ et al. Myocardial revascularisation before abdominal aortic aneurysmorrhaphy: effect of coronary angioplasty. *Mayo Clinic Proceedings* 1993; **68**: 637–641.

20 Gagnon RM, Dumont G, Sestier F et al. The role of coronary angioplasty in patients with associated noncardiac medical and surgical condidtions. *Canadian Journal of Cardiology* 1990; **6**: 287–292.

21 Huber KC, Evans MA, Bresnahan JF, Gibbons RJ, Holmes DR. Outcome of noncardiac operations in patients with severe coronary artery disease successfully treated preoperatively with coronary angioplasty. *Mayo Clinic Proceedings* 1992; **67**: 15–21.

22 Sutton-Tyrell K, Rihal C, Burek K et al. Long-term prognostic value of cerebral and lower extremity atherosclerosis in patients undergoing coronary revascularisation in the Bypass Angioplasty Revascularisation Study (BARI). *Circulation* 1996; **94**: I–175 (abstract).

23 Cohen MC. The role of the cardiology consultant: putting it all together. *Progress in Cardiovascular Disease* 1998; **40**: 419–440.

24 Fleisher LA, Barash PG. Preoperative cardiac evaluation for non-cardiac surgery: a functional approach. *Anesthesia and Analgesia* 1992; **74**: 586–598.

25 McPhail N, Calvin JE, Shariatmadar A, Barber GG, Scobie TK. The use of preoperative exercise testing to predict cardiac complications following arterial reconstruction. *Journal of Vascular Surgery* 1988; **7**: 60–68.

26 Cutler BS, Wheeler HB, Paraskos JA, Cardullo PA. Applicability and interpretation of electrocardiographic stress testing in patients with peripheral vascular disease. *American Journal of Surgery* 1981; **141**: 501–506.

27 Paul SD, Eagle KA, Kuntz KM, Young JR, Hertzer NR. Concordance of preoperative clinical risk with angiographic severity of coronary artery disease in patients undergoing vascular surgery. *Circulation* 1996; **94**: 1561–1566.

28 Hertzer NR, Young JR, Beven EG et al. Late results of coronary bypass in patients with peripheral vascular disease, II: five-year survival according to sex, hypertension and diabetes. *Cleveland Clinic Journal of Medicine* 1987; **54**: 15–23.

29 Hlatky MA, Boineau RE, Higginbotham MB et al. A brief self-admistered questionnaire to determine functional capacity (the Duke Activity Status Index). *American Journal of Cardiology* 1989; **64**: 651–654.

30 Mantha S, Roizen MF, Barnard J, Thisted RA, Ellis JE, Foss J. Relative effectiveness of four preoperative tests for predicting adverse cardiac outcomes after vascular surgery: a meta-analysis. *Anesthesia and Analgesia* 1994; **79**: 422–433.

31 Huber KC, Evans MA, Bresnahan JF, Gibbons RJ, Holmes DR. Outcome of non-cardiac operations in patients with severe coronary artery disease successfully treated pre-operatively with coronary angioplasty. *Mayo Clinic Proceedings* 1993; **67**: 15–21.

32 Urbinati S, DiPasquale G, Andreoli A et al. Preoperative noninvasive coronary risk stratification in candidates for carotid endarterectomy. *Stroke* 1994; **25**: 2022–2027.

33 Naylor AR, Thompson MM, Varty K, Sayers RD, London NJM, Bell PRF. Provision of training in carotid surgery

does not compromise patient safety. *British Journal of Surgery* 1988; **85**: 939–942.

34 Ryan TJ, Anderson JL, Antman EM *et al*. ACC/AHA guidelines for the management of patients with acute myocardial infarction. *Journal of the American College of Cardiology* 1996; **28**: 1328–1428.

35 Campeau L. Grading of angina pectoris. *Circulation* 1976; **54**: 522–523.

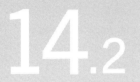

14.2

When is preoperative cardiac evaluation advisable?

Michael Belkin (USA)

Mark W Sebastian (USA)

INTRODUCTION

The effectiveness of CEA in the prevention of stroke is now well established.[36,37] Atherosclerosis, however, is a systemic disease and associated coronary artery disease is prevalent in patients undergoing carotid surgery. A great deal of attention in the vascular literature has been focused on the perioperative evaluation and management of coronary artery disease in patients undergoing vascular surgery. Remarkably, less attention has been focused on the evaluation of coronary artery disease in patients undergoing CEA rather than other vascular operations. This is despite the fact that perioperative myocardial infarction remains a major contributor to perioperative and late deaths after CEA.

A number of factors have been responsible for the decreased emphasis on perioperative cardiac evaluation of carotid patients. These include the perception that CEA is a focused surgical procedure without the hemodynamic stress associated with larger vascular reconstructions. Some authors have advocated that the performance of this operation under regional anesthesia also decreases cardiac stress, morbidity, and mortality.[38,39] Furthermore, CEA is unusual in that it is the only major vascular reconstructive procedure that may be easily and effectively combined with CABG. The ability to combine these procedures can occasionally simplify the complex staging process for patients who have concurrent severe disease in both systems.

In this chapter, we will review the impact of coronary artery disease on patients undergoing CEA. The unique aspects of CEA which differentiate it from other major vascular reconstructive procedures will be addressed. The incidence of coronary artery

disease in patients undergoing CEA is reviewed in detail and the impact of coronary artery disease on perioperative morbidity and mortality, as well as late survival, is discussed. Finally, our approach to cardiac evaluation, risk factor modification, and the staging of surgical procedures is reviewed. The underlying theme of evaluating and treating atherosclerosis as a systemic disease with the vascular surgeon serving as the vascular specialist for the whole patient is developed and stressed.

UNIQUE ASPECTS OF CAROTID ENDARTERECTOMY

Hemodynamic Stresses

Unlike many vascular surgical operations which involve major surgical incisions, significant blood loss, and major intravascular volume shifts, CEA is a more isolated surgical procedure, performed through a small incision with minimal blood loss. Routine discharge from the hospital on the first postoperative day testifies to how well tolerated this surgical procedure is in the vast majority of patients. Despite these relative advantages, there are unique potential hemodynamic stresses associated with CEA which differentiate it from other vascular surgical procedures. Chief among these stresses is the significant lability of blood pressure which many CEA patients suffer, resulting in significant hypotension and hypertension. All experienced vascular surgeons have occasionally witnessed a patient suffering profound bradycardia or broad swings in blood pressure necessitating alternating treatment with vasodilators and vasoconstrictors. A number of theories have been proposed to explain this significant lability in blood pressure. The most widely accepted theory relates to the baroreceptors, which are located within the adventitia of the internal carotid artery at the carotid bifurcation. These baroreceptors send impulses to the carotid sinus nerve, which runs between the external and internal carotid arteries to the glossopharyngeal nerve, which in turn affects blood pressure centers within the medulla oblongata. It has been theorized that direct surgical stimulation of the baroreceptors, as well as the increased stretch imparted to the baroreceptors as the endarterectomized vessel is reperfused, results in increased stimulation, resulting in bradycardia and peripheral vasodilatation, thereby resulting in hypotension.[40,41] When significant bradycardia and hypotension occur intraoperatively, infiltration along the carotid sinus nerve with 1% lidocaine is helpful in reversing both immediate and postoperative hypotension.[42]

Perioperative hypertension tends to be a more difficult problem. In addition to the cardiac stresses imparted by elevated systolic blood pressures, hemorrhagic complications within the wound and intracranial bleeding are increased in this setting.[43] A number of poorly understood factors may contribute to this significant perioperative hypertension. Unrecognized damage to the carotid sinus nerve during the carotid dissection may decrease impulses to the medulla, erroneously suggesting hypotension, and resulting in hypertensive compensation.[42,44] Abnormalities in cerebral autoregulation, resulting from the sudden increased perfusion from a chronically stenosed vessel, may contribute to the hypertension, as may the release of renin from the central nervous system.[45] Although wide swings in perioperative blood pressure must be controlled with vasodilators (sodium nitroprusside, nitroglycerin) or vasopressors (phenylephrine, epinephrine), the need for significant pressor therapy may contribute to postoperative myocardial ischemia and infarction.[38]

Regional Anesthesia
Advocates of CEA under regional anesthesia suggest a number of advantages over general anesthesia.[38,39] These include shorter operative time, a decreased need for intraluminal shunting, less lability of blood pressure, decreased need for the

surgical intensive care unit, and decreased cardiopulmonary morbidity. This issue is discussed in more detail in Chapter 16. A careful review of the literature, however, does not suggest any significant advantage in decreasing cardiac morbidity or mortality when regional anesthesia is compared to general anesthesia. A large comparative series identified a 2.9% myocardial infarction rate for general anesthesia versus a 0.7% rate for cervical anesthesia, a trend which did not reach statistical significance.[39] Similarly, the cardiac death rate of 0.8% for general anesthesia did not differ from the 0.3% death rate for regional anesthesia. Another large series from advocates of carotid endarterectomy using regional anesthesia at New York University also failed to identify significant differences in perioperative myocardial infarction or cardiac death rate based on anesthetic technique.[46] In the most recent series over the past decade, the perioperative myocardial infarction rate was 0.6% for regional anesthesia versus 1.2% for general anesthesia, with perioperative cardiac death rates of 0.9% in each group.

Although the application of regional anesthesia has offered potential advantages in terms of cardiac morbidity and mortality in the past, recent advances in general anesthetic techniques have effectively eliminated significant differences in the modern literature.

Combined Carotid Endarterectomy and Coronary Artery Bypass Surgery
The ability to combine the CEA with coronary bypass surgery offers a unique alternative in patients who present with severe symptomatic carotid artery occlusive disease and unstable coronary artery disease. The advantages and limitations of this combined approach are discussed in Chapter 6. More difficult to determine, however, is the appropriate application of this combined approach in patients who have asymptomatic carotid stenosis or unstable coronary artery disease. A collective review of the literature has identified a 5.6% stroke rate for the combined operation.[47] This is certainly a higher stroke rate than would commonly be encountered under the conditions of CEA alone or coronary artery bypass surgery in the absence of CEA. Whether or

not the stroke morbidity and mortality rates of the combined procedures would be less than the additive morbidity and mortality of the procedures performed separately is the subject of intense debate and awaits resolution through a large prospective randomized trial. On our service, we tend to treat the carotid and coronary disease on their own merits. Thus, we prefer to combine the procedures for patients who have high-grade symptomatic carotid stenosis and unstable symptoms of angina. We would also consider CEA for patients with asymptomatic bilateral high-grade stenosis when coronary artery bypass surgery is warranted. The overall cardiac morbidity and mortality of carotid artery surgery (reviewed below) has become sufficiently low that we would not recommend the surgical treatment of coronary artery disease to 'get the patient through' carotid surgery.

In summary, it is best to approach the surgical treatment of carotid and coronary artery disease based on their individual merits. In selected cases, it may prove to be more cost-effective and convenient, and potentially safer to combine these procedures.

INCIDENCE OF CORONARY ARTERY DISEASE IN PATIENTS UNDERGOING CAROTID ENDARTERECTOMY

Large series of CEA patients have revealed a significant incidence of coronary artery disease as well as risk factors for atherosclerosis. As seen in Table 14.3, a history of myocardial infarction is present in 18–24% of patients.[37,47,48] Similarly, 17–22% of patients have a history of angina. Over 50% of patients have a significant history of tobacco abuse and the North American Symptomatic Carotid Endarterectomy Trial (NASCET) trial demonstrated that 37% of patients were currently active smokers.[37] Similarly, 28% of the surgical patients in the Asymptomatic Carotid Atherosclerosis Study (ACAS) trial were also currently active smokers.[36] Diabetes is present in 17–20% of patients, with documented hyperlipidemia in 12–21% of patients. Hypertension is common, occurring in approximately 60% of patients undergoing CEA.

Perhaps the best indicator of the true incidence of coronary artery disease in patients undergoing CEA comes from the seminal work of Hertzer and

Table 14.3
Coronary artery disease and risk factors

Risk factor	CAD prevalence		
	Mackey et al.[48]	Rizzo et al.[47]	NASCET[37]
History of myocardial infarction	24.3%	19%	18%
Angina	21.3%	17%	17%
Current cigarette use			37%
Significant smoking history	62.1%	48%	
Diabetes	20.5%	18%	17%
Hyperlipidemia	12.1%	16%	21%
Hypertension	62.2%	59%	60%

NASCET, North American Symptomatic Carotid Endarterectomy Trial; CAD, coronary artery disease

colleagues from the Cleveland Clinic.[49] In the early 1980s, these authors performed routine coronary angiography prospectively on 506 patients who presented for CEA. Sixty percent of the patients had a clinical history of coronary artery disease, including a past myocardial infarction, angina pectoris, or electrocardiogram changes. As demonstrated in Table 14.4, among patients with clinically suspected coronary artery disease, 35.6% were found to have severe correctable coronary artery disease and 9.8% were found to have severe, inoperable coronary artery disease. Perhaps more remarkable, however, was the finding that among patients with no clinical evidence of coronary artery disease, 16% were found to have severe correctable coronary artery disease and 1.5% were found to have severe inoperable coronary artery disease. Only 13.5% of patients with no clinically suspected coronary artery disease had normal coronary arteries. Inoperable disease was particularly common (14%) among those patients with diabetes.

Another prospective study used exercise thallium-

201 myocardial scintigraphy to evaluate prospectively the incidence of coronary artery disease in patients with cerebrovascular occlusive disease.[50] Ninety-four percent of patients who were clinically suspected to have coronary artery disease were found to have positive exercise thallium stress tests. Similar to Hertzer's findings, however, a full 41% of patients without clinically suspected coronary artery disease had positive exercise thallium stress tests.

In summary, a significant percentage of patients presenting for CEA will have a clinical history of coronary artery disease or significant risk factors for the same. More importantly, however, both non-invasive studies and prospectively applied coronary arteriography have confirmed a high incidence of significant coronary artery disease in patients who have no clinical indicators of coronary artery stenosis.

SHORT- AND LONG-TERM CARDIAC MORBIDITY AND MORTALITY AFTER CAROTID ENDARTERECTOMY

Despite the high incidence of documented coronary artery disease in patients undergoing CEA, the perioperative cardiac morbidity and mortality have been acceptably low. Table 14.5 reviews a large series of patients undergoing CEA from the late 1970s through the early 1990s.[38,48,51,52] Over this time interval, cardiac morbidity and mortality rates remained remarkably stable. The overall incidence of myocardial infarction ranged from 1.5% to 4% with fatal perioperative myocardial infarctions occurring in 0.4–0.9% of cases. Patients with clinical evidence of coronary artery disease (prior myocardial infarction, angina, or electrocardiogram changes) had a significantly poorer outcome than those with no evidence of clinically overt coronary artery disease, suffering a 5.9% incidence of myocardial infarction (range 2.9–6.1%) with a 2.7% fatal myocardial infarction rate (range 0.9–2.9%). Conversely, patients with no clinically

Table 14.4
Prospective angiography of 506 patients presenting for carotid endarterectomy

	No clinical CAD	Clinical CAD
Normal coronary arteries	13.5%	2.9%
Mild to moderate CAD	46.5%	16.9%
Advanced compensated CAD	22.5%	35.6%
Severe surgically correctable CAD	16%	37%
Severe inoperable CAD	1.5%	9.8%

CAD, coronary artery disease.
Reproduced with permission from Hertzer et al.[49]

Table 14.5
Perioperative cardiac morbidity and mortality

Author	Total group			Clinical CAD			No overt CAD		
	No.	Total No. of MI	No. of fatal MI	No.	Total No. of MI	No. of fatal MI	No.	Total No. of MI	No. of fatal MI
Ennix et al.[51]	1391	21 (1.5)	13 (0.9)	85	11 (2.9)	11 (2.9)	1306	10 (0.8)	2 (0.2)
Riles et al.[38]	683	16 (2.3)	5 (0.7)	284	14 (4.9)	5 (1.8)	399	2 (0.5)	0 (0.0)
Yeager et al.[52]	249	10 (4.0)	1 (0.4)	114	7 (6.1)	1 (0.9)	139	3 (2.2)	0 (0.0)
Mackey et al.[48]	614	16 (2.6)	5 (0.8)	324	14 (4.3)	5 (1.5)	290	2 (0.7)	0 (0.0)
Total	2937	63 (2.2)	23 (0.8)	807	46 (5.7)	22 (2.7)	2134	17 (0.8)	2 (0.1)

MI, myocardial infarction; CAD, coronary artery disease.

overt evidence of coronary artery disease had only a 0.8% incidence of perioperative myocardial infarction (range 0.5–2.2%) with only a 0.1% fatal myocardial infarction rate (range 0–0.2%). The perioperative cardiac morbidity and mortality from the recent NASCET trial was similar to that of these large single-institution studies, with a 0.9% myocardial infarction rate and a 0.3% ischemic cardiac death rate.[37] Although the vast majority of patients enjoy a smooth perioperative course without cardiac complications, the 5.7% incidence of myocardial infarctions and 2.7% incidence of fatal cardiac complications in patients with clinical evidence of coronary artery disease is quite sobering.

Although the incidence of perioperative cardiac complications has been the most closely scrutinized parameter among vascular surgeons, the long-term impact of coronary artery disease on late survival after CEA is extremely important. A number of studies have determined that approximately 30–60% of late deaths after CEA are attributable to coronary artery disease.[48,52,53] Table 14.6 demonstrates the long-term survival of patients after CEA.[48,54–56] The 5-year survival rates of 72–78% are clearly lower than the 93% expected 5-year survival of age-matched controls. Similarly, the 36–64% 10-year survivals are lower than the 80% expected 10-year survival of age-matched normal individuals.

Table 14.6
Late survival after carotid endarterectomy

	5-year	10-year	Cardiac death
Mackey et al.[48]	77%	48%	36.4%
Hertzer et al.[54]	71.6%	42.5%	37%
Lord[55]	78%	64%	
Bernstein and Dilley[56]	73.3%	36.6%	
Age-matched population	93%	80%	5%

Adapted with permission from Mackey et al.[48]

Clearly, coronary artery disease impacts severely on the long-term morbidity and mortality of patients after CEA. It is essential for vascular surgeons to focus on atherosclerosis as a systemic disease requiring effective management strategies and risk factor modification in order to maximize both quality of life and survival. To take the short-term view of minimal evaluation and intervention to simply 'get the patient through' the perioperative period fails to seize a major opportunity to impact on the long-term well-being of our patients.

EVALUATION AND MANAGEMENT OF CORONARY ARTERY DISEASE IN PATIENTS UNDERGOING CAROTID ENDARTERECTOMY

Rationale

Given the high incidence of coronary artery disease in patients undergoing CEA and the appreciable cardiac morbidity and mortality of this operation, we believe that all patients undergoing elective CEA should undergo a preoperative cardiac evaluation. On our service, patients undergoing elective CEA are evaluated preoperatively by cardiologists from the vascular medicine service. Routine preoperative evaluation of all patients undergoing peripheral vascular reconstructions, including CEA, offers several advantages.

The most important advantage is the preoperative identification of the important minority of patients who are at high risk for cardiac complications based on their past history or presenting characteristics. These patients undergo further cardiac testing with either Persantine–Sestamibi myocardial scintigraphy or ambulatory Holter monitoring for myocardial ischemia. Patients with positive stress tests undergo optimization of their medical regimen in preparation for their surgery. Only a small minority of patients, such as those with unstable angina, are referred on for coronary angiography for possible coronary revascularization. It is clearly unnecessary to subject patients to coronary revascularization for the express purpose of getting them through CEA in a safe manner. Coronary revascularization should be recommended based on the degree of coronary artery disease, independent of the need for CEA. When patients are identified as having significant coronary artery disease and appreciable risk of cardiac morbidity or mortality, surgeons should be very cautious in recommending CEA for asymptomatic stenosis. Although the ACAS trial showed a statistically significant benefit to patients treated with CEA for high-grade asymptomatic carotid stenosis, it should be remembered that the benefits of CEA over medical management were relatively modest and clearly dependent upon the less than 3% perioperative morbidity and mortality which were achieved in that study.[36] Furthermore, high-risk patients with significant coronary artery disease were excluded from enrollment in the ACAS trial. The significant but modest benefits of CEA for asymptomatic stenosis could clearly be eliminated if the procedure were applied to a series of patients at excessive risk for cardiac morbidity and mortality.

The second goal of the cardiac evaluation is to allow preoperative adjustments in the patient's medical regimen in order to minimize perioperative risk. Optimization of the medical regimen generally involves the addition or modification of appropriate cardiac medications, including the establishment of an effective beta-blockade regimen. The utility of routine beta-blockade on cardiovascular morbidity and mortality after non-cardiac surgery has been established, not only during the perioperative period but over the first 2 years after surgery.[57,58] Based on preoperative and ambulatory Holter monitoring for cardiac ischemia, we and others have demonstrated the relationship between perioperative tachycardia and myocardial ischemia.[59,60] The use of oral as well as intravenous beta-blockade may be directed at maintaining the heart rate below the threshold value of tachycardia which results in cardiac ischemia. Patients with a recent history of a myocardial infarction should have elective CEA (primarily that performed for asymptomatic carotid stenosis) delayed until 3–6 months after the myocardial infarction. This is based on the well-established data which have identified a reinfarction rate of approximately 10% when surgery is performed within 3 months of an infarction, decreasing to 5% 3–6 months after infarction.[61,62]

The third benefit of perioperative cardiac evaluation constitutes the aggressive risk factor modification programs which can be instituted in these patients who suffer from diffuse atherosclerotic occlusive disease. The patients are counseled in

smoking cessation and are often started on pharmacologic aids as well as enrolled in appropriate support programs. All patients are evaluated for hyperlipidemia and treated using the appropriate dietary counseling as well as pharmacologic cholesterol-lowering agents, when indicated. Effective lifestyle modification and the establishment of appropriate long-term medical regimens constitute the best potential measures we can offer patients for limiting long-term morbidity and improving long-term survival.

Algorithm for Cardiology Evaluation of Patients Presenting for Elective Carotid Endarterectomy

Our algorithm for the evaluation of patients presenting for elective carotid endarterectomy is outlined in Fig. 14.1. All patients undergo initial evaluation by their cardiologist after the indication for CEA has been established. Patients who are found to be low-risk based on their electrocardiogram, history, and physical examination and who demonstrate a good exercise tolerance have no further testing. Their medical regimens are optimized and they are placed on a program of risk factor modification, including smoking cessation and a lipid-lowering program. They then proceed to surgery with the usual vascular precautions.

Patients who are deemed to be moderate- to high-risk based on their initial evaluation undergo further non-invasive cardiology testing. A number of tests are available, including exercise stress testing, dipyridamole myocardial scintigraphy, echocardiography with or without stress, or Holter monitoring for ischemia. All these tests are of proven utility and the choice depends on the local expertise within an institution. Patients who are found to be low-risk based on this non-invasive testing undergo optimization of their medical regimens and risk factor modification and proceed to surgery. Patients who are deemed high-risk based on their non-invasive cardiology testing are evaluated for indications for coronary revascularization. Those patients who do not have independent indications for coronary revascularization, such as class III–IV angina, or left ventricular ischemic dysfunction, undergo an aggressive program of medical optimization and risk

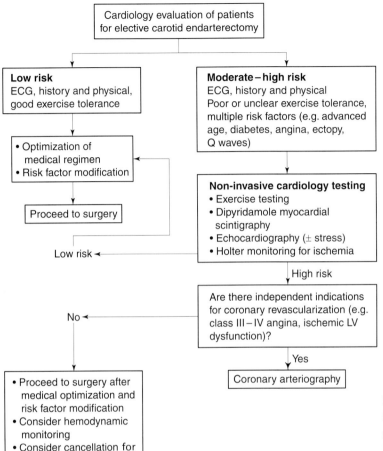

Fig. 14.1
Cardiology evaluation of patients for elective carotid endarterectomy. ECG, electrocardiogram; LV, left ventricular.

factor modification. These patients are the subgroup who may benefit from intensive perioperative hemodynamic monitoring. Consideration for cancellation of surgery for patients with asymptomatic carotid stenosis is appropriate in this subgroup.

Those patients who do have independent indications for coronary revascularization undergo coronary arteriography. If coronary arteriography does not reveal an indication for coronary reconstruction, patients may be considered for surgery with the precautions outlined above. Conversely, patients who have an indication for coronary revascularization will be referred for CABG. The staging of the CEA as a prior, simultaneous, or post-CABG procedure is individualized based on the presentation and degree of disease.

REFERENCES

36 Executive Committee for the Asymptomatic Carotid Atherosclerosis Study. Endarterectomy for asymptomatic carotid artery stenosis. *Journal of the American Medical Association* 1995; **273**: 1421–1428.

37 North American Symptomatic Carotid Endarterectomy Trial Collaborators. Beneficial effect of carotid endarterectomy in symptomatic patients with highgrade stenosis. *New England Journal of Medicine* 1991; **266**: 3289–3294.

38 Riles TS, Kopelman 1, Imparato AM. Myocardial infarction following carotid endarterectomy. A review of 683 operations. *Surgery* 1979; **85**: 249–252.

39 Allen BT, Anderson CB, Rubin BG *et al*. The influence of

anesthetic technique on perioperative complications after carotid endarterectomy. *Journal of Vascular Surgery* 1994; **19**: 834–843.

40 Bove EL, Fry WJ, Gross WS, Stanley JC. Hypotension and hypertension as consequences of baroreceptor dysfunction following carotid endarterectomy. *Surgery* 1979; **85**: 633–637.

41 Tarlow E, Schmidek H, Scott RM, Wepsic JG, Ojemann RG. Reflex hypotension following carotid endarterectomy: mechanism and management. *Journal of Neurosurgery* 1973; **39**: 323–327.

42 Angell-James JE, Lumley JSP. The effects of carotid endarterectomy on the mechanical properties of the carotid sinus and carotid sinus nerve activity in atherosclerotic patients. *British Journal of Surgery* 1974; **61**: 805–810.

43 Towne JB, Bernhard VM. The relationship of post operative hypertension to complications following carotid endarterectomy. *Surgery* 1980; **88**: 575–580.

44 Cafferata HT, Merchant RF, Depalma RG. Avoidance of post carotid endarterectomy hypertension. *Annals of Surgery* 1982; **196**: 465–472.

45 Smith B. Hypertension following carotid endarterectomy: the role of cerebral renin production. *Journal of Vascular Surgery* 1984; **1**: 623–627.

46 Rockman CB, Riles TS, Gold M *et al*. A comparison of regional and general anesthesia in patients undergoing carotid endarterectomy. *Journal of Vascular Surgery* 1996; **24**: 946–956.

47 Rizzo RJ, Whittemore AD, Couper GS *et al*. Combined carotid and coronary revascularization: the preferred approach to the severe vasculopath. *Annals of Thoracic Surgery* 1992; **54**: 1099–1109.

48 Mackey WC, O'Donnell TF, Callow AD. Cardiac risk in patients undergoing carotid endarterectomy: impact on perioperative and long term mortality. *Journal of Vascular Surgery* 1990; **11**: 226–234.

49 Hertzer NR, Young JR, Beven EG *et al*. Coronary angiography in 506 patients with extracranial cerebrovascular disease. *Archives of Internal Medicine* 1985; **145**: 849–852.

50 Rokey R, Rolak LA, Harati Y, Kutka N, Verani MS. Coronary artery disease in patients with cerebrovascular disease: a prospective study. *Annals of Neurology* 1984; **16**: 50–55.

51 Ennix CL, Lawrie GM, Morris GC *et al*. Improved results in patients with symptomatic coronary artery disease. An analysis of 1546 consecutive carotid operations. *Stroke* 1979; **10**: 122–125.

52 Yeager RA, Moneta GL, McConnell DB, Neuwelt EA, Taylor LM, Porter JM. Analysis of risk factors for myocardial infarction following carotid endarterectomy. *Archives of Surgery* 1989; **124**: 1142–1145.

53 Hertzer NR, Lees CD. Fatal myocardial infarction following carotid endarterectomy. Three hundred thirty-five patients followed 6–11 years after operation. *Annals of Surgery* 1981; **194**: 212–218.

54 Hertzer NR, Arison R. Cumulative stroke and 10-year survival after carotid endarterectomy. *Journal of Vascular Surgery* 1985; **2**: 661–668.

55 Lord RSA. Late survival after carotid endarterectomy for transient ischemic attacks. *Journal of Vascular Surgery* 1984; **1**: 512–519.

56 Bernstein EF, Dilley RB. Late results of carotid endarterectomy for amaurosis fugax. *Journal of Vascular Surgery* 1987; **6**: 333–340.

57 Mangano D. Effect of atenolol on mortality and cardiovascular morbidity after non-cardiac surgery. *New England Journal of Medicine* 1996; **335**: 1713–1720.

58 Pasternak PF, Imparato AM, Baumann FG *et al*. The hemodynamics of beta blockade in patients undergoing abdominal aortic aneurysm repair. *Circulation* 1987; **76**: 1111–1117.

59 McCann RL, Clements FN. Silent myocardial ischemia in patients undergoing peripheral vascular surgery: incidence and association with perioperative cardiac morbidity and mortality. *Journal of Vascular Surgery* 1989; **9**: 583–587.

60 Raby KE, Goldman L, Creager MA *et al*. Correlation between preoperative ischemia and major cardiac events after peripheral vascular surgery. *New England Journal of Medicine* 1989; **321**: 1296–1300.

61 Wells PH, Kaplan JA. Optimal management of patients with ischemic heart disease for noncardiac surgery by complementary anesthesiologist and cardiologist interaction. *American Heart Journal* 1981; **102**: 1029–1037.

62 Rao Tik, El-Etr AA. Myocardial reinfarction following anesthesia in patients with recent acute myocardial infarction. *Anesthesia and Analgesia* 1981; **60**: 271–290.

14.3 Editorial Comment

KEY POINTS

1 Coronary artery disease (CAD) affects over 90% of CEA patients and severe CAD affects 82% of CEA patients with symptoms and signs of CAD and 40% of CEA patients with no symptoms or signs of CAD.

2 Overall, < 5% of CEAs are complicated by myocardial infarction (MI) and < 1% by fatal MI. In patients with signs and symptoms of CAD, up to 2.5% will die from perioperative MI.

3 CAD is a major determinant of long-term survival post-CEA. About 50% of deaths at any interval after CEA are attributable to CAD.

4 A thorough cardiac history and physical examination together with chest X-ray and electrocardiogram ECG are mandatory prior to CEA. Further tests are reserved for those patients with positive findings on initial risk assessment.

5 Formal preoperative cardiologic assessment is useful for
- identifying those at highest risk for perioperative cardiac complications;
- optimizing perioperative medical management of CAD;
- long-term follow-up and risk factor management.

6 Formal preoperative cardiologic assessment is advised in patients with poorly compensated congestive cardiac failure, recent MI, severe or unstable angina, angina associated with dyspnea or syncope, significant arrhythmias or conduction blocks or anyone with recurrent angina after coronary bypass or angioplasty.

COMMENT

Given the prevalence of CAD in CEA patients and its impact on both short- and long-term outcome, clinical assessment of CAD is mandatory in all potential CEA patients. In those centers which do not have access to vascular medicine specialists, this assessment will be carried out by the vascular surgeon, the referring physician/neurologist, or the anesthesiologist. Each should review the clinical and ECG data in order to stratify operative risk. Patients with no signs or symptoms of CAD and with a normal or mildly abnormal ECG can undergo CEA without formal cardiological assessment. Those at highest risk (severe congestive cardiac failure, unstable angina, recent MI) should be assessed and appropriately treated prior to surgery or be disqualified as a CEA candidate. Obviously the indications for the contemplated CEA will have a bearing on the decision to proceed or not. Patients deemed at intermediate risk (stable angina, distant MI, diabetes, mild compensated congestive failure, multiple additional risk factors for CAD) are a heterogeneous group. The evaluation of patients in this group is complex and controversial. In the elective setting, evocative stress testing is useful to stratify risk further, although the optimal use of data derived from such studies is unknown. Coronary revascularization prior to, or in conjunction with, CEA is best reserved for patients with compelling indications for bypass or percutaneous transluminal coronary angioplasty. Positive stress studies mandate increased vigilance throughout the perioperative period but one should probably assume that *all* CEA patients have significant coronary artery disease and manage them accordingly.

15.1

What does optimal medical therapy really entail?
Peter RD Humphrey (Europe)

INTRODUCTION

No apology is made for emphasizing that the most important aspect of medical management is to take a detailed, careful history of the presenting complaint. This will usually alert the clinician to other conditions which may mimic a stroke or transient ischaemic attack (TIA).[1] In our cerebrovascular clinics, up to 24 new patients are seen each week. At the most, only 3 or 4 will be candidates for carotid endarterectomy (CEA).

The remainder will require medical treatment because they have appropriate symptoms but a carotid stenosis of less than 70%, vascular pathology due to other causes or a non-vascular aetiology for their symptoms. Many will have no serious problems whatsoever and a lot of time is, thereafter, spent 'undiagnosing' TIAs and reassuring people that nothing serious has happened.[2] However, on occasions it may be necessary to exclude one of the more unusual causes of stroke or TIA (Table 15.1).

The benefits of involving a neurologist within the multidisciplinary team have been discussed elsewhere. Whilst not a universally held opinion, my view is that most patients should be initially assessed by a neurologist or stroke physician and those who might benefit from CEA are then referred on to the vascular surgeon for operation. This is analogous to the relationship between the cardiologist and the cardiac surgeon in the assessment of cardiac conditions such as angina. Team work, including primary care, is the essence of good management for TIA and minor stroke.[3]

INVESTIGATIONS

Once a diagnosis of TIA or stroke has been made, appropriate investigations can be planned. The principles underlying the use of ultrasound, angiography and computed tomography (CT) are dealt with elsewhere and will not be discussed further. There is, perhaps, a misconception that the most important function of a cerebral vascular clinic is the identification of patients suitable for CEA. However, irrespective of the need for surgery, every patient requires management of risk factors and the institution of appropriate antiplatelet therapy.

Routinely Performed Investigations

In practice, a number of relatively simple investigations should be routinely performed (Table 15.2). These include a full blood count to exclude polycythaemia, anaemia, thrombocytosis and sickle-cell disease. Similarly, the ESR or plasma viscosity should be checked to exclude an underlying vasculitis, although a moderately raised ESR is not uncommon in atherosclerotic vascular disease. Should the ESR or plasma viscosity be significantly elevated, the clinician should be alerted to the possibility of an unusual cause of the stroke or TIA and more discriminatory investigations performed (see below). Blood should also be taken to exclude diabetes mellitus and hyperlipidaemia. I would not normally test for the presence of autoantibodies, but would consider this in younger – especially female – patients. A chest X-ray should be performed to exclude lung malignancy and evidence of subclinical heart failure. Patients should also have an electrocardiogram (ECG) to look for evidence of ischaemic heart disease, left ventricular hypertrophy and heart block as well as any other occult rhythm disturbances.

Selectively Performed Investigations

Twenty-four-hour ECG monitoring is rarely useful

Table 15.1
Unusual causes of stroke or transient ischaemic attack

Large-artery disease
Carotid and vertebral dissection
Fibromuscular dysplasia
Radiotherapy
Homocystinuria
Moya-moya disease
Takayasu's arteritis

Vasculitis
Drug abuse
Cerebral lupus
Polyarteritis nodosa
Wegener's granulomatosis
Sarcoidosis
Behçet's disease
Isolated angiitis of the nervous system
Zoster arteritis

Small-artery disease
Hypertension-associated vasculopathy
Migraine

Cardiogenic embolism
Valvular heart disease
Prosthetic heart valves
Atrial fibrillation
Acute myocardial infarction
Left ventricular dyskinesia/aneurysm
Dilated cardiomyopathy
Atrial septal defect, including PFO
Bacterial endocarditis
Libman–Sachs endocarditis
Atrial myxoma

Others
CADASIL
MELAS
Inheritable disorders of connective tissue
Fabry's disease
Pregnancy

Thrombophilia
Protein C and S deficiency
Antithrombin III deficiency
Hyperfibrinogenaemia
Myeloproliferative disorders
Hyperviscosity syndromes
Antiphospholipid syndrome
Sickle-cell disease

Venous infarction

Reproduced with permission from Martin *et al.*[3]

unless there is a suggestion of paroxysmal atrial fibrillation. Routine requests for echocardigraphy are unnecessary as the yield in patients with no clinical history or signs of heart disease is very low. For the general population, echocardiography is best reserved for those with abnormal cardiac findings suggestive of valvular heart disease, if there is evidence of recent myocardial infarction and/or a left ventricular aneurysm either clinically or on ECG or chest X-ray. I would, however, perform echocardiography in younger stroke patients if there were:

1   no other obvious cause for their symptoms (e.g. dissection);

Table 15.2
Planning of investigations

Routine	Selected patients
Full blood count	Transthoracic echocardiography
ESR/plasma viscosity	24-h ECG
Blood sugar	Thrombophilia screen
Urea and electrolytes	Autoantibodies
Chest X-ray	Lupus anticoagulant, anticardiolipin antibodies
ECG	Complement
	Serology for syphilis/HIV
	Drug abuse screen
	Haemoglobin electrophoresis
	Screening tests for homocystinuria
	Screening tests for mitochondrial cytopathy
	Methionine loading test
	Muscle biopsy
	Lumbar puncture
	Brain/meningeal biopsy
	Skin biopsy
	DNA analysis

ESR, erythrocyte sedimentation rate; ECG, electrocardiogram; HIV, human immunodeficiency virus.

2 multiple vascular territory strokes without any alternative explanation;
3 serological evidence of systemic lupus erythematosus or the antiphospholipid syndrome.

A variety of other tests will occasionally be necessary in those in whom atherosclerosis is unlikely to be the explanation for their symptoms (Table 15.1). A detailed description of the investigation and management of each of these rare conditions is beyond the scope of this chapter. Possible investigations for this group of patients are summarized in Table 15.2 and these investigations should be targeted appropriately.

ANTIPLATELET THERAPY

Aspirin remains the standard treatment.[4] It is important to emphasize that aspirin only reduces the risk of any subsequent stroke or myocardial event by about 20%. There is much debate about the optimum dose, with some clinicians using as much as 1300 mg/day and others as little as 37.5 mg day. All of these doses are probably equally effective, although there is no doubt that the side-effects of aspirin are more common with the higher doses. The number of people in randomized trials with the smaller doses (75 mg or less) is relatively small and therefore the confidence limits for the efficacy of these doses are wider than for larger doses. My preference is for 150–300 mg/day. In practice, a daily dose of 300 mg has a more rapid mode of action than the smaller doses when antiplatelet therapy is being initiated. However, if 150–300 mg is not tolerated by the patient, I use doses of 37.5–75 mg.

Ticlopidine is an alternative antiplatelet agent;[5] the daily dose is 250 mg b.d. Unfortunately, serious side-effects, including diarrhoea, skin rash and neutropenia, in about 10% of patients tends to limit its clinical usefulness. Accordingly, regular blood tests are necessary for the first 6 months, particularly to prevent neutropenia.

Clopidogrel is as effective as ticlopidine but is generally free of serious side-effects.[6] The single daily dose is 75 mg and, now marketed, it is very likely to replace ticlopidine. Some authors consider that ticlopidine and clopidogrel are more clinically effective antiplatelet agents than aspirin and that they should be preferentially used in all patients. However, the overall confidence limits for the efficacy of all three agents overlaps and aspirin is significantly cheaper. It therefore seems sensible to start with aspirin as the initial antiplatelet agent. There is no doubt that clopidogrel will become the drug of second choice, and it should be considered in patients who are aspirin insensitive or intolerant.

The European Stroke Prevention Study 2 has suggested that the combination of aspirin and dipyridamole confers a better antiplatelet activity than either agent on its own.[7] Some reservations remain about the methodology of this trial, but dipyridamole plus aspirin remains an alternative to clopidogrel.[8]

ANTICOAGULATION

Anticoagulation reduces the risk of stroke by over 60% in patients with atrial fibrillation.[9] In these patients, the international normalized ratio (INR) should be kept between 2 and 3.5. The risks of anticoagulation rise steeply as the INR exceeds 4.

The role of warfarin versus aspirin in the treatment of patients with TIA has recently been assessed in the SPIRIT study.[10] Unfortunately, the complication rate on warfarin was such that the study was terminated early. This may be partly because the level of anticoagulation was considered excessive by some (recommended INR 3–4.4). In view of this, a new study is underway (ESPRIT) which is using lower-dose anticoagulation regimens.

Thus, at present, there is no evidence to support the *routine* use of warfarin in the management of patients with TIA or minor stroke other than those with proven atrial fibrillation. However, I might consider using warfarin or heparin in patients with no significant carotid disease who present with frequent TIAs (more than one a month) not controlled by antiplatelet therapy, although there are no good randomized data for this practice. In this situation I would tend to give anticoagulation for 3–6

months and then switch back to antiplatelet therapy alone.

If the symptoms fail to settle on these regimes, the diagnosis should be carefully reassessed and the possibility of an unusual underlying cause considered. Embolic TIAs rarely fail to settle on one of the above regimes. Haemodynamic TIAs, although rare, clearly require an entirely different method of treatment with a surgical procedure to improve cerebral blood flow, e.g. external CEA, subclavian angioplasty or extracranial–intracranial bypass, if a routine CEA is not an option.

RISK FACTOR MANAGEMENT

Medical treatment and risk factor advice should not be left to the most junior member of the surgical team who otherwise sees well patients in the postoperative clinic. It is essential that careful practical guidelines are given for a patient's long-term health. It seems a shame to carry out a delicate and precise operation, only for the patient to succumb to some other, possibly avoidable, vascular event in the next few years.

Blood Pressure

Good blood pressure control remains the cornerstone of managing cerebrovascular disease. It alone will do more to prevent stroke than aspirin, CEA or any other treatment available to us at present.[11] Despite increased awareness of the benefits of optimization of correctable risk factors, evidence suggests that these are not well controlled in most cases.[12,13] For example, up to 40% of known hypertensives were not having their blood pressure actively managed before their stroke and only 54% of those on antihypertensive therapy had a documented diastolic blood pressure reading of < 90 mmHg before the acute event.[14]

A detailed discussion of the precise choice of drug therapy is beyond the scope of this article. Most cases of hypertension are best managed in the primary-care setting, but hypertension clinics are now usually available in most hospitals for those with poorly controlled hypertension. However, it is essential that patients do not undergo CEA with untreated hypertension, as this will invariably increase the risk of perioperative cardiac and cerebrovascular complications. As a general rule, drug therapy, weight loss and reducing salt intake comprise the main treatments for controlling high blood pressure. I think it is worthwhile giving patients and family doctors an exact level to aim for; e.g. for those under 50 years of age, the ideal blood pressure should be less than 150/95 mmHg, while for those aged over 70 years, the figure is 170/100 mmHg.

Diabetes Mellitus

To date, there is no clear evidence that rigorous control of glycaemia reduces the long-term risk of stroke. However, the UK Prospective Diabetes Study Group[15] has shown that tight control of blood pressure (< 150/85mmHg) in type 2 diabetics was associated with a 44% reduction in the risk of stroke as compared to patients randomized to less tight control of blood pressure (< 180/105mmHg). Because 40–60% of type 2 diabetics also have hypertension, this study has reinforced the importance of careful blood pressure management.

Smoking

Stopping smoking reduces the risk of further vascular events by about 50%.[16]

Cholesterol

Greater attention is now being directed towards the treatment of hyperlipidaemia, mainly with a view to preventing myocardial infarction. Although a stroke physician is naturally trying to reduce the long-term risk of stroke, it is important to remember that most TIA/stroke patients will ultimately die of ischaemic heart disease.

The most recent lipid-lowering studies leave no doubt that cholesterol reduction reduces the risk of late ischaemic events and that, in addition to reducing the risk of myocardial infarction, a programme of cholesterol reduction will also reduce the risk of late stroke.[17,18]

In my practice, the treatment of choice is one of the statins. These are easy to administer and are well tolerated with only very occasional muscle and liver side-effects. As a general rule, therefore, all patients with symptomatic cerebral vascular disease and who have a total cholesterol in excess of 5.0 mmol/l should be considered for treatment.

CONCLUSIONS

In summary, the purpose of cerebral vascular clinics is not simply to identify patients who are suitable for CEA. All patients should undergo a number of routine baseline investigations which identify unsuspected risk factors that will also need correction. More complex investigations should be targeted to those patients whose clinical features are not typical of atherosclerotic disease.

All patients should receive antiplatelet therapy. Aspirin is the first choice, with clopidogrel perhaps kept in reserve for those who are aspirin insensitive or intolerant. There is no evidence that routine anticoagulation is of any benefit in stroke prevention other than in those patients with atrial fibrillation. Blood pressure control is the single most important risk factor to be corrected, especially in diabetics. All symptomatic patients with a total cholesterol > 5.0 mmol/l should be considered for treatment with a statin. Finally, the management of risk factors should not be the duty of the most junior member of the team.

REFERENCES

1 Warlow CP, Dennis MS, Van Gijn J et al. Is it a vascular event? Transient ischaemic attack or stroke. In: Warlow CP (ed.) Stroke: A Practical Guide to Management, pp. 25–79. Blackwell Science, 1996.

2 Martin PJ, Young G, Enevoldson TP, Humphrey PRD. Overdiagnosis of TIA and minor stroke: experience at a regional neurovascular clinic. Quarterly Journal of Medicine 1997; 90: 759–763.

3 Martin PJ, Enevoldson TP, Humphrey PRD. Causes of ischaemic stroke in the young. Postgraduate Medical Journal 1997; 73: 8–16.

4 Antiplatelet Trialists' Collaboration. Collaborative overview of randomised trials of antiplatelet therapy. British Medical Journal 1994; 308: 81–106.

5 Ticlopidine editorial. Lancet 1991; 337: 450–460.

6 CAPRIE Steering Committee. A randomised blinded trial of clopidogrel versus aspirin in patients at risk of ischaemic events (CAPRIE). Lancet 1996; 348: 1329–1339.

7 Diener H, Cunha L, Forbes C, Sivenius J, Smets P, Lowenthal A. European Stroke Prevention Study (ESPS) 2. Dipyridamole and acetylsalicylic acid in the secondary

prevention of stroke. *Journal of Neurological Science* 1996; **143**: 1–13.

8 Davis SM, Donnan GA. Secondary prevention for stroke after CAPRIE and ESPS-2. *Cerebrovascular Disease* 1998; **8**: 73–77.

9 European Atrial Fibrillation Study Group. Secondary prevention in non-rheumatic atrial fibrillation after transient ischaemic attack or minor stroke. *Lancet* 1993; **342**: 1255–1262.

10 Algra A, Franke CL, Koehler PJJ *et al*. A randomised trial of anticoagulants versus aspirin after cerebral ischaemia of presumed arterial origin. *Annals of Neurology* 1997; **42**: 857–865.

11 Dennis M, Warlow C. Strategy for stroke. *British Medical Journal* 1991; **303**: 636–638.

12 Payne JN, Milner PC, Saul C, Bowns IR, Hannay DR, Ramsay LE. Local confidential inquiry into avoidable factors in death from stroke and hypertensive disease. *British Medical Journal* 1993; **307**: 1027–1030.

13 Campbell NC, Thain J, Deans HG, Ritchie LD, Rawles JM. Secondary prevention in coronary heart disease; baseline survey of provision in general practice. *British Medical Journal* 1998; **316**: 1430–1434.

14 Kalra L, Perez I, Melbourn A. Stroke risk management: changes in mainstream practice. *Stroke* 1998; **29**: 53–57.

15 UK Prospective Diabetes Study Group. Tight blood pressure control and risk of macrovascular and microvascular complications in type 2 diabetes. *British Medical Journal* 1998; **317**: 703–713.

16 Wannamethee SG, Shaper AG, Whincup PH, Walker M. Smoking cessation and the risks of stroke in middle aged men. *Journal of the American Medical Association* 1995; **274**: 155–160.

17 Crouse JR, Byington RP, Hoen HN, Furberg CD. Reductase inhibitor monotherapy and stroke prevention. *Archives of Internal Medicine* 1997; **157**: 1305–1310.

18 Rosendorff C. Statins for prevention of stroke. *Lancet* 1998; **351**: 1002–1003.

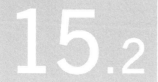

15.2

What does optimal medical therapy really entail?
Louis R Caplan (USA)
Brian Silver (USA)

INTRODUCTION
Aggressive medical therapy and risk factor management are the cornerstones of treatment for stroke-prone atherosclerotic patients. This chapter will discuss four aspects of medical management:

1 medical and risk factor management applicable to all patients with carotid disease;
2 medical management of asymptomatic patients with carotid disease;
3 medical management of patients with TIA and stroke;
4 medical management of CEA patients in the perioperative period.

TREATMENT APPLICABLE TO ALL PATIENTS WITH CAROTID DISEASE
Disease of the internal carotid artery is almost always atherosclerotic in origin. Plaques arise on the posterior surface of the common carotid and opposite the flow divider at the bifurcation. These plaques gradually increase in size and may crack and ulcerate as they progress. Carotid disease is one manifestation of generalized atherosclerosis. Patients with carotid disease have a high prevalence of coronary and peripheral arterial disease. They also have the major risk factors for these diseases – hypertension and hypercholesterolemia.

The advent of high-quality extracranial duplex ultrasound has given clinicians a means for non-invasively imaging the atherosclerotic plaque to follow its progression or regression. The progression or regression of plaques in the carotid bifurcation may mirror plaque evolution in other vascular beds, most notably the coronary arteries. It should always be kept in mind that death in patients with carotid atherosclerosis is most frequently due to myocardial infarction and not stroke. Modification of atherosclerotic risk factors in patients with carotid disease is, therefore, critical not only for stroke prevention but also for prevention of premature cardiac death. In the setting of an acute neurologic presentation, clinicians often lose sight of the critical importance of risk factor modification. The acute neurologic event may represent a real opportunity to intervene and alter the long-term natural history of the atherosclerotic process.

Excessive use of alcohol, hypertension, homocysteinemia, and smoking have been directly linked to carotid disease.[19] Other risk factors, such as diabetes, obesity, lack of exercise, and fibrinogen levels, have been linked to stroke in general but not specifically to carotid disease.[19] More recent studies have correlated the level of cholesterol (especially low high-density lipoproteins (HDL)) with the severity of carotid disease and with increased intimal–medial thickness of the carotid artery as measured by duplex ultrasound. Drugs that lower cholesterol and improve the balance of HDL and low-density lipoproteins (LDL), especially reductase inhibitors, have been shown to slow the progression of carotid plaques and decrease the incidence of TIAs and strokes even in patients with normal cholesterol levels.[20]

Fibrinogen may also play an important role in the pathogenesis of carotid artery-related atherothrombotic neurologic events. Fibrinogen contributes significantly to whole blood viscosity and is a potent activating agent in both the intrinsic and extrinsic cascades. Unfortunately, there are few substances known to reduce fibrinogen levels. Omega-3 fish oils, ticlopidine, atromid, and

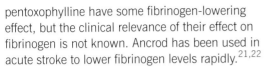

pentoxophylline have some fibrinogen-lowering effect, but the clinical relevance of their effect on fibrinogen is not known. Ancrod has been used in acute stroke to lower fibrinogen levels rapidly.[21,22]

Elevated homocysteine levels are probably an important risk factor for premature atherosclerosis.[23] Young patients presenting with symptomatic atherosclerosis should be evaluated for homocysteinemia, especially in the absence of other significant risk factors. In addition, in older patients, homocysteinemia may act synergistically with other risk factors in atherogenesis and disease progression. Prescription of folic acid, vitamin B_6, or restriction of dietary methionine should be helpful in patients with high homocysteine levels.

Aspirin (650 mg of enteric coated aspirin daily) is appropriate for all patients with carotid disease. In patients intolerant of aspirin, clopidogrel or omega-3 oils (1–2 g eicosopentanoic acid daily) are useful. Although a recent European study suggests a potentiating effect when dipyridamole is used with aspirin, several previous negative trials cast doubt on this finding.[24] With the advent of clopidogrel, the role of ticlopidine is less well defined.

MEDICAL MANAGEMENT OF THE PATIENT WITH ASYMPTOMATIC CAROTID DISEASE

A careful history and neurologic examination may be revealing in these patients.[25] Careful questioning often elicits symptoms of retinal or brain ischemia. Abnormalities – even subtle ones – on neurologic examination can also provide evidence for brain infarction. Both high-quality duplex ultrasound and transcranial Doppler are critical for the adequate assessment of patients presenting with asymptomatic carotid disease. Both degree of stenosis and carotid plaque morphology are accurately assessed by duplex and are known to correlate with disease progression and the occurrence of strokes and TIAs.[26,27] Transcranial Doppler can provide important data on the effect of the cervical carotid lesion on intracranial hemodynamics and on coexistent intracranial stenoses. The significance of transcranial Doppler-detected emboli in asymptomatic patients remains uncertain. Emboli detection might be used to monitor the effectiveness of antiplatelet or

antithrombotic regimens in these patients. Large numbers of emboli persisting despite medical therapy might be an indication for more aggressive medical therapy or for surgery in selected patients.

Brain-imaging studies may be useful in selected asymptomatic patients, especially those whose neurologic exam is not normal. CT scans or magnetic resonance images often show infarcts appropriate for the carotid territory in patients with no history of a neurologic event. These patients may have suffered symptoms which they did not consider significant at the time (transient clumsiness or difficulty finding the right ward) and have subsequently forgotten. Such silent infarcts are indicative of end-organ damage related to the carotid pathology and in selected patients constitute an indication for surgical or interventional therapy. Magnetic resonance imaging may come to replace CT scanning since magnetic resonance can also provide reasonable vascular images without contrast administration. While magnetic resonance angiography should not be used as a screen for carotid disease, it may be helpful to confirm duplex findings, especially when an experienced duplex technician is not available or the duplex is suboptimal.

Tight carotid stenosis, progression of stenosis, low plaque echodensity, silent brain infarction, and a large number of transcranial Doppler-detected microemboli are probably indications for more aggressive therapy than simple risk factor reduction and aspirin. CEA, carotid angioplasty with stenting, other antiplatelet agents (ticlopidine or clopidogrel), and full anticoagulation are possible more aggressive alternatives. Red (erythrocyte fibrin) clots are most apt to occur and embolize in patients with tight stenosis and ulceration. Anticoagulants are probably more effective than antiplatelet agents in preventing red clots. Anticoagulants are especially important in patients with severe intracranial disease and in those with severe carotid disease who are not candidates for surgical or interventional therapy.

In asymptomatic patients with moderate to severe carotid stenosis, aggressive risk factor control, including the use of reductase inhibitors for lipid control, antiplatelet therapy, patient education regarding TIAs, and close follow-up with serial duplex studies to detect lesion progression are the mainstays of therapy. The pros and cons of surgery for asymptomatic stenosis should be discussed. When there is significant disease progression or when ischemic symptoms occur, surgery is indicated, though more aggressive medical therapy may be tried in those at especially high surgical risk or who refuse surgery.

MEDICAL THERAPY FOR PATIENTS WITH TIAs AND STROKES

Patients with severe carotid disease and TIA should undergo CEA as soon as feasible. Patients with acute stroke might best be served by delaying surgery for several weeks, especially if the stroke results in a large defect on CT or MRI. (See Chapter 4 for an indepth discussion of this controversial topic.) Obviously, patients who develop further ischemic symptoms while awaiting surgery should proceed to endarterectomy without delay. Patients with stroke related to acute carotid occlusion are not candidates for surgery, except in the rare instances when the occlusion occurs during angiography and surgery can be carried out very promptly, or when there is good reconstitution of the distal cervical internal carotid. In the vast majority of patients with carotid occlusion-related stroke, medical therapy, bedrest with the patient flat for several days, careful blood pressure maintenance initially and when the patient is allowed up, and therapeutic anticoagulation with heparin converted to coumadin for approximately 12 weeks constitute the safest course. Fresh thrombi are poorly organized and non-adherent. They have a tendency to propagate or embolize. The period of anticoagulation is designed to cover this period and allow the thrombus to organize and adhere. In addition, collateral circulation increases during this period.

In all stroke patients, blood pressure management is critical. Protection of viable brain tissue depends on the maintenance of flow in collateral arteries. If the blood pressure is not excessively high (< 175/95 mmHg), it is usually most prudent to leave it alone unless there is evidence for hemorrhage into the infarct. If the blood pressure is low or demonstrates postural drops, liberal fluid administration by mouth or intravenously is

necessary both to increase plasma volume and decrease blood viscosity. Occasionally, vasopressors are necessary to protect the collateral supply.

Systemic thrombolysis is rarely effective in patients with acute internal carotid occlusion. Intra-arterial thrombolysis may play a role in highly selected patients with acute carotid occlusion. Passage of catheters through cervical carotid thrombi into the intracranial vessels can allow direct administration of lytic agents to the intracranial thrombi. Once these clots are dissolved, the cervical carotid lesion can be managed with further lytic therapy followed by endarterectomy or angioplasty/stenting.[28] Intervention early in the course of the stroke is essential for safe and effective thrombolytic therapy. It is not currently known which stroke patients are most likely to benefit from this aggressive approach. In the absence of clear treatment guidelines, optimization of collateral flow and anticoagulation are the safest means of minimizing the stroke deficit in the vast majority of patients. In patients with severe stroke deficits, anticoagulation is used only after hemorrhage is ruled out. In highly selected patients with large regions of hypodensity on CT scan or NEU, a decompressive craniectomy can be life-saving and is often followed by a gratifying recovery.[29]

MEDICAL THERAPY OF THE ENDARTERECTOMY PATIENT IN THE PERIOPERATIVE PERIOD

CEA is often followed by a variable period of blood pressure lability. Most often the blood pressure is elevated, though occasionally it runs quite low. Patients who are significantly hypertensive preoperatively are especially apt to have worsening of their hypertension in the early postoperative period. Uncontrolled hypertension in the perioperative period can contribute to the hyperperfusion syndrome. Severe headache, progressive worsening of hypertension, seizures, brain edema, and brain hemorrhage may result in early postoperative death in severe cases of post-endarterectomy hyperperfusion.[30] In some cases, hyperperfusion syndrome may have a more insidious onset developing up to a week after surgery. It is therefore imperative that all endarterectomy patients, and especially those with significant preoperative hypertension, have their blood pressure monitored for at least 7 days postoperatively. Significant postoperative hypertension, especially when associated with headache, is an indication for readmission to the hospital and aggressive blood pressure reduction, usually in a monitored unit.

In all endarterectomy patients, risk factor control and aspirin therapy are important. The patients should be followed lifelong, not only for their contralateral carotid disease, but also, and more importantly, for their coronary disease. Since most CEA patients die not from stroke but from coronary disease, a work-up for coronary disease, if not carried out preoperatively, is warranted.

REFERENCES

19 Fine-Edelstein JS, Wolf PA, O'Leary DH *et al*. Precursors of extracranial carotid atherosclerosis in the Framingham Study. *Neurology* 1994; **44**: 1046–1050.

20 Crouse JR, Byington RP, Hoen HM, Furberg CD. Reductase inhibitor monotherapy and stroke prevention. *Archives of Internal Medicine* 1997; **157**: 1305–1310.

21 Ancrod Study Investigators. Ancrod for the treatment of acute ischemic brain infarction. *Stroke* 1994; **25**: 1755–1759.

22 Atkinson RP. Ancord in the treatment of acute ischemic stroke. *Drugs* 1997; **54** (Suppl. 3): 100–108.

23 Selhub J, Jacques PF, Bostom AG *et al*. Association between plasma homocysteine concentrations and extracranial carotid artery stenosis. *New England Journal of Medicine* 1995; **332**: 286–291.

24 European Stroke Prevention Study Group. European stroke prevention study: principal endpoints. *Lancet* 1987; **2**: 1351–1354.

25 Caplan LR. A 79 year old musician with asymptomatic carotid artery disease. *Journal of the American Medical Association* 1995; **274**: 1383–1389.

26 Geroulakos G, Hobson RW, Nicolaides A. Ultrasonographic carotid plaque morphology in predicting stroke risk. *British Journal of Surgery* 1996; **83**: 582–587.

27 Golledge J, Cuming R, Ellis M, Davies AH, Greenhalgh RM. Carotid plaque characteristics and presenting symptoms. *British Journal of Surgery* 1997; **84**: 1697–1701.

28 Barnwell SL, Clark WM, Nguyen J *et al*. Safety and efficacy of delayed intra-arterial urokinase therapy with mechanical clot disruption for thromboembolic stroke. *American Journal of Neuroradiology* 1994; **15**: 1817–1822.

29 Hacke W, Schwab S, DeGeorgia M. Intensive care of acute ischemic stroke. *Cerebrovascular Disease* 1995; **5**: 385–392.

30 Breen JC, Caplan LR, DeWitt LD *et al*. Brain edema after carotid surgery. *Neurology* 1996; **46**: 175–181.

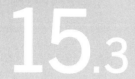

15.3 Editorial Comment

KEY POINTS

1 The randomized trials of CEA recognized the critical importance of risk factor and medical management by mandating best medical therapy for all study subjects.
2 Aspirin alone does not constitute best medical therapy.
3 Risk factor management is an essential but often neglected aspect of care.
4 Antiplatelet therapy is indicated for all stroke-prone patients.

The principal risk factors to be controlled include hypertension, hyperlipidemia, diabetes, and tobacco use.

The threshold levels for hypertension management and target blood pressure are controversial and age-dependent. In the UK and US respectively, blood pressures of $\leq 160/90$ and $\leq 140/90$ mmHg are considered appropriate targets, although, especially in carotid patients, these are often not met. It is generally accepted, however, that the lower the blood pressure, the lower the stroke risk.

Similarly, it is quite likely that there is a linear relationship between blood lipid levels and stroke risk. The emergence of the statin drugs has greatly facilitated hyperlipidemia control.

While there is no doubt that diabetes is a significant risk factor for stroke, it is unclear that tight glycemic control using currently available methods alters this risk. On the other hand, hyperglycemia in stroke victims is associated with worse outcomes.

While smoking cessation is associated with as much as a 50% reduction in stroke risk, it is a goal that is difficult to achieve for most patients. Evidence suggests that patients highly motivated to improve their overall health can quit smoking without the aid of unproven adjunctive therapy.

Given the disappointing results of various trials of therapeutic intervention after acute stroke, prevention is clearly the preferred strategy. Optimization of risk factors and medical preventive therapy should never be assumed or delegated to the most junior surgical team member. This task should be undertaken by dedicated medical specialists.

Part Three Operative Care

16.1

What evidence is there that regional anesthesia confers any benefit over general anesthesia?

Michael Horrocks (Europe)

INTRODUCTION

Over the past few years there has been increasing interest in the role of local or locoregional anaesthesia (LA) as an alternative to general anaesthesia (GA) during carotid endarterectomy (CEA). As the complication rate following CEA has gradually fallen, every effort has been made to try and reduce the risk of perioperative stroke and death even further. A recent meta-analysis[1] has suggested that there may well be a benefit in terms of a reduction in the risk of death and/or stroke if CEA is done under regional anaesthesia rather than GA. In addition, there is increasing evidence that CEA under LA may be associated with a reduced length of hospital stay, reduced requirements for blood pressure control and enhanced patient preference.[2]

ADVANTAGES OF GENERAL ANAESTHESIA

Most vascular surgeons would probably concede that having the patient asleep, quiet and stable is the ideal way to perform CEA. This means that the surgeon can take as long as needed to do the operation and that he or she can perform any additional procedures that are required, there is no difficulty in extending the operation either proximally or distally and there is ample opportunity to teach younger colleagues. In addition, some GA agents may reduce cerebral metabolic oxygen requirements and increase cerebral blood flow whilst conferring a degree of neuroprotection.[3]

DISADVANTAGES OF GENERAL ANAESTHESIA

The main problem with GA is that there is no precise knowledge as to what is happening to the brain during carotid cross-clamping. Thus, for those

surgeons who adopt the practice of selective shunting, some indirect or direct method of assessing cerebral blood flow or neuronal function is necessary. There are a number of techniques for assessing neuronal function and/or cerebral blood flow, including stump pressure measurement, transcranial Doppler ultrasound, near infra-red spectroscopy, electroencephalography and evoked potentials, but none has been shown to be absolutely reliable in predicting the outcome of cross-clamping. This is largely because individual patients vary in their susceptibility to reduced cerebral blood flow, particularly if there is an area of infarction with a surrounding ischaemic penumbra. In addition, although GA may be associated with some degree of cerebral protection, patients may be less haemodynamically stable under GA: their blood pressure often falls and they require therapeutic blood pressure elevation by the anaesthetist in order to maintain the cerebral collateral circulation.[4]

One way of avoiding the problem of hypoperfusion during carotid artery cross-clamping is routinely to insert a shunt. It is well-recognized, however, that shunt insertion is not without its problems and that dissection, mural emboli and air emboli can occur.[5] In addition, in patients with small arteries (usually women) the shunt may be too large and injudicious attempts to force the shunt into a small internal carotid artery may cause damage. Shunts also occasionally come out of the carotid artery during the procedure, requiring urgent reinsertion.

Selective shunting, a policy which is widely advocated, requires strict criteria for shunt insertion. Preoperative tasks such as carotid compression (the Matas test) and observing thereafter whether a neurological deficit occurs in the awake patient are unreliable, and preoperative assessment by angiography (i.e. looking at patterns of cross-over flow in the brain) has also been shown to be unreliable.

Intraoperative assessment, such as stump pressure measurement and changes in middle cerebral artery velocity (MCAV) using transcranial Doppler, whilst appearing to indicate good or poor collateral flow, may well be flawed.[6] It has been observed that, when patients have been operated on under local anaesthesia, there is often a poor correlation between these observations and whether or not the patient stays awake or develops a neurological deficit during carotid clamping.[7] In practice, shunts seem to be required in only 10–15% of patients who are operated upon under LA as opposed to approximately 50% of those under GA.[2,7]

ADVANTAGES OF LOCAL ANAESTHESIA

The obvious advantage of LA is that the patient remains awake and cooperative during the procedure. This enables the surgeon or anaesthetist continuously to monitor the patient's cerebral function as the patient can talk, can explain to the surgeon how he or she feels and can be observed moving the arms and legs. It is common practice to give the patient a squeaky ball or toy to hold in the contralateral hand during the operation so that he or she can elicit a noise by moving the fingers, thus confirming movement and control of the hand hidden under the drapes.

Other advantages conferred by LA appear to be patient preference, a much more stable postoperative course, earlier recovery and earlier discharge.[2]

Further advantages of LA, particularly if a long-acting local anaesthetic such as Marcain is used, is that, should the patient develop a wound haematoma in the early postoperative period, it is usually possible to take the patient back to theatre, evacuate the haematoma and deal with the bleeding source under the same local anaesthetic as was originally used for the operation. This is clearly not possible after 4–5 h have elapsed, but most haematomas occur in the first 2–4 h following operation and can be dealt with

in this way. Trying to reanaesthetize a patient under GA can be hazardous as intubation may be difficult in the presence of an expanding haematoma in the neck.

DISADVANTAGES OF LOCAL ANAESTHESIA

The main disadvantages of LA relate to the possible interreaction between surgeon and patient, with the potential for the patient becoming disturbed or uncomfortable during the procedure. A good regional block is essential to provide an area of dense anaesthesia in the region of the neck so that the patient will not feel the procedure at all. At the first sign of any discomfort by the patient, it is wise to extend a local block by infiltration in the wound, followed by a short period of waiting whilst the anaesthetic takes effect. This has the disadvantage that it may slightly delay the operation, although in experienced hands there is little difference between LA and GA in the time taken for the procedure (personal observations).

A good pre-med is essential in order to relieve anxiety and make the patient relaxed during the procedure. It may occasionally be necessary to sedate an overanxious patient by using intravenous anxiolytic but is clearly important not to oversedate the patient as neurological response may be difficult to assess.

Like all techniques, CEA under LA requires practice and experience and there is inevitably a learning curve related to the anaesthetic technique as well as to the operation itself. With care and practice, however, these potential disadvantages can be easily overcome, resulting in a swift and easy technique which takes no longer than GA and may even reduce the operative time because there is no need to insert or remove an indwelling shunt in any patient.

WHAT IS THE EVIDENCE?

The Cochrane Collaboration has recently reviewed 17 non-randomized studies (5970 patients) and three randomized trials (143 patients) with respect to early outcome.[1] In the randomized trials (Table 16.1), there were too few end-points in the small number of patients and there was no overall difference in the risk of death, any stroke or myocardial infarction within 30 days of operation.[1]

There was, however, a small but significant reduction in the incidence of neck haematoma formation and, as might be expected, a significant decrease in the number of arteries shunted in patients undergoing CEA under LA. The evidence relating to changes in blood pressure is conflicting. In each of the randomized studies, blood pressure fell following induction of GA. In the study of Forssell et al.,[8] hypotension requiring treatment in the perioperative period was significantly more likely to be encountered in GA patients (25%) than in LA patients (7%), whilst Pluskwa et al.,[9] and Prough et al.[10] observed that hypotension was more commonly encountered in the early postoperative period in patients undergoing surgery with LA.

Table 16.1
Summary of outcomes in an overview of the randomized trials of endarterectomy under general versus locoregional anaesthesia

Outcome	CEA under LA	CEA under GA
Death	0%	1.3%
Any stroke	5.1%	4.0%
Stroke or death	5.1%	5.3%
Myocardial infarction	2.5%	1.3%
Neck haematoma	1.88%	10.9%*
Arteries shunted	8.9%	45%*

CEA, carotid endarterectomy; LA, Locoregional anaesthesia, GA, general anaesthesia.
*$P < 0.05$.
Adapted from Tangkanakul et al.[1] with permission.

In an overview of the non-randomized trials (Table 16.2), surgery under LA was associated with a 40–50% relative risk reduction in operative stroke and/or death, a 60% reduction in the relative risk of perioperative myocardial infarction or pulmonary complications and a significant reduction in the requirement for shunting. Although not always cited as an end-point, surgery under LA was associated with one day less in the intensive therapy unit and two fewer days in hospital.[1]

Table 16.2
Summary of outcomes in an overview of the non-randomized trials of endarterectomy under general versus locoregional anaesthesia

Outcome	CEA under LA	CEA under GA
Death	0.8%	1.1%
Any stroke	2.0%	5.3%*
Stroke or death	2.2%	6.1%*
Myocardial infarction	0.6%	1.3%*
Neck haematoma	2.4%	2.9%
Pulmonary complications	0.7%	0.9%*
Cranial nerve injury	3.4%	5.5%
Arteries shunted	10.8%	44.3%*

*$P < 0.05$.
Adapted from Tangkanakul et al.[1] with permission. CEA, carotid endarterectomy; LA, locoregional anaesthesia; GA, general anaesthesia.

OPERATIVE TECHNIQUE

Administration of Local Anaesthetic

LA is best administered in the anaesthetic room once the patient's invasive monitoring has been set up. It is important to have electrocardiogram and blood pressure monitoring as, occasionally, patients may react to the local anaesthetic and become hypertensive and tachycardic.

It is helpful to have the neck marked out as shown in Figure 16.1, with the anterior border of sternomastoid clearly marked from the suprasternal notch to the mastoid process. It is also helpful to have the angle of the jaw marked so that this can be clearly avoided, reducing the risk of damage to the mandibular branch of the facial nerve.

A total of 30 ml 0.5% Marcain with adrenaline is used for the locoregional block. The tips of the transverse processes of C_2, C_3 and C_4 are marked and a spinal needle is inserted on to the tip of each transverse process and approximately 4 ml local anaesthetic is infiltrated. This is usually sufficient to give a dense anterior cervical block. It is wise to give

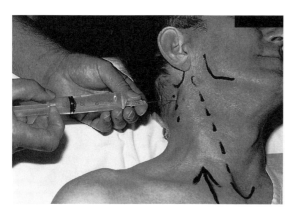

Fig. 16.1
Neck marked out for local anaesthetic, with spinal needle inserted to block C_2.

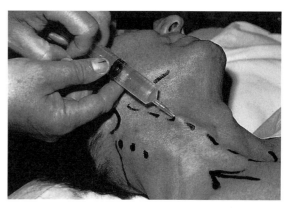

Fig. 16.2
Infiltration of the skin wound with local anaesthetic.

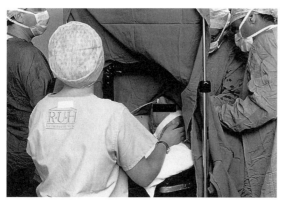

Fig. 16.3
View from the head end, with the assistant talking to the patient during the operation.

a further 15 ml along the line of the incision in the subcutaneous plane in order to provide good skin anaesthesia and also to reduce the amount of subcutaneous oozing (Fig. 16.2).

Setting up the Patient for Operation

It is important to set the patient up on the operating table in a comfortable position so that he or she does not become restless during the operation. Care should be taken to ensure that all pressure points are well padded and supported and that there is adequate access to reach all the limbs for assessment. It is routine practice to ask the patient

to empty the bladder before going to the operating theatre and it is advisable to ask the anaesthetist not to give too much intravenous fluid during the operation, as this may produce an unwanted diuresis and full bladder. Should the patient develop a full bladder, then in the male patient a bottle can be placed to allow him to pass urine. In the female patient it may be necessary to pass a temporary urethral catheter. However, these complications do not normally arise with good preoperative organization.

Dealing With a Restless Patient during Operation

Patients may become restless during the procedure for a variety of reasons. One of the commonest causes that I found initially was oversedation of the patient before starting the procedure. This made the patient disoriented and slightly confused and this was generally unhelpful. An oral pre-med of temazepam 20 mg (30 mg for very heavy patients) seems to be adequate and intravenous sedation is now rarely required. Should the patient become uncomfortable during the procedure, then a further infiltration with local anaesthetic and a few minutes' pause to allow the patient to settle down is very important.

The key person during the operation is the nurse or technologist, who sits with the patient on the opposite side of the operating table behind the drapes and talks to and assesses the patient continually during the procedure (Fig. 16.3).

Engaging the patient in conversation and giving constant reassurance is a valuable way of reducing anxiety. In my experience of more than 100 CEAs under local anaesthesia, I have not had to convert a patient to GA and it has always been possible to complete the operation without undue haste. Should it be necessary to extend the endarterectomy above and behind the posterior belly of digastric, it is usually possible to do so with further infiltration of local anaesthetic. Obvious care needs to be taken with extension up to the level of the styloid process, but otherwise the operation proceeds as if the patient were under GA. The cervical block with Marcain will last for up to 6 h, so there is usually no problem with the additional time required for anastomosing a patch. It is clearly sensible to have an anaesthetist present in the operating theatre during this time. Occasionally patients may start to cough during the procedure and may have difficulty in clearing the airway. Having an experienced person to aspirate the airway and reassure the patient can prevent any unnecessary distress.

There is a group of patients who appear to become slightly disoriented and confused following cross-clamping. If there is no simple cause for this, such as wound discomfort, and the patient does do not settle with simple reassurance, then sometimes insertion of a carotid shunt may improve the situation. It is likely that these patients are suffering from frontal lobe hypoperfusion and, on occasions, the response to shunting has been quite dramatic, with the patient becoming settled and stable, thus allowing the operation to proceed.

Normally, the requirement for a shunt is much more obvious, in that patients develop a contralateral hemiparesis or become uncooperative or unrousable. The response to insertion of a shunt in these cases is usually quite dramatic.

The time at which the patient may become hypoxic is extremely variable. There are patients who appear to become unconscious immediately following cross-clamping and this is reversed with the insertion of a shunt. However, there are others who become subtly less cooperative as the operation proceeds and who may then suddenly become disengaged in conversation or unresponsive. This can occur up to 20 min following cross-clamping, so the patient must be constantly monitored. It is clearly important to have a trained observer to monitor the patient's cerebral function. If there is any doubt, then a shunt should be inserted. This does not pose any more difficulties than under GA but results in most operations being done without a shunt, allowing much easier access, particularly to the top end of the internal carotid artery.

Abandoning Endarterectomy under Local Anaesthesia

It has been my experience that it is never necessary to abandon CEA under LA. Clearly, if a patient became so agitated and failed to respond to normal sedation despite shunt insertion and reassurance, and the operation became impossible, then conversion might be required. It would seem sensible to have an anaesthetist present in theatre throughout the operation with the appropriate instrumentation and drugs available for induction and intubation. In experienced hands, however, this does not appear to be required and management as above appears to be sufficient to manage all patients under LA. The confidence of the operating team, the administration of an adequate pre-med and constant reassurance during LA appear to be more than sufficient to enable the operation to be performed regularly under LA without resort to GA.

It is often felt that some patients, possibly those from certain cultural backgrounds, are not appropriate for regional anaesthesia. It is the author's experience that all patients can be encouraged to go through this operation under LA with good results. The practice of recruiting a patient who has previously had the operation under LA to talk to an anxious patient appears to be an effective and successful way of giving reassurance.

REFERENCES

1 Tangkanakul C, Counsell C, Warlow CP. Local versus general anaesthesia in carotid endarterectomy: a systematic review of the evidence. *European Journal of Vascular and Endovascular Surgery* 1997; **13**: 491–499.

2 John CR, Budd JS, Horrocks M. Carotid endarterectomy – unexpected benefits of local anaesthesia *British Journal of Surgery* (in press).

3 Campkin TV, Turner JM. Anaesthesia for the surgery of cerebral arterial insufficiency. In: Campkin TV, Turner JM (eds) *Neurosurgical Anaesthesia and Intensive Care,* pp. 222–236. London: Butterworths, 1986.

4 Luosto R, Ketonon P, Mattila S, Takkunem O, Eerola S. Local anaesthesia in carotid surgery. *Scandinavian Journal of Thoracic and Cardiovascular Surgery* 1984; **18**: 133–137.

5 Halsey JH. Risks and benefits of shunting in carotid endarterectomy. *Stroke* 1992; **23**: 1583–1587.

6 Hobson RW, Wright CB, Sublett JW, Fedde W, Rich NM. Carotid artery back pressure and endarterectomy under regional anaesthesia. *Archives of Surgery* 1974; **109**: 680–687.

7 Benjamin ME, Silva MB, Watt C *et al.* Awake patient monitoring to determine the need for shunting during carotid endarterectomy. *Surgery* 1993; **114**: 673–679.

8 Forssell C, Takolander R, Bergqvist D, Johansson A, Persson NH. Local versus general anaesthesia in carotid surgery: a prospective randomised study. *European Journal of Vascular Surgery* 1989; **3**: 503–509.

9 Pluskwa F, Bonnet F, Abhay K *et al.* Blood pressure profiles during carotid endarterectomy: comparing flunitrazepan/fentanyl/nitrous oxide with epidural anaesthesia. *Annales Françaises d'Anesthesie Reanimation* 1989; **8**: 26–32.

10 Prough DS, Scuderi PE, McWhorter JM, Balestrieri FJ, Davis CH, Stullken EH. Haemodynamic status following regional and general anaesthesia for carotid endarterectomy. *Journal of Neurosurgical Anesthesiology* 1989; **1**: 35–40.

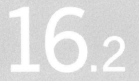

16.2

What evidence is there that regional anesthesia confers any benefit over general anesthesia?

Caron B Rockman (USA)

Thomas S Riles (USA)

The optimal anesthetic management for CEA has remained a matter for debate for more than three decades. The techniques of local and cervical block anesthesia for carotid surgery have been described and used since before 1962.[11] The initial reason for using regional or local anesthesia rather than GA at our institution and others in the early 1960s was to observe directly the neurologic status of the patient during carotid clamping. The observation that a small number of patients were intolerant to clamping of the internal carotid artery, and therefore required a shunt for cerebral protection during the endarterectomy, led to a dilemma when performing surgery with the patient under GA. To ensure that unconscious patients would not have a stroke while the operation was being performed, one of two methods could be used: a shunt could either be used routinely, or some monitoring technique could be devised to differentiate patients at risk for cerebral ischemia during carotid clamping. Therefore, shunting could be performed selectively.

Although excellent results have been achieved with GA and a variety of monitoring approaches, historically no single technique has correlated well with the direct observation of the conscious patient.[12–15] All of the direct methods (electroencephalography (EEG), evoked potential responses) and indirect methods (carotid stump pressure, transcranial Doppler ultrasound, jugular venous oxygen tension) of detecting cerebral ischemia during carotid clamping have been found to lack either sensitivity or specificity when compared with the neurologic status of the awake patient. EEG, for example, may lead to as high as a 20–25% incidence of intraluminal shunting;[12] the rate of selective shunting in a similar population of

conscious patients has been reported to be as low as 7%.[15] Conversely, perioperative strokes have clearly occurred in the absence of any detectable EEG changes.

Historically, regional anesthetic was an essential tool to aid in the development and evaluation of these various cerebral monitoring techniques and protective measures.[15] However, as experience and expertise grew with carotid shunting and with cerebral monitoring with the patient under GA, some surgeons concluded that keeping the patient awake was unnecessary in most cases.[16]

Although advocates of each anesthetic technique often use perioperative stroke rates to support their positions, it has become increasingly clear that these perioperative neurologic complications are more often related to etiologies other than clamping ischemia, and include postoperative thrombosis at the endarterectomy site, intraoperative embolization, and reperfusion injury.[15,17] Operating on the conscious patient has been crucial in allowing accurate differentiation between the various mechanisms of perioperative stroke, especially the distinction between clamping ischemia and non-specific cerebral embolization.[12–15] The causes of perioperative stroke have been analyzed in detail at our institution, and only 15% of all perioperative strokes have been found to be definitively related to cerebral ischemia during clamping. Because the inability to monitor directly the patient's neurologic status during clamping is inextricably related to the anesthetic method used, presumably only those strokes that are caused specifically by clamping ischemia should vary with the anesthetic route. None the less, experienced surgeons at major centers for carotid surgery have demonstrated excellent results with both GA and regional anesthesia. With perioperative complication rates of less than 2.0% becoming the standard, comparisons using perioperative stroke and death as the end-points may only be meaningful with thousands of patients being randomized and prospectively studied.

Regional anesthesia clearly has been the preferred technique when performing CEA at our institution for more than 30 years.[17] Recently there has been a renewed focus on regional anesthesia for additional reasons. As regional anesthesia has come to be preferred for lower-extremity vascular reconstructions, several investigators have argued that this technique for CEA will similarly decrease operative time, length of hospital stay, and hospital costs – issues that have received increased attention in current times. In light of the recent resurgence of interest in regional anesthesia, we shall try to answer the question: What evidence is there that regional anesthesia is superior to GA?

Advocates have reasoned that, among several advantages of regional anesthesia, neurologic complications should be less frequent, because with regional anesthesia the need for shunting can be most accurately assessed.[12–15,18–31] Thus, manifestations of intraoperative cerebral ischemia can be treated immediately. In addition, patients who have coronary and pulmonary disease should seemingly fare better without endotracheal intubation and GA.

Of nine relatively recent reports in the literature that specifically compare local or regional anesthesia with GA for carotid surgery, six found no discernible differences in perioperative strokes or death on the basis of anesthetic technique.[23–31] However, two reports did detect an increased rate of perioperative stroke in the GA group.[26,29] Three studies revealed an increased incidence of cardiopulmonary complications or myocardial infarction in patients who underwent surgery under GA.[23,27,30] Most dramatically, Peitzman et al. demonstrated a significantly increased incidence of non-neurologic complications among those patients who received GA when compared with those who received regional anesthesia (12.9% vs 2.8%).[27] These findings are in conflict with those of several excellent series reported in the literature that demonstrate equally low neurologic and cardiopulmonary complication rates with GA using various forms of intracerebral monitoring (Fig. 16.4).[32–36]

A recent meta-analysis has attempted a review of 17 non-randomized and 3 randomized studies comparing regional with general anesthesia, encompassing a total of approximately 6000 patients.[37] This review found that non-randomized studies suggested that local anesthesia may be associated with significant reductions in the odds of stroke, death, myocardial infarction, and pulmonary complications. However, it was also concluded that there were far too few data from any randomized trials to confirm these findings.

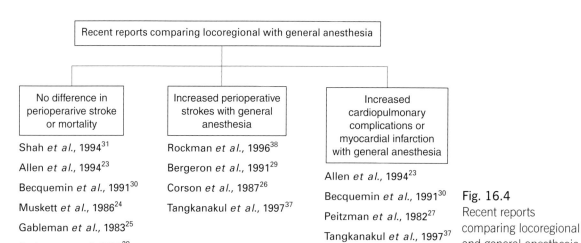

Fig. 16.4 Recent reports comparing locoregional and general anesthesia.

A recent review of this topic at our institution reported results with regional anesthesia for carotid surgery over a 30-year period.[28] Of the 3975 CEAs performed, regional anesthesia was used in 3382 (85.1%). The remaining 593 operations were performed with the patient under GA (14.9%). All patients who required GA underwent operation with an empirically placed intra-arterial shunt. All awake patients who demonstrated signs of ischemia with test clamping of the internal carotid artery (convulsions, loss of consciousness, aphasia, extremity weakness, confusion, slowing of mentation) were selectively treated with intra-arterial shunting during endarterectomy. Regional anesthesia was used in 86.9% of patients who underwent surgery for asymptomatic high-grade stenosis, 88.4% of patients who had preoperative transient ischemic attacks or amaurosis fugax, and 82.4% of patients who had preoperative strokes. Patients who underwent surgery under regional anesthesia were compared with those who received GA with respect to preoperative risk factors, intraoperative courses, and perioperative complications. There were no significant differences in the incidences of hypertension, coronary artery disease, diabetes mellitus, smoking history, or age of these two populations.

In comparing operative indications, there was a statistically significant increase in the proportion of patients who received GA for which the surgical indication was stroke when compared with the regional anesthesia cases (36.1% vs 26.4%; $P < 0.001$). Conversely, there was a corresponding decreased percentage of patients who received GA for which the surgical indication was a transient ischemic attack (46.6% vs 56.6%; $P < 0.001$). There was, in addition, a statistically significant higher frequency of contralateral total occlusion in the GA group (21.8% vs 15.4%). Intra-arterial shunting was used in 372 (11.0%) of the operations that were performed with the patient under regional anesthesia. The overall frequencies of complications were perioperative stroke in 2.2%, myocardial infarction in 1.7%, and death in 1.5%. There was an increased rate of perioperative stroke (3.2% vs 2.0%) and perioperative mortality (2.0% vs 1.4%) in the GA group, although these results were not statistically significant (Table 16.3 and 16.4).

The entire group was broken down into three subgroups on the basis of the year of operation in order to examine recent trends (1962–1974, 1975–1984, and 1985–1994). In the last 10 years (1985–1994) there was a statistically higher incidence of perioperative stroke in the cases receiving GA (3.2% vs 1.2%; $P < 0.01$).

Table 16.3
Comparison of locoregional with general anesthesia at New York University Medical Center (1962–1994)

	General anesthesia ($n = 593$)	Regional anesthesia ($n = 3382$)	P value
Surgical indications			
Asymptomatic	17.3%	18.0%	NS
Transient ischemic attack	46.6%	55.6%	<0.001
Stroke	36.1%	26.4%	<0.001
Contralateral occlusion	21.8%	15.4%	<0.001
Intraoperative management			
Shunt utilized	100.0%	11.0%	
Perioperative complications			
Stroke	3.2%	2.0%	NS
Myocardial infarction	1.7%	1.7%	NS
Mortality	2.0%	1.4%	NS

Table 16.4
Comparison of locoregional with general anesthesia at New York University Medical Center (1992–1997)

	General anesthesia (n = 593)	Regional anesthesia (n = 3382)	P value
Patient characteristics			
Coronary disease	44.7%	46.4%	NS
Diabetes mellitus	22.0%	24.2%	NS
Smoking	39.2%	31.3%	< 0.03
Hypertension	62.8%	60.9%	NS
Surgical indications			
Asymptomatic	32.7%	50.7%	< 0.0001
Transient ischemic attack	35.9%	33.8%	NS
Stroke	31.3%	15.4%	< 0.0001
Contralateral occlusion	22.8%	11.7%	< 0.0001
Perioperative complications			
Stroke	4.6%	1.7%	< 0.02
Myocardial infarction	1.8%	0.5%	0.055
Mortality	0.9%	0.7%	NS

Univariate analysis performed for the entire 32-year period revealed that only hypertension ($P < 0.02$) and a history of preoperative stroke ($P < 0.001$) were found to be associated with perioperative stroke. The use of GA was nearly statistically significant in this regard ($P = 0.057$). These three factors were then entered into a multivariate analysis, which identified only a history of preoperative stroke as an independent predictor of perioperative stroke. A similar analysis was performed for the most recent 10-year period (1985–1994). By univariate analysis in this subgroup, the use of a GA ($P < 0.02$) and a history of preoperative stroke ($P < 0.01$) were found to be significantly associated with perioperative stroke. A multivariate analysis was again performed, which once more identified only a history of preoperative stroke to be independently associated with perioperative stroke.

In our current series the risk of myocardial infarction was identical between the two anesthetic groups. A trend toward increased perioperative mortality rates was noted in the GA group (2.0% vs 1.4%), although this increase did not reach statistical significance. The same was true of

perioperative strokes (3.2% vs 2.0%) over the entire 32-year period. In the most recent 10 years, however, the difference in perioperative stroke rates between the two anesthetic groups did reach statistical significance (3.2% vs 1.2%; $P < 0.01$). Unfortunately, it is evident that the two patient populations did not have equivalent risk factors; those who underwent surgery under GA appear to be a group at increased risk for perioperative stroke, having a higher incidence of contralateral total occlusion and preoperative stroke. Although it is possible that the differences found are a result of the anesthetic method used, the significant differences in the risk factors of the patient populations are likely to be at least partially responsible for the higher incidence of perioperative stroke found with operations performed with the patient under GA.

To explain the higher complication rate with GA in recent years entirely on the selection of patients may, however, be overly simplistic. Likewise, to conclude that in earlier years there was no significant difference between the techniques may be open to criticism. Because the overall incidence of complications is very low, in some instances the outcome of a single case may determine the

16.2

What evidence is there that regional anesthesia confers any benefit over general anesthesia?

statistical significance. Without a detailed analysis of the causes of the complications, it is hazardous to assume that the choice of anesthetic was the only determining factor. In their enthusiasm to defend or oppose the use of regional anesthesia for carotid surgery, many authors have looked at perioperative complications as a measure to compare.

A more recent review was conducted for CEAs performed for the years 1992–1997. This revealed a significantly higher perioperative stroke rate among the GA cases as opposed to the regional anesthesia cases (4.6% vs 1.7%; $P < 0.02$).

Regional anesthesia with selective shunting has obviously been, and currently still is, the preferred method of carotid surgery at our institution. In our practice there are no absolute contraindications to regional anesthesia. If a patient expresses a strong preference for GA, an effort is made to accommodate the patient's wishes. Claustrophobia, neurologic disorders, including stroke, and language barriers have been relative contraindications to regional anesthesia if these factors make cooperation and communication difficult. The trend toward using GA for patients who have contralateral occlusion and prior stroke, in recent years has come from the earlier observation that these patients are more likely to require a shunt. The feeling among some surgeons is that, if a shunt is likely to be necessary anyway, there is no particular reason to monitor cerebral function; this belief is likely to be somewhat responsible for the increased use of GA in these patients. However, we are not suggesting that GA is superior for these patients; in fact, the opposite may be true. These are simply cases in which the operating surgeon would feel uncomfortable performing the operation without a shunt in place during carotid clamping.

CONCLUSIONS

Only a randomized prospective trial could absolutely determine the small, but possibly clinically significant, differences between regional anesthesia and GA. Although the data reported from our institution and elsewhere do not definitively prove that regional anesthesia reduces the rate of adverse events after CEA, there are certainly suggestions that it may reduce both neurologic and cardiopulmonary complications. Additionally, we believe that there are useful and important advantages to this technique that are unrelated to the issue of perioperative complications. No specialized equipment or intraoperative monitoring of cerebral function is required. The need for intra-arterial shunting appears to us from our own experience and from the available reported data to be most accurately assessed with the patient awake; this may make some anatomically difficult cases more manageable in that a prophylactic shunt may not be absolutely necessary. Assessment of the neurologic status of the patient after surgery and in the recovery room is simplified without the after-effects of GA.

We conclude that regional anesthesia can be safely used for CEA in the vast majority of patients, with good clinical results. Unexpected conversion to GA during the course of surgery occurs in approximately 3% of cases, based on a recent prospective study of this topic at our institution. The incidence of serious complications related to the administration of the anesthetic itself is extremely low. Although the data in our series clearly suggest that regional anesthesia may be better than GA with regard to perioperative stroke, patient selection may account for these differences. Even if used only selectively, however, we believe that the ability to perform carotid surgery under regional anesthesia is crucial and should be a part of the armamentarium of skills of every vascular surgeon.

REFERENCES

11 Spencer FC, Elsemann B. Technique of carotid endarterectomy. *Surgery, Gynecology and Obstetrics* 1962; **115**: 115–117.

12 Imparato AM. Cerebral protection during anesthesia for carotid and vertebral surgery. In: Bernstein EF, Callow AD, Nicolaides AN *et al.* (eds) *Cerebral Revascularisation*, pp. 405–505. London: Med-Orion, 1993.

13 Imparato AM. Carotid endarterectomy: indications and techniques for carotid surgery. In: Haimovici H, Ascer E, Hollier LH *et al.* (eds) *Haimovici's Vascular Surgery*, 4th edn, pp. 913–937. Boston: Blackwell Science, 1996.

14 Imparato AM, Riles TS, Ramirez AA, Lamparello PJ, Mintzer R. Anaesthetic management in carotid artery

surgery. *Australia and New Zealand Journal of Surgery* 1985; **55**: 315–319.

15 Imparato AM, Ramirez A, Riles TS, Mintzer R. Cerebral protection in carotid surgery. *Archives of Surgery* 1982; **117**: 1073–1078.

16 Riles TS, Gold M. Alternatives to general anesthesia for carotid endarterectomy. In: Moore WS (ed.) *Surgery for Cerebrovascular Disease*, 2nd edn, pp. 338–341. Philadelphia: WB Saunders, 1996.

17 Riles TS, Imparato AM, Jacobowitz GR *et al.* The cause of perioperative stroke after carotid endarterectomy. *Journal of Vascular Surgery* 1994; **19**: 206–216.

18 Connolly JE. Carotid endarterectomy in the awake patient. *American Journal of Surgery* 1985; **150**: 159–165.

19 Donato AT, Hill SL. Carotid arterial surgery using local anesthesia: a private practice retrospective study. *American Surgeon* 1992; **58**: 446–450.

20 Hafner CD, Evans WE. Carotid endarterectomy with local anesthesia: results and advantages. *Journal of Vascular Surgery* 1988; **7**: 232–239.

21 Rich NM, Hobson RW II. Carotid endarterectomy under regional anesthesia. *American Surgeon* 1975; **41**: 253–258.

22 Benjamin ME, Silva MB, Watt C. Awake patient monitoring to determine the need for shunting during carotid endarterectomy. *Surgery* 1993; **114**: 673–681.

23 Allen BT, Anderson CB, Rubin BG *et al.* The influence of anesthetic technique on perioperative complications after carotid endarterectomy. *Journal of Vascular Surgery* 1994; **19**: 834–843.

24 Muskett A, McGreevy J, Miller M. Detailed comparison of regional and general anesthesia for carotid endarterectomy. *American Journal of Surgery* 1986; **152**: 691–694.

25 Gableman CG, Gann DS, Ashworth CJ. One hundred consecutive carotid reconstructions: local versus general anesthesia. *American Journal of Surgery* 1983; **145**: 477–482.

26 Corson JD, Chang BB, Shah DM. The influence of anesthetic choice on carotid endarterectomy outcome. *Archives of Surgery* 1987; **122**: 807–812.

27 Peitzman AB, Webster MW, Loubeau JM. Carotid endarterectomy under regional (conductive) anesthesia. *Annals of Surgery* 1982; **196**: 59–64.

28 Andersen CA, Rich NM, Collins GJ, McDonald PT. Carotid endarterectomy: regional versus general anesthesia. *American Surgeon* 1980; **46**: 323–327.

29 Bergeron P, Benichou H, Rudondy P, Jausseran JM, Gerdani M, Courbier R. Stroke prevention during carotid surgery in high risk patients (value of transcranial Doppler and local anesthesia). *Journal of Cardiovascular Surgery (Torino)* 1991; **32**: 713–719.

30 Becquemin JP, Paris E, Valverde A, Pluskwa F, Melliere D. Carotid surgery. Is regional anesthesia always appropriate? *Journal of Cardiovascular Surgery (Torino)* 1991; **32**: 592–598.

31 Shah DM, Darling RC III, Chang BB, Bock DEM, Paty PSK, Leather RP. Carotid endarterectomy in awake patients: its safety, acceptability, and outcome. *Journal of Vascular Surgery* 1994; **19**: 1015–1020.

32 Callow AD, Matsumoto G, Baker D *et al.* Protection of the high risk carotid endarterectomy patient by continuous electroencephalography. *Journal of Cardiovascular Surgery (Torino)* 1978; **19**: 55–64.

33 Hertzer NR, Avellone JC, Farrel CJ *et al.* The risk of vascular surgery in a metropolitan community. *Journal of Vascular Surgery* 1984; **1**: 13–21.

34 Fode NC, Sundt TM Jr, Robertson JT, Peerless SF, Shields CB. Multicenter retrospective review of results and complications of carotid endarterectomy in 1981. *Stroke* 1986; **17**: 370–374.

35 Moore WS, Yee JM, Hall AD. Collateral cerebral blood pressure: an index of tolerance to temporary carotid occlusion. *Archives of Surgery* 1973; **106**: 520–523.

36 Towne JB, Bernhard VM. Neurologic deficit following carotid endarterectomy. *Surgery, Gynecology and Obstetrics* 1982; **154**: 849–852.

37 Tangkanakul C, Counsell CE, Warlow CP. Local versus general anaesthesia in carotid endarterectomy: a systematic review of the evidence. *European Journal of Vascular and Endovascular Surgery* 1997; **13**: 491–499.

38 Rockman CB, Riles TS, Gold M *et al.* A comparison of regional and general anesthesia in patients undergoing carotid endarterectomy. *Journal of Vascular Surgery* 1996; **24**: 946–956.

16.3 Editorial Comment

KEY POINTS

1   CEA can be performed under regional anesthesia without compromising outcome.
2   For those who advocate selective shunting, CEA under regional anesthesia is the only way of accurately predicting who needs to be shunted.
3   CEA under regional anesthesia will not protect against stroke due to technical error unless some other method of quality control assessment is employed.
4   Not all patients will be suitable for CEA under regional anesthesia and an anesthesiologist must always be present to intubate patients if necessary.
5   There is no clear evidence, to date, that CEA under regional anesthesia is safer than general anesthesia and associated with reduced cardiovascular risk. This can only be answered by a properly designed randomized trial.

COMMENT

For those surgeons who adopt a policy of selective shunting, CEA under regional anesthesia is the *only* method capable of predicting accurately which patients need a shunt. For those who routinely shunt their patients, awake testing will warn of shunt malfunction, but this can also be achieved with transcranial Doppler or other modalities. However, reliance on awake testing is no substitute for obsessional surgical technique because clamp ischemia is a relatively rare cause of operation related stroke. Awake testing, while noting that some adverse event has occurred, will not prevent a thromboembolic stroke, which is the principal cause of operative morbidity.

The overview suggests that CEA under regional anesthesia may be associated with important benefits over general anesthesia (reduced cardiovascular and pulmonary morbidity, reduced hospital stay) which merit further assessment. This overview is, however, slightly unusual in that it was largely based on the results of non-randomized (often retrospective) studies rather than on outcomes after randomized trials. The fact that bias may be present through differences in presentation (LA patients tended to be asymptomatic) and use of antiplatelet agents was recognized by the authors. Moreover, not all patients will be suitable for CEA under regional anesthesia and many surgeons may simply find the experience too stressful.

Apart from predisposing towards earlier discharge, one of the most important benefits of CEA under regional anesthesia may be greater cardiovascular stability throughout the perioperative period. Unfortunately, to date, the evidence appears contradictory and no firm conclusions can be drawn in the absence of a large, randomized trial, which now seems inevitable.

What steps can I take to minimize inadvertent cranial nerve injury?

Torben V Schroeder (Europe)

Niels Levi (Europe)

INTRODUCTION

The stroke rate and operative mortality associated with carotid endarterectomy have been thoroughly documented and a 5–7% perioperative stroke and death rate was reported in the European Carotid Surgery Trial (ECST), and the North American Symptomatic Carotid Endarterectomy Trial (NASCET).[1,2]

In contrast, the incidence of injury to the cranial nerves has received relatively little attention.[3,4] The reported incidence of cranial nerve paresis following carotid endarterectomy varies from less than 5% to more than 50%, depending on whether the study · was conducted prospectively or retrospectively and on the sensitivity of the investigative method.[5–14]

The incidence of cranial nerve injuries from various studies is given in Table 17.1. Disregarding the frequently injured cutaneous sensory cervical nerves (Fig. 17.1), the cranial nerves which are at potential risk include VII, IX, X, XI and XII (Fig. 17.2).

GENERAL CONSIDERATIONS

A thorough understanding of both normal and abnormal anatomy is essential for the surgeon as well as the assistant.[15,16] As a general rule, no nerves crossing the bifurcation should be divided and, with care, it is usually possible to complete the procedure when anomalous anatomy is encountered (Fig. 17.3; see plate section). Careful handling of tissues, particularly during retraction, can avoid stretching of the nerves and so reduce the incidence of neuropraxia.[17] Although most cranial nerve palsies are usually transient, they can delay the patient's recovery and may increase the overall morbidity.[17–19]

Retractors should be placed with great care and should not be placed too deep within the tracheo-oesophageal groove and any self-retaining retraction of cutaneous flaps should be minimized.[16,17] Transection injuries should be rare, provided the normal and anomalous courses of the cranial nerves are recognized.[4] Sharp dissection close to the arterial wall will also lessen the risk of nerve injuries.[16] Precise bipolar electrocautery and carefully placed ligatures are important parts of the surgical technique. If bleeding occurs during the procedure, the vessels should not be grasped blindly with clamps.[16]

Because the surgeon's technique is important, it is possible that a learning curve may exist,[20] though the literature on this point is conflicting. Krupski et al. examined 300 operations performed by three categories of surgeons with varying experience and found no difference in the frequency of cranial nerve injury.[21] In contrast, Forssell et al. found that experienced surgeons had a lower incidence of nerve injury when compared to trainees, although the relationship was complex and may have been related to the varying use of a shunt and patch closure.[16] Prolonged clamp time was associated with an increased incidence of cranial nerve injury (presumably reflecting complex or high lesions) but the presence of postoperative haematoma and reoperation for bleeding had no association.[16]

CRANIAL NERVE ANATOMY

Vagus Nerve

The vagus nerve has the most extensive distribution of all the cranial nerves, innervating the heart and a

Table 17.1
Cranial nerve injuries in carotid surgery in prospective studies

Author	Year	No. op	VII (%)	IX (%)	Xr (%)	Xs (%)	XI (%)	XII (%)	Total (%)	
Hertzer[25]	1980	240	2.5		5.8	2.1		5.4	16	
Liapis et al.[9]	1981	40	5.0		27.0			20.0	53	
Evans et al.[35]	1982	128		1.5	35.0			11.0	47	
Astor et al.[17]	1983	133			5.9	1.3		5.8	14	
Dehn and Taylor[15]	1983	43			25.0			5.0	30	
Schmidt et al.[13]	1983	109	2.8		3.7			8.3	12	
Forssell et al.[37]	1985	162	0.6	1.2	3.1			10.5	17	
Weiss et al.[23]	1987	536	6.2	0.4	3.7			8.9	20	
Roger and Root[36]	1988	433	0.5	0.2	1.2			1.2	3	
Aldoori and Baird[5]	1988	52	5.8		5.8			15.8	25	
Forssell et al.[16]	1995	665	0.3	0.3	1.2	0.5	0.2	10.7	11	
Schauber et al.[18]	1997	183	1.1		7.7			4.4	14.2	Transient
					0.6			0.6	1.1	Permanent
Zanetti et al.[19]	1998	187	12		7		0	4	14	Transient
			1		1		0	0.5	2.5	Permanent

VII, mandibular branch of the facial nerve; IX, glossopharyngeal nerve; Xr, recurrent laryngeal nerve; Xs, superior laryngeal nerve; XI, accessory nerve; XII, hypoglossal nerve.
Adapted from Forssell et al.[20] with permission.

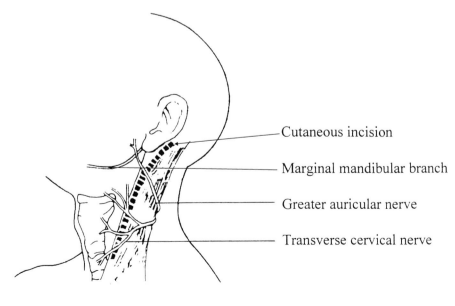

— Cutaneous incision

— Marginal mandibular branch

— Greater auricular nerve

— Transverse cervical nerve

Fig. 17.1
Frequently injured cutaneous sensory cervical nerves during carotid surgery.

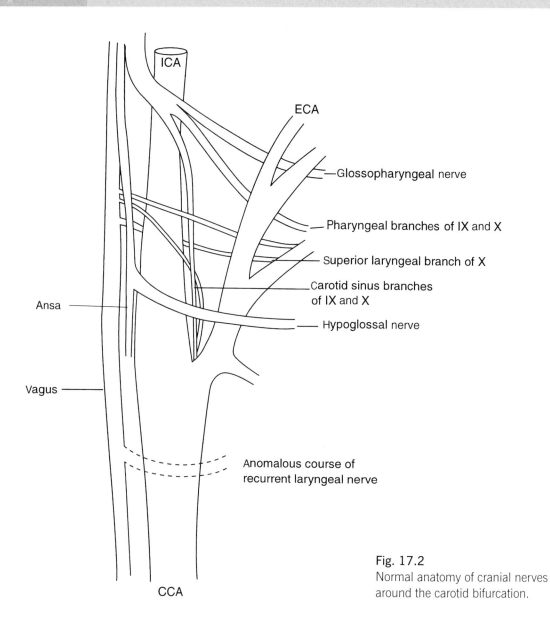

ICA

ECA

—Glossopharyngeal nerve

— Pharyngeal branches of IX and X

— Superior laryngeal branch of X

Carotid sinus branches of IX and X

— Hypoglossal nerve

Ansa

Vagus

Anomalous course of recurrent laryngeal nerve

CCA

Fig. 17.2
Normal anatomy of cranial nerves around the carotid bifurcation.

major component of the respiratory and alimentary tracts. The vagus nerve is usually identified posterior to the common carotid artery within the carotid sheath, but it can be found anterior and lateral to the artery or medial to the internal jugular vein.[4] In either position, it may be injured during injudicious dissection, by excessive retraction, or by compression within the proximal vascular clamp.[3] Although injury to the vagus nerve itself can cause significant problems, a number of important branches must also be considered.

Recurrent laryngeal nerve
The recurrent laryngeal nerve branches from the medial fibres of the vagus nerve within the mediastinum, loops around the subclavian artery on the right side and the aortic arch on the left side and lies in the tracheo-oesophageal groove, where it is concealed by the strap muscles.[4,20] The recurrent

laryngeal nerve is generally well removed from the operative field. Injury to either the vagus nerve or the recurrent laryngeal nerve produces paralysis of the ipsilateral vocal cord causing hoarseness and loss of an effective cough mechanism.[4] Bilateral recurrent laryngeal nerve injuries may be life-threatening because of airway obstruction.[4,22] Therefore bilateral carotid procedures must be staged with an intervening laryngoscopy to document vocal cord function. The same caution should also apply to patients who have undergone previous thyroid surgery. On rare occasions, a non-recurrent laryngeal nerve may emerge from the vagus, passing medially and behind the carotid bifurcation. In this situation, it is at greater risk of injury.

Superior laryngeal nerve

Another important (but often unrecognized) branch of the vagus is the superior laryngeal nerve. This originates from the nodose ganglion and passes obliquely down to the upper aspect of the larynx. It lies posterior to both the internal and external carotid arteries before terminating in an external branch to the cricothyroid muscle and the inferior pharyngeal constrictor as well as an internal branch for sensory innervation of the laryngeal mucosa.[3,4]

Injury to the superior laryngeal nerve leads to voice fatigue and inability of high-pitch phonation, both of which may be significant disabilities to vocalists or public speakers.[4,23] Minor swallowing problems may also occur as a result of injury to the internal branch. However, the deficits are generally transient.[24] The superior laryngeal nerve is small in comparison to the size of the vagus or hypoglossal nerves, and the vasa nervorum on its surface are helpful in its identification.[4]

The superior laryngeal nerve may be injured by compression within the distal internal carotid clamp or by manipulation of its terminal branches, particularly during isolation of the proximal part of the superior thyroid artery.[3,18] The diagnosis may be hard to make, thus the incidence is almost certainly underreported.[5,15,24]

Hypoglossal Nerve

The other frequently injured nerve is the hypoglossal nerve. The hypoglossal nerve descends into the neck in a relatively constant position medial to the internal carotid artery. About 3–5cm above the carotid bifurcation it crosses the bifurcation to enter the base of the tongue.[23,25] It may, however, cross the bifurcation in a lower position and can be quite adherent to adjacent structures. Identification during preliminary dissection is mandatory. The hypoglossal nerve is invariably tethered by its descending branch, which eventually joins the cervical nerves to form the ansa cervicalis, and also by the occipital artery and by the sternomastoid artery and vein.[26] The descending branch of the ansa supplies motor function to the omohyoid muscle, but transection has little, if any, clinical impact.[23,24]

The 12th cranial nerve supplies all the intrinsic and extrinsic muscles of the tongue, with the exception of palatoglossus. Division of the hypoglossal nerve causes ipsilateral paralysis and wasting of the muscles of the tongue and this is detected clinically by deviation of the protruded tongue to the affected side.

Unilateral paralysis is disturbing to the patient through difficulties in speech, mastication and swallowing.[20] Bilateral injuries can be potentially life-threatening through upper-airway obstruction.[20,26–28]

Injury to the hypoglossal nerve is well documented and is more commonly due to overzealous retraction than to division of the nerve trunk, especially in those subjects with a high carotid bifurcation.[15] Considering the frequency with which the nerve is retracted it is surprising that the incidence of neuropraxia is so low. The use of a transverse skin incision may increase the likelihood of this injury occurring because of the reduced access associated with this approach.[15] Atraumatic mobilization of the hypoglossal nerve (avoiding cautery or blind clamping) may be easier if the descending hypoglossal nerve (the superior limb of ansa cervicalis) and restrictive arterial branches are divided.[26] The hypoglossal nerve is often surrounded by several small veins which should be ligated and divided electively because application of clamps to control unexpected venous bleeding may injure the nerve itself.[26]

Glossopharyngeal Nerve

The glossopharyngeal nerve contains sensory fibres for the pharynx and the posterior one-third of the tongue. It also supplies motor fibres to the stylopharyngeus muscle, the middle pharyngeal constrictor, the tensor muscle of the soft palate and secretomotor fibres to the parotid gland. The glossopharyngeal nerve exits the skull via the jugular foramen and is located between the internal jugular vein and the internal carotid artery. The nerve then descends (deep to the styloid process and its associated muscles) and passes in front of the internal carotid artery (Fig. 17.2) and then anteriorly, where it lies upon the stylopharyngeus muscle before entering the pharyngeal constrictors.

Although glossopharyngeal nerve trauma is rare unless the internal carotid lesion is exceedingly high,[25,29,30] its symptoms are amongst the most serious of all cranial nerve deficits.[25] Solid food becomes difficult to swallow because of middle constrictor paralysis. Oral fluids are tolerated even more poorly because of nasopharyngeal reflux.[25] It is therefore essential that high carotid dissections are performed with extreme care. The mandibular subluxation technique provides a marked increase in exposure of the internal carotid artery up to the base of the skull and it has been advocated in this situation.[31,32]

Most glossopharyngeal nerve palsies are transient. In practice, therefore, the patient can be hydrated intravenously for 48–72h. If the palsy persists thereafter, a fine-bore feeding tube should be passed and enteral feeding continued until recovery has occurred.

Accessory Nerve

The accessory nerve lies anterior to the most distal portion of the internal carotid artery, and is therefore not normally encountered during a standard carotid endarterectomy and injuries are therefore rare. Potential mechanisms of injury in its more peripheral passage include extensive traction, oedema, haematoma or entrapment in scar tissue.[20,33,34]

Facial Nerve

The mandibular branch of the facial nerve passes parallel to the ramus of the mandible between the platysma and the deep cervical fascia.[23] Injury is manifested by drooping of the corner of the mouth and limited mobility of half of the lower lip and may be confused with a central facial paresis.[23] Whilst this injury imposes little in the way of functional disability, it is cosmetically unsatisfactory to most patients.[4] The nerve may be transected if the upper section of the skin incision extends too far anteriorly. An incision made beyond the angle of the mandible towards the mastoid process will safely avoid the marginal branch.[18,23] Liberal and long-standing use of self-retaining retractors may also injure the nerve by squeezing the tissue between the wound and the jaw.

Cervical Sympathetic Plexus

Horner's syndrome may occur if the superior cervical sympathetic chain is transected during mobilization of the internal carotid artery above the level of the digastric muscle. This injury is extremely rare but usually avoidable.[25]

CONCLUSIONS

As with many other complications, it is impossible to devise a foolproof method to avoid cranial nerve injury. However, more than 80% are transient. The key to their prevention is a thorough understanding of the patterns of normal and abnormal anatomy and extreme caution should be exercised before dividing any nerves that traverse the bifurcation. The risk of cranial nerve injury is increased in complex cases and, in particular, during operations for high carotid lesions. Any patient who has a history of previous thyroid surgery or contralateral carotid endarterectomy must undergo formal assessment of vocal cord function. A bilateral recurrent laryngeal nerve injury can be fatal.

REFERENCES

1 European Carotid Surgery Trial, triallists collaborative group. MCR European Carotid Surgery Trial: interim results for symptomatic patients with severe (70–99%) or with mild (0–29%) carotid stenosis. *Lancet* 1991; **337**: 1235–1243.

2 North American Symptomatic Carotid Endarterectomy Trial Collaborators. Beneficial effect of carotid endarterectomy in symptomatic patients with high grade carotid stenosis. *New England Journal of Medicine* 1991; **325**: 445–453.

3 Hertzer NR. Non-stroke complication of carotis endarterectomy. In: Bernhard VM, Towne J (eds) *Complications in Vascular Surgery*. Orlando, FL: Grune & Stratton, 1980

4 Hertzer NR, Feldman BJ, Beven EG, Tucker HM. A prospective study of the incidence of injury of the cranial nerves during carotid endarterectomy. *Surgery, Gynecology and Obstetrics* 1980; **151**: 781–784.

5 Aldoori MI, Baird RN. Local neurological complication during carotid endarterectomy. *Journal of Cardiovascular Surgery* 1988; **29**: 432–436.

6 Coyle KA, Smith III RB, Gray BC *et al*. Treatment of recurrent cerebrovascular disease. *Annals of Surgery* 1995; **221**: 517–524.

7 Knight FW, Yeager RM, Morris DM. Cranial nerve injuries during carotid endarterectomy. *American Journal of Surgery* 1987; **154**: 529–532.

8 Liapis CD. Cranial nerve injury. *European Journal of Vascular and Endovascular Surgery* 1996; **12**: 257.

9 Liapis CD, Satiani B, Florence CL, Evans WE. Motor speech malfunction following carotid endarterectomy. *Surgery* 1981; **89**: 56–59.

10 Maniglia AJ, Han P. Cranial nerve injuries following carotid endarterectomy: An analysis of 336 procedures. *Head & Neck Surgery* 1991; 13: 121–124.

11 Palmer JB, Holloway AM, Tanaka E. Detecting lower motor neuron dysfunction of the pharynx and larynx with electromyography. *Archives of Physical Medicine and Rehabilitation* 1991; **72**: 214–218.

12 Papachristou E, Dragojevic D. Cranial nerve injury associated with surgery of the carotid system. *Vascular Surgery* 1993; **27**: 431–436.

13 Schmidt D, Zuschneid W, Kaiser M. Cranial nerve injury during carotid arterial reconstruction. *Journal of Neurology* 1983; **230**: 131–135.

14 Theodotou B, Mahaley MS. Injury of the peripheral cranial nerves during carotid endarterectomy. *Stroke* 1985; **16**: 894–895.

15 Dehn TCB, Taylor GW. Cranial and cervical nerve damage associated with carotid endarterectomy. *British Journal of Surgery 1983;* **70**: 365–368.

16 Forssell C, Kitzing P, Bergqvist D. Cranial nerve injuries after carotid artery surgery. A prospective study of 663 operations. *European Journal of Vascular and Endovascular Surgery* 1995; **10**: 445–449.

17 Astor FC, Santilli P, Tucker HM. Incidence of cranial nerve dysfunction following carotid endarterectomy. *Head & Neck Surgery* 1983; **6**: 660–663.

18 Schauber MD, Fontenelle LJ, Solomon JW, Hanson TL. Cranial/cervical nerve dysfunction after carotid endarterectomy. *Journal of Vascular Surgery* 1997; **25**: 481–487.

19 Zanetti S, Parente B, De Rango P *et al*. Role of surgical techniques and operative findings in cranial and cervical injuries during carotid endarterectomy. *European Journal of Vascular and Endovascular Surgery* 1998; **15**: 528–531.

20 Forssell C, Bergqvist D, Bergentz SE. Peripheral nerve injuries in carotid artery surgery. In: Greenhalgh RM, Hollier LH (eds) *Surgery for Stroke*, pp. 217–234. London: WB Saunders, 1993.

21 Krupski WC, Effeney DJ, Goldstone J *et al*. Carotid endarterectomy in a metropolitan community: comparison of results from three institutions. *Surgery* 1985; **98**: 492–498.

22 Welch EL, Geary JE. Vocal cord paralysis following carotid endarterectomy. *Journal of Cardiovascular Surgery* 1979; **20**: 393–394.

23 Weiss K, Kramar R, Firt P. Cranial and cervical nerve injuries: local complication of carotid artery surgery. *Journal of Cardiovascular Surgery* 1987; **28**: 171–175.

24 Verta MJ, Applebaum EL, McClusky DA, Yao JST, Bergan JJ. Cranial nerve injury during carotid endarterectomy. *Annals of Surgery* 1977; **185**: 192–195.

25 Hertzer NR. Postoperative management and complication following carotid endarterectomy. In: Rutherford F (ed.) *Vascular Surgery*. London: WB Saunders, 1995.

26 Imparato AM, Bracco A, Kim GE, Bergmann L. The hypoglossal nerve in carotid arterial reconstructions. *Stroke* 1972; **3**: 576–578.

27 Bageant TE, Tondini D, Lysons D. Bilateral hypoglossal nerve palsy following a second carotid endarterectomy. *Anesthesiology* 1975; **43**: 595–596.

28 Levelle JP, Martinez OA. Airway obstruction after bilateral carotid endarterectomy. *Anesthesiology* 1985; **63**: 220–222.

29 Rosenbloom M, Friedman SG, Lamparello PJ, Riles N, Imparato AM. Glossopharyngeal nerve injury complicating carotid endarterectomy. *Journal of Vascular Surgery* 1987; **5**: 469–471.

30 Sandmann W, Hennerici M, Aulich A, Kniemeyer H, Kremer KW. Progress in carotid artery surgery at the base of the skull. *Journal of Vascular Surgery* 1984; **1**: 727–733.

31 Fisher DF, Clagett GP, Parker JI *et al*. Mandibular subluxation for high carotid exposure. *Journal of Vascular Surgery* 1984; **1**: 727–733.

32 Frim DM, Padwa B, Buckley D, Crowell RM, Ogilvy CS. Mandibular subluxation as an adjunct to exposure of the distal internal carotid artery in endarterectomy surgery. *Journal of Neurosurgery* 1995; **83**: 926–928.

33 Swann KW, Heros RC. Accessory nerve palsy following carotid endarterectomy. *Journal of Neurosurgery* 1985; **63**: 630–632.

34 Sweeney PJ, Wilbourn AJ. Spinal accessory (11th) nerve palsy following carotid endarterectomy. *Neurology* 1992; **42**: 674–675.

35 Evans WE, Mendelowitz DS, Liapis C, Wolfe V, Florence C.

Motor speech deficit following carotid endarterectomy. *Annals of Surgery* 1982; **196**: 461–464.

36 Roger W, Root HD. Cranial nerve injuries after carotid artery endarterectomy. *Southern Medical Journal* 1988; **81**: 1006–1009.

37 Forssell C, Takolander R, Bergqvist D, Bergentz SE, Gramming P, Kitzing P. Cranial nerve injuries associated with carotid endarterectomy. *Acta Chirurgica Scandmavica* 1985; **151**: 1595–1598.

What steps can I take to minimize inadvertent cranial nerve injury?

James M Estes (USA)

INTRODUCTION

The Asymptomatic Carotid Atherosclerosis Study (ACAS) demonstrated that carotid endarterectomy (CEA) can be performed with stroke and death rates below 2%. However, the incidence of cranial nerve injury as a result of CEA is 4–17%, depending on how carefully patients are examined.[38–41]

Cranial nerve injury can result in substantial morbidity for patients. Surgeons performing CEA therefore need to be aware of the potential for injury and how to avoid it. It is especially important to avoid preventable morbidity now that interventional alternatives for treating carotid atherosclerosis are competing with CEA.

Strategies for preventing nerve injury focus on an understanding of normal and anomalous anatomic relationships, identification of nerves, and on techniques of dissection that avoid putting neural structures at risk. The latter point is particularly important during reoperative carotid surgery.

VAGUS NERVE

The vagus nerve is nearly always identified during primary CEA. It tends to lie directly posterior to the common carotid artery within the carotid sheath but may also take a more lateral or even anterior course along the common carotid artery (Fig. 17.4). It emerges from the skull base through the jugular foramen and then travels posteriorly to the internal carotid artery. The vagus nerve is the most commonly injured cranial nerve during CEA, and this injury is usually detected as dysfunction of a vagal branch – the recurrent laryngeal nerve. Hertzer et al. documented a 6% incidence of recurrent nerve injury in a prospective series of 240 CEAs.[42] 29% of

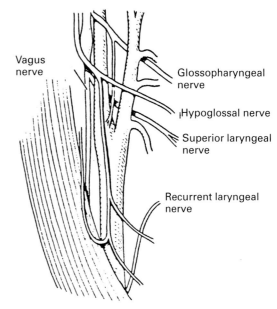

Fig. 17.4
Anatomic relationship of cranial nerves and the carotid artery. Modified from Astor et al.[45] with permission.

those injured had no symptoms and were only recognized with direct laryngoscopy. A more recent retrospective review by Schauber et al. identified the risk of recurrent nerve injury at 8%.[41]

The vagus nerve is at risk during several stages of the procedure. Extensive atherosclerosis often creates a fibrotic reaction in the tissues immediately adjacent to the carotid bulb. Dissection of the bulb along its anterolateral aspect may be in close proximity to the vagus nerve, which may not be readily seen within the perivascular fibrosis. Injury at this point can be prevented by staying within the tissue plane immediately adjacent to the artery and relying on both sharp and blunt dissection. One must be careful to avoid undue manipulation of the bulb during this maneuver to prevent disruption of plaque. In symptomatic patients the author completes mobilization of the bulb after the internal carotid artery has been clamped.

The most likely mechanism of injury to the vagus nerve is entrapment in the proximal or distal clamp. If one positions the proximal clamp so that the tips pass beyond the posterior extent of the common carotid artery, entrapment of the nerve within carotid sheath tissue is possible. This can be avoided by complete circumferential dissection of the common carotid artery proximal to the proposed site of clamping. Using a vascular tape passed around the vessel as a handle, the artery is elevated as the clamp is applied with full visualization of the tips. Entrapment of the vagus nerve can also occur as the distal internal carotid artery is clamped, particularly when high exposure is needed and the tips of the clamp are poorly visualized.

The recurrent laryngeal nerve is also directly at risk for injury. It branches off the vagus near the root of the neck, passes around the subclavian artery on the right and the aortic arch on the left, and then travels distally in the tracheoesophageal groove to enter the larynx where it innervates the vocal cord adductors. Rarely, a non-recurrent laryngeal nerve will be present: this takes a direct route to the larynx by passing obliquely behind the carotid artery. The recurrent laryngeal nerve may be damaged by self-retaining retractors placed in the tracheoesophageal groove, by clamp injury of a non-recurrent branch, or by injudicious use of monopolar electrocautery in close proximity to the vagal trunk.

Consequences of vagal nerve injury in the neck are mainly recognized by their impact on larnygeal innervation. Unilateral injury can result in hoarseness of voice and mild swallowing difficulties. Bilateral injury or unilateral injury with contralateral cord paralysis is a devastating complication that can cause acute airway obstruction requiring emergent tracheostomy. Recurrent laryngeal nerve injury is diagnosed using direct or indirect laryngoscopy during phonation.

The implications of recurrent nerve injury are especially important for those patients who require bilateral CEA. The author does not endorse simultaneous bilateral CEA due to the life-threatening nature of bilateral recurrent nerve injury. Rather, a staged approach with interval assessment of vocal cord function using direct fiberoptic laryngoscopy is recommended.

SUPERIOR LARYNGEAL NERVE

The superior laryngeal nerve is a proximal branch of the vagus exiting the nerve trunk as it passes under the digastric muscle. It passes medially and deep to the external carotid artery before it enters the larynx to innervate the cricothyroid muscle (external branch) and supply sensation to the piriform sinus mucosa (internal branch). Based on its anatomic location, it is at high risk for injury during CEA (Fig. 17.4).

The superior laryngeal nerve is at risk during more extensive dissection of the internal or external carotid artery. This occurs during distal exposure of the internal carotid artery or repair of a persistent intimal flap after eversion endarterectomy of the external carotid artery. In order to gain the more distal exposure of the vessels required for repair, the superior laryngeal nerve can easily be divided or incorporated in a loop as it passes under the vessels.

Awareness of the anatomic relationships can help prevent injury to the superior laryngeal nerve and its branches. Isolation of the superior thyroid artery should be done carefully to avoid incorporating or damaging the nerve, which may pass directly posteriorly. In addition, if more distal external or internal carotid artery exposure is required, dissection should be confined to the plane immediately adjacent to the vessels. Injury to the superior laryngeal nerve may not be readily apparent unless the patient performs occupational use of the voice. In such cases, injury will be manifest by fatigability and difficulty achieving high pitch.

HYPOGLOSSAL NERVE

Injury to the hypoglossal nerve is the most common cranial nerve injury that causes significant morbidity. This structure is especially at risk due to its anatomic location in proximity to the internal carotid artery

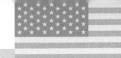

(Fig. 17.4). Older studies have identified a 5–17% risk of hypoglossal nerve injury during CEA.[38,40] More recent accounts have documented a 5% risk.[41,42] In all series, approximately 80% of these injuries are transient.

The hypoglossal nerve exits the skull base at the hypoglossal canal and passes along the anterolateral aspect of the internal carotid artery. It crosses over the anterior surface of the vessel and enters the floor of the mouth to innervate the myoglossus muscle. A branch of the hypoglossal nerve takes off as it crosses the internal carotid artery to contribute to the trunk of the ansa cervicalis, which courses inferiorly over the anterior surface of the carotid artery.

The hypoglossal nerve is most vulnerable to injury during exposure of the distal portion of the carotid bifurcation. The nerve lies parallel and in close proximity to the facial vein. The posterior sweep of an instrument around the facial vein can easily ensnare the nerve and create the potential for inadvertent ligation and division. This can be avoided by more complete dissection of the common facial vein and inspection of its posterior aspect before isolation and division.

The hypoglossal nerve is also at risk during exposure of the distal internal carotid artery. Maneuvers to gain high carotid exposure include mobilization of the hypoglossal nerve. By ligating the small sternomastoid artery and vein that tether the nerve over the internal carotid artery, one can free this structure and allow it to advance anteriorly and superiorly. Further exposure is gained by separating the vagus nerve posteriorly and the hypoglossal nerve anterolaterally. Careful dissection under direct vision in a bloodless field will help avoid nerve injury during these maneuvers. One should also avoid using monopolar cautery in this area due to the proximity of major nerve trunks.

The use of a hand-held retractor to displace the digastric muscle facilitates high carotid exposure. Entrapment of the hypoglossal nerve in the retractor blade can cause a temporary neuropraxia that may take several weeks or months to resolve.

Division of the hypoglossal nerve leads to permanent paralysis of the ipsilateral myoglossus muscle. Although this is not a medically serious condition, it does result in a moderate degree of disability. Patients have difficulty masticating in the ipsilateral part of the mouth due to inability to sweep food from the buccal surface. In addition, speech is slurred and dysarthric-sounding, as if the patient had had a stroke. Fortunately, after a period of 3–6 months, adaptation occurs from hypertrophy of the contralateral myoglossus muscle and masticatory function returns to normal.

GLOSSOPHARYNGEAL NERVE

The glossopharyngeal nerve is not usually identified during routine CEA. However, exposure of the distal internal carotid artery or dissection near the skull base can put this structure at risk. The glossopharyngeal nerve emerges from the skull base through the jugular foramen (Fig. 17.4). It then passes posteriorly and medially to the distal internal carotid artery where it innervates the pharyngeal constrictor muscles.

As the glossopharyngeal nerve exits the jugular foramen, it spirals around the stylopharyngeus muscle. The styloid process projects from the base of the skull just lateral to the jugular foramen and lies directly anterior to the nerve. Division of the stylohyoid muscle or resection of the styloid process risks injury to the glossopharyngeal nerve. This maneuver is often recommended to enhance difficult distal exposure of the internal carotid artery. Resection of the styloid process should only be performed when adequate skull base exposure is obtained, ideally through preoperative mandibular subluxation with dental wires. In addition, when mobilizing the distal internal carotid artery posteriorly one must dissect under direct visualization to avoid injury to the glossopharyngeal nerve.

Although uncommon, division of the glossopharyngeal nerve leads to substantial disability.[43] The resulting hemiparalysis and discoordination of pharyngeal musculature cause significant dysphagia, which may require temporary or permanent enteral tube feeding.

SPINAL ACCESSORY NERVE

The spinal accessory nerve emerges from the skull base through the jugular foramen and passes anteriorly and then laterally to the jugular vein. It

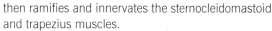
then ramifies and innervates the sternocleidomastoid and trapezius muscles.

The accessory nerve is rarely visualized during routine CEA. Consequently, injuries to this structure are extremely unusual. Tucker *et al.* reviewed an experience of 850 CEAs and identified 4 patients with accessory nerve injury (0.5%).[44] Three of these patients had normal nerve function postoperatively and later developed accessory nerve palsies.

The spinal accessory nerve is not generally at risk for injury during routine CEA. However, this structure can be injured during other vascular exposures in the neck. Specifically, exposure of the vertebral artery in the C_1–C_2 interspace requires dissection lateral to the jugular vein and directly exposes the accessory nerve. The usual methods of gentle isolation and avoidance of traction will prevent injury in these cases.

MARGINAL MANDIBULAR NERVE

The mandibular and cervical branches form the lower divisions of the facial nerve. The mandibular branch innervates the intrinsic facial muscles of the lower lip and chin, while the cervical branch supplies the platysma. The mandibular branch passes along the lower edge of the masseter muscle and adjacent to the facial artery near the inferior edge of the mandible. Although not exposed during CEA using the traditional oblique incision, the mandibular branch may be injured during injudicious retraction of the upper wound edge.

Injury to the mandibular branch of the facial nerve results in lower facial assymmetry due to impaired depression of the lateral lip and chin ipsilateral to the incision. The inexperienced observer could confuse this finding with an early postoperative neurologic event. By asking the patient to show the teeth, ipsilateral weakness of the corner of the mouth can clearly be seen. These injuries are almost always due to traction on the nerve and will resolve with time.

GREATER AURICULAR NERVE

The greater auricular nerve is not a cranial nerve but rather a cutaneous sensory nerve supplying the skin of the lower pinna and mastoid area. It is frequently encountered and purposely divided during the skin incision for CEA. The nerve is usually identified at the superior pole of the incision crossing obliquely.

Division or injury causes altered sensation to the skin around the upper portion of the incision. Affected patients may complain of annoying paresthesia or hypersensitivity in this area. Frequently the nerve can be mobilized along the upper posterior edge of the incision, thereby obviating the need for division. In order to prevent these minor but troubling symptoms after an otherwise successful operation, it is worth the extra few minutes that it takes to perform this maneuver.

CONCLUSION

CEA is a safe procedure in the hands of well-trained vascular surgeons. Unfortunately, cranial nerve injury occurs in up to 14% of patients. Injury is usually associated with minor temporary symptoms but can also lead to severe permanent disability and even death. An awareness of anatomy and its variations, careful dissection in a bloodless field, and attention to detail can minimize these risks. Avoidance of even minor nerve injury has become more important as use of conventional CEA is now being challenged by endovascular therapies that are free of the risk of direct nerve damage.

REFERENCES

38 Ranson JH, Imparato AM, Clauss RH, Reed GE, Hass WK. Factors in the mortality and morbidity associated with surgical treatment of cerebrovascular insufficiency. *Circulation* 1969; **39** (Suppl 5): 1269–1274.

39 DeWeese JA, Rob CG, Satran R *et al*. Surgical treatment for occlusive disease of the carotid artery. *Annals of Surgery* 1968; **168**: 85–94.

40 DeWeese JA, Rob CG, Satran R *et al*. Results of carotid endarterectomies for transient ischemic attacks 5 years later. *Annals of Surgery* 1973; **178**: 258–264.

41 Schauber MD, Fontenelle LJ, Solomon JW, Hanson TL. Cranial/cervical nerve dysfunction after carotid endarterectomy. *Journal of Vascular Surgery* 1997; **25**: 481–487.

42 Hertzer NR, Feldman BJ, Beven EG, Tucker HM. A prospective study of the incidence of injury to the cranial

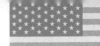

nerves during carotid endarterectomy. *Surgery, Gynecology and Obstetrics* 1980; **151**: 781–784.

43 Rosenbloom M, Friedman SG, Lamparello PJ, Riles TS, Imparato AM. Glossopharyngeal nerve injury complicating carotid endarterectomy. *Journal of Vascular Surgery* 1987; **5**: 469–471.

44 Tucker JA, Gee W, Nicholas GG, McDonald KM, Goodreau JJ. Accessory nerve injury during carotid endarterectomy. *Journal of Vascular Surgery* 1987; **5**: 440–445.

45 Astor FC, Santilli P, Tucker HM. Incidence of cranial nerve dysfunction following carotid endarterectomy. *Head and Neck Surgery* 1983; **6**: 660–663.

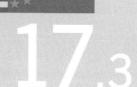

17.3 Editorial Comment

KEY POINTS

1 Cranial nerve injury complicates approximately 11% of CEAs.
2 Although most endarterectomy-associated cranial nerve palsies are transient, they can be associated with significant morbidity.
3 The key to minimizing the risk of injury is a thorough knowledge of both normal and anomalous anatomy.
4 With the exception of the ansa cervicalis, all nerves traversing the carotid arteries should be preserved and handled with great care.
5 Re-do carotid operations and high carotid exposures are associated with the highest risk for nerve injury. In addition, the injuries occurring in this setting tend to be more significant.

Cranial nerve injuries are usually considered to be a less significant complication of CEA when compared to stroke or cardiac morbidity. Some surgeons do not discuss these injuries in obtaining informed consent. These injuries can, however, be quite significant and a source of medicolegal action. The potential for nerve injury must be discussed in detail with the patient preoperatively.

The emergence of angioplasty/stenting as a potential low-risk alternative to CEA has highlighted the need for prevention of cranial nerve injury.

The authors agree that dissection in the axis of the carotid, especially high in the neck, should be carried out in the plane immediately adjacent to the artery. The facial vein is divided only after inspection of its entire circumference and especially its posterior surface. Similarly, clamps should be applied to vascular structures only under direct vision. Cautery should not be used in immediate proximity to neural structures. In the advent of venous bleeding from the superior portion of the wound, the head of the table should be elevated and gentle pressure applied. Precise control of small bleeding veins should then be possible. Indiscriminate clamping without precision greatly increases the risk of cranial nerve injury.

Common scenarios for cranial nerve injury are injury to the vagus at the time of common or internal carotid clamping. Great care should be taken not to catch the vagus in the tip of the proximal or distal clamps. High exposure of the internal carotid often requires extensive mobilization and retraction of the hypoglossal nerve. A ligature placed on the divided descending branch of the ansa cervicalis can provide gentle retraction of the hypoglossal without the excessive tension often associated with elastic loops encircling the nerve.

In the editors' experience, injuries to the glossopharyngeal nerve are devastating, especially when combined with hypoglossal injuries. Because of the risk of aspiration in this setting, fine-bore tube feedings may be necessary pending return of function.

An absolute requirement in patients with a history of contralateral CEA or prior major neck surgery is assessment of cranial nerve function, which must include laryngoscopy. It is important to note that patients with a permanent vocal cord palsy may have few symptoms. Bilateral cord palsies can result in sudden airway obstruction and death.

In those patients with a known contralateral cord palsy, endarterectomy should be approached with caution. If the indication for surgery is compelling, preoperative ear, nose and throat assessment with a view toward vocal cord fixation is appropriate.

18.1

What practical steps can I take if I (a) know preoperatively that the lesion extends very high or (b) unexpectedly encounter a high lesion at operation?

Peter RF Bell (Europe)

INTRODUCTION

The most essential practical step in dealing with high carotid disease is to be prepared and forewarned. In other words, planning is paramount. This is of particular significance as current practice is increasingly moving towards a policy of non-invasive assessment prior to carotid endarterectomy (CEA), with angiography being reserved for selected patients. Whilst reliance on preoperative duplex has important clinical and cost-effective benefits, there is always the potential risk that a surgeon may encounter unexpected high disease at operation.

DISTAL DISEASE ANTICIPATED PREOPERATIVELY

The actual incidence of so-called high lesions is relatively small, only about 5% of patients undergoing CEA being affected.[1] Distal (high) disease is defined radiologically as being present if the upper limit of the stenosis lies above a line drawn between the tip of the mastoid process and the angle of the mandible.[2] In practical operative terms, high disease is perhaps best defined as being present when it extends above the level of the digastric muscle.

It is fundamentally important that the technologist performing the preoperative duplex scan is experienced and able to warn the surgeon that a high lesion is probably present. In our institution, 97% of CEAs are currently performed without angiography but the commonest single reason for performing an angiogram has been an inability to image the upper limits of the disease.[3] Once alerted to the possibility of high disease, adjustments can be made to both anaesthetic and operative practice.

The first stage in planning the operation in a patient with suspected distal disease is to undertake a careful review of the patient's history. For example, if the patient were asymptomatic, the presence of high disease might militate against performing the operation because first, the overall risk will be significantly higher than that reported in the randomized trials; second, CEA only reduces the annual risk of stroke by 1% in asymptomatic patients; and third, CEA does not appear to prevent disabling stroke in these individuals.[4] In addition, it is important to inform the patient that the risks of a cranial nerve injury, especially to the glossopharyngeal and hypoglossal nerves, are increased.

The next step is to decide whether mandibular subluxation or disarticulation is needed.[1,5–7] Although both will increase access, neither it without risk and I would not normally recommend them. In the last 800 CEAs performed in our unit we have not performed either of these manoeuvres.

There are, however, a number of useful practical steps that the surgeon can take preoperatively which will facilitate distal access. The first is to ask the anaesthetist to intubate the patient through the nose. The absence of an orotracheal tube opens up the angle between the mastoid process and the mandible and this can be further improved by taping the patient's chin to the semicircular metal head guard that we use to protect the transcranial Doppler probe. If it is felt that mandibular subluxation will be necessary, it is important to involve appropriate colleagues (e.g. a maxillofacial specialist) in the preoperative planning of the procedure. This is not a decision that can be readily taken once the operation has started.

The patient is otherwise positioned in the usual way, with the head on a ring, a sandbag under the shoulders and the head turned away from the side of the operation. The transcranial Doppler probe is applied to obtain information about flow in the middle cerebral artery. Further details about operative technique will be summarized in the next section.

UNEXPECTED HIGH DISEASE AT OPERATION

The operative approach in this situation is essentially the same as when the extent of the disease is anticipated from the outset. The problem now, however, is that the surgeon may be faced with operating in relatively unfamiliar territory. The bifurcation is dissected out in the normal way and, once the external carotid artery has been dissected free, a loop is placed around it which is then used to pull the bifurcation gently downwards (Fig. 18.1). The vagus and hypoglossal nerves will have been identified earlier and mobilized.

The first step in achieving distal access is to divide the descending branch of the hypoglossal nerve and then to ligate and divide the small artery and vein that invariably tether the hypoglossal nerve (Fig. 18.1). It is important not to apply diathermy to

the small tethering veins which often cover the nerve as this usually causes irritating venous bleeding and inadvertent cranial nerve injury may occur. These thin-walled veins should be ligated or clipped. The digastric muscle can then be divided if necessary.

Gentle palpation of the carotid artery at this point will give the operator an idea of whether or not the distal disease will be a problem. A hard artery with a plaque continuing upwards means that further dissection should take place until a segment of soft internal carotid artery can be palpated. The hypoglossal nerve will need to be mobilized further. The presence of a rubber sling around the nerve will facilitate distal dissection around the nerve but care is required to minimize a traction injury. Alternatively, a tie placed on the divided descendens branch of the hypoglossal nerve will allow the nerve to be kept out of the way of dissection whilst minimizing the risks of a traction injury.

In the upper reaches of the neck the vagus and hypoglossal nerves are closely related and the surgeon must apply meticulous dissection techniques. The vagus nerve will also need to be separated from the internal carotid artery higher up in the neck. If access is still not satisfactory, the styloid process can be fractured using the surgeon's finger and moved aside; this will allow a further centimetre or two of the artery to be mobilized.

Using these various manoeuvres, the vast majority of cases can be dealt with. It is best to stop the dissection at the point where a reasonably soft piece of artery can be palpated. The patient should then be heparinized and a Pruitt–Inahara shunt inserted. The use of a Pruitt shunt, which can be pushed up into the highest reaches of the carotid artery, permits greater access while the distal carotid artery is being mobilized. In this situation, the Javid shunt is often impractical because the distal holding clamp impedes access.

The plaque should then be inspected and the artery opened as high as necessary along the front of the Pruitt shunt. By dislocating the Pruitt shunt anteriorly it is possible to see the posterior wall of the internal carotid artery, which is the part which normally carries a tongue of posterior atheroma (Fig. 18.2). More often than not, this tongue is not

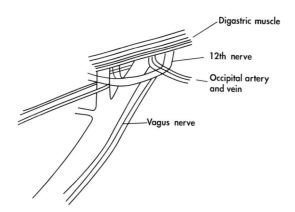

Digastric muscle

12th nerve

Occipital artery and vein

Vagus nerve

Fig. 18.1
Traction on the external carotid artery and division of the occipital artery, which tethers the hypoglossal nerve, improve access to the upper reaches of the internal carotid artery.

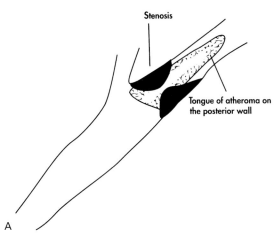

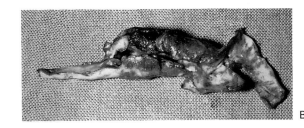

A   B

Fig. 18.2
(A) Tongue of atheroma extending cranially on the posterior wall of the carotid artery above the stenosis.
(B) Operative specimen illustrating the distal extent of the tongue of plaque.

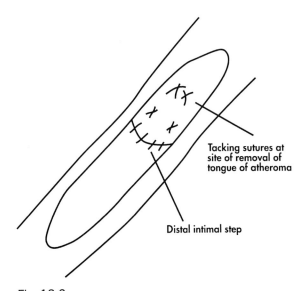

Fig. 18.3
The tongue has been removed without attempting to remove the intima on either side of it. Both the distal intimal step and the residual intima adjacent to the tongue should be tacked down.

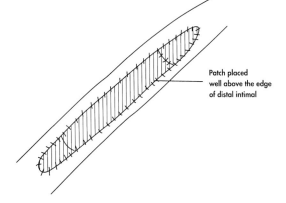

Fig. 18.4
A patch of Dacron or groin saphenous vein should be used to close the arteriotomy, which should extend well above the area where the endarterectomy has ended.

visible on either preoperative duplex or angiography as it tends not to project into the lumen.

It should now be possible to visualize how high this tongue of atheroma extends and to decide if one can get above it. As before, the Pruitt shunt facilitates distal dissection and abolishes the risk of uncontrolled bleeding from an inadvertent breach of the vessel wall. Within the limited access available in the upper reaches of the carotid artery, bleeding will rapidly obscure vision and increases the risks of the procedure. A further practical tip is to ensure that the distal limb of the shunt is well up the distal

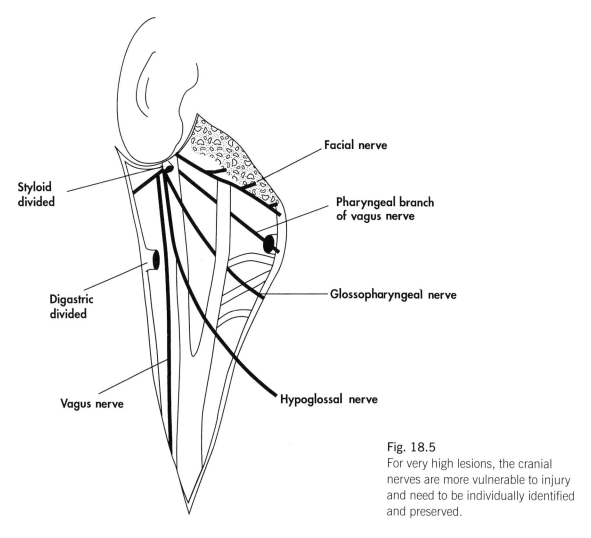

Styloid divided

Facial nerve

Pharyngeal branch of vagus nerve

Digastric divided

Glossopharyngeal nerve

Vagus nerve

Hypoglossal nerve

Fig. 18.5
For very high lesions, the cranial nerves are more vulnerable to injury and need to be individually identified and preserved.

internal carotid artery. If it were inadvertently to slip out at this stage, it might be difficult to replace.

If at this point the distal intimal step is relatively thin (<2 mm), I tack it down and do not perform any further distal dissection. If there is still a significant tongue of plaque, the surgeon will soon notice that it can be readily removed, leaving the intima intact on either side. Attempts to try and endarterectomize the intima increase the risk of taking the dissection too high and of not being able to see the distal edge. In this situation, the safest course of action is simply to remove the posterior tongue of plaque and then tack down the remaining intimal edge (Fig. 18.3).

If there is still significant distal disease, a decision has to be made between the increased risks of going even higher and the risks of leaving part of the plaque behind with a patch to cover the edge of the plaque (Fig. 18.4).

The glossopharyngeal nerve must be identified and protected (Fig. 18.5). This is essential as the effects of permanent damage are catastrophic for the patient.[2] In this situation, I think that the best course of action is to leave part of the plaque remaining and cover it with a patch (Fig. 18.4). The edge does not occupy the entire circumference of the artery and can be shaped with scissors to present a relatively unobtrusive edge. It does, of course, have to be tacked down with 7–0 suture, and this is not usually a problem. What is important, however, is that the artery should be closed with a patch to cover the step that may be left. Removing the tongue of plaque blindly is, in my opinion, not to be recommended. However, if the plaque is still circumferential then this is not really an option and further dissection is necessary. In that event, the incision should be carried up on either side of the tragus of the ear. The facial nerve, which should be formally identified, is then slung and pulled cranially.

If this approach is taken it is usually possible to deal with most cases without the need for extensive skull-based procedures. An alternative option if the plaque goes high and there is by now a long endarterectomy zone, is to divide the internal carotid artery and insert a reversed end-to-end vein. This does, however, expose the patient to a higher risk of restenosis and any such patient will require long-term duplex surveillance.

CONCLUSIONS

High carotid disease is fortunately rare but most surgeons have relatively little experience of distal exposure and reconstruction. The key to ensuring an optimal outcome is therefore to identify these patients preoperatively. This will allow for adjustments to operative and anaesthetic technique. In some situations, it might even be an indication not to operate on the patient. When faced with unexpected high disease at operation, the measures outlined will usually enable the procedure to be completed. However, sometimes it may be more judicious to leave a small portion of the distal plaque and patch the lumen.

REFERENCES

1 Ernst CB, Dossa C, Shephard AD. Mandibular subluxation for exposure of the distal internal carotid artery. In: Greenhalgh RM, Hollier L (eds) *Surgery for Stroke*, pp. 199–204. London: WB Saunders, 1993.
2 Blaisdell WF, Clauss RH, Galbraith G *et al*. Joint study of extracranial arterial occlusion. *Journal of the American Medical Association* 1969; **209**: 1889–1895.
3 Loftus IM, McCarthy MJ, Pau H *et al*. Carotid endarterectomy without angiography does not compromise operative outcome. *European Journal of Vascular and Endovascular Surgery* 1998; **16**: 489–493.
4 Executive Committee for the Asymptomatic Carotid Atherosclerosis Study. Endarterectomy for asymptomatic carotid artery stenosis. *Journal of the American Medical Association* 1995; **273**: 1421–1428.
5 Dossa C, Shapero A, Wolford G *et al*. Distal internal carotid exposure: a simplified technique for temporary mandibular subluxation. *Journal of Vascular Surgery* 1990; **12**: 319–325.
6 Fisch U, Oldring D, Seaning A. Surgical therapy of internal carotid artery lesions of the skull base and temporal bone. *Otolaryngology, Head and Neck Surgery* 1980; **88**: 548–554.
7 Shaha A, Phillips T, Scalea T *et al*. Exposure of the internal carotid artery near the skull base: the posterolateral anatomic approach. *Journal of Vascular Surgery* 1998; **8**: 618–622.

18.2

What practical steps can I take if I (a) know preoperatively that the lesion extends very high or (b) unexpectedly encounter a high lesion at operation?

Alexander D Shepard (USA)

Peter S Dovgan (USA)

INTRODUCTION

Most atherosclerotic carotid artery lesions are located at the bifurcation and proximal internal carotid artery (ICA) and are therefore accessible through the standard anterior sternocleidomastoid approach. Approximately 1–2% of patients undergoing CEA, however, require exposure of the more distal ICA. In addition, other disease processes, including radiation changes, loops and kinks, fibromuscular dysplasia, dissection, aneurysmal degeneration, trauma, and carotid body tumors can frequently involve this segment of the ICA. Exposure of the ICA above the superior aspect of the second cervical vertebral body, although uncommon, requires familiarity with adjuvant surgical maneuvers and cephalad cervical anatomy. Potential complications of exposure at this level and above include injuries to the cranial nerves, parotid gland, and the temporomandibular joint (TMJ). In order to maintain the excellent results now established for CEA and other carotid operations, a thorough understanding of access to the cephalad portions of the extracranial ICA is important.

WHAT STEPS SHOULD BE TAKEN UPON PREOPERATIVE DETECTION OF A HIGH ICA LESION?

Identification of a distal ICA lesion during preoperative evaluation should alert the surgeon to the need for extended exposure to complete a successful procedure. In accordance with the definition of the surgically inaccessible portion of the ICA by the Joint Study of Extracranial Arterial Occlusion, distal lesions are classically described as those cephalad to a line drawn between the tip of the mastoid process and the angle of the mandible

(Fig. 18.6).[8] Anatomically, this corresponds to the level of the upper border of the second cervical vertebral body on a lateral angiographic view. When duplex imaging suggests a carotid lesion extending above this level we routinely employ cerebral angiography to define the location of the bifurcation and the distal end-point of the plaque. Preoperative angiography allows for a planned stepwise approach to surgical exposure of the distal extracranial ICA and consideration for the use of certain adjunctive maneuvers.

Standard CEA exposure through an incision along the anterior border of the sternocleidomastoid provides access to the ICA up to the level of the interspace between the first and second cervical vertebral bodies. Another centimeter or so of ICA can be exposed by division of the posterior belly of the digastric. When faced with a lesion above this point we consider use of temporary ipsilateral mandibular condyle subluxation. A decision to proceed with mandibular subluxation (MS) is based not only on the level of exposure required but also on the patient's local anatomy. In short, obese, heavily joweled patients we may use MS for any lesion approaching the upper border of the second cervical vertebra, while in patients with long, slender necks, we will avoid MS unless the lesion is well above the mid-portion of the first cervical vertebra.

Subluxation is always performed in conjunction with an oral surgeon. Stabilization of the subluxed mandible requires intraoral fixation, which is facilitated by nasotracheal intubation; provision for MS must therefore be made prior to initiation of the neck dissection.[9,10] The diagonal wiring method described for stabilization of the subluxed mandible is safe, quick, and independent of the patient's

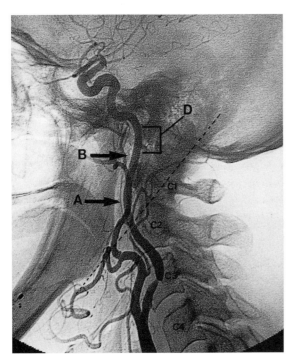

Fig. 18.6
Lateral carotid digital subtraction angiogram with landmarks. Hatched line delineates the border between internal carotid artery (ICA) which is easily accessible and that which is difficult to expose. A, level of ICA exposure available with diagastric division only; B, superior border of C_1, the distal-most exposure provided by mandibular subluxation, diagastric division, styloid musculature division, and styloidectomy; D, the last centimeter of the extracranial ICA, inaccessible in most situations without mastoidectomy.

dentition status.[9] In brief, general anesthesia is induced with nasotracheal intubation, and Ivy loop wiring performed around the ipsilateral mandibular bicuspid/cuspid teeth and the contralateral maxillary bicuspid/cuspid teeth. The ipsilateral mandibular condyle is then subluxed by grasping the body of the mandible and gently pulling the jaw forward and toward the contralateral side. This temporary subluxation is maintained by twisting the positioned wires together. Steinmann pins drilled through the oral mucosa into the ipsilateral mandible and contralateral maxilla can serve as fixation points in patients with poor or absent dentition.

Mandibular subluxation provides extended anterior translational movement of the mandibular condyle, but is not associated with the TMJ disabilities caused by mandibular dislocation. The anterior movement provided by subluxation is an exaggeration of normal jaw motion. Exposure of the distal ICA is improved as a result of changing the shape of the space bounded by the posterior border of the mandibular ramus and anterior border of the sternocleidomastoid muscle, from a narrow vertically oriented triangle to a wider trapezoid. This change in shape allows exposure of another 1.5–2.0 cm of distal ICA (Fig. 18.7).

Operative Technique

Carotid dissection starts with a standard longitudinal incision anterior to the stenocleidomastoid muscle; retroauricular extension of the incision may be necessary. The common carotid artery is exposed and controlled with elastic tubing to allow atraumatic traction and control as necessary. As dissection is carried distally the hypoglossal nerve is identified and carefully mobilized. Subluxation usually distorts the course of this nerve, stretching it anteriorly so that it assumes a more cephalad and horizontal orientation than usual. Complete mobilization of the bend and proximal vertical portion of the hypoglossal nerve is essential for distal ICA exposure. The descendens hypoglossi branch of the nerve is divided just below the main trunk. The sternomastoid artery, a small branch of the external carotid artery to the sternocleidomastoid, is invariably present at the genu of the hypoglossal nerve and requires careful ligation and division for adequate nerve mobilization. Dissection along the vertical portion of the nerve exposes many small, delicate crossing veins which can result in troublesome bleeding if not carefully ligated and divided.

Following complete mobilization of the hypoglossal nerve, ICA dissection proceeds distally, leaving the nerve in place. Division of the posterior belly of the digastric muscle as well as the underlying, crossing occipital artery exposes an additional 1–1.5 cm of vessel. Like the hypoglossal nerve, the course of the digastric is distorted and slightly more cephalad when MS is used. Exposure

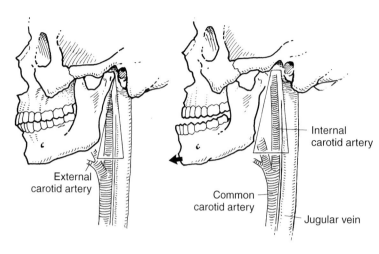

Fig. 18.7
Subluxation of the mandible opens up the space posterior to the mandible and anterior to the sternocleidomastoid. Expanding this space from a narrow vertically oriented triangle to a trapezoid improves exposure just enough to allow unencumbered dissection of the distal internal carotid artery. Modified from Fisher et al.[10] with permission.

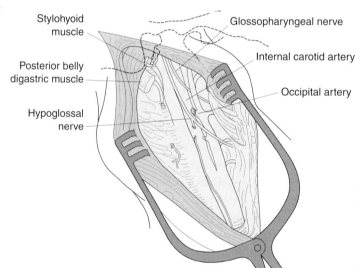

Fig. 18.8
Exposure of distal right internal carotid artery (ICA) obtained after mandibular subluxation, division of posterior belly of diagastric muscle and styloid muscles, and ligation/division of occipital artery. The styloid process can be excised for additional exposure. Modified from Dossa et al.[9] with permission.

of the ICA beyond this point is difficult without MS or some other adjunctive technique. Subluxation widens the operative field to allow reasonably unencumbered dissection of another 1.5–2 cm of artery. Access above this level is impeded by the styloid musculature (styloglossus, stylopharyngeus, and stylohyoid) and ligaments as well as the styloid process itself. Division of these structures at their attachment to the styloid process along with styloidectomy or fracture can provide another 4–5 mm of exposure. The styloid can easily be pushed out of the way posteriorly by fracturing it with the tip of the operator's index finger. Care must

be taken at this level to identify and preserve the glossopharyngeal nerve to avoid inadvertent injury. The course of this nerve as it runs from posterior to anterior is superficial to the ICA and deep to branches of the external carotid artery. It is most commonly found at the level of the tip of the styloid process (Fig. 18.8).

Although arterial exposure close to the skull base can be readily obtained with this approach, distal control can still be problematic within the resulting confined space. Use of small microvascular occluding clips (e.g. of the Heifetz or Yasargil variety) is helpful. In addition, the length of vessel available for suturing can be increased by avoiding application of a clamp altogether and obtaining distal control with an intraluminal balloon occlusion catheter (no. 3 Fr) or a balloon-tipped shunt. Obviously, great care must be taken when inflating such balloons within the intracranial ICA because of the well-recognized fragility of this vessel.

This sequence of subluxation, digastric division, and styloid fracture provides exposure to all but the distal-most 1 cm of extracranial ICA – a level defined radiographically as just above the superior border of the first cervical vertebral (Fig. 18.6). Access to more distal ICA, either at the skull base or within the carotid canal requires mastoidectomy – a time-consuming, complex, and morbid procedure frequently associated with conductive hearing loss as well as facial nerve injury.[11] These associated problems have led some surgeons to advocate ICA ligation, if deemed safe, when dealing with the rare lesion at this level. Other approaches described for distal extracranial ICA exposure include a variety of mandibulotomies, sternocleidomastoid division near the mastoid, and resection of adjacent bony and soft-tissue structures.[12,13] None of these approaches, however, can improve upon the exposure outlined above, and all are time-consuming and associated with their own complications.[14]

The use of unilateral MS, with or without styloid fracture, has provided us with adequate exposure for carotid surgery in every case encountered on the Vascular Surgery Service at Henry Ford Hospital over the last 13 years. Our diagonal wiring technique for stabilizing the subluxed mandible has proved easy, quick, and safe. TMJ problems are unusual with MS. The occasional patient with TMJ pain had complete resolution of symptoms within a few days, and no patient has complained of problems on long-term follow-up. Care must be taken during the subluxation maneuver, however, to avoid condylar dislocation into the infratemporal fossa, which risks injury to the TMJ and greatly increases the chance for problems.

A word of caution regarding the use of rigid mechanical retraction devices with MS is also in order. Subluxation exposes the main trunk of the facial nerve to inadvertent injury by distorting the normal anatomy. Placement of an unyielding, right-angle retractor in the upper margin of the wound for long periods of time can result in a compressive neuropraxia of this nerve. We have had two such patients, both of whom required prolonged distal ICA exposure for repair of complex lesions. Although nerve function recovered completely in both cases, one within 1 week and the other by 6 months, the potential for permanent disability was obviously of great concern for both patient and surgeon. We have avoided this problem in subsequent cases by releasing pressure from the retractor at regular intervals during the procedure.

WHAT STEPS SHOULD BE TAKEN UPON ENCOUNTERING A HIGH LESION DURING CAROTID SURGERY?

Duplex examination of the carotid is now used with increasing frequency as the sole preoperative imaging study prior to endarterectomy. It thus seems intuitive that even the experienced carotid surgeon will occasionally be faced with unexpected cephalad extension of ICA plaque beyond the reaches of standard exposure.

When an unexpected high lesion is encountered, the skin incision is extended to the posterior auricular area as needed. As outlined above, division of the posterior belly of the digastric and occipital artery extends exposure another 1–1.5 cm and allows dissection of the suprahypoglossal ICA. Further distal exposure is largely limited by the ramus of the mandible anteriorly and the edge of the sternocleidomastoid posteriorly. It is still possible to divide the styloid musculature in some patients, particularly those with slender necks, but without adjunctive measures, dissection in this cramped space is difficult. Division of the sternocleidomastoid near its insertion on the mastoid may be of some help in this situation, but can be cosmetically deforming. Although MS can still be performed, fixation of the subluxed mandible to allow more than a few minutes of manual distraction is not possible without a very talented and enterprising oral surgeon.

Recently the use of an oral Molt mouth prop or rubber bite block to produce physiologic MS has been described.[15] This technique is based on the normal wide opening of the jaw being associated with anterior displacement of the mandibular condyles on to the articular eminences of the zygomas to an extent nearly equal to that for MS. With this approach the mandible is pulled anteriorly and maximally opened manually and then held in place with one of these devices. This technique does not need the preoperative planning that subluxation requires, or nasotracheal intubation; it therefore has the potential for use intraoperatively where more distal ICA exposure is unexpectedly required. Similar to subluxation, the use of this approach has not been associated with any significant TMJ complications. We have not yet found an instance to employ this novel technique.

In very rare situations distal exposure of the ICA above the target lesion may not be possible. In this setting the surgeon should be prepared to proceed with ICA ligation. An ICA stump pressure can be measured and, if greater than 70 mmHg systolic, provides reasonable assurance that the intracranial collateral circulation is adequate to avoid neurologic sequelae with ICA ligation.[16] With lower pressures,

consideration should be given to other revascularization techniques, including extracranial–intracranial bypass.

CONCLUSIONS

- Preoperative identification of a high lesion allows the necessary planning for temporary unilateral MS, which widens the distal end of the operative field for improved access to the suprahypoglossal ICA.
- ICA exposure to a level just above the first cervical vertebra can be obtained using MS and stepwise dissection, including hypoglossal nerve mobilization, digastric division, occipital artery ligation, styloid musculature transection, and styloidectomy or fracture.
- ICA exposure within a centimeter of the skull base requires mastoidectomy.
- The outlined approach can facilitate exposure in the unexpected high lesion, though provision for intraoperative MS is problematic; an oral prop or bite block has been reported to help.

REFERENCES

8 Blaisdell WF, Clauss RF, Galbraith G, Imparato AM, Wylie EJ. Joint study of extracranial arterial occlusion. *Journal of the American Medical Association* 1969; **209**: 1889–1895.

9 Dossa C, Shepard AD, Wolford DG, Reddy DJ, Ernst CB. Distal internal carotid exposure: a simplified technique for temporary mandibular subluxation. *Journal of Vascular Surgery* 1990; **12**: 319–325.

10 Fisher DF Jr, Clagett GP, Parker JI et al. Mandibular subluxation for high carotid exposure. *Journal of Vascular Surgery* 1984; **1**: 727–733.

11 Purdue GF, Pellegrini RV, Arena S. Aneurysms of the high internal carotid artery: a new approach. *Surgery* 1981; **2**: 268–270.

12 Shaha A, Phillips T, Scalea T et al. Exposure of the internal carotid artery near the skull base: the posterolateral anatomic approach. *Journal of Vascular Surgery* 1988; **8**: 618–622.

13 Dichtel WJ, Miller RH, Feliciano DV, Woodson GE, Hurt J. Lateral mandibulotomy: a technique of exposure of the penetrating injuries of the internal carotid artery at the base of the skull. *Laryngoscope* 1984; **94**: 1140–1144.

14 Mock CN, Lilly MP, McRae RG, Carney WI. Selection of the approach to the distal internal carotid artery from the second cervical vertebra to the base of the skull. *Journal of Vascular Surgery* 1991; **13**: 846–853.

15 Coll DP, Lerardi R, Mermer RW, Matsumoto T, Kerstein MD. Exposure of the distal internal carotid artery: a simplified approach. *Journal of the American College of Surgeons* 1998; **186**: 92–95.

16 Ehrenfeld WK, Stoney RJ, Wylie EJ. Relation of carotid stump pressure to safety of carotid artery ligation. *Surgery* 1983; **93**: 299–305.

18.3 Editorial Comment

KEY POINTS

1 Preoperative identification of the high carotid lesion is critical so that appropriate planning for high exposure is carried out.
2 Surgeons should remain aware of the potential for undiagnosed high disease in this era of increased reliance on duplex as the sole preoperative imaging modality.
3 In the presence of known high disease, nasotracheal intubation is the simplest method of improving distal access. Access will be further improved when nasotracheal intubation is combined with mandibular subluxation.
4 Surgeons familiar with mandibular subluxation have found it to be simple and relatively free from morbidity. This is preferable to mandibular dislocation or osteotomy.
5 Intraoperative means for facilitating distal exposure include: hypoglossal mobilization, digastric division, occipital artery ligation, styloid musculature transection, and styloidectomy or fracture. Complete mobilization to the skull base requires mastoidectomy, which is associated with significant morbidity.

The key to safe management of patients with high carotid disease is their preoperative identification. Vascular laboratory staff should routinely identify distal plaque extent. If there is a question regarding upper extent of the plaque, angiography should be performed. If, on the lateral angiogram, the plaque extends above a line drawn between the mandibular angle and the mastoid tip, arrangements for nasotracheal intubation and/or mandibular subluxation should be made. This is especially important since, once the operation has started, mandibular subluxation is impractical. In addition, the preoperative diagnosis of high disease is an important predictor of increased perioperative risk (stroke and cranial nerve injury), which must be discussed with the patient. The presence of a very high lesion might also influence the decision for or against surgery, especially in patients with asymptomatic disease.

What is the optimal perioperative antithrombotic regimen?

David Bergqvist (Europe)

INTRODUCTION

Several factors increase the risk of thrombotic complications after carotid endarterectomy (CEA), the most dramatic being permanent stroke and fatal myocardial infarction. The surgical trauma itself renders the patient prone to develop thrombosis, primarily because the reconstructed area is locally thrombogenic.

The thrombotic process is, however, multifactorial and it is therefore not easy to optimize the methodology of studies designed to modify this process. For example, counteracting the local thrombogenicity after CEA is the high-volume blood flow which is usually present after reconstruction of the stenosed area.

WHAT SHOULD BE PREVENTED?

Permanent Stroke

It is most important to prevent permanent stroke, which occurs in 3–5% of patients.[1–3] The highest risk is observed during the first 6–12 months after surgery. Thereafter, the risk falls to around 1% per year, which is slightly less than that observed in the normal population.

Restenosis

This is a complex process in which smooth-muscle cells play an integral role. The incidence of developing a restenosis in excess of 50% is reported to range between 5% and 20%.[4–10] This great variation in frequency may in part be due to the lack of uniform criteria to define restenosis and the use of proportional rather than actuarial data. There seems, however, to be no correlation between the occurrence of restenosis and the development of

neurological events.[10,11] The development of restenosis *per se* seems to be a benign clinical process.

Death

The 30-day mortality after CEA is about 1%.[1–3] Long-term survival after CEA, however, is very much dependent on the presence of coronary artery disease.[12] Ischaemic heart disease is the principal cause of late death after CEA and patients with no clinical evidence of ischaemic heart disease can expect a survival similar to that of a matched control population.[12]

Venous Thromboembolism

The frequency of venous thromboembolism after CEA has not been systematically studied. However, the risk of fatal pulmonary embolism appears to be small. There are no studies on the prophylactic effect of heparin or any of the low-molecular-weight heparins on outcome.

PREOPERATIVE PHARMACOTHERAPY

As can be seen from Fig. 19.1, the aim of adjuvant therapy is to decrease the initial complication rate as much as possible. As soon as the decision has been made to operate, the procedure should be performed without undue delay. In the European Carotid Surgery Trial (ECST), 50% of patients were operated upon within 14 days and 95% within 70 days.[3] Although stroke whilst awaiting surgery was rare (0.3% in the ECST), patients must be protected against neurological events occurring during the waiting period.

In a meta-analysis, antiplatelet therapy has been shown to reduce the risk of stroke by 23% in

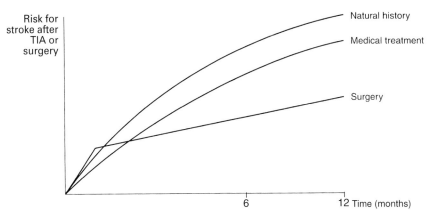

Fig. 19.1
Surgical complications are most frequent in the first 6–12 months. For carotid endarterectomy to be beneficial, it is important that complications should be reduced to a minimum, so that the break-even point compared to conservative treatment is reached as soon as possible. TIA, transient ischaemic attack.

patients with a history of transient ischaemic attack (TIA) or stroke as compared with placebo.[13] The optimal dose of aspirin remains controversial,[14] but the American Health Association recommends 325mg daily.[15] Lower doses are associated with fewer side-effects and, in Sweden, 75mg or 160mg are the preferred dosages.

In the second European Stroke Prevention Study, the combination of aspirin (25mg twice daily) and dipyridamole (200mg twice daily) was more effective than either agent alone, which in turn was more effective than placebo in reducing stroke and/or death after stroke or TIA.[16] Duplex or angiography were not routinely performed, so we do not know if patients with a severe stenosis showed better or worse results as compared with the remainder.

Ticlopidine has also been shown to be effective in reducing the risk of secondary stroke but the safety profile is not as good as with aspirin.[17,18] The commonest side-effect is diarrhoea but the most serious complication is neutropenia. A further alternative is clopidogrel, which acts in a similar manner to ticlopidine. It is associated with few side-effects and will probably become the second agent of choice.

PERIOPERATIVE PHARMACOTHERAPY

Anticoagulation and Antiplatelet Therapy
Any patient who is on oral anticoagulants preoperatively should have this medication withdrawn about two days before surgery in order to lessen the risk of bleeding. If the indication for anticoagulation was 'hard' (e.g. certain types of prosthetic heart valve replacement), the patient should be systemically heparinized while the warfarin therapy is withdrawn. The half-life of intravenous heparin is about 90min and therefore the infusion should be stopped about 2h preoperatively. Otherwise antiplatelet therapy should not be withdrawn during the operative period.

Intraoperative Anticoagulation
During cross-clamping, most vascular surgeons systemically heparinize their patients, although the dose varies between centres. However, few centres check to see whether the dose is therapeutic. Heparin acts by inhibiting coagulation by reversible binding to antithrombin, promoting the inactivation of thrombin and inhibiting the activation of prothrombin.

I would only use heparin (usually 5000iu) if I was inserting a shunt. The administration of heparin, especially if the patient is on aspirin therapy, may contribute to an increased risk of postoperative bleeding and wound haematoma formation. Haematomas in the neck region may expand rapidly, causing respiratory symptoms, and may even be life-threatening.

Heparin can be instantaneously reversed by protamine, which is routinely used by 26% of surgeons in Europe and 54% of surgeons in the US.[19] In a recent randomized study, protamine administration was associated with significantly less wound drainage (median 35 vs 68.5ml).[20] However, the study was stopped prematurely because of an increased incidence of postoperative thrombotic occlusions in patients receiving protamine. A similar association has been reported elsewhere.[21] Thus, although the practice of heparin reversal is quite common, it should be used with caution because of the potential risk of carotid artery thrombosis. There are preliminary experimental data supporting the combined use of heparin and aspirin to prevent acute carotid thrombosis,[22] but this observation needs confirmation in further clinical studies. The half-life of heparin is between 1 and 2h and so it is rarely necessary to repeat the dose.

In a small number of patients, heparin can predispose to venous and arterial thromboses through enhanced platelet aggregation which then leads to a state of thrombocytopenia. Heparin-induced thrombocytopenia is a rare phenomenon and it is poorly understood. There are four subtypes (acute onset, early onset, delayed onset and combined onset). During the intraoperative period, the acute-onset type is the only one that may give rise to trouble because platelet aggregation and thrombocytopenia can occur within minutes of administering the heparin.[23] This is therefore impossible to predict but the diagnosis should, at least, be considered in any patient who suffers an on-table carotid thrombosis. However, if a patient about to undergo CEA is known to have this type of heparin sensitivity, he or she should be given intravenous dextran during the period of carotid clamping.

Early Postoperative Pharmacotherapy

Aspirin should be continued during this period, although the role of perioperative antiplatelet substances at the time of surgery has not been comprehensively investigated. In the North American Symptomatic Carotid Endarterectomy Trial (NASCET),[2] a retrospective analysis showed a tendency towards lower perioperative stroke rates when higher doses of aspirin were used.[24] The results were, however, based on non-randomized data. Results from the Mayo Asymptomatic Carotid Endarterectomy Study and the Antiplatelet Trialists' Collaboration suggest that aspirin therapy is associated with a reduced rate of perioperative coronary artery events.[13]

The early-onset (2–4 days) subtype of heparin-induced thrombocytopenia can also predispose towards carotid thrombosis in the early postoperative period. Although it is important to exclude underlying technical error as the cause of the thrombosis, this diagnosis should at least be considered and excluded so that susceptible patients can avoid being given heparin in the future (e.g. during contralateral endarterectomy, peripheral vascular reconstruction, angioplasty or coronary heart surgery).

A number of studies have now shown that sustained embolization in the first few hours after CEA is highly predictive of thromboembolic stroke.[25,26] In addition, preliminary evidence suggests that the progression towards stroke may be arrested by administering intravenous dextran to these high-risk patients.[25] Dextran is a plasma volume expander with antithrombotic properties, and it has been used extensively in vascular surgical practice in Scandinavia.[27] The role of dextran in this situation has been reviewed elsewhere and will not be discussed further in this section.

LONG-TERM PHARMACOTHERAPY

Prevention of Thromboembolic Symptoms from the Operated Side

Studies based on the uptake of [111]indium-labelled platelets on endarterectomy sites and its inhibition by aspirin have been the catalyst for five randomized prospective trials (Table 19.1). All except the study by Kretschmer et al.[28] were double-blind using placebo.

In the multicentre study by Fields et al.[29] randomization was made postoperatively (day 5 was intended and 60–70% were randomized within 1 week of surgery). The primary end-points were mortality, cerebral infarction and retinal infarction and there was no difference between the placebo and aspirin (1300mg daily) groups over a 24-month period. However, if deaths from causes other than cerebral and retinal infarction were excluded from analysis, there was a significant difference in favour of aspirin.

Table 19.1
Randomized prospective trials

	No. of patients		Follow-up time (months)	Daily dose of ASA (mg)	Start of prophylaxis	No. of events	
	Control	ASA				Control	ASA
Fields et al.[29]	60	65	24	1300	+ 5 days	8	8
Boysen et al.[30]	151	150	25	50–100	+ 1 week to 3 months	39	39
Kretschmer et al.[28]	34	32	Life table, 60	1000	− 2 days	11	4
Harker et al.[31]	80	83	12	975	− 1 day	5	6
Lindblad et al.[32]	115	117	6	75	− 1 day	24	15

ASA, acetysalicylic acid.
+ postoperatively; − preoperatively.

The study by Boysen et al.[30] used a very low dose of aspirin (50mg), but some patients had up to 100mg. The mean treatment period was 21 months and the end-points were TIA, amaurosis fugax, retinal infarction, stroke, myocardial infarction, vascular death and non-vascular death. The relative risk reduction with aspirin for the combined-outcome TIA, stroke, myocardial infarction and vascular death was 11% (but the 95% confidence limits were −38% to +48%!). Just as in the study by Fields et al.,[29] aspirin was started relatively late in the postoperative period (between 1 week and 3 months), which may therefore confound meaningful interpretation of the findings.

The study by Kretschmer et al.[28] was initiated because of the results from a retrospective analysis in 252 patients where it was shown that patients given up to 3500mg aspirin per day showed a significantly prolonged survival, primarily through a reduction in the incidence of cardiac death. The primary end-point in the prospective trial, where 1000mg acetylsalicylic acid (ASA) was started 2 days prior to surgery, was also survival. This study did show a significant benefit in favour of aspirin but the sample size was small (total 66 patients).

The primary aim in the study by Harker et al.[31] was to evaluate the effect of aspirin (325mg daily) plus dipyridamole (75mg daily) on ipsilateral cerebral ischaemic symptoms and the prevention of restenosis. Treatment was started 12h preoperatively and continued for 12 months. Aspirin was found to confer no benefit in terms of restenosis or in the prevention of late neurological events.

In the study by Lindblad et al.,[32] the daily dose of aspirin was low (75mg), with the end-points being cerebrovascular events (stroke with or without recovery within 1 week, TIA, amaurosis fugax) and death. There was a significant difference in favour of aspirin concerning stroke without recovery ($P < 0.01$) within the 6-month period (Table 19.2). However, the overall difference in neurological end-points did not reach statistical significance, although the relative risk reduction was 39%.

Thus, the methodology and aspirin dose of these five studies differ considerably and we still do not know the optimal study conditions. In addition to clinical benefit, the problem associated with bleeding complications must also be considered when discussing the choice and dose of aspirin therapy. In none of the studies summarized in Table 19.1 were there any significant differences between groups with respect to perioperative haemorrhagic complications. None the less, there is a significant dose-related increase in bleeding time associated with aspirin use. Most of the antiplatelet effect of aspirin is obtained at doses of 50mg daily and at 100mg all thromboxane A_2 seems to be effectively blocked. Although it has been difficult to relate the effect to dosage, there is evidence that fewer side-effects are seen with low doses.

Table 19.2
Events in the study on low-dose acetylsalicylic acid (ASA: 75mg daily) by Lindblad et al.[32]

	Placebo (n = 117)	ASA (n = 115)	P
Stroke without restitution	11	2	0.01
Minor stroke/TIA/ amaurosis fugax	7	11	0.75
Contralateral stroke	5	1	0.12
Death	10	4	0.11
Cerebrovascular death	10	2	0.08

TIA, transient ischaemic attack.

Thus, there is a consensus towards the use of long-term antiplatelet therapy in CEA patients to reduce the risk of late neurological and cardiological events.[33]

Prevention of Restenosis

In view of the fact that there is relatively little correlation between restenosis and the onset of late neurological symptoms, it may be of little clinical relevance to discuss preventive measures aimed at reducing restenosis. This is all the more so because we still know little about the pathophysiological mechanisms causing a recurrent stenosis.

There are several strategies aimed at preventing restenosis, some being purely technical, such as the role of patch closure. Regarding the potential link between early platelet activation, thrombosis and the risks of late restenosis, therapeutic platelet inhibition may be of value, but there will almost certainly be other substances worth evaluating, such as growth factor inhibitors, agents with an effect on vasospasm or even heparin.

Retrospective studies suggest that routine antiplatelet therapy does *not* reduce the frequency of recurrent carotid artery stenosis. In our prospective randomized study on low-dose aspirin (75mg daily)

versus placebo, we did not find any difference between the groups with regard to the incidence of recurrent carotid stenosis or on progression of arteriosclerosis on the contralateral side.[10,32] A similar lack of effect was observed when 975mg aspirin was combined with 225mg dipyridamole daily for 1 year.[31] This lack of effect on neointimal hyperplasia is also supported by experimental data from primates.[34]

Prevention of Other Cardiovascular Symptoms and Mortality

Extrapolating the data from studies dealing with the effect of antiplatelet agents on secondary prevention as a whole, there does seem to be a beneficial effect.[28] The relative risk reduction regarding stroke, myocardial infarction and vascular death compared with placebo is around 25–30%. Although the primary aim of CEA is stroke prevention, most of our patients will ultimately die from cardiac causes and preventing this outcome is probably the principal role for postoperative aspirin therapy.

CONCLUSIONS

Antiplatelet therapy is indicated in all patients undergoing CEA and it should not be stopped during the perioperative period. Alternative antiplatelet agents such as clopidogrel or ticlopidine are now available for those who are either aspirin insensitive or intolerant. Patients on oral anticoagulation should have this stopped 2 days preoperatively. If necessary, systemic heparin therapy should be administered during this period. Heparin therapy is an effective intraoperative anticoagulant but its overall effect varies. In practice, the dose can only be tailored to individual needs if the appropriate therapeutic tests are made. Heparin very rarely causes thrombocytopenia, but this should be considered in those with carotid thrombosis and no obvious underlying technical error. In those with suspected heparin-induced thrombocytopenia, intravenous dextran can be used during carotid clamping. For those patients with sustained embolization in the early postoperative period, intravenous dextran may prevent progression towards thrombotic stroke. Antiplatelet therapy should be continued long-term, if only to reduce the risks of myocardial infarction.

REFERENCES

1 ECST. European Carotid Surgery Trialists Collaborative Group: MRC European Carotid Surgery Trial: interim results for symptomatic patients with severe (70–90%) or with mild (0–29%) carotid stenosis. *Lancet* 1991; **337**: 721–729.

2 NASCET. North American Symptomatic Carotid Endarterectomy Trial Collaborators: Beneficial effect of carotid endarterectomy in symptomatic patients with high-grade carotid stenosis. *New England Journal of Medicine* 1991; **325**: 445–453.

3 Randomised trial of endarterectomy for recently symptomatic carotid stenosis: final results of the MRC European Carotid Surgery Trial (ECST). *Lancet* 1998; **351**: 1379–1387.

4 Thomas M, Otis SM, Rush M *et al*. Recurrent carotid artery stenosis following endarterectomy. *Annals of Surgery* 1984; **200**: 74–79.

5 O'Donnell TF, Callow AD, Scott G *et al*. Ultrasound characteristics of recurrent carotid disease: hypothesis explaining the low incidence of symptomatic recurrence. *Journal of Vascular Surgery* 1985; **2**: 375–381.

6 Nichols SC, Phillips DJ, Bergelin RO *et al*. Carotid endarterectomy. Relationship of outcome to early restenosis. *Journal of Vascular Surgery* 1985; **2**: 375–381.

7 Sanders EACM, Hoeneveld H, Eikelboom BJ *et al*. Residual lesions and early recurrent stenosis after carotid endarterectomy. A serial follow-up study with duplex scanning and intravenous digital subtraction angiography. *Journal of Vascular Surgery* 1987; **5**: 731–737.

8 Eikelboom BC, Ackerstaff GA, Hoeneveld H *et al*. Benefits of carotid patching: a randomized study. *Journal of Vascular Surgery* 1988; **7**: 240–247.

9 Knudsen L, Sillesen H, Schroeder T, Buchardt Hansen HJ. Eight to ten years follow-up after carotid endarterectomy: clinical evaluation and doppler examination of patients operated on between 1978–1980. *European Journal of Vascular Surgery* 1990; **4**: 259–264.

10 Hansen F, Lindblad B, Persson NH, Bergqvist D. Can current stenosis after carotid endarterectomy be prevented by low-dose acetylsalicylic acid? A double-blind randomised and placebo-controlled study. *European Journal of Vascular Surgery* 1993; **7**: 380–385.

11 Golledge J, Cuming R, Ellis M *et al*. Clinical follow-up rather than duplex surveillance after carotid endarterectomy. *Journal of Vascular Surgery* 1997; **25**: 55–63.

12 Forssell C, Takolander R, Bergqvist D *et al*. Long-term results after carotid artery surgery. *European Journal of Vascular Surgery* 1988; **2**: 93–98.

13 ATC. Antiplatelet Trialists' Collaboration. Collaborative overview of randomised trials of antiplatelet therapy I: Prevention of death, myocardial infarction, and stroke by prolonged antiplatelet therapy in various categories of patients. *British Medical Journal* 1994; **308**: 81–106.

14 Cohen S. Antiplatelet drugs in patients with carotid bifurcation disease. *Seminars in Vascular Surgery* 1995; **8**: 2–10.

15 Guidelines for the management of transient ischaemic attacks. From Ad Hoc committee on Guidelines for the Management of Transient Ischemic Attacks of the Stroke Council of the American Heart Association. *Stroke* 1994; **25**: 1320–1335.

16 Diener HC, Cunha L, Forbes C *et al*. European stroke prevention study 2. Dipyridamole and acetylsalicylic acid in the secondary prevention of stroke. *Journal of Neurological Science* 1996; **143**: 1–13.

17 Gent M, Easton JD, Hachinski VC and the CATS group. The Canadian American Ticlopidine Study (CATS) in thromboembolic stroke. *Lancet* 1989; **i**: 1215–1220.

18 Hass WK, Easton JD, Adams HP *et al*. for the Ticlopidine Aspirin Stroke Study Group. A randomized trial comparing ticlopidine hydrochloride with aspirin for the prevention of stroke in high-risk patients. *New England Journal of Medicine* 1989; **321**: 501–507.

19 Wakefield TW, Lindblad B, Stanley TJ *et al*. Heparin and protamine use in peripheral vascular surgery: a comparison between surgeons of the Society for Vascular Surgery and the European Society for Vascular Surgery. *European Journal of Vascular Surgery* 1994; **8**: 193–198.

20 Fearn SJ, Parry AD, Picton AJ *et al*. Should heparin be reversed after carotid endarterectomy? A randomised prospective trial. *European Journal of Vascular and Endovascular Surgery* 1997; **13**: 394–397.

21 Mauney MC, Buchanan SA, Lawrence WA *et al*. Stroke rate is markedly reduced after carotid endarterectomy by avoidance of protamine. *Journal of Vascular Surgery* 1995; **22**: 264–270.

22 Huang Z-S, Teng C-M, Lee T-K *et al*. Combined use of aspirin and heparin inhibits in vivo acute carotid thrombosis. *Stroke* 1993; **24**: 829–838.

23 Atkinson JLD, Sundt TM, Kazmier FJ, Bowie EJW. Heparin induced thrombocytopaenia and hypercoagulability in ischaemic stroke. In: Meyer FB (ed.) *Sundt's Occlusive Cerebrovascular Disease*: pp. 280–285. London: WB Saunders, 1994.

24 Dyken ML, Barnett HJM, Easton JD *et al*. Low dose aspirin and stroke. *Stroke* 1992; **23**: 1395–1399.

25 Lennard N, Smith J, Dumville J *et al*. Prevention of postoperative thrombotic stroke after carotid endarterectomy: the role of transcranial Doppler ultrasound. *Journal of Vascular Surgery* 1997; **26**: 579–584.

26 Levi CR, Roberts AK, Fell G *et al*. Transcranial Doppler microembolus detection in the identification of patients at high risk of perioperative stroke. *European Journal of Vascular and Endovascular Surgery* 1997; **14**: 170–176.

27 Bergqvist D. Dextran. In: Verstraete M, Fuster V, Topol E (eds) *Cardiovascular Thrombosis: Thrombocardiology and Thromboneurology*, 2nd edn, pp. 235–250. Philadelphia: Lippincott-Raven, 1998.

28 Kretschmer G, Pratschner T, Prager M *et al*. Antiplatelet treatment prolongs survival after carotid bifurcation endarterectomy. *Annals of Surgery* 1990; **211**: 317–322.

29 Fields WS, Lemak NA, Frankowski RF, Hardy RJ. Controlled trial of aspirin in cerebral ischemia. Part II: surgical group. *Stroke* 1978; **9**: 309–319.

30 Boysen G, Soelberg Sørensen P, Juhler M *et al*. Danish very-low-dose aspirin after carotid endarterectomy trial. *Stroke* 1988; **19**: 1211–1215.

31 Harker L, Bernstein E, Dilley R *et al*. Failure of aspirin plus

dipyridamole to prevent restenosis after carotid endarterectomy. *Annals of Internal Medicine* 1992; **116**: 731–736.

32 Lindblad B, Persson NH, Takolander R, Bergqvist D. Does acetylsalicylic acid prevent stroke after carotid surgery? A double-blind placebo controlled randomized trial. *Stroke* 1993; **24**: 1125–1128.

33 Büller J, Feinberg WM, Castaldo JE *et al*. Guidelines for carotid endarterectomy. A statement for health care professionals from a special writing group of the stroke council, American Heart Association. *Stroke* 1998; **29**: 554–562.

34 Bush HL, Jakubowski JA, Sentessi JM. Early healing after carotid endarterectomy: effect of high- and low-dose aspirin on thrombosis and early neointimal hyperplasia in nonhuman primate model. *Journal of Vascular Surgery* 1988; **7**: 275–283.

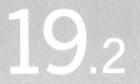

What is the optimal perioperative antithrombotic regimen?

Mark W Sebastian (USA)

Michael S Conte (USA)

Perioperative anticoagulation for patients undergoing CEA has involved many agents, including heparin, warfarin, antiplatelet therapy, and low-molecular-weight dextran. Few indications are based on prospective randomized trials. Current therapeutic recommendations for patients with carotid disease must consider the varied definitions of critical stenosis within the literature, as reflected in the Asymptomatic Carotid Atherosclerosis Study (ACAS), NASCET and ECST trials. Although these trials have identified subsets of patients at high risk for stroke, the disparate manner of measuring degree of carotid stenosis contributes to a lack of consistency within the literature. Evolving research interest in the contribution of plaque morphology and plaque degeneration to the progression from asymptomatic to symptomatic carotid disease may eventually play a major role in defining those patients likely to benefit from antithrombotic therapy. Major areas of current interest center around optimal aspirin dosing, the roles of heparin and warfarin, and a resurgent interest in low-molecular-weight dextran.

PREOPERATIVE CONSIDERATIONS

There are several categories of patients who are candidates for CEA and may be considered for antithrombotic therapy preoperatively. These include:

1 asymptomatic patients with known high-grade stenosis;
2 patients experiencing TIAs with ipsilateral critical carotid stenosis;
3 patients with fixed or progressive neurologic deficit and known high-grade ipsilateral carotid stenosis;

4 patients with preocclusive carotid stenosis (the arteriographic string sign).

Patients with known high-grade atherosclerotic lesions of the carotid bifurcation at risk for embolic stroke have traditionally been placed on aspirin. This includes asymptomatic patients, and patients exhibiting TIA symptoms with referable ipsilateral lesions.[35–37] Although this pharmacologic therapy is ubiquitous within the literature, scientifically based guidelines for the use of aspirin for stroke prevention in patients with carotid atherosclerosis have not been clearly established. The data and dosage recommendations stem for the most part from the Antiplatelet Therapy Trialists' reports[38–40] and other meta-analyses.[36] These studies have documented a clear association between aspirin therapy and a global reduction in severe cardiovascular events (including stroke) in heterogeneous populations of patients with atherosclerotic disease.

The role of antiplatelet therapy in patients with TIAs, minor strokes, unstable angina or myocardial infarction was analyzed in the first meta-analysis of the Antiplatelet Trialists' Collaboration involving 29 000 patients.[38] This analysis reported a 27% reduction in risk of non-fatal stroke. The benefit was similar regardless of agent, dose used, or type of ischemic stroke (i.e. cardiac vs non-cardiac etiology). A second meta-analysis involving over 100 000 patients revealed a similar benefit, with 23% risk reduction for non-fatal stroke.[39] A number of studies have evaluated antiplatelet agents in the more specific setting of TIA or minor stroke of non-cardiac origin. Meta-analysis of these trials suggests a modest protective effect at best.[36] In addition, a wide range of aspirin dosages employed in the source studies prevents firm conclusions about an optimal regimen. In the absence of conclusive data, many practitioners employ standard aspirin dosing of 325mg daily. There is some evidence to suggest that symptomatic patients with carotid atherosclerosis should be treated with higher (e.g. 650mg daily) doses.

The role of alternative or adjunctive antiplatelet agents is still being defined. There appears to be minimal or no additional benefit to sulfinpyrazone or dipyridamole combinations with aspirin. Aspirin, ticlopidine,[41] and clopidogrel[42] are known to reduce the risk of stroke, but the benefit of these other agents over aspirin alone is modest. There may be some benefit to combination therapy but firm evidence is not yet available. Presently cost, compliance, and side-effect profiles assume a predominant role, generally favoring aspirin as sole therapy for patients who can tolerate the drug. Newer antiplatelet agents, in particular the oral glycoprotein IIb/IIIa inhibitors, have yet to be evaluated in patients with cerebrovascular disease.

The clinical scenario of multiple repetitive or crescendo TIA with an ipsilateral high-grade carotid lesion is treated more aggressively. Aspirin remains the first line of therapy. Patients experiencing breakthrough symptoms while on aspirin are usually anticoagulated with heparin after radiologic exclusion of intracranial hemorrhage, and undergo CEA urgently. This management approach has not been validated by scientific study, but rests on the observation that causative lesions are not infrequently found to harbor a significant component of fresh thrombus complicating a degenerated plaque.

Special considerations apply to the less common scenario of progressive neurologic deficit or stroke in evolution. Rapid assessment of the brain parenchyma and vascular system is essential. If imaging studies (ultrasound or angiography) strongly suggest acute thrombus in the extracranial carotid, urgent heparinization and surgical exploration are strongly considered. Contraindications to an aggressive approach include impaired consciousness, large cerebral infarct or any hemorrhagic component by computed tomography (CT) or magnetic resonance imaging (MRI), marked hypertension, or stable deficit more than 24h old. Patients presenting within several hours of onset should also be considered for possible thrombolytic therapy in the absence of contraindications.

The role for anticoagulation in acute stroke remains controversial and is centered around the differentiation between hemorrhagic and ischemic origins for the neurologic deficit. Once the diagnosis of non-hemorrhagic infarction has been established, evaluation of the heart and proximal arterial tree (aortic arch, carotid arteries) is indicated. Patients with cardiac disorders and probable cardioembolic events are anticoagulated with heparin and coumadin, as a primary preventive measure against future events. The role of heparinization in the setting of acute cerebrovascular accident related to atheroembolism from the carotid bifurcation is uncertain. The primary pathophysiologic considerations are to reduce the extent of thrombosis (and infarction) for a progressing stroke, and the prevention of recurrent events. There is no evidence to support routine use of anticoagulation in patients presenting with fixed deficits of greater than 24h duration. The role of coumadin anticoagulation in stroke prevention is even less well defined. A randomized controlled trial of warfarin versus placebo in patients with TIAs or small fixed stroke revealed no clear-cut benefit from warfarin therapy.[43] Patients with fixed stroke and high-grade carotid lesions are considered for early or delayed CEA depending on their clinical and neurologic status. Although data within the literature suggest that there is no increased risk of bleeding or stroke extension from heparin therapy in these patients preoperatively, antiplatelet therapy alone appears to be adequate.

There are no documented benefits for heparinization with preocclusive carotid lesions, although patients presenting in symptomatic fashion with string signs, or critical 99% stenosis, who have this diagnosis confirmed by arteriogram, are usually maintained on heparin before undergoing CEA on an urgent basis. Patients with asymptomatic string sign present a unique subset in whom the role of endarterectomy remains somewhat uncertain, and most often would be treated with aspirin alone prior to possible CEA. Warfarin has been proposed as a sole treatment for these patients but is of unproven value.

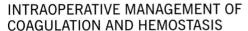
INTRAOPERATIVE MANAGEMENT OF COAGULATION AND HEMOSTASIS

Intraoperative considerations for anticoagulation in patients undergoing CEA center around coexistent bleeding diatheses, concurrent medications, anticipated length of procedure, and contralateral disease. Essentially all patients are prescribed antiplatelet therapy preoperatively, and generally this should not be discontinued prior to surgery. Maintenance of intraoperative antiplatelet activity is important given the potential for platelet interactions with the post-endarterectomy arterial surface and prosthetic patch. Occasionally physicians will instruct their patients to stop aspirin 1–2 weeks prior to surgery, as is often done for other major general surgical procedures. Low-molecular-weight dextran may be used as an intraoperative antiplatelet agent in patients not on aspirin at the time of endarterectomy.

While major carotid and extremity vascular reconstructions in patients on aspirin are clearly safe, less is known about multiple drug combinations, which should be viewed with caution. Anecdotal evidence in patients treated with both aspirin and ticlopidine (e.g. for coronary stenting) has suggested that intraoperative bleeding may be significantly increased.

Maintenance of adequate heparin anticoagulation during the period of carotid clamping is essential. The activated clotting time may be utilized to confirm adequate intraoperative heparinization.[44] Alternatively, the proper heparin dose may be calculated using the patient's weight. Our standard protocol for intraoperative anticoagulation consists of 60–70iu heparin per kilogram given as a bolus injection. Thus, for most patients, a dose of 5000u heparin intravenously 2min before carotid clamping is appropriate. Due to the generally abbreviated length of cross-clamp time for CEA, a single bolus injection of heparin is normally all that is required.

Protamine reversal after intraoperative heparinization should be considered only in the presence of excessive coagulopathic intraoperative bleeding. The routine reversal of heparin is not recommended. Although the heparin–protamine complex is known to cause leukopenia, thrombocytopenia, complement activation, and

respiratory insufficiency due to pulmonary vasoconstriction, the role of protamine in platelet activation and thrombosis is not well known. The best data concerning protamine use in CEA come from retrospective series. In one such paper 155 patients had no heparin reversal and 193 received protamine. All patients survived to discharge. No patients in the group receiving no protamine suffered strokes, whereas 5 patients in the group receiving protamine suffered strokes.[45]

The presence of platelet aggregates intraoperatively or a particularly roughened tunica media after endarterectomy may prompt the institution of intravenous low-molecular-weight dextran therapy for additional antiplatelet effect in synergy with aspirin. Intraoperative use of dextran was initially evaluated in the literature as an adjunct for difficult peripheral bypass surgery.[46] In the US dextran is most often used during CEA if there is evidence of increased platelet activity or concern over the character of the endarterectomized surface. Patients are premedicated with Promit® to minimize antigenic reactions to dextran. This is usually followed by a loading dose of 50–100ml dextran 40, then a standard continuous intravenous infusion of 25–50ml/h. This therapy is continued for 24h and overlaps with the resumption of oral aspirin. Major contraindications include known sensitivity to the drug, renal insufficiency, and patients at risk for volume overload.

Recent reports suggest that an expanded use of perioperative dextran in CEA should be considered. A study designed to determine the incidence of particulate embolization after CEA utilized dextran 40 and transcranial Doppler to monitor embolization.[47] One hundred patients underwent CEA with transcranial Doppler monitoring. Standard heparin therapy was employed and the arteriotomies were closed with Dacron patches. A transcranial Doppler (TCD) probe was positioned to monitor blood flow in the middle carotid artery on the operated side. Patients found to have 25 or more emboli on the operative side were begun on dextran 40 infusion. In the 5 patients in whom dextran 40 therapy was instituted, TCD-detected emboli decreased dramatically.

Optimal anticoagulation for CEA must also consider the potential increased risk of suture line bleeding (and associated increase in operative time), particularly in the setting of prosthetic patching. There are data within the literature suggesting that recurrent carotid stenosis can be minimized by carotid patching.[48–51] This may be particularly relevant for smaller-caliber arteries and female patients. There is no consensus about the optimal patch material, with vein, polytetrafluoroethylene, and Dacron all routinely employed by surgeons in the US. At the authors' institution, Dacron patches (filamentous or collagen-coated) are selectively employed. We have not perceived any elevated risk of suture line bleeding associated with our protocol for antiplatelet therapy and intraoperative heparin, without routine protamine use, in patients undergoing CEA with Dacron patch angioplasty.

Patients who require multiple drug antiplatelet therapy, more aggressive anticoagulation (e.g. combined coronary bypass–CEA patients) or who have significant coagulopathic bleeding intraoperatively, have a small-diameter closed suction drain placed within the operative field, which is generally discontinued on their first postoperative morning.

POSTOPERATIVE CONSIDERATIONS

Special considerations apply to the patient who awakens in the recovery room or in the operating room with a new neurologic deficit. The primary surgical decision is whether to return to the operating room immediately for re-exploration or to obtain an emergent imaging study to assess patency of the carotid artery. Urgent heparinization is appropriate in this setting unless there is evidence for a hemorrhagic stroke. The surgical management of early carotid thrombosis consists of thrombectomy, revision of technical defects, and usually patch angioplasty. A heparin bolus is readministered, and

may be followed postoperatively by either continuous heparin administration or dextran, depending on operative findings and surgeon's preference.

Following CEA, most patients are continued on antiplatelet therapy long-term as primary prevention of combined atherosclerotic morbidity. The optimal aspirin dose for long-term treatment is still undergoing study primarily in trials examining the prevention of myocardial infarction. At this time in the US, 325mg enteric-coated aspirin once a day for life is the most common regimen. Although aspirin is the most commonly used agent for preoperative, intraoperative, and postoperative anticoagulation, there are many subsets of patients for whom the optimal antithrombotic regimen remains to be defined. The role of the newer antiplatelet agents (ticlopidine, clopidogrel, and oral glycoprotein IIa/IIIb inhibitors) in high-risk subgroups awaits definition.

CONCLUSIONS

Management of the coagulation system and platelet activity in patients undergoing CEA should incorporate the following:

- Antiplatelet therapy (usually aspirin) in all patients should be continued preoperatively up to the day of surgery, and resumed postoperatively for life if tolerated.
- Consider preoperative heparinization in patients with crescendo TIA, stroke in evolution, or arteriographic carotid string sign.
- Use standard intraoperative heparin dosing and avoid protamine reversal.
- Low-molecular-weight dextran should be used for intraoperative platelet aggregation or particularly high-risk residual flow surfaces.
- Keep a low threshold for placing a closed suction drain for 24h postoperatively.

REFERENCES

35 Gorelick PB. Stroke prevention. *Archives of Neurology* 1995; **52**: 347–355.
36 Barnett JM, Eliasziw M, Meldrum HE. Drugs and surgery in the prevention of ischemic stroke. *New England Journal of Medicine* 1995; **332**: 238–248.
37 Rance C, Hecker H, Creutzig A *et al*. Dose-dependent effect of aspirin on carotid atherosclerosis. *Circulation* 1993; **87**: 1873–1879.

38 Antiplatelet Trialists' Collaboration. Secondary prevention of vascular disease by prolonged antiplatelet treatment. *British Medical Journal* 1988; **296**: 320–331.
39 Antiplatelet Trialists' Collaboration. Collaborative overview of randomised trials of antiplatelet therapy-1: Prevention of death, myocardial infarction, and stroke by prolonged antiplatelet therapy in various categories of patients. *British Medical Journal* 1994; **308**: 81–106.

40 Antiplatelet Trialists' Collaboration. Collaborative overview of randomised trials of antiplatelet therapy-II: Maintenance of vascular graft or arterial patency by antiplatelet therapy. *British Medical Journal* 1994; **308**: 159–168.

41 Hass WK, Easton JD, Adams HP Jr *et al*. A randomized trial comparing ticlopidine hydrochloride with aspirin for the prevention of stroke in high-risk patients. *New England Journal of Medicine* 1989; **321**: 501–507.

42 CAPRIE Steering Committee. A randomised, blinded, trial of clopidrogel versus aspirin in patients at risk of ischemic events (CAPRIE). *Lancet* 1996; **348**: 1329–1339.

43 Genton E, Barnett HJM, Fields WS, Gent M, Hoak JC. Cerebral ischemia: the role of thrombosis and of antithrombotic therapy. *Stroke* 1977; **8**: 150–175.

44 Fernandez F, Hnuyen P, Van Ryn J, Ofosu FA. Hemorrhagic doses of heparin and other glycosaminoglycans. *Thrombosis Research* 1986; **43**: 491–495.

45 Mauney M, Buchanan S, Lawrence A *et al*. Stroke rate is markedly reduced after carotid endarterectomy by avoidance of protamine. *Journal of Vascular Surgery* 1995; **22**: 264–270.

46 Rutherford RB, Jones DN, Bergentz SE. The efficacy of dextran 40 in preventing early postoperative thrombosis following difficult lower extremity bypass. *Journal of Vascular Surgery* 1984; **1**: 765–773.

47 Lennard N, Smith J, Dumville J *et al*. Prevention of postoperative thrombotic stroke after carotid endarterectomy: the role of transcranial Doppler ultrasound. *Journal of Vascular Surgery* 1997; **26**: 579–584.

48 Deriu GP, Ballotta E, Bonavina G *et al*. The rationale for patch-grafts in carotid endarterectomy. Early and long-term follow-up. *Stroke* 1984; **15**: 972–979.

49 Eikelboom BC, Ackerstaff RG, Hoeneveld H. Benefits of carotid patching: a randomized study. *Journal of Vascular Surgery* 1988; **5**: 241–247.

50 Ranaboldo CJ. Randomized controlled trial of patch angioplasty for carotid endarterectomy. *British Journal of Surgery* 1993; **14**: 1528–1530.

51 AbuRahma AF, Robinson PA, Saiedy S, Kahn JH, Boland JP. Prospective randomized trial of carotid endarterectomy with primary closure and patch angioplasty with saphenous vein, jugular vein, and polytetrafluoroethylene: long-term follow-up. *Journal of Vascular Surgery* 1998; **27**: 222–232.

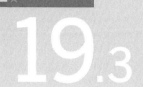

19.3 Editorial Comment

Aspirin is universally accepted as the optimal antiplatelet agent for the prevention of stroke and myocardial infarction in patients awaiting CEA, although it seems remarkable that the optimal dose remains unknown! Similarly, the contention that all patients are equally sensitive to aspirin has never been proven. It is possible that some patients undergo CEA with suboptimal antiplatelet activity. The role of the newer agents, ticlopidine and clopidogrel, has yet to be clearly defined, although they obviously have a role in those intolerant of or insensitive to aspirin. They may also play a role in the management of the young arteriopath in whom maximal antiplatelet protection is warranted. Aspirin should be continued right up to the day of surgery. The safety of the newer agents in the immediate preoperative period is not well established. Intravenous heparin may be necessary preoperatively in selected patients with unstable neurologic presentation (stroke in evolution, crescendo TIAs) or with preocclusive carotid lesions.

Intraoperatively, heparin is used (usually 5000u) just prior to carotid clamping in virtually all cases, Professor Bergqvist's comments notwithstanding. Because of the brevity of cross-clamping in most carotid operations, more exact tailoring of the dose and ACT monitoring of effect seem unnecessary. Protamine reversal has been shown to be associated with an increased risk for perioperative stroke and is increasingly discouraged. When wound oozing seems excessive, the use of a suction drain for 12–24h seems far preferable to the use of protamine.

Low-molecular-weight dextran (LMWD) probably plays a role in decreasing platelet adherence to the endarterectomized surface, and by TCD has been shown to decrease the frequency of microemboli occurring in the immediate postoperative period. This agent may be administered intravenously, after administration of Promit® to prevent anaphylaxis. Alternatively, irrigation of the endarterectomized surface with LMWD, just prior to completion of the arteriotomy closure, may help to prevent subsequent platelet adherence. Intravenous use of LMWD has some risk (anaphylaxis, fluid overload, acute renal failure). LMWD is not a substitute for aspirin,

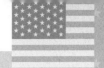

although it can be very helpful in the rare patient who comes to the operating room on no antiplatelet therapy or who cannot receive heparin.

Postoperatively, aspirin is accepted as appropriate therapy for most patients because of its efficacy in the prevention of neurologic events and myocardial infarction. Heparin is not used postoperatively except in patients returned to the operating room for early postoperative carotid thrombosis.

There is no evidence to support routine warfarin anticoagulation postoperatively, but it may have a role in patients with recurrent TIAs and intracranial lesions. Cardiac embolic sources are most often treated with warfarin agents.

ADDENDUM

A review of the outcomes in NASCET suggested that perioperative complications were higher in patients receiving < 600mg of aspirin daily. However, a subsequent randomized trial (> 2800 CEAs) has shown that the risk of stroke, myocardial infarction and death were significantly lower at 30 days and 90 days in patients receiving low dose aspirin (80–325mg daily) as compared with higher doses (650–1300mg daily). (Taylor DW, Barnett HJM, Haynes RB *et al*. Low dose and high dose acetylsalicylic acid for patients undergoing carotid endarterectomy: a randomized trial. *Lancet* 1999; **353**: 2179–2184.)

Should all patients be shunted? If not, how can I predict which patients will require a shunt?

Jonathan D Beard (Europe)

INTRODUCTION

Haemodynamic failure comprises 20% of all strokes apparent upon recovery from anaesthesia.[1] Shunts aim to reduce this risk by maintaining cerebral perfusion during carotid artery cross-clamping. Studies during carotid endarterectomy[2] and in animals[3] have shown that a fall in cerebral blood flow below 15–20ml/100g brain tissue per min results in rapid paralysis of neuronal activity and permanent damage within 15–30min. This equates to a carotid blood flow of about 75–100ml/min. The normal cerebral hemisphere can withstand ipsilateral carotid occlusion due to cross-cerebral flow from the other extracranial vessels via the circle of Willis. However, disease frequently affects these vessels and the circle of Willis may be congenitally incomplete.

Due to loss of autoregulation, areas of previous cerebral infarction and those compromised by a recent embolus have an increased risk of ischaemia.[4] This explains why the risk of intraoperative stroke reaches its highest in patients with a combination of previous cerebral infarction and contralateral carotid or vertebral disease.[5] Furthermore, adequate ipsilateral carotid blood flow of over 100ml/min can occur even in the presence of a severe 90% stenosis.[6] Therefore, cross-clamping such an artery may cause cerebral ischaemia, especially when it also involves the external carotid, which can act as an important collateral.

TO SHUNT OR NOT TO SHUNT?

Few aspects of carotid surgery create more controversy than the use of an intraluminal shunt. Like most areas of controversy, this implies a wealth of personal dogma and a dearth of comparative studies (see below). Proponents fall into three camps: those who routinely shunt, those who never do and those who use a shunt selectively.

Advocates of routine shunting argue that adherence to this policy reduces the risk of intraoperative stroke for the reasons outlined above. Thompson et al. have produced the best morbidity and mortality figures yet reported by using a shunt in all cases, although the differences remain small.[7] Proponents of routine shunting claim that they benefit from plenty of time for a thorough endarterectomy and that it facilitates the training of junior surgeons.[8] In support of this argument, the European Carotid Surgery Trial (ECST) reported better results for those operations that lasted for more than 1h.[9] Routine shunt use also ensures familiarity with shunt insertion, which can prove vital in a difficult situation.

Shunts held in place by balloons avoid the need for clamps, which can limit access and injure vessels (Fig. 20.1). Shunts can also act as a useful stent that reduces the risk of creating a stenosis when repairing the apex of the arteriotomy.

Opponents reply that performing the operation without a shunt seems just as safe and many large personal series have been reported to support this stance.[10,11] They claim that a shunt may make the procedure more difficult, because of impaired access, and that it unnecessarily prolongs the operation time.[12] Shunt complications, such as air embolism, plaque embolism, intimal dissection, acute carotid occlusion and restenosis due to intimal damage, have all been reported.[13,14] However, accurate data on these risks seem limited and anecdotal.

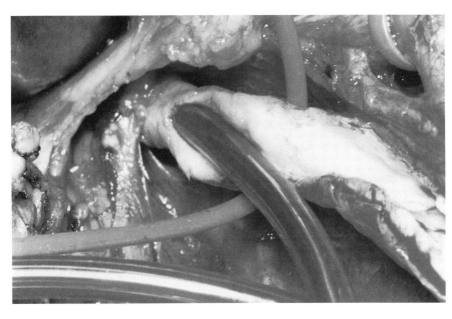

Fig. 20.1
Pruitt–Inahara shunt inserted into the distal carotid artery. The balloon avoids the need for a distal clamp, which can interfere with access in high lesions.

Many surgeons pursue a selective policy of only shunting those patients who seem at most risk of developing cerebral ischaemia during carotid cross-clamping.[15] They argue that this avoids many of the potential risks associated with routine shunting and that it saves unnecessary expenditure. However, compared to the overall cost of the procedure, the actual cost of the shunt seems small. The main problem with adopting a policy of selective shunting pivots around how to identify which patients need a shunt. Table 20.1 summarizes a number of methods for predicting those at greatest risk of suffering haemodynamic failure during carotid cross-clamping. Unfortunately, apart from awake testing, none of these methods are infallible.

Studies have shown that both electroencephalogram (EEG) monitoring and carotid stump pressures seem normal in 6–30% of those who develop neurological signs under local anaesthesia and are abnormal in 3–11% of those with no signs of ischaemia.[16–18] Many of these techniques also require additional technology and expert interpretation, which works out considerably more expensive than routinely using a shunt.

However, transcranial Doppler (TCD) seems the most practical and reliable method overall. Some authors suggest that a middle carotid artery velocity

Table 20.1

Methods for determining patients at risk of haemodynamic failure

Preoperative criteria, including a history of previous, contralateral carotid occlusion or impaired carbon dioxide reactivity
Carotid stump back-pressure measurement
Transcranial Doppler monitoring of middle cerebral artery velocity
Measurement of cerebral perfusion by intra-arterial ^{133}xenon, ^{99}technetium-hexamethyl propylene amine oxime or near-infrared spectroscopy
Indirect assessment of neurological activity by electroencephalography or somatosensory evoked potentials
Watching for the development of a neurological deficit in those undergoing carotid endarterectomy under local/regional anaesthesia

(MCAV) of less than 30cm/s or a clamp/preclamp ratio of less than 0.6 indicates the need for a shunt.[19] However, any reduction in flow on clamping carries a slight risk and some would advocate the use of a shunt in all such cases as being the safest policy. TCD detects changes in cerebral blood flow more quickly than EEG or somatosensory evoked potentials (SEP) [20] and also provides information about emboli.[21] It therefore acts as a useful monitor, even in routine shunt cases. Some consider awake monitoring as more accurate than TCD or electrocardiogram (ECG). However, the awake patient cannot monitor all cerebral activity, especially higher cortical functions such as memory which may be affected by silent emboli.[22]

Clinical practice reflects this lack of agreement about shunting. A recent survey of British vascular surgeons found that 40% always or often used a shunt and 60% rarely or never did.[23] An earlier study from North America showed that about one-third of surgeons routinely used a shunt, one-third never did and one-third used them selectively.[24]

RANDOMIZED TRIALS?

Performing a randomized controlled trial seems the best way of determining the risks and benefits of shunting. The Cochrane group have recently performed a systematic review of the available data.[25] They identified two trials (total 590 patients) in which routine shunting was compared with no shunting,[26,27] both of which seemed well conducted. There seemed a promising but non-significant 25% reduction in both deaths and strokes within 30 days of surgery in favour of routine shunting. The small number of outcome events means that a trial with the power to confirm this finding would require approximately 5000 patients.

There were, however, flaws in both of these trials. In the first,[26] the shunted group had more severe disease in the contralateral carotid artery, which might have biased the results against shunting. In the second, the shunted group had patching performed more frequently than primary closure (57% vs 39%), which might have biased the results towards shunting. More importantly, there were 10 patients randomized to no-shunting who were subsequently shunted because neuromonitoring showed evidence of ipsilateral ischaemia. Thus, to date, there is no randomized trial evidence to guide practice.

WHICH SHUNT?

We now have numerous shunt designs available for use, ranging from simple tubes held in position with Silastic slings, tapered shunts (e.g. the Javid) which are held in position with special clamps and shunts which are held in position by proximal and distal balloons (e.g. the Pruitt–Inahara).

According to Poiseuille's law, volume flow

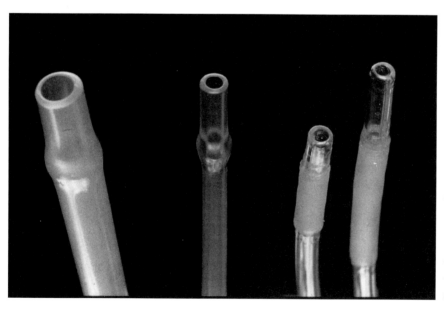

Fig. 20.2
Proximal and distal ends of the Javid (left) and Pruitt (right) shunts. The tapered Javid shunt takes advantage of the larger-diameter common carotid artery but it has a thick wall, which makes it stiffer. The Pruitt–Inahara shunt has no taper and slightly thinner walls, although the balloons add to the overall thickness.

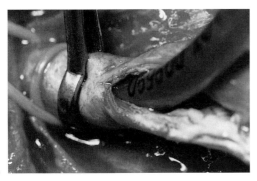 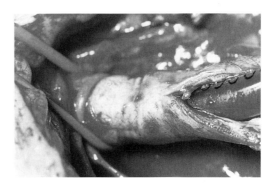

A   B

Fig. 20.3
Damage to the distal internal carotid artery caused by a Javid clamp (A), clearly seen after removal of the clamp (B).

capacity depends largely on the internal diameter of the shunt. The size of the distal internal carotid artery constrains the external diameter, and shunts larger than 10FG may not fit into a small distal internal carotid artery. Many shunts fail to provide a sufficiently adequate flow of blood to guarantee cerebral perfusion, in some cases reducing flow to the equivalent of a 95% stenosis.[28]

The Javid and Pruitt–Inahara shunts have become the most commonly used shunts in clinical practice. Both have given good results in extensive personal series,[8,29] yet they possess different characteristics. The Javid shunt is 32cm in length and tapers from 17FG proximally to 10FG distally. External clamps hold the fusiform swellings at each end of the shunt in position. The Pruitt–Inahara shunt has the same length as the Javid, but has an internal lumen of 10FG. It uses inflatable balloons at each end to hold it in position (Fig. 20.2).

The small lumen of the Pruitt shunt reduces the blood flow capacity to less than half that of the Javid but it has more flexibility and the balloons cause less trauma. The Javid clamps can interfere with access to the distal internal carotid artery (because a distal retaining clamp has to be used) and may damage the vessel wall (Fig. 20.3). A randomized trial of the two shunts in 163 carotid endarterectomies performed at Sheffield has shown lower MCAV in the

Pruitt group but more emboli on declamping in the Javid group.[30] Overall, there was a trend towards more disabling strokes in the Javid group, although this did not reach significance, probably due to insufficient power of the study to answer this question.

CONCLUSIONS

In summary, the available evidence suggests that either routine shunting or selective shunting is preferable to a policy of routine no-shunting. Awake monitoring under local/regional anaesthetic seems the most reliable method of predicting who needs a shunt during carotid clamping. For those who prefer to perform carotid endarterectomy under general anaesthesia, TCD is probably the most practical method of monitoring and also gives valuable information about cerebral emboli. Just because a shunt has been inserted does not mean that it is working. It is imperative that some form of monitoring (e.g. TCD) is used to ensure optimal shunt function. We cannot assume that a safe level of cerebral blood flow reduction exists, especially in the presence of reduced perfusion in the ischaemic penumbra surrounding an area of infarction. Despite the disadvantage of a lower flow capacity, the Pruitt–Inahara shunt causes less vessel wall injury, which may result in fewer embolic storkes.

REFERENCES

1 Krul JMJ, van Gyn J, Ackerstaff RGA, Eikelboom BC, Theodorides T, Bermeulen FE. Site and pathogenesis of infarcts associated with carotid endarterectomy. *Stroke* 1989; **20**: 324–328.

2 Sundt TM, Sharbrough FW, Anderson RE, Michenfelder JD. Cerebral blood flow measurements and electroencephalograms during carotid endarterectomy. *Journal of Neurosurgery* 1974; **41**: 310–320.

3 Branston NM, Symon L, Crockard HA, Pasztor E. Relationship between the cortical evoked potential and local cortical blood flow following acute middle cerebral artery occlusion in the baboon. *Experiments in Neurology* 1974; **45**: 195–205.

4 Fieschi CA, Agnoli A, Battistini N. Derangement of regional blood flow and of its regulatory mechanisms in acute cerebrovascular lesions. *Neurology* 1968; **7**: 1166–1179.

5 Naylor AR, Merrick MV, Ruckley CV. Risk factors for intra-operative neurological deficit during carotid endarterectomy. *European Journal of Vascular Surgery* 1991; **5**: 33–39.

6 Beard JD. Blood flow in carotid shunts. In: Greenhalgh RM, Hollier LH (eds) *Surgery for Stroke*, pp. 167–182. London: WB Saunders, 1993.

7 Thompson JE, Austin DJ, Patman RD. Carotid endarterectomy for cerebrovascular insufficiency: long-term results in 592 patients followed up to 13 years. *Annals of Surgery* 1970; **172**: 663–679.

8 Javid H, Julian OC, Dye WS *et al.* Seventeen-year experience with routine shunting in carotid surgery. *World Journal of Surgery* 1979; **3**: 167–177.

9 European Carotid Surgery Trialists' Collaborative Group. MRC European carotid surgery trial: interim results for symptomatic patients with severe (70–99%) or with mild (0–29%) carotid stenosis. *Lancet* 1991; **337**: 1235–1243.

10 Ott DA, Cooley DA, Chapa L, Coelho A. Carotid endarterectomy without temporary intraluminal shunt: study of 309 consecutive operations. *Annals of Surgery* 1980; **191**: 708–714.

11 Reddy K, West M, Anderson B. Carotid endarterectomy without indwelling shunts and intraoperative electrophysiologic monitoring. *Canadian Journal of Neurological Science* 1987; **14**: 131–135.

12 Green RM, Messick WJ, Ricotta JJ *et al.* Benefits, shortcomings and costs of EEG monitoring. *Annals of Surgery* 1985; **201**: 785–792.

13 Halsey JH. Risks and benefits of shunting in carotid endarterectomy. *Stroke* 1992; **23**: 1583–1587.

14 Ouriel K, Green RM. Clinical and technical factors influencing recurrent carotid stenosis and occlusion after endarterectomy. *Journal of Vascular Surgery* 1987; **5**: 702–706.

15 Sundt TM. The ischemic tolerance of neural tissue and the need for monitoring and selective shunting during carotid endarterectomy. *Stroke* 1983; **14**: 93–98.

16 Evans WE, Hayes JP, Waltke EA, Vermilion BD. Optimal cerebral monitoring during carotid endarterectomy: neurologic response under local anaesthetic. *Journal of Vascular Surgery* 1985; **2**: 775–777.

17 Benjamin ME, Silva MB, Watt C, McCaffrey MT, Burford-Foggs A, Flinn WR. Awake patient monitoring to determine the need for shunting during carotid endarterectomy. *Surgery* 1993; **114**: 673–681.

18 Connolly JE, Jack HM, Stemmer EA. Improved results with carotid endarterectomy. *Annals of Surgery* 1977; **186**: 334–342.

19 Jorgensen LG, Schroeder TV. Transcranial Doppler for carotid endarterectomy. *European Journal of Vascular and Endovascular Surgery* 1996; **12**: 1–2.

20 Arnold M, Sturzenegger M, Shaffler L, Seila RW. Continuous intraoperative monitoring of middle cerebral artery blood flow velocities and electroencephalography during carotid endarterectomy. *Stroke* 1997; **28**: 1345–1350.

21 Ackerstaff RGA, Jansen C, Moll FL, Vermeulen FEE, Hamerlinjck RPHM, Mansen HW. The significance of microemboli detection by means of transcranial Doppler ultrasonography monitoring in carotid endarterectomy. *Journal of Vascular Surgery* 1995; **21**: 963–969.

22 Sise MJ, Sedwitz MM, Rowley WR. Prospective analysis of carotid endarterectomy and silent cerebral infarction in 97 patients. *Stroke* 1989; **20**: 329–332.

23 Murie JA, John TG, Morris PJ. Carotid endarterectomy in Great Britain and Ireland: practice between 1984 and 1992. *British Journal of Surgery* 1994; **81**: 827–831.

24 Fode NC, Sundt TM, Robertson JT, Peerless SJ, Shields CB. Multicenter retrospective review of results and complications of carotid endarterectomy in 1981. *Stroke* 1986; **17**: 370–375.

25 Counsell C, Salinas R, Naylor R, Warlow C. Routine or selective carotid artery shunting during carotid endarterectomy and the different methods of monitoring in selective shunting. In: Warlow C, Van Gijn J, Sandercock P, Candelise L, Langhorne P (eds) *Stroke Module of the Cochrane Database of Systematic Reviews* (updated 01.12.97). Available in the Cochrane Library (database on disk and CD-ROM). The Cochrane Collaboration; issue 1. Oxford: Update Software; 1998. Updated quarterly.

26 Gumerlock MK, Neuwelt EA. Carotid endarterectomy: to shunt or not to shunt? *Stroke* 1988; **19**: 1485–1490.

27 Sandmann WF *et al.* In: Veith FJ (ed.) *Current Critical Problems in Vascular Surgery*, vol. 5, pp. 434–440. St Louis, MO: Quality Medical Publishing 1993.

28 Gee W, McDonald KM, Kaupp HA. Carotid endarterectomy shunting: effectiveness determined by operative ocular pneumoplethysmography. *Archives of Surgery* 1979; **114**: 720–721.

29 Pruitt JC. 1009 consecutive carotid endarterectomies using local anaesthesia, EEG and selective shunting with Pruitt-Inahara shunt. *Contemporary Surgery* 1983; **23**: 49–59.

30 Wilkinson JM, Rochester JR, Sivaguru A, Cameron IC, Fisher R, Beard JD. Middle cerebral artery blood velocity, embolisation and neurological outcome during carotid endarterectomy: a prospective comparison of the Javid and Pruitt-Inahara shunts. *European Journal of Vascular and Endovascular Surgery* 1997; **14**: 399–402.

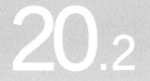

20.2 Should all patients be shunted? If not, how can I predict which patients will require a shunt?

Allen D Hamdan (USA)

Frank W LoGerfo (USA)

The methodology and indications for cerebral monitoring and protection during carotid endarterectomy (CEA) remain controversial. Although there is vigorous argument from several perspectives, most surgeons will agree that in some cases the presence of an indwelling shunt will prevent the development of postoperative stroke. The underlying rationale for cerebral monitoring is to determine the subgroup of patients most likely to benefit from the cerebral protection afforded by shunt placement. The basis for cerebral protection is to prevent strokes due to inadequate intraoperative cerebral perfusion.

Technical errors and embolization are probably the cause of most perioperative strokes – possibly up to 65%.[31] Vessel thrombosis is often due to a technical error or, more rarely, a hypercoagulable state and not likely related to the method of cerebral monitoring employed. Embolization can occur during the dissection and isolation of the vessels alone or as a consequence of an intimal flap and can result with any technique. Intracerebral hemorrhage is an uncommon, highly morbid cause of stroke, but other than a possible role for hypertension the mechanism is unclear. Probably the only cause of stroke that can be impacted upon by the method of cerebral protection is intraoperative hypoperfusion ischemia.

To evaluate the utility of shunts we must identify the number of strokes that would be prevented by shunting, versus strokes, if any, that are caused by the shunting process itself. Valid data comparing different methods of cerebral monitoring are somewhat difficult to obtain because the overall stroke rate is low and only a fraction of these are potentially preventable by cerebral protection. In addition, this discussion deals only with clinical strokes. Studies have shown that computed tomographic scans will identify a number of silent infarcts before and after CEA that have no apparent clinical manifestations.[32] To determine the value of each method, this information would also be helpful.

In general, most patients have sufficient cerebral collateral flow to permit clamping of the carotid artery during CEA.[33] Ischemia can result when intracerebral blood flow to a particular area of the brain cannot meet the metabolic needs of the tissue, eventually causing infarction. This is most likely to occur in patients with decreased intracerebral collateral flow and increased intracerebral atherosclerotic disease. The overall problem of trying to gauge which patient is at high risk for hypoperfusion ischemia is that there is no clinical factor, test, or combination of factors that will predict this reliably. In general, patients with a contralateral carotid artery occlusion will be at higher risk but in some series 80% will tolerate carotid artery clamping without a detectable detriment in cerebral function.[34] Another study showed that this group may be safely operated on without a shunt.[35] In contrast, the patient with a completely patent contralateral artery would be assumed to be safe. In one series there were 15 patients who had significant ipsilateral carotid stenosis but who were currently asymptomatic. All had previously undergone contralateral CEA for a symptomatic lesions and at that original operation did not develop signs of ischemia upon clamping. Nine (60%) of this group, however, developed ischemia upon clamping during the second operation.[36] This emphasizes how inaccurate preoperative clinical status is in predicting which patients will tolerate cross-clamping by EEG criteria.

Intraoperative testing using carotid artery stump pressure (the pressure that is due to collateral circulation when the common carotid artery (CCA) and external carotid artery are clamped) is another common measure used to determine which patients will tolerate clamping.[37] The problem with this criterion is that patients can become ischemic by EEG with pressures of 70mmHg and not be ischemic with pressures below the accepted threshold of 25mmHg. Attempts to refine this by taking into account the mean arterial pressure and developing a stump pressure index have generally not improved the reliability. It is true, however, that there is a decrease in perioperative stroke rates when comparing groups with high stump pressures to those with low stump pressures.[38]

There are essentially four different approaches to performing CEA with regard to cerebral monitoring and/or protection:

1 general anesthesia with no shunt;
2 general anesthesia with continuous EEG monitoring, TCD or carotid stump pressure, shunting only those patients in whom changes are noted or thresholds are met – selective shunting;
3 regional anesthesia (cervical block), shunting only those patients who experience a change in neurologic status – clinical shunting;
4 general anesthesia plus shunting in all patients – routine shunting.

NO SHUNTING WITH GENERAL ANESTHESIA

This method relies on the data suggesting that few patients are at risk for 'shunt-preventable' strokes. The argument is that shunt placement can cause strokes in some cases and thus the risks outweigh the benefits. Large series have been reported without the use of shunts, with very acceptable results.[39] The main problem with this method is that some strokes are preventable with cerebral protection from a shunt and thus in a sense these are being allowed to occur. An advantage is that there is no shunt in place to interfere with the endarterectomy and there are no concerns about possible shunt complications, which might include stroke, albeit rare.

SELECTIVE SHUNTING WITH USE OF EEG

With selective shunting only a small percentage – 10–20% – of patients will require a shunt to prevent hypoperfusion ischemia during carotid cross-clamping. In this model EEG changes are used as the gold standard to identify ongoing cerebral hypoperfusion. EEG however is not 100% sensitive or specific in identifying critical cerebral ischemia.

The normal value of cerebral blood flow is 50ml/100g per min. Blood flow required to maintain a normal EEG is greater than 15ml/100g per min. Less than 10ml/100g per min will always produce rapid changes in EEG and probably less than 8ml/100g per min will result in infarction.[40] Intraoperative hypotension alone can result in EEG changes that can be corrected with simple normalization of blood pressure. Also the reverse can occur, when placement of a shunt with augmentation of cerebral blood flow does not restore the EEG to baseline.[41]

In 449 patients with a normal EEG during CEA and thus no shunt, 3 patients still developed strokes. In that series EEG failed to detect ischemia in 3 of 15, or 20%, of perioperative strokes.[36] In addition, changes do not always occur immediately upon clamping and can manifest more than 3 min later, a point which is very disruptive for precise shunt placement. Other series have confirmed the insensitivity of EEG in predicting stroke, with the false-negative rate as high as 50%.[38] However, it appears to be reliable in identifying a shunt that has become malpositioned or kinked, noted by sudden repeat EEG changes after previous normalization after shunting.[33]

Another factor to be considered when using EEG is that it requires equipment and interpretation, often by a neurologist, adds significant cost, and mandates specific skills by the anesthesiologist. Anesthesia must be at a depth that does not induce slow-wave activity, but maintains normovolemia, normocapnia and normal temperature as well as the mean arterial pressure in the upper portion of that particular patient's range. It is reliable as a measure of cortical function but notoriously poor for subcortical areas.[41]

In general, surgeons who use EEG with selective shunting as their technique for cerebral monitoring

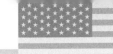

and protection will achieve acceptable postoperative complication rates. However, EEG can be inaccurate, expensive, insensitive, and unreliable in detecting ischemia or predicting perioperative stroke.

CLINICAL SHUNTING WITH USE OF REGIONAL ANESTHESIA

This technique is based on the theory that a change in mental status of the awake patient upon cross-clamping, i.e., inability to speak or to move the contralateral side, is a harbinger of a stroke and thus mandates shunt placement. There is a surprising lack of correlation between these clinical signs and EEG changes. Studies revealed that 23–30% of patients who developed a clear-cut clinical change upon clamping did not show any EEG changes at all and that in 3–11% EEG changes developed in the absence of any clinical change.[42,43] These results have been used to argue that clinical changes in the awake patient are the most sensitive measure of cerebral ischemia upon cross-clamping. However, although this is probably an accurate statement, the fraction of patients with clinical changes who would suffer an intraoperative stroke is not known since these patients are always shunted.

Regional anesthesia and clinical shunting is an accurate and safe way to perform CEA. It requires special expertise from the anesthesiologist or the surgeon, and all patients will not submit to regional anesthesia. During the operation the patient's responsiveness must be frequently assessed and in a sedated patient this can sometimes be difficult to detect promptly. It also allows for the development of a particularly dangerous situation where a patient becomes uncooperative at a critical point during the endarterectomy and must be emergently converted to general anesthesia. In addition, it has never been clearly shown that general anesthesia carries a higher cardiac morbidity than regional anesthesia.

ROUTINE SHUNTING WITH GENERAL ANESTHESIA

Opponents of this method argue that placement of shunts can cause intimal injuries, embolization, and difficulty in visualizing the end-point of the endarterectomy, and that there may be a lower incidence of stroke due to technical errors in patients who are not shunted.[35] Reports documenting shunt-induced technical errors are from EEG-selective series in which only those manifesting EEG changes are shunted. Of this group, the ECG changes will not resolve in some patients with proper shunt placement and they usually develop a stroke. It is unlikely that stroke in this group is due to the shunt but occurs in spite of the shunt. The remainder of patients – those with normalized EEG after shunting – are selected out as a very high risk group, probably with poor collateral flow and/or intracerebral atherosclerosis and thus are exactly the people who have the greatest potential to benefit from the shunt. A concern is that, if the surgeon is not completely prepared at all times for possible shunting, the sudden development of EEG changes may result in a hurried, forced attempt to place the shunt under less than ideal conditions, possibly raising the risks of technical errors seen in the EEG-selected group.

Table 20.2
Routine shunting leads to a low rate of shunt-induced problems

n	Institution	Stroke/death rate (%)	Shunt method
128	Medical College of Georgia[35]	2.4	None
342	Netherlands[45]	2.6	None
1924	Cleveland Clinic[46]	2.3	Routine
1001	NEDH*	1.6	Routine/regional
150	Brigham and Women's[33]	1.4	EEG
562	University of Rochester[36]	2.7	EEG
1145	Mayo Clinic[40]	3.5	EEG
709	Northwestern[38]	2.8	EEG/stump pressure
134	St Anthony[43]	0.7	Regional
81	Chicago Institute of Neurology.[42]	2.4	Regional

*Unpublished results.

Routine shunting in experienced hands leads to a low rate of shunt-induced problems, and a low rate of stroke and death, and is a cost-effective procedure (Table 20.2). The objection to this method is that shunts are placed in at least 80% of patients who 'do not need it.' However, the key point is in the conduct of the procedure. Wide exposure with special attention to the distal internal carotid artery is mandated. To achieve this exposure, it is often necessary to divide the sternocleidomastoid branch of the occipital artery to allow complete mobilization and preservation of the hypoglossal nerve. In some instances the posterior belly of the digastric muscle will be partly divided. Thus, the surgeon is never in the position where he or she must emergently shunt a patient with inadequate distal exposure. This situation can be hazardous, especially in the case where EEG or clinical changes develop several minutes after clamping – an inopportune time during the operation. Routine shunting avoids the need for test clamping of the CCA, which alone can cause embolic stroke. Use of general anesthesia also obviates the need to intubate urgently an unstable patient during CEA under regional anesthesia.[44]

In our institution, data from 1001 consecutive CEAs without the use of EEG were examined (unpublished). The stroke rate was 1.4% and the mortality rate 0.2%, giving a combined stroke and death rate of 1.6%. The series includes regional anesthesia with clinical shunting but the majority of CEAs were performed under general anesthesia with routine shunting. Currently we almost exclusively use general anesthesia with routine shunting and frequent patching.

In conclusion, there are a number of different methods which surgeons employ that result in very low stroke and death rates from CEA. We have found, as have others, that routine use of a shunt under general anesthesia without EEG monitoring results in a stroke and death rate as good as or better than other approaches to cerebral protection. It is safe, straightforward, and cost-effective.

REFERENCES

31 Riles TS, Imparato AM, Jacobowitz GR et al. The cause of perioperative stroke after carotid endarterectomy. Journal of Vascular Surgery 1994; 19: 206–216.

32 Berguer R, Sieggreen MY, Lazo M, Hodakowski BA. The silent brain infarct in carotid surgery. Journal of Vascular Surgery 1986; 3: 442–447.

33 Whittemore AD, Kaufman JL, Kohler TR, Mannick JA. Routine electroencephalographic (EEG) monitoring during carotid endarterectomy. Annals of Surgery 1982; 197: 707–713.

34 Lawrence PF, Alves JC, Jicha DJ et al. Incidence, timing, and causes of cerebral ischemia during carotid endarterectomy with regional anesthesia. Journal of Vascular Surgery 1998; 27: 329–337.

35 Whitney EG, Brophy CM, Kahn EM, Whitney DG. Inadequate cerebral perfusion is an unlikely cause of perioperative stroke. Annals of Vascular Surgery 1997; 11: 109–114.

36 Green RM, Messick WJ, Ricotta JJ et al. Benefits, shortcomings and costs of EEG monitoring. Annals of Surgery 1985; 201: 785–792.

37 Harada RN, Comerota AJ, Good GM et al. Stump pressure, electroencephalographic changes and the contralateral carotid artery: another look at selective shunting. American Journal of Surgery 1995; 170: 148–153.

38 McCarthy WJ, Park AE, Koushanpour E et al. Carotid endarterectomy: lessons from intraoperative monitoring – a decade of experience. Annals of Surgery 1996; 224: 297–307.

39 Baker WH. Diagnosis and Treatment of Carotid Artery Disease. Mt Kisco, NY: Futura, 1979.

40 Sundt TM Jr, Sharbrough FW, Piepgras DG et al. Correlation of cerebral blood flow and electroencephalographic changes during carotid endarterectomy. Mayo Clinic Proceedings 1981; 56: 533–543.

41 Plestis KA, Loubser P, Mizrahi EM et al. Continuous electroencephalographic monitoring and selective shunting reduces neurologic morbidity rates in carotid endarterectomy. Journal of Vascular Surgery 1997; 25: 620–628.

42 Benjamin ME, Silva MB Jr, Watt C et al. Awake patient monitoring to determine the need for shunting during carotid endarterectomy. Surgery 1993; 114: 673–681.

43 Evans WE, Hayes JP, Waltke EA, Vermilion BD. Optimal cerebral monitoring during carotid endarterectomy: neurologic response under local anesthesia. Journal of Vascular Surgery 1985; 2: 775–777.

44 LoGerfo FW, Jepsen SJ. Role of carotid shunting during carotid endarterectomy. In: Ernst CB, Stanley JC (eds) Current Therapy in Vascular Surgery, II, pp. 81–84. London: Mosby, 1990.

45 Boontje AH. Carotid endarterectomy without a temporary indwelling shunt: results and analysis of back pressure measurements. Cardiovascular Surgery 1994; 2: 549–554.

46 Hertzer NR, O'Hara PJ, Mascha EJ et al. Early outcome assessment for 2228 consecutive carotid endarterectomy procedures: the Cleveland Clinic experience from 1989 to 1995. Journal of Vascular Surgery 1997; 26: 1–10.

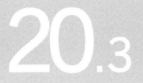

20.3 Editorial Comment

On both sides of the Atlantic there is significant uncertainty and controversy surrounding the optimal means of cerebral monitoring and protection. As Beard so appropriately states; 'like most areas of controversy, this implies a wealth of personal dogma and a dearth of comparative studies.' Because intraoperative stroke is unusual, and because only a small percentage of intraoperative strokes will be related to preventable hypoperfusion, the design of comparative studies with meaningful statistical power is very difficult. Compounding this difficulty is the lack of any reliable means of determining which intraoperative strokes were in fact related to hypoperfusion and which were related to emboli.

It appears that the practice of never shunting is becoming obsolete and that almost all modern carotid surgeons are either selective or routine shunters. Speed in performance of the operation is not a safe or effective means of cerebral protection. The controversies then lie in the areas of routine versus selective shunting and, for the selective shunters, in the optimal means of cerebral monitoring. The arguments in favor of routine shunting are straightforward. Routine use of a shunt confers facility with shunt placement obviates the need for expensive and potentially confusing monitoring procedures, and yields state-of-the-art results in the hands of its proponents. Selective shunters counter that the shunt is unnecessary in 80–90% of cases, is awkward and potentially traumatic to place, is constantly obstructing the exposure, especially at the distal end-point, and is associated with a small number of shunt-related embolic strokes. There is truth in both arguments. At the risk of sliding down the slippery slope of relativism and abrogating our responsibility to arrive at a best practice, the editors feel that either stance is reasonable as long as the associated stroke morbidity results are consistent with international norms (< 2% for asymptomatic patients and < 4% for symptomatic patients).

The controversy over the optimal means for cerebral monitoring in carotid patients is likewise impossible to resolve with evidence-based reasoning. TCD, EEG, and awake-patient monitoring all have their strengths and weaknesses. TCD detects both deficient flow and emboli and is useful for both intraoperative and postoperative monitoring. The correlation of TCD findings with clinically relevant ischemia or emboli is not well established. Expensive equipment and significant expertise in signal interpretation are required. EEG is now well standardized but is imperfect in both specificity and sensitivity in the detection of cortical events. It is especially poor in detection of subcortical or brainstem events. Like TCD, EEG requires expensive equipment and significant technical expertise. Awake-patient monitoring, by contrast, is inexpensive and requires no special technical

expertise. It is not, however, uniformly applicable since many patients cannot tolerate the procedure under regional anesthesia. In addition, the cardiac stress (for patient and surgeon) associated with the need for sudden conversion to general anesthesia in an agitated, disoriented, and uncooperative, or oversedated, barely breathing patient should not be underestimated. Again, no technique is perfect, although many surgeons have reported superb results using strict adherence to each of these protocols.

21.1 How can I achieve the optimal flow surface and distal end-point following carotid endarterectomy?

Nicholas JM London (Europe)

INTRODUCTION

The optimal flow surface after carotid endarterectomy (CEA) should no longer contain any embolic source, should not be flow-limiting and should be minimally thrombogenic. In addition, it is essential that the endarterectomized artery is not left too thin because of the risk of pseudoaneurysm formation.

The optimal distal end-point therefore represents a compromise between continuing the endarterectomy until relatively normal intima is obtained, yet not continuing so high that the operation becomes needlessly and/or dangerously compromised.

WHAT IS THE OPTIMAL ENDARTERECTOMY PLANE?

The atheromatous process is usually confined to the intima and therefore the optimal endarterectomy plane should be between the diseased intima and the media. Dissection in a plane superficial to this (i.e. within the atheroma itself) is unsatisfactory and risks leaving layers of the plaque attached to the media. Conversely, dissection deep to the media risks leaving the arterial wall too thin and the exposed collagen-rich adventitia may be more thrombogenic.

It is essential that, before beginning the endarterectomy, the surgeon clearly displays its cranial extent. In order to do this, the arteriotomy may need to be extended. The point at which to stop the cranial extent of the endarterectomy can be a difficult decision. However, the surgeon should remember that the purpose of CEA is not primarily to produce a 'beautifully clean artery' but rather to remove all embolic sources. Obsessive cleanliness

risks dangerously thinning the arterial wall and continuing the endarterectomy needlessly high. Thus, it does not matter if the cranial extent of the endarterectomy stops at a point where there is still some firmly adherent but thin intimal disease because this does not pose an embolic risk and, if a patch is used, it will not cause narrowing.

An important principle is that, if the endarterectomy plane proves difficult to identify at first, the surgeon should initially perform the endarterectomy in a more superficial plane. This is because it always possible to repeat the endarterectomy in a slightly deeper plane having started more superficially. However, if the endarterectomy plane is initially too deep and damage to the wall occurs, then some form of arterial repair or bypass may become inevitable.

One of the most important practical tips is to perform the operation under loupe magnification. This greatly facilitates the procedure and contributes towards achieving the optimal end-result. The technique that I use for finding the endarterectomy plane is to hold the adventitia with a pair of DeBakey forceps (finer forceps may damage the adventitia) and, whilst applying traction, use the tapered end of a Watson–Cheyne dissector to develop a plane between the diseased intima and media. The dissection is started at the bifurcation of the common carotid artery (CCA) where the atheromatous process is most marked. This is often facilitated by the presence of calcification within the plaque. The plane is then developed proximally down the CCA for 2–3cm, at which point I would gently insinuate the dissector across the whole width of the artery so that it appeared on the other side. I then cut down on the dissector with a scalpel blade, thereby transecting the diseased intima and defining the proximal end-point.

The endarterectomized atheroma is then held with forceps and the endarterectomy continued distally up to the origin of the external carotid artery (ECA). The atheroma around the origin of the ECA is freed and the atheroma within the ECA removed.

The endarterectomy is then continued distally and, once the cranial end-point has been reached, the specimen is carefully divided with curved microscissors which are laid flat against the arterial wall. This should leave a clean, smooth distal intimal step.

HOW SHOULD I REMOVE INTIMAL FLAPS AND FRAGMENTS?

Immediately following endarterectomy, the surface will be relatively smooth but will still contain a number of fragments. Although these are often termed intimal flaps, they usually comprise strips of circular muscle derived from the media. Most can be removed by firm stroking movements with a pledget, taking care to avoid direct contact with the residual intimal steps. Thereafter, most of the remaining fragments can be removed by radial (circumferential) stripping using a pair of fine Adson forceps. Great care should be taken to avoid axial (longitudinal) stripping of these fragments as this can lead to the plane of dissection deepening. Any fragments that are resistant to removal should be transected at their base using the microscissors.

If, during the course of this phase, the wall becomes focally weakened or damaged, a few interrupted 7–0 Prolene sutures will usually be sufficient to restore the integrity of the endarterectomized wall. Finally, the endarterectomy zone is examined whilst heparinized saline is sprayed through a cannula, which should elevate and display any residual intimal fragments. These can then be removed radially or transected.

TACKING SUTURES?

To my knowledge, no randomized trials have addressed the issue of whether to tack down the proximal and/or distal intimal steps. I routinely tack down both the proximal and distal intimal steps in the belief that, if one is trying to achieve a stroke rate

of 1–2%, everything possible must be done to minimize the risk of inadvertent technical error.

The rationale underlying tacking down the distal intimal step is to minimize the risk of subintimal dissection and secondary thrombus formation. Because this is done routinely, I tend to find that, in those situations where the intima is very thin, one is already experienced at avoiding any 'cheese-wiring' by the suture and the potential difficulty is reduced.

I accept that the same rationale may not necessarily apply to the proximal intimal step but retrograde dissection or oscillation of the proximal flap has been described and it is therefore possible that platelet aggregates might develop beneath a non-adherent proximal step and act as a source of embolization.[1]

PROXIMAL DISEASE EXTENSION?

For the most part, the preoperative duplex and/or angiographic studies will have identified those patients with significant proximal disease extension. However, every now and again the surgeon will encounter a patient with mural disease. In the majority, no action need be taken other then partially extending the arteriotomy over this segment prior to tacking and patching. In a few patients, however, the presence of confluent, and occasionally ulcerative, mural disease with loose overlying debris can be worrying. In this situation, the aim should be to achieve a balance between removing the soft ulcerated plaques whilst leaving the firmer solid areas of disease. In practice, the surgeon will get into more trouble by trying obsessively to achieve an entirely smooth proximal endarterectomy zone than if mural disease is simply covered with a patch.

THE POSTERIOR TONGUE OF DISTAL PLAQUE?

It is not uncommon to find a posterior tongue of plaque which extends above the distal limits of the stenosis. These are often not evident on preoperative duplex or angiographic studies because they are not usually flow-limiting. At operation, they become manifest by displaying a posterior segment of atheromatous mural disease (protruding into the media and adventitia) whilst the intima on either side is usually very thin and adherent.

In practice, there are three possible ways of dealing with this problem. The first is simply to extend the arteriotomy and patch this area. Although this may be acceptable in those cases where the intimal thickness is < 2 mm, the tongue is often thicker than this and runs the risk of secondary stenosis formation, thrombus deposition or distal dissection. The second option is to continue with the plane of dissection until the narrow tongue is removed. In practice, this can be difficult because the intima on either side of the tongue is thin and adherent to the underlying media. Consequently, the surgeon may end up with a distal endarterectomy zone that is damaged or dangerously thinned. The third option – and my preferred one, should the first option not be possible – would be simply to remove the posterior tongue and leave the intima on either side intact. Here the plaque can be carefully removed whilst transecting the junction with the filmy adjacent intima using curved microscissors. At the end, the posterior crescent of intima can be tacked down with interrupted 7–0 Prolene sutures.

REDUNDANCY OF THE CAROTID BIFURCATION?

It is difficult to define redundancy of the bifurcation and it is therefore worth considering why redundancy might be problematic. The endarterectomy zone after CEA is potentially thrombogenic and the surgeon should therefore do everything possible to optimize flow across its surface.

The problem of redundancy or kinking can arise in a number of situations. The first follows the functional elongation of the carotid bifurcation after removal of the plaque (Fig. 21.1). This is particularly accentuated if the bifurcation is excessively mobilized and when the original plaque volume was considerable. The second scenario arises when there is natural kinking or looping of the distal internal carotid artery (ICA). Thus, following restoration of flow, the bifurcation may become sufficiently redundant that angulation occurs and this may thereafter compromise flow and predispose towards thrombosis.

There are no evidence-based guidelines to aid surgeons regarding formal shortening of the carotid

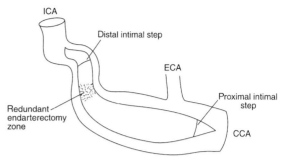

Fig. 21.1
Redundancy of the proximal internal carotid artery (ICA) after endarterectomy. ECA, external carotid artery; CCA, common carotid artery.

artery, but there are a number of different scenarios that merit discussion.

The coiled carotid artery can be a particular problem. Although the coiling may not have caused any problems prior to endarterectomy, it is often necessary to mobilize the coil in order to perform the operation. Moreover, the coil usually retains a 'memory' and cannot be readily straightened out without compromising the integrity of the reconstruction. In practice, if the coil is so distal that it does not impinge on either the shunt lumen or the actual endarterectomy, I would leave it alone. However, if the coil impedes flow in the shunt or if it is immediately above the endarterectomy zone, some form of secondary intervention is necessary. In those situations where there is marked coiling, it may not be possible formally to shorten the ICA and an end-to-end vein bypass may be the preferable option (Fig. 21.2). In our experience this has only been necessary in 3% of all CEAs performed in our unit. An alternative would be formally to resect the looped segment and re-anastomose the two ends (see below).

With regard to redundancy or elongation of the carotid artery, the surgeon must estimate whether he or she thinks that, on restoration of flow, this will cause significant angulation. If it is felt that angulation will occur, then some form of shortening should be performed.

There are a number of techniques for shortening an endarterectomized carotid artery prior to patching. In the first, a section of the endarterectomized ICA is resected and the vessel

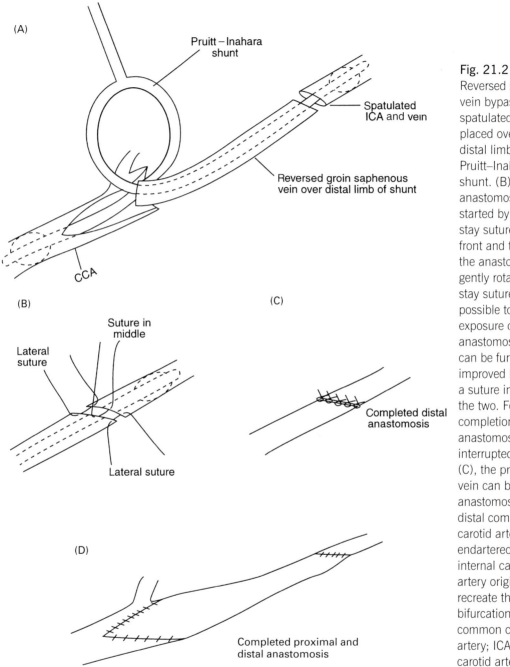

(A)

Pruitt – Inahara shunt

Spatulated ICA and vein

Reversed groin saphenous vein over distal limb of shunt

CCA

(B)

Suture in middle

Lateral suture

Lateral suture

(C)

Completed distal anastomosis

(D)

Completed proximal and distal anastomosis

Fig. 21.2
Reversed saphenous vein bypass. (A) The spatulated vein is placed over the distal limb of the Pruitt–Inahara shunt. (B) The distal anastomosis is then started by placing stay sutures at the front and the back of the anastomosis. By gently rotating the stay sutures, it is possible to gain good exposure of the anastomosis, which can be further improved by placing a suture in between the two. Following completion of the anastomosis with interrupted sutures (C), the proximal vein can be anastomosed to the distal common carotid artery and endarterectomized internal carotid artery origin to recreate the bifurcation (D). CCA, common carotid artery; ICA, internal carotid artery.

re-anastomosed (Fig. 21.3). In practice, there is usually a disparity between the diameter of the distal artery to be reanastomosed and the proximal endarterectomy zone. In addition, the distal artery may be very thin and

friable, thereby predisposing to suture tearing. My preferred option is to perform an eversion plication (Fig. 21.4). The principal advantage of this is that the residual wall is effectively strengthened and the distal

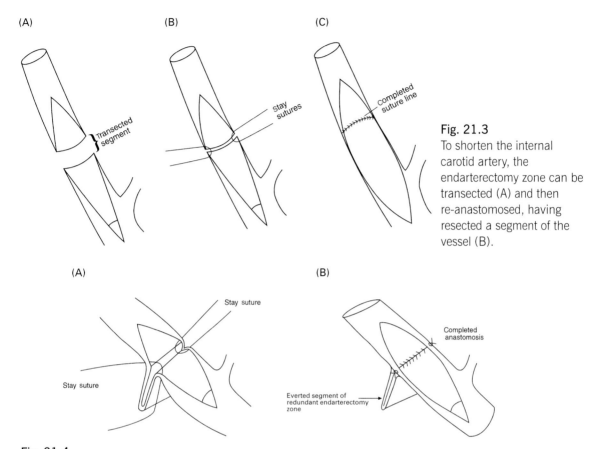

(A)   (B)   (C)

Transected segment

Stay sutures

Completed suture line

Fig. 21.3
To shorten the internal carotid artery, the endarterectomy zone can be transected (A) and then re-anastomosed, having resected a segment of the vessel (B).

(A)   (B)

Stay suture

Stay suture

Completed anastomosis

Everted segment of redundant endarterectomy zone

Fig. 21.4
Eversion plication of the internal carotid artery. (A) A segment of redundant endarterectomy zone is everted and stay sutures are placed at the edges. The stay sutures should be carefully positioned so that, when they are pulled laterally, the distal intimal step is incorporated into the eversion. The eversion is then completed by either a running suture (B) or, alternatively, externally placed interrupted sutures through the everted segment only will complete the internal anastomosis.

intimal step is usually buried within the plication. A further option which has not, as yet, become established in the UK, is eversion endarterectomy (see below).

ENDARTERECTOMY ZONE TOO THIN?

The recognition of an endarterectomy zone that is dangerously thinned and prone to pseudoaneurysm formation is difficult. Upon completion of the endarterectomy, I place a pair of forceps behind the endarterectomized distal ICA. If I can easily visualize them through the posterior wall, I would repair the distal ICA by either resection or plication (see above).

I prefer not to perform a vein bypass in this situation because approximately one-third of such bypasses develop localized stenoses as a consequence of intimal hyperplasia. This incidence is far higher than that observed during standard endarterectomy and warrants serial postoperative surveillance imaging by duplex, because stenoses can seriously threaten graft patency. On the other hand, I would always favour a carotid vein bypass to resection or plication under tension.

CAROTID BYPASS?

The protocol for our unit requires us to perform

carotid bypass only when either a standard endarterectomy or plication is deemed inappropriate or unsafe. In practice, we only consider it in patients with marked coiling of the ICA or if there is any question of tension following plication.

I perform a carotid bypass using reversed long saphenous vein obtained from the upper thigh. This operation is facilitated by placing the vein graft over the distal limb of the shunt (Fig. 21.2), which then not only acts as a stent for closure, but also ensures continuing cerebral perfusion. If, however, access is difficult and middle carotid artery (MCA) velocities were satisfactory, I do not struggle unnecessarily to use the shunt at all costs. I have, on occasion, placed the shunt into the ECA, thereby raising the MCA velocities to such an extent that I have been happy to perform the bypass without a shunt in the ICA.

The distal ICA anastomosis is performed first. Interrupted stay sutures are placed anteriorly and posteriorly between the spatulated ends of the vein and ICA and then a further suture is placed in between the two (Fig. 21.2). These sutures can then be used to rotate the distal anastomosis gently to allow insertion of interrupted sutures between these.

The proximal anastomosis can then be performed. If, at completion of the endarterectomy, the CCA up to the level of the bifurcation is narrow but not too thin, I consider an end-to-end anastomosis between the transected CCA and the vein graft. The disadvantage is that the ECA must be sacrificed. The second approach, which is currently the preferred option in the unit, reimplants the vein graft on to the distal CCA and proximal ICA so as to reconstruct the bifurcation (Fig. 21.2). In this way, flow in the ECA can also be restored whilst maintaining the anatomic integrity of the carotid bifurcation. A third option is to oversew the proximal ICA and then anastomose the vein graft end-to-side to the common carotid artery.

EXTERNAL CAROTID ENDARTERECTOMY?

In my opinion, CEA performed to cure ICA embolization does not require formal endarterectomy of the ECA. However, I routinely perform eversion endarterectomy of the ECA origin to remove any material that may potentially embolize into the ICA. At the end of the procedure, it is important to inspect the origin of the ECA and ensure there are no residual intimal flaps.

If the operation of CEA is being performed specifically to deal with ECA embolization such as may occur when the ICA is occluded and the patient has ipsilateral embolic symptoms secondary to a stenosed ECA, then I consider a formal ECA endarterectomy.[2–4] In addition, if I had to ligate the ICA for any reason and the ECA origin was diseased, I would formally perform an ECA endarterectomy and patch.

EVERSION ENDARTERECTOMY?

Broadly speaking, there are two techniques for ICA endarterectomy. The standard method has been described above. However, the original description by DeBakey et al.[5] involved transection of the CCA with eversion endarterectomy of the proximal CCA, ICA and ECA. A variation on this technique has been described by Raithel and Kasprzak[6] and involves disconnection of the ICA from the CCA and eversion endarterectomy of the ICA followed by endarterectomy of the carotid bifurcation and ECA. The ICA can then be shortened to size and re-anastomosed to the CCA to prevent kinking. Prior to re-anastomosing the ICA to the CCA, angioscopy is performed to assess the intraluminal structures. In approximately 20% of cases the ICA has to be revised because of intimal flaps.[6]

In theory, the potential advantages of eversion CEA are that, because there is no longitudinal arteriotomy (the only incision is transverse), there is no need for patching and because the operation can be performed rapidly, there is a reduced need for intraluminal shunts.

In my view, the main disadvantage of eversion ICA endarterectomy is that the distal endarterectomy point is completely uncontrolled and therefore there must always be a risk of intimal flaps (as noted on angioscopy by Raithel and Kasprzak in 20% of cases). In addition, any technique which requires speed raises the spectre of technical error and thus is not an effective teaching tool. In my opinion, every stage of CEA should be carefully and precisely performed and everything possible should be done to minimize the risk of stroke. I would stress again that if one is trying to achieve stroke rates as low as 1 or 2%, it is vital that everything possible is done to minimize technical error. The eversion endarterectomy technique cannot minimize error because of the lack of visualization and precise control of the distal endarterectomy point. Moreover, a shunt cannot be inserted until the endarterectomy phase has been completed.

QUALITY CONTROL?

The most important aspect of quality control is that the surgeon should design the operative approach and technique so that every stage of the operation can be performed carefully under direct vision and in a sequence that minimizes the risks of technical

error and intraoperative embolization. It is also important that the carotid surgeon realizes that, despite his or her best efforts, errors will occur and they must be detected before blood flow to the brain is restored.

I stress that it is important that these errors are detected *before* restoring blood flow to the brain. This is because, if there is thrombus at the endarterectomy site at the time of clamp release, this will immediately embolize; techniques to assess quality control after restoration of flow cannot detect this because it may already be in the brain. A summary of monitoring and quality control methods during carotid surgery has been presented elsewhere.

REFERENCES

1 Padayachee TS, Brooks MD, Modaresi KB, Arnold AJ, Seld GW, Taylor PR. Intra-operative high resolution duplex imaging during carotid endarterectomy: Which abnormalities require surgical correction? *European Journal of Vascular and Endovascular Surgery* 1998; **15**: 387–393.

2 Rush DS, Holloway WO, Fogartie JE Jr, Fine JG, Haynes JL. The safety efficacy, and durability of external carotid endarterectomy. *Journal of Vascular Surgery* 1992; **16**: 407–411.

3 Nicolosi A, Klinger D, Bandyk D, Towne J. External carotid endarterectomy in the treatment of symptomatic patients with internal carotid artery occlusion. *Annals of Vascular Surgery* 1988; **2**: 336–339.

4 Gertler JP, Cambria RP. The role of external carotid endarterectomy in the treatment of ipsilateral internal carotid occlusion: collective review. *Journal of Vascular Surgery* 1987; **6**: 158–167.

5 DeBakey ME, Crawford ES, Cooley DA, Morris JC Jr. Surgical considerations of occlusive disease of innominate, carotid, subclavian and vertebral arteries. *Annals of Surgery* 1959; **149**: 690–710.

6 Raithel D, Kasprzak P. Angioscopy after carotid endarterectomy. *Annales Chirurgicales et Gynécologie* 1992; **81**: 192–195.

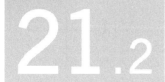

21.2

How can I achieve the optimal flow surface and distal end-point following carotid endarterectomy?

Joseph P Archie, Jr (USA)

INTRODUCTION

CEA can be a treacherous and unforgiving operation. The degree of difficulty is infrequently predicted by preoperative imaging studies. The surgeon must not only be knowledgeable, experienced, and technically proficient, but must also recognize that he or she will be operating with incomplete information on the extent of disease and degree of difficulty. An easy CEA is an afterthought. In addition to patient selection, intraoperative decisions and technique are the primary determinants of outcome. Given proper selection of patients, other perceived operative risk factors, such as contralateral carotid occlusion, prior stroke, and the necessity for use of a shunt are minor issues.

Except for adverse events related to occult coronary disease and the rare occurrence of hyperperfusion syndrome, the outcome of CEA is almost completely determined by the surgeon. While some may argue with this view, any surgeon who considers perioperative stroke and/or internal carotid thrombosis to be an acceptable or unpreventable complication is fooling him- or herself.

CAROTID GEOMETRY, HEMODYNAMICS, AND OPTIMAL RECONSTRUCTION

The normal extracranial carotid bifurcation geometry and blood flow distribution contribute to atherogenesis. Zarins *et al.*[7] have quantitatively correlated zones of blood flow separation and low wall shear stresses with intimal thickening and plaque in the carotid bulb. Both theoretical solutions to the fluid flow equations and experimental models clearly illustrate that the normal carotid bifurcation is a focus of severely abnormal hemodynamics.[8–11] Arterial blood flow in a relatively normal CCA is

laminar, unidirectional, and does not contain primary or secondary disturbed flow components. This undisturbed flow pattern changes abruptly in a normal carotid bulb or sinus. The major region of disturbed flow is in the posterior lateral wall of the internal carotid bulb opposite the bifurcation or flow divider. This is characterized by recirculation during late systole and throughout diastole, with vortex formation and propagation down the internal carotid with each cardiac cycle.

There are several reasons for this. The carotid bifurcation is not symmetric like the distal aorta. Both the geometry and flow requirements of the internal and external carotid are quite different. These two factors play a major role in producing adverse hemodynamic events. There is a change in geometry from the circular cross-section of the common carotid to an eccentric, elliptical one just proximal to the bifurcation, the common carotid component of the carotid sinus. The bulb segment of the internal carotid is unlike that found in other bifurcating arteries and further disturbs the flow patterns. There is a great deal of variability in the geometry of human carotid bifurcations. The location, size, and shape of the bulb, as well as the angle of incidence between the ICA and ECA are quite variable.[12,13]

The second cause of disturbed flow in the carotid bulb – variability in the distribution of internal and external carotid flow – has to date not been investigated. Not only is there an unequal distribution of average volume flow to the internal and external carotids, usually taken on average between 60% and 75% to the internal and 25% and 40% in the external, but the relative distribution changes throughout each cardiac cycle. The temporal flow variation throughout a cardiac cycle in the internal carotid is similar to that of arteries supplying other solid organs such as the kidney and liver, namely, a relatively high diastolic component. In contrast, the temporal flow profile in the external carotid is similar to that of an artery supplying a resting extremity; the diastolic component is small. This relative redistribution of blood flow during each pulse is significant enough to produce flow disturbances at the bifurcation and further amplify those caused by the unusual geometry.

The hemodynamic disturbances produced in the carotid bulb are believed to be one of the major factors leading to intimal thickening, atherosclerosis, myointimal proliferation, and thrombus formation in or on walls. The zones of recirculation and low shear near walls are associated with prolonged blood particle transit times and an increased propensity and opportunity for mass transport into and platelet deposition on surfaces.

Given these adverse hemodynamic events in the normal carotid with each cardiac cycle, the optimal carotid reconstruction after a complete endarterectomy would be to eliminate the bifurcation and the carotid bulb and to construct a smooth, gradually tapered transition from the CCA to the uniform-diameter distal ICA. This could be achieved by obliterating the orifice of the ECA and either patch reconstruction or an interposition graft properly matched and configured to the ICA and CCA. While this approach is occasionally taken in reoperations or in severely diseased arteries, it is unlikely to become standard or to be given a clinical trial.

The next best solution is as complete an endarterectomy as possible and a reconstruction that eliminates the carotid bulb, minimizes tortuosity or kinking, and provides a smoothly tapered transition from the CCA to the ICA. It has been shown by computational methods that the carotid geometry that minimizes flow disturbances, vortex formation, low wall shear stress, and high wall shear stress gradients has a low bifurcation angle and no bulb in the common or internal carotid.[9] While it is possible to reconstruct an endarterectomized carotid artery so that the origin of the proximal ICA has essentially the same diameter as its more distal segment, this may not be advisable. All or part (if a vein patch is used)

of the reconstructed walls are thrombogenic surfaces on which platelets rapidly adhere, the process of wall thickening and repair soon begins, and some degree of narrowing will occur. Thus, it is advisable to maintain the bulb segment of the CCA and provide a gradual transition in the diameter of the ICA from its origin to the downstream uniform diameter.

Currently, one of the most controversial issues regarding CEA is the method of reconstruction. Both primary closure and patching have been utilized with satisfactory results. Thompson[14] obtained satisfactory outcomes by current standards with primary closure two decades ago. Sundt,[15] working in the same timeframe, found that he could significantly reduce the incidence of perioperative stroke and internal carotid thrombosis from 4% to 1% by patch reconstruction with an autologous greater saphenous vein. Based on the above hemodynamic considerations, the carotid reconstruction, whether by primary closure or patch reconstruction, should eliminate the bulb and result in a smooth gradually tapered transition from the larger diameter of the bifurcation to the smaller-diameter distal ICA. Patches, when used, should not simply widen the bulb and proximal ICA but rather should aid in the achievement of this tapered transition.

Most surgeons agree that primary closure is acceptable and appropriate when the arteriotomy necessary to obtain a complete internal carotid end-point does not extend beyond the bulb. However, in my experience this occurs in only approximately 4% of operations.[16] Primary closure of an arteriotomy that extends beyond the bulb results in some degree of stenosis, as illustrated in Figure 21.5. It has been shown that such a primary closure produces an approximately 15% stenosis.[17] Even precisely done with optical magnification and fine sutures, it is difficult to close a longitudinal arteriotomy in a

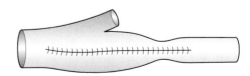

Fig. 21.5
Result of primary closure of an arteriotomy that extends cephalad to the carotid bulb.

uniform-diameter artery without producing some degree of stenosis. This is consistent with simple calculations. If 1mm suture bites are taken in a 5mm-diameter ICA, the resulting circumference is reduced by 2mm, giving a 13% diameter stenosis and a 24% area stenosis. If the suture bites are 1.5mm, the resulting stenosis is 19% diameter and 35% area stenosis. If a 4mm-diameter artery is primarily closed with 1mm suture bites, the stenosis is 16% diameter and 29% area. Closure of a 4mm artery with 1.5mm bites results in a 24% diameter and a 42% area stenosis. Clearly, primary closure of arteriotomies that extend beyond the carotid bulb into small-diameter ICAs may produce significant residual stenosis.

Recent meta-analysis of six published prospective randomized trials of primary closure versus patch reconstruction strongly supports patching, even though taken individually they send a mixed message.[18,19] Patching gives two to four times lower incidence of early postoperative thrombosis ($P = 0.001$, power = 0.99), perioperative stroke ($P = 0.008$, power = 0.83) and > 50% restenosis at 1 year ($P < 0.001$, power = 0.99) than does primary closure.[19] The issues surrounding primary versus patch closure are covered in more detail in Chapter 22.

RESIDUAL DISEASE AND TECHNICAL DEFECTS

Residual disease and technical defects are associated with perioperative stroke, restenosis, and late stroke.[20–22] The incidence of significant residual defects in the ICA or CCA is reported to be between 5% and 14%.[23–26] The etiology and types of residual defects include clamp injury to the CCA and ICA, kinking at the distal end of a patch angioplasty, kinking of the internal carotid distal to a patch, intimal dissection and/or flaps at the internal carotid end-point, residual atheroma with or without tack sutures at the internal carotid end-point, primary closure of an arteriotomy that extends beyond the carotid bulb, too wide a patch reconstruction, and an endarterectomy-produced proximal end-point common carotid step. The incidence of stroke after CEA is reported to be 1.6–3% per year.[22,27,28] Many of these strokes may be preventable if retained

disease and technical defects are eliminated or corrected. The importance of optimizing the primary operation cannot be overemphasized.

The major objective in performing endarterectomy is to obtain a smooth, feathered and complete end-point in the internal carotid. Failure to do so means a less than optimal flow surface. At best, residual defects produce flow disturbances that may abate with time as the defect smooths out and, at worst, cause thrombotic occlusion, distal embolization, or restenosis. My experience with approximately 2000 CEAs is that a complete internal carotid end-point can be obtained in 98%. Of these, only 4% of complete end-points were obtained within the carotid bulb. Put another way, the arteriotomy necessary to obtain a complete internal carotid end-point extends beyond the bulb into the uniform-diameter distal segment in 96% of operations. Failure to obtain adequate exposure and extend the arteriotomy to achieve an acceptable end-point is a technical error. Possible results of incomplete end-points are illustrated in Fig. 21.6. These include retained atherosclerotic plaque, intimal flaps of residual plaque, and attempted damage control with tack sutures.

One component of contemporary CEA is frequent use of internal carotid end-point tack sutures. The necessity for doing this means that a feathered complete endarterectomy was not obtained. The residual defect – either intimal dissection, flaps, or

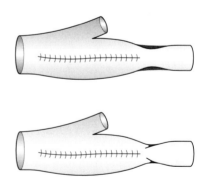

Fig. 21.6
Internal carotid end-point defects when the arteriotomy is limited to the carotid bulb. Top: retained plaque with or without tack sutures; bottom: residual flaps or dissection.

retained atheroma – is secured with fine sutures. While this may occasionally be necessary, the concept of more than rarely using this technique is flawed. Most surgeons who utilize patch angioplasty reconstruction do so because the arteriotomy required to obtain a complete end-point extends beyond the bulb. With an adequate endarterectomy through an arteriotomy extending above all gross disease, tacking should be required rarely (2% in my experience).[16] Anything more than occasional tacking translates into retained disease or a focal defect, both of which produce some degree of adverse hemodynamics and their possible consequences.

It is rare that a complete, feathered proximal end-point is obtained in the CCA. Eccentric or concentric common carotid steps or shelves > 2mm in depth are occasionally associated with both early postoperative emboli production and significant late restenosis at this location.[29] Common carotid steps 1mm or more produce significant flow disruption with recirculation zones just distal to the step; vortex formation, and secondary flow phenomena.[30] Several methods of smoothing out this residual defect have been recommended, including eversion plication,[29] which also serves to cover the exposed, highly thrombogenic diseased media and intima, and sharp beveling of the step.[31]

The technique of management of the external carotid during CEA is infrequently considered. However, flaps and thrombosis of the external carotid have been incriminated in distal embolization into the internal carotid and strokes. It is often difficult to obtain a complete end-point in the external carotid utilizing the usual partial eversion – a blind technique. I have found that early after standard primary CEA approximately 28% of external carotids have > 50% residual stenosis. In addition, repair of intraoperatively identified severe defects in the external carotid had a similarly poor outcome. Ascer et al.[32] found that simple division at the orifice of the external carotid gave satisfactory results.

While patching helps to insure satisfactory geometry and an adequate end-point, it is not without its pitfalls. In a 1988 editorial Imparato[33] clearly stated that the goal of patch angioplasty is not to enlarge the carotid bulb but rather to allow an adequate arteriotomy to remove the plaque and provide a hemodynamically optimal reconstruction. It is now recognized that there is approximately 10% dilatation in carotid bulb diameters in the first year after patch reconstruction with vein and synthetic materials.[34,35] Intraoperative pre- and post-endarterectomy measurements confirm that patch reconstruction can be routinely performed without increasing the diameter of the carotid bulb.[36] The key is to tailor each reconstruction so that the resulting geometry is a smooth axial transition in internal carotid diameter from the common carotid to the uniform-diameter distal segment.

Four major hemodynamic defects are possible. First, a correctly tailored patch reconstruction in a redundant endarterectomized artery can result in kinking of the ICA distal to the patch. The tapered geometry of patch reconstruction produces an axially straight reconstruction, but if there is redundancy, coiling, or tortuosity of the endarterectomized segment, this will be transmitted and amplified distally, as illustrated in Fig. 21.7 (top). This is a commonly recognized problem with patch reconstruction of long arteriotomies. The defect can be modified somewhat by suturing the artery to adjacent tissue but this is generally unsatisfactory. The best way to prevent this problem is shortening of the endarterectomized segment prior to reconstruction, as described below.

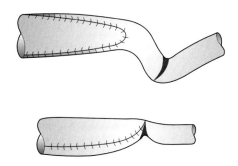

Fig. 21.7
Kinks in patched internal carotid arteries produced by (top) redundant endarterectomized segments and/or long arteriotomies with resulting transfer of length cephalad, and (bottom) too wide a patch toe relative to the normal internal carotid diameter.

Second, if the distal end of the patch is too wide relative to the ICA diameter a kink is produced at the distal end of the patch, as illustrated in Fig. 21.7 (bottom). The problem is a sudden successive change from a tapering circular cross-section of the distal patch segment to an eccentric elliptical one at the tip of the patch to the circular one just distal to the patch. Simple calculations for a 5mm diameter ICA and a 4mm wide patch tip give a circumference at the end of the patch that is 25% greater than that of the more distal normal ICA. However, the cross-sectional area of the eccentric lumen at the tip of the patch is only 30–60% (depending on the major and minor axes of the ellipse) of the internal carotid area, representing constituting a 40–70% stenosis, as well as an abrupt geometry change. This is one of the major unrecognized technical errors of patch reconstruction.

Third, too wide a patch body produces a bulb-like geometry that is subject to the same adverse hemodynamics as the normal carotid. An optimally reconstructed artery does not have an internal carotid bulb. The distal common carotid of an optimal reconstruction has an elliptical geometry that is more circular (lower eccentricity) than that of the pre-endarterectomy artery but has nearly the same cross-sectional area.[36] Further, there is no internal carotid bulging or bulb. Failure to eliminate the bulb by too wide a patch results in excessive posterior wall mural thrombus formation.[37]

Fourth and finally, the proximal end of patch reconstruction should begin 3–7mm proximal to the common carotid step. This allows for a gradual transition into the bulb segment of the common carotid and may decrease the probability of a recurrent stenosis at the step.[29]

RECOMMENDED TECHNIQUE

Adequate exposure of the CCA and ICA prior to clamping is paramount to obtaining optimal endarterectomy end-points. The extent of disease is only occasionally determined by preoperative imaging studies. The CCA should be exposed and palpated proximally in order to place an occlusion device below the major component of disease. Determination of the extent of atheroma in the ICA can occasionally be difficult. Observation of the proximal ICA is helpful, as one can frequently see a change in color of the artery at the end of the anterior lateral wall plaque. However, many internal carotids have a tongue of plaque that extends up the posterior inferior wall but is sometimes spiral. Gentle palpation of the apparently normal more distal segment of ICA with a fine vascular forceps will usually identify a tongue and its distal extent. A good rule of thumb is to expose the ICA approximately 1cm distal to the highest identifiable disease.

My experience is that in approximately half of the operations the hypoglossal nerve must be reflected anterior medially to obtain adequate exposure of the internal carotid. This is done by dividing and ligating the small artery and vein that pass over the nerve and reflecting the ansa hypoglossi anteriorly along with the hypoglossal. In approximately 20% of cases it is helpful to divide the belly of the diagastric muscle. I frequently use 3–0 silk retraction sutures in adjacent tissue to maintain the tunnel-like distal exposure. If a shunt is to be used, slightly more exposure is needed proximally and distally. I have used elastic vessel loops on the common carotid, superior thyroid and main trunk of the ECA for two decades without an identified complication due to vessel injury. On the ICA I use a very soft special bulldog clamp (Codman 37–1062) with a 5–6mm arm. Having two or more with different spring occlusion thresholds on hand is helpful as the internal carotid back-pressure is usually less than 50mmHg and a very soft clamp often suffices. If a non-balloon-type shunt is used, vessel loops work nicely on both the CCA and ICA.

After systemic heparinization, occlusion and longitudinal (axial) arteriotomy, the endarterectomy is begun in the deep media of the proximal bulb segment. I use a blunt-end, curved right-angle clamp to create the proximal dissection end-point and divide the plaque sharply at the proximal end with a coronary artery scissors. This invariably creates an eccentric or occasionally a concentric radial step 3–4mm distal to the origin of the arteriotomy. The step can be trimmed, but by the nature of dividing the media and intima, a small radial dissection is created in the deep media. If the step or part thereof is > 2mm in thickness I repair it by eversion plication prior to reconstruction, as described below. The endarterectomy is then carried to the orifice of the ECA where a partial eversion and blind endarterectomy are performed on the ECA. If the plaque disease in the ICA is limited to the internal carotid bulb, care should be taken at this point when pulling down on the external carotid plaque. Pulling on the external carotid plaque invariably continues the endarterectomy well into the internal carotid bulb and may spoil an opportunity to obtain a finely taped end-point there.

The deep endarterectomy is then carefully and meticulously carried into the internal carotid. At some point, usually anteriorly at one edge of the arteriotomy, the plaque thins and the feathering process begins. Occasionally this can be initiated by cutting the thin, slightly elevated intima at the edge of the arteriotomy and then circumferentially or obliquely carefully developing a feathered end-point. If a tongue of plaque is present it is gently endarterectomized. The thin almost transparent inner endothelial layer, probably endothelium, does not have a tendency to separate or divide circumferentially. I use a fine ophthalmologic scissors to trim this layer when it does not break cleanly. If the tongue of plaque extends beyond the distal most obtainable arteriotomy it is advisable to stop 3–4mm short of the end of the arteriotomy, sharply transect the tongue, bevel it, and use tack sutures to secure it. With adequate prior exposure this should occur in fewer than 3% of cases. The reason for securing the retained disease proximal to the end of the arteriotomy is to allow the defect to preside within the transition section of patch reconstruction, not at the distal end. Under no circumstances should a blind endarterectomy of the internal carotid be attempted. While this may result in an adequate end-point, it may also result in retained disease, flaps or dissection with the resulting chance of thrombosis, embolization, or restenosis. The endarterectomy surface is then inspected and loose media removed. Heparin saline irrigation of this surface is thought to reduce later platelet deposition.

Two adjunctive procedures should be considered. If the retained common carotid step is > 2mm eversion, plication reconstruction with 6–0 polyethylene suture is advisable.[29] The second adjunctive technique to be considered is shortening the endarterectomized internal carotid segment. The decision to do so is based on judgment and not quantitatively determined. As described previously, a patched redundant segment may produce a kink just past the distal end of the patch. If the segment is redundant it is advisable to shorten it. The simplest method of doing so is eversion plication with a running 6–0 polypropylene suture.[16]

Primary closure is advisable when the arteriotomy necessary to obtain a feathered complete internal carotid end-point does not extend beyond the bulb. The sutures should be placed so as to eliminate the carotid bulb. Depending on the bulb size as evaluated prior to occlusion, progressively deeper sutures are taken in the mid-segment of the closure. The combination of a primary closure and common carotid step repair has occurred only once in my experience. In most cases where patch reconstruction is utilized, the patch must be tailored to the native artery to give a hemodynamically smooth bifurcation and transition in diameter of the internal carotid. The technique of achieving this is somewhat different for tissue and synthetic patches.

The technique of using a vein patch to produce a uniformly tapered, hemodynamically optimal reconstruction requires accurate suture placement in the patch so as to produce a result similar to that illustrated in Fig. 21.8. Vein patches are difficult to trim to accurate shape because of their elasticity. It is advisable to trim longitudinally veins with distended diameters of 5mm or more, as large veins have more than ample material to construct a patch. Using a vein patch I take deep sutures in the lateral

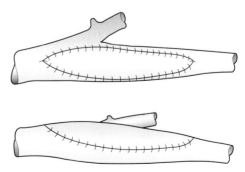

Fig. 21.8
(Top) Anterior and (bottom) lateral views of a hemodynamically optimal patch reconstruction.

endarterectomized wall, thereby increasing the percentage of flow surface that has intact endothelium. That is, I use more vein than I would synthetic material in the reconstruction. I use a continuous 6–0 polypropylene suture for the anastomosis, beginning distally with four end-point sutures parachuted in and a transitional U stitch on the side. While some surgeons use three or more individual sutures at the end-point, I believe that a continuous suture technique allows the anastomosis to smooth out when arterial pressure is restored. The tapering of the internal carotid bulb, its resulting diameter, and the diameter of the common carotid bulb are determined by the depth of bites into the endarterectomized arterial wall and the vein patch. As mentioned above, the resulting bulb diameters should be equivalent to or smaller than the preoperative ones. At the common carotid end a more blunt taper of the patch is used. Because the arteriotomy required to obtain an accurate common carotid end-point extends 3–5 mm caudad, the patch extends over the common carotid step and helps to diffuse adverse hemodynamic effects, even if the step is not repaired.

Synthetic patch materials commonly used are woven and knitted Dacron and polytetrafluoroethylene (PTFE). Several precut 8mm wide collagen-treated knitted Dacron patches are commercially available. The technique of using a synthetic patch is slightly different from that of vein. Synthetic patches should be cut accurately to match the artery with a finely tapered distal end and a more bluntly cut V at the common carotid end. This is because, unlike vein patches, it is difficult to tailor the shape and width of a synthetic patch with sutures. The resulting geometry should be similar with both synthetic and vein patches.[35]

Two other techniques, interposition grafting and eversion endarterectomy, require consideration. End-to-end grafting from the CCA to the ICA is frequently used in reoperations. I have used vein interposition grafting for a primary CEA only seven times. This is a good technique when the internal CEA segment is quite long and the endarterectomized surface is in poor condition with an uneven 'raw hamburger'

appearance. Interposition grafting is another way of managing a retained tongue of plaque.[16] The luxury of having harvested a 5–6mm diameter greater saphenous vein makes this technique possible. When using saphenous vein for a patch, I harvest it first but do not prepare it for a patch until the final decision about reconstruction is made. While interposition grafting gives an excellent hemodynamic result with no bulb, there are no large series documenting its outcome when used for primary CEA. When performing interposition grafting I bevel the distal anastomosis at approximately 45° and tailor the proximal anastomosis from the origin of the ICA caudad and anteriorly, and use the proximal vein segment to complete the closure similar to a vein patch on the common carotid arteriotomy.

Eversion endarterectomy requires transection of the CCA or ICA. While I have no experience with this method, others report satisfactory early outcomes. This method preserves the internal carotid bulb and accordingly results in a flow surface with the original geometry that contributed to development of the disease being treated. A second concern is the re-anastomosis zone, particularly if it is at the origin of the internal carotid. I have found that suture lines used in this location for shortening are associated with early restenosis.

CONFIRMATION OF ADEQUATE HEMODYNAMICS

I have used continuous-wave Doppler for over two decades to interrogate the arteries after restoring flow. While vein patch reconstructions are easily examined, synthetic patched arteries are more difficult because of acoustic interference. However, the probe can be placed superiorly or laterally to check the patch end-points. By far the most commonly identified defect is in the ECA. If the flow impairment is severe I isolate the ECA and repair it. While it is difficult to make a technical error with patch angioplasty, I have occasionally noted a kink distal to the patch due to more redundancy than anticipated, or a kink at the cephalad end of the patch because the patch is too wide relative to the normal artery diameter. These defects should be immediately repaired.

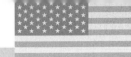

CONCLUSIONS

The objective of CEA is a hemodynamically sound geometry that minimizes blood flow disturbances known to be associated with thrombus formation – excessive myointimal hyperplasia, recurrent atherosclerosis, and distal embolization. Achieving this requires as complete an endarterectomy as possible and a reconstruction that is hemodynamically optimal. A complete internal carotid end-point is mandatory and obtainable in over 97% of operations. To achieve this requires an endarterectomy that extends beyond the carotid bulb in approximately 96% of cases. In these cases, patch reconstruction provides the opportunity to eliminate the adverse hemodynamics of primary closure and the carotid bulb by constructing a gradual transition in diameter from the CCA to the uniform-diameter more distal internal carotid. Primary closure should be limited to the approximately 4% of cases when a complete finely feathered end-point is obtained in the bulb segment.

REFERENCES

7 Zarins CK, Giddens DP, Bharadvaj BK *et al*. Carotid bifurcation atherosclerosis. Quantitative correlation of plaque localization with flow velocity profiles and wall shear stress. *Circulation Research* 1983; **53**: 502–514.

8 Perktold K, Resch M. Numerical flow studies in human carotid bifurcations: basic discussion of the geometric factor in atherogenesis. *Journal of Biomedical Engineering* 1990; **12**: 111–123.

9 Wells DR, Archie JP, Kleinstreuer C. The effect of carotid artery geometry on the magnitude and distribution of wall shear stress gradients. *Journal of Vascular Surgery* 1996; **23**: 667–678.

10 Ku DN, Giddens DP. Pulsatile flow in a model carotid bifurcation. *Arteriosclerosis* 1983; **3**: 31–39.

11 Ku DN, Giddens DP. Laser Doppler anemometer measurements of pulsatile flow in a model carotid bifurcation. *Journal of Biomechanics* 1987; **20**: 407–421.

12 Boyd JD. Observations on the human carotid sinus and its nerve supply. Anatomischer Anzeiger 1937; **8**: 386–389.

13 Forster FK, Chikos PM, Frazier JS. Geometric modeling of the carotid bifurcation in humans: implications in ultrasonic Doppler and radiologic investigation. *Journal of Clinical Ultrasound* 1985; **13**: 385–391.

14 Thompson JE. Review: Carotid endarterectomy, 1982. State of the art. *British Journal of Surgery* 1983; **70**: 371–376.

15 Sundt TM. *Occlusive Cerebrovascular Disease*, pp. 197–198. Philadelphia, PA: WB Saunders, 1987.

16 Archie JP. Carotid endarterectomy with reconstruction techniques tailored to operative findings. *Journal of Vascular Surgery* 1993; **17**: 141–151.

17 Fietsan R, Ranval T, Cohn S *et al*. Hemodynamic effect of primary closure versus patch angioplasty of the carotid artery. *Annals of Vascular Surgery* 1992; **6**: 443–449.

18 Counsell CE, Salinas R, Naylor R, Warlow CP. A systematic review of the randomized trials of carotid patch angioplasty in carotid endarterectomy. *European Journal of Vascular and Endovascular Surgery* 1997; **13**: 345–354.

19 Archie JP. Prospective randomized trials of carotid endarterectomy with primary closure and patch reconstruction: the problem is power. *Journal of Vascular Surgery* 1997; **25**: 1118–1119.

20 Jackson MR, D'Addio J, Gillespie DL, O'Donnell SD. The fate of residual defects following carotid endarterectomy detected by early postoperative duplex ultrasound. *American Journal of Surgery* 1996; **172**: 184–187.

21 Reilly LM, Okuhn SP, Rapp JH *et al*. Recurrent carotid stenosis: a consequence of local or systemic factors: the influence of unrepaired technical defects. *Journal of Vascular Surgery* 1990; **11**: 448–460.

22 Avramovic JR, Fletcher JP. The incidence of recurrent stenosis after carotid endarterectomy and its relationship to neurological events. *Journal of Cardiovascular Surgery* 1992; **33**: 54–58.

23 Zierier RE, Bandyk DF, Thiele BL. Intraoperative assessment of carotid endarterectomy. *Journal of Vascular Surgery* 1984; **1**: 73–83.

24 Courbier R, Jausseran J, Reggi M *et al*. Routine intraoperative carotid angiography; its impact on operative morbidity and carotid restenosis. *Journal of Vascular Surgery* 1986; **3**: 343–350.

25 Cato R, Bandyk D, Karp D *et al*. Duplex scanning after carotid reconstruction: a comparison of intraoperative and postoperative results. *Journal of Vascular Technology* 1991; **15**: 61–65.

26 Kinney EV, Seabrook GR, Kinney LY *et al*. The importance of intraoperative detection of residual flow abnormalities after carotid artery endarterectomy. *Journal of Vascular Surgery* 1993; **17**: 912–923.

27 Washburn WK, Mackey WC, Belkin M, O'Donnell TF Jr. Late stroke after carotid endarterectomy: the role of recurrent stenosis. *Journal of Vascular Surgery* 1992; **15**: 1032–1037.

28 Barnett HJM, Taylor DW, Haynes RB *et al*. Beneficial effect of carotid endarterectomy in symptomatic patients with high-grade carotid stenosis. *New England Journal of Medicine* 1991; **325**: 334–353.

29 Archie JP. The endarterectomy produced common carotid artery step. A harbinger of early emboli and late restenosis. *Journal of Vascular Surgery* 1996; **23**: 932–939.

30 Hyun S, Kleinstreuer C, Archie JP. Computational flow analysis in tubular sudden expansions with implications to the development of thrombosis and stenosis. *Journal of Biomechanics* (in press).

31 Stoney RJ. Regarding the endarterectomy produced

common carotid artery step: a harbinger of early emboli and late restenosis. *Journal of Vascular Surgery* 1997; **25**: 958–959.

32 Ascer E, Gennavo M, Pollina RM *et al*. The natural history of the external carotid artery after carotid endarterectomy. Implications for management. *Journal of Vascular Surgery* 1996; **23**: 582–586.

33 Imparato AM. The role of patch angioplasty after carotid endarterectomy. *Journal of Vascular Surgery* 1988; **7**: 715–716.

34 Lord RSA, Raj TB, Stary DL *et al*. Comparison of saphenous vein patch, polytetrafluoroethylene patch, and direct arteriotomy closure after carotid endarterectomy. Part 1: perioperative results. *Journal of Vascular Surgery* 1989; **9**: 521–529.

35 Archie JP. Early and late geometric changes after carotid endasrterectomy patch reconstruction. *Journal of Vascular Surgery* 1991; **14**: 258–266.

36 Archie JP. Geometric dimension changes with carotid endarterectomy reconstruction. *Journal of Vascular Surgery* 1997; **25**: 488–498.

37 Jackson BL, Gupta AK, Bandyk DF *et al*. Anatomic patterns of carotid endarterectomy healing. *American Journal of Surgery* 1996; **172**: 188–190.

21.3 Editorial Comment

Both authors appropriately emphasize that the outcome of CEA is virtually always determined in the operating room by the responsible surgeon. Superior operative technique and fastidious attention to detail are of utmost importance if perioperative stroke rates are to be minimized. As Dr Archie so aptly states: 'Any surgeon who considers perioperative stroke and/or internal carotid thrombosis to be an acceptable or unpreventable complication is fooling him- or herself.' Drs Archie and London agree on several critical technical points. Adequate exposure of the carotid is essential so that the arteriotomy can be extended above the plaque and the internal carotid end-point clearly visualized. Both stress the importance of complete endarterectomy with removal of all plaque up to a fine feathered end-point with a minimal step. Neither is an advocate of eversion endarterectomy, although others have described good results with this technique. Restoration of a smooth tapered transition between the bulb and ICA is essential and facilitated by patching in most cases. Patches should be carefully tailored to avoid making the bulb region too bulbous. Kinks which result from carotid redundancy should be prevented by selective use of eversion plication or, when necessary, resection of a short length of endarterectomized internal carotid. With plication or resection, patching is always essential to insure preservation of luminal diameter and a smooth tapered transition from the bulb to the ICA

The authors differ in their practices with respect to tacking. Clearly, all carotid surgeons should be familiar with the technique of tacking the distal end-point. The frequency with which tacking sutures are placed is a matter of individual judgment. Liberal heparin saline irrigation helps to determine the adequacy of the end-point and flow surface by identifying lifting at the end-point. If the step-up seems excessive or the end-point lifts, additional strands of circumferentially oriented smooth-muscle fibers are removed until the end-point is more satisfactory or interrupted tacking sutures are placed through part or all of the circumference. Tacking is helpful when the endarterectomy cannot be extended further cephalad, but tacking is not a substitute for complete endarterectomy.

Dr London addresses the appropriate depth of the endarterectomy plane. In practice this cannot be standardized. The appropriate endarterectomy plane is that which removes all atheromatous plaque and loose circular smooth-muscle fibers. In the rare instance where excessive thinning of the wall may compromise arterial integrity, eversion plication or even vein bypass may be necessary. As the distal end-point is approached, the plane should become more superficial to achieve a

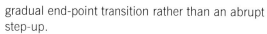

gradual end-point transition rather than an abrupt step-up.

The key to achieving the lowest perioperative stroke risk is obsessive attention to detail. This not an operation for the 'smash and grab' approach. In the European Carotid Surgery Trial, the highest operative stroke rates were noted in the shortest operations.

22.1 Should all patients be patched? If not, how should I select which patients to patch?

Hakan Parsson (Europe)

David Bergqvist (Europe)

INTRODUCTION

The randomized trials have clearly established the effectiveness of carotid endarterectomy (CEA) in the management of selected patients with carotid artery disease.[1–3] The overall results, however, might be influenced by different surgical techniques adopted during the procedure.

The postoperative risks are critically dependent upon achieving a smooth endarterectomized surface, a smooth and tapered distal end-point and precise closure. However, while there is general consensus regarding the first two aims, controversy persists regarding the optimal method for arteriotomy closure.[4]

RATIONALE FOR PATCHING

The use of a patch, as opposed to primary suture, has been suggested to improve haemodynamics whilst providing a beneficial increase in the calibre of the endarterectomized segment and particularly its most distal aspect.[5] Patch closure may also provide an increase in internal carotid bulb length and a more rounded common carotid bulb.[6] Animal study models tend to show the persistence of a mild local stenosis with non-turbulent flow as compared with patching where no flow disturbance is found.[7] Larger-sized patches may, however, be associated with a significant increase in turbulence and a transverse width of 5–10mm seems to be ideal in terms of achieving optimal flow patterns. Patch closure, intuitively, facilitates closure in small or unusually thin arteries by allowing for more accurate, safe placement of sutures without causing narrowing. If a vein patch is used, the provision of endothelialized tissue should, theoretically at least, reduce the risks of thrombosis and neointimal hyperplasia.

The main concerns regarding patch closure include prolonged carotid occlusion time and other complications directly associated with the patch material itself. The additional clamping and/or shunt time associated with patching has been estimated to be about 10min[8] but the evidence to date does not show any increased perioperative risk associated with haemodynamic failure.

EARLY POSTOPERATIVE STROKE

Several studies have reported that routine patching is associated with a decreased incidence of early carotid thrombosis and thrombotic stroke.[8–10] However, a major problem in these studies is the low overall statistical power due to:

1 small sample size;
2 the incorporation of serial rather than randomized data;
3 the small number of adverse end-points;
4 different selection criteria;
5 the use of different patch materials.

Two recent meta-analyses of the available randomized trials (Table 22.1) have demonstrated that routine primary closure is associated with a three-to fourfold excess risk of early postoperative stroke or carotid thrombosis.[11,12] However, the results of meta-analyses must still be interpreted with caution due to the varying methodology and the small number of important outcome events.[12] In particular, meaningful interpretation is frustrated by incomplete follow-up and the fact that many of the studies randomized carotid arteries rather than patients. Accordingly, because 5–10% of patients underwent bilateral procedures, some may have

Table 22.1
Summary of the findings of a meta-analysis of the randomized trials of routine patching versus primary closure

	Routine patching	Primary closure	Odds ratio of increased risk with primary closure
30-day outcomes			
Ipsilateral stroke	1.3%	3.9%	2.9 (95% CI 1.3–6.7)
All strokes	1.6%	4.2%	2.6 (95% CI 1.1–6.7)
Carotid thrombosis	0.3%	3.9%	5.9 (95% CI 2.2–17)
Long-term outcomes			
Ipsilateral stroke	1.6%	4.4%	2.6 (95% CI 1.1–6.3)
All strokes	2.2%	5.9%	2.6 (95% CI 1.2–5.9)
50–100% restenosis	4.5%	13%	3.1 (95% CI 1.9–5.3)

Adapted from Counsell *et al.*[12] with permission. CI, confidence interval.

been patched on one occasion and primarily closed on others.

All of the randomized trials have concentrated on comparing primary closure with patching. None, however, has compared selective patching with routine patch closure. Accordingly, we do not know whether patching is preferable in certain situations, such as in patients with a small-calibre internal carotid artery (ICA: < 4mm) or those with an unusually long arteriotomy. However, the results from the meta-analyses have not found any evidence to support a policy of routine primary closure.

LONG-TERM OUTCOME

Significant recurrent carotid artery stenosis (> 50%) or occlusion occurs in 0–15% of patients within 5 years of surgery.[13] However, only a minority of these patients will suffer any neurological sequelae. Accordingly, the number of patients with symptomatic restenoses requiring re-do carotid artery surgery is low compared to the incidence of restenosis. Nevertheless, the contribution of late restenosis to ipsilateral neurological events during long-term follow-up remains an important but controversial subject.

Data from the literature are conflicting with regard to the exact relationship between recurrent stenosis

and symptoms, but a severe (> 80%) restenosis seems to be associated with a higher rate (22%) of ipsilateral events.[14] Several studies have now documented that patch closure is associated with a reduced risk of restenosis and stroke.[9,10,15] The meta-analysis shows that primary closure was associated with a nearly threefold increase in the risk of late ipsilateral stroke (Table 22.1) and a threefold excess risk of a 50–100% recurrent stenosis.[12]

In addition to the role of patching, it is important to remember that other risk factors such as smoking, hypercholesterolaemia and a relatively young age (< 60 years) contribute to an increased risk of recurrent disease and the specific influence of these factors has to be addressed as well. Moreover, it is important to consider the pathological process in patients with recurrent disease; for example, is it due to deposition of thrombus secondary to localized turbulence, neointimal hyperplasia or true atherosclerosis?

It is often difficult to establish the true cause of a restenosis or occlusion unless the patient undergoes reoperation and the plaque is sent for histological examination. Generally speaking, early recurrence (within 6 months) may be due to laminated thrombus formation or neointimal hyperplasia.

Stenoses occurring between 6 and 12 months are almost exclusively due to hyperplasia, whilst recurrences after 24 months tend to be due to true atherosclerosis.

Analysis of the plaque structure by duplex occasionally shows a laminated appearance suggesting thrombus deposition. These lesions are subject to remodeling and even spontaneous regression. The difference between a stenosis due to initial perioperative failure as opposed to true recurrent disease also needs to be addressed. By definition, recurrent disease is present only if the abnormality was not detected on the immediate postoperative duplex examination.

SELECTIVE PATCHING

The concept of selective patching is based on the assumption that only certain patients really need a patch. Intuitively, these include patients with a narrow ICA or an arteriotomy that extends long into the ICA. However, several authors have noted an increased risk of restenosis in women as well as a shorter recurrence interval in this group and that patching was associated with a reduced long-term risk.[15] This difference in women has been attributed to the fact that women have a smaller average ICA diameter (4.9 ± 0.6mm) as compared with 5.3 ± 0.7mm in men.[6]

Thus, if one were to adopt a policy of selective patching on the basis of an ICA diameter ″ 5mm, approximately 50% of patients would qualify for patch repair. If the threshold were reduced to ″ 4mm, only 9% of women and 3% of men would be patched.[6]

One study has partially addressed this problem by having a protocol of compulsory patching if the ICA diameter was < 5mm or if the arteriotomy extended more than 3cm beyond the origin of the ICA.[16] The results demonstrated a similar rate of perioperative complications as compared to those patients who had an ICA of > 5mm and were randomized to closure with vein patch. Paradoxically, long-term follow-up demonstrated a lower restenosis rate in the group of patients with a < 5mm ICA and obligate patching as compared to the group with > 5mm ICA and who were randomized to vein patch!

VEIN OR PROSTHETIC?

Vein
The choice of patch material is a further controversial issue. Autologous vein confers several advantages over synthetic materials. The principal advantages of using vein include the provision of endothelialized tissue and a less thrombogenic surface.[7] In addition, vein confers greater resistance against infection. The disadvantages of using vein include the risk of early rupture, harvest site complications, aneurysmal dilatation and the fact that the vein cannot be used in the future for other reconstructions.

Central vein patch rupture is associated with a high risk of stroke or death and affects 0.5–1% of patients. Evidence suggests that saphenous vein harvested from the ankle carries a significantly higher risk of rupture when compared to vein harvested from the groin. The reason for this is probably related to the different histological structure of the vein at the two locations and the lower burst strength associated with ankle saphenous vein.[17] It is accepted, however, that other factors such as age and diabetes might also reduce the strength of the distal saphenous vein. The rupture almost always occurs within the first postoperative week and may even occur within the first 24h, which would indicate a primary defect in the wall rather than a degenerative process.

Progressive dilatation of a patch not only carries the risk of rupture but also creates the possibility of turbulent flow and subsequent deposition of thrombus material. Usually these dilatations are asymptomatic but early postoperative formation of thrombus carries the risk of embolization and encroachment on the lumen. The problem is not helped by the lack of a definition of aneurysm formation, but a diameter of the common carotid artery or the bifurcation which is more than twice its intraoperative diameter has been proposed.[8]

Other complications associated with the use of autogenous vein include those related to the harvesting of the vein. Wound-healing problems with prolonged oozing from the wound as well as skin necrosis contribute towards increased morbidity and prolonged hospital stay. This may be partly due to the increased risk of infection in groin wounds at the best of times, but if the harvesting and closure of the wound are delegated to an unsupervised junior member of the team, then increased wound complications are inevitable. In view of this, alternative sources of vein have been tried, including the facial, external and internal jugular veins, which seem to produce equivalent results to groin saphenous vein.

The final disadvantage of using groin saphenous vein is the fact that it becomes unavailable for use in peripheral vascular or cardiac reconstructions. Evidence suggests, however, that this is only applicable in about 15% of patients undergoing CEA.[18]

Prosthetic

A number of synthetic patches are now available. The advantages of prosthetic patches include immediate access, avoidance of groin wound complications and the fact that the vein is still available for other uses in the future. Many different materials have been evaluated but only Dacron and expanded polytetrafluoroethylene (ePTFE) have gained widespread use. The early Dacron patches were rather thick and often required pre-clotting, but the newer, thinner patches with either collagen or fluoroethylene impregnation have been a major advance.[19,20]

The principal alternative to Dacron is ePTFE. PTFE patches are thin and flexible but they are prone to suture hole bleeding. However, the use of sutures with a needle versus suture ratio of 1:1, topical haemostatic agents and careful intraoperative monitoring of heparin anticoagulation should reduce this in the future.

The main concerns with the use of prosthetic patches are the risk of infection and enhanced thrombosis. Prosthetic patch infection affects 1% of patients and is a catastrophic complication. The diagnosis and management of this condition are detailed elsewhere in this text.

Enhanced thrombogenicity is the second area of concern amongst surgeons. There is a perception that prosthetic patches are more thrombogenic than vein patches, although the meta-analyses do not support this.[12] Similarly, while experimental studies have demonstrated that ePTFE has a lower thrombogenicity when compared to Dacron, this has not been borne out in clinical practice.[11]

Despite these reservations, results from studies comparing synthetic versus vein patches suggest no major difference in either early or late outcome. In particular, the meta-analyses show no evidence that the risk of vein rupture exceeds the risk of prosthetic patch infection or that restenosis (symptomatic or asymptomatic) is related to the choice of patch material.[12]

CONCLUSIONS

Although accurate interpretation of the meta-analyses is confounded by certain well-recognized methodological problems, evidence suggests that early and late stroke and restenosis rates are probably higher in patients whose arteriotomies are closed primarily. Thus, overall, there appears to be more evidence supporting a policy of selective or routine patching as opposed to routine primary closure. No randomized trial data are available to indicate whether a policy of selective patching is preferable to routine patching. There is no evidence to suggest that the type of patch (vein or prosthetic) alters early and long-term outcomes. In particular, the incidence of vein patch rupture is about the same as the incidence of prosthetic patch infection.

REFERENCES

1 North American Symptomatic Carotid Endarterectomy Trial Collaborators. Beneficial effect of carotid endarterectomy in symptomatic patients with high-grade carotid stenosis. *New England Journal of Medicine* 1991; **325**: 445–453.
2 European Carotid Surgery Trialists' Collaborative Group. MRC European Carotid Surgery Trial: interim results. *Lancet* 1991; **337**: 1235–1243.
3 European Carotid Surgery Trialists' Collaborative Group. Randomized trial of endarterectomy for recently symptomatic carotid stenosis: final results of the MRC European Carotid Surgery Trial (ECST). *Lancet* 1998; **351**: 1379–1387.
4 Murie JA, John TG, Morris PJ. Carotid endarterectomy in Great Britain and Ireland: practice between 1984

and 1992. *British Journal of Surgery* 1994; **81**: 827–831.

5 Imparato AM, Baumann FG. Consequences of hemodynamic alterations on the vessel wall after revascularization. In: Bernhard VM, Towne JB (eds) *Complications in Vascular Surgery*, pp. 107–131. New York: Grune and Stratton, 1980.

6 Archie JP. Geometric dimension changes with carotid endarterectomy reconstruction. *Journal of Vascular Surgery* 1997; **25**: 488–498.

7 Fietsan B, Ranval T, Conn S *et al*. Hemodynamic effect of primary closure versus patch angioplasty of the carotid artery. *Annals of Vascular Surgery* 1992; **6**: 443–449.

8 Lord RSA, Raj B, Stary DL *et al*. Comparison of saphenous vein patch, polytetrafluoroethylene patch and direct arteriotomy closure after carotid endarterectomy. Part I. Perioperative results. *Journal of Vascular Surgery* 1989; **9**: 5210–5219.

9 Ranaboldo CJ, Barros D'Sa ABB, Bell PRF *et al*. Randomized controlled trial of patch angioplasty for carotid endarterectomy. *British Journal of Surgery* 1993; **80**: 1528–1530.

10 AbuRhama AF, Robinson PA, Saiedy S *et al*. Prospective randomized trial of carotid endarterectomy with primary closure and patch angioplasty with saphenous vein, jugular vein and polytetrafluoroethylene: long term follow-up. *Journal of Vascular Surgery* 1998; **27**: 222–234.

11 Archie JP. Patching with carotid endarterectomy: when to do it and what to use. *Seminars in Vascular Surgery* 1998; **11**: 24–29.

12 Counsell CE, Salinas R, Naylor R, Warlow CP. A systematic review of the randomised trials of carotid patch angioplasty in carotid endarterectomy. *European Journal of Endovascular Surgery* 1997; **13**: 345–354.

13 Ricotta JJ, O'Brien MS, DeWeese JA. Natural history of recurrent and residual stenosis after carotid endarterectomy: implications for postoperative surveillance and surgical management. *Surgery* 1992; **112**: 656–663.

14 Toursarkissian B, Rubin BG. Recurrent carotid artery stenosis. *Journal of the American College of Surgeons* 1997; **184**: 93–98.

15 Eickelboom BC, Ackerstaff RGA, Hoeneveld H *et al*. Benefits of carotid patching: a randomized study. *Journal of Vascular Surgery* 1988; **7**: 240–247.

16 Clagett PG, Paterson CB, Fisher DF *et al*. Vein patch versus primary closure for carotid endarterectomy. *Journal of Vascular Surgery* 1989; **9**: 213–223.

17 Archie JP, Green JJ. Saphenous vein rupture pressure, rupture stress and carotid endarterectomy vein patch reconstruction. *Surgery* 1990; **107**: 389–396.

18 De Vries AC, Riles TS, Lamparello PJ *et al*. Should proximal saphenous vein be used for carotid patch angioplasty? *European Journal of Vascular Surgery* 1990; **4**: 301–304.

19 Rhee RY, Gloviczki P, Cambria RA, Miller VM. Experimental evaluation of bleeding complications, thrombogenicity and neointimal characteristics of prosthetic patch materials used for carotid angioplasty. *Cardiovascular Surgery* 1996; **4**: 746–752.

20 Hirt SW, Aoki M, Demertzis S *et al*. Comparative in vivo study on the healing qualities of four different presealed vascular prostheses. *Journal of Vascular Surgery* 1993; **17**: 538–545.

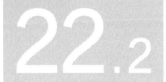

Should all patients be patched? If not, how should I select which patients to patch?
Hugh A Gelabert (USA)

INTRODUCTION
The publication of the Asymptomatic Carotid Atherosclerosis Study ACAS trial[21] marks the completion of a remarkable period of prospective randomized study of CEA. Several large multicenter studies have scientifically validated the benefit of endarterectomy[22–25] in both symptomatic and asymptomatic patients. These studies have demonstrated conclusively that CEA reduces the risk of stroke in the years following the procedure. Following the completion of these trials, awareness of the significance of safety and durability has spurred interest in technical issues such as the utility of carotid patch angioplasty closure of the endarterectomy site.

Recurrent stenosis is a significant problem reducing the long-term benefit of CEA. Recurrent stenosis is believed to increase the risk of TIA and stroke in the late postoperative period. While proponents of patch closure hold that routine application of patch angioplasty to CEA will reduce the incidence of restenosis and, by extension, the number of postoperative neurologic events, the benefit of patch closure is widely debated.

Primary closure of a carotid arteriotomy is the technique in which a single suture line is used to approximate the adjacent walls of the artery following completion of the endarterectomy. This has long been the standard approach to carotid repair. It has the advantages of simplicity, ease, and rapidity, and does not expose the patient to the potential complications of patch closure. Patch angioplasty is the technique where closure of the arterial defect is augmented by the inclusion of a patch. The patch may consist of either autogenous vein or synthetic material (usually either Dacron or PTFE).

The self-evident rationale for patch closure is to avoid narrowing the arterial lumen in the course of arteriotomy closure. Should the arterial lumen be inadvertently narrowed, several significant problems may arise. In the early postoperative period, embolic events or even arterial thrombosis may result in stroke. In the later postoperative period, the narrowed closure may be identified as a residual stenosis and may predispose to the development of a significant postoperative stenosis, possibly resulting in the need for reoperation.

RECURRENT STENOSIS: INCIDENCE AND RISK FACTORS
The incidence of recurrent stenosis has been reported to be between 2% and 31%, though reports in recent years suggest it to be between 2% and 7.0%[26,27] (Table 22.2). The rate of reoperation for recurrent stenosis is reported to be from 0 to 4%. Several factors account for these discrepancies. There is a lack of consensus as to what exactly is a recurrent stenosis. Some authors will consider any evidence of a lesion, such as an abnormal B-mode image, sufficient to diagnose recurrent stenosis. Others consider any lesion causing more than 30% reduction of lumen diameter a recurrent stenosis.[28,29] The most common criterion is a lesion with hemodynamic impact – one causing more than 50% reduction of the arterial lumen. Yet another criterion exists for defining a recurrent stenosis: lumen reduction greater than 80%.[30] This standard has been adopted by those who argue that lesser stenoses do not pose significant risk and are not preocclusive.

Another significant problem in assessing the true incidence of restenosis is the lack of distinction

Table 22.2
Reported late complications of recurrent stenosis

Author	Year	Number of cases	Recurrent stenosis (%)	Late Occlusion	Symptoms CVA	TIA
Nicholls et al.[36]	1985	145		1	1	
Hertzer et al.[29]	1987	917	31	4		
Sanders et al.[31]	1987	109	8	1		
Eikelboom et al.[37]	1988	129	11	3		
Healey	1989	301	21	2	1	
Clagett et al.[28]	1989	152	12.9	11	4	
Salenius et al.[38]	1989	257	13	5		
Reilly et al.[34]	1990	131	18	8		
Mattes et al.[51]	1993	409	10.8	7	1	1
Hansen	1993	232	9.2	4		
Myers	1993	163	9.8	0		
Gelabert	1994	268	11	0		
De Letter et al.[27]	1994	129	27	0		
Katz et al.[56]	1994	100	3.9	0		

CVA, cerebrovascular accident; TIA, transient ischemic attack.

between residual lesions and recurrent stenoses in many reports. This distinction can only be made when intraoperative or early postoperative studies are performed to insure the adequacy of the endarterectomy. Sanders and associates[31] noted that half of the post-endarterectomy stenoses identified at 12 months were residual lesions. Ricotta et al.[30] reported that half of the severe (> 80%) recurrent lesions identified in their study were in fact residual lesions which had progressed. Bandyk et al.[32] observed the impact of residual stenosis on the outcome of CEA. Patients with no residual lesions had a 9% incidence of recurrent stenosis 24 months after operation, while those who demonstrated hemodynamic evidence of a residual defect had a 21% incidence of restenosis at 24 months after surgery. Sawchuck et al.[33] noted that not all residual lesions result in recurrent stenosis. Reilly et al.[34] noted that the presence of residual defects increased the risk of recurrent stenosis.

In addition to the local factors described above, several systemic factors influence the risk for restenosis. Gender has been considered one of the strongest risk factors for recurrent stenosis. Clagett et al.[28,35] noted that recurrent stenosis occurred more frequently in women. Similar findings were recorded by Nicholls and colleagues.[36] Eikelboom and associates[37] observed recurrent stenosis in 55% of women who underwent primary closure, whereas it occurred in only 11% of men treated in the same manner. On the other hand, Salenius and colleagues[38] noted that restenosis occurred in 16% of men and only 8% of women.

Diabetes and smoking have been considered significant risk factors predisposing to the development of recurrent stenosis.[28,35] Diabetes was the only risk factor associated with an increased risk of restenosis in the group reported by Atnip and colleagues.[39] The study consisted of 184 consecutive endarterectomies over a period of 5 years. During this time recurrent stenosis was observed in 11 arteries. The only statistically significant risk factor for recurrence among their patients was the presence of diabetes. Lipid abnormalities have also been implicated in recurrent stenosis by two groups. Salenius *et al.*[38] observed a statistically significant decrease in the occurrence of restenosis in patients with high levels of high-density lipoproteins, low cholesterol, and low triglycerides. Those whose high-density lipoprotein was low, and whose cholesterol and triglycerides were high, appeared to be at increased risk of restenosis. Reilly *et al.*[34] also observed a detrimental effect of elevated cholesterol.

PRIMARY CLOSURE vs PATCH CLOSURE

The principal advantage of primary arterial closure is simplicity. This in turn yields secondary benefits such as shortened surgical time, lower potential for infectious complications, and elimination of aneurysmal complications following endarterectomy. Since the primary closure requires one suture line, this closure of the arteriotomy is accomplished in about half the time required to complete a patch closure. By shortening the duration of surgery, the patient is exposed to less anesthesia. A shorter operation reduces the potential for wound contamination. The potential for wound sepsis is further reduced by avoidance of a foreign body within the wound.

Primary closure may itself give rise to several problems if done incorrectly or in poorly selected patients. Primary closure of a small artery will result in a stenosis. This predisposes to thrombosis and postoperative stroke. Use of primary closure in patients who may be considered at increased risk of carotid restenosis may result in an increased incidence of intimal hyperplasia and increased risk of late occlusion or stroke. Of particular concern would be patients with small arteries and patients whose risk factors include cigarette smoking, diabetes, and/or hyperlipidemia.

Advocates of routine patch closure note several benefits of this technique. The use of a patch closure allows for a greater margin of error in the suturing of the endarterectomized arterial wall. Difficulties with the endarterectomy end-point may be partially corrected by use of a patch. Small arteries will be less likely to be narrowed in the course of repair. Thus, the incidence of early postoperative complications such as TIA, stroke, arterial occlusion,

and embolization might be reduced. Proponents of routine patch closure also hold that recurrent stenosis should be reduced. This, in turn, leads to a reduction in late occlusions, late neurological events, and late reoperations for significant restenosis.

Routine patch closure does present problems which may detract from its proposed benefits. Large patches inappropriately tailored to the artery may result in an iatrogenic pseudoaneurysm.[40] This in turn may predispose to complications which attend a pseudoaneurysm: expansion, thrombus within the arterial lumen, embolization, and stroke. Ultimately, arterial expansion may lead to disruption of the arterial wall.[41–49] A second concern with patch closure is the incidence of prosthetic graft infection[50] (Fig. 22.1). While rare, prosthetic patch infection carries a significant risk and obligates a second operation for removal of the infected prosthesis and reconstruction with autologous tissue. For a complete discussion of the management of the infected prosthetic patch, see Chapter 30.

Economic analysis of routine patch closure calls into question its cost-effectiveness.[51] In calculating the added expense associated with a patch closure, several elements must be considered: the cost of the

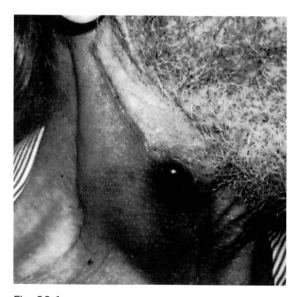

Fig. 22.1
Wound abscess in a patient who underwent carotid endarterectomy with prosthetic patching.

Table 22.3
Patch angioplasty compared to primary closure in non-randomized studies with more than 1-year follow-up

Author	Year	n	Mean follow-up (months)	Restenosis (%) No patch	Patch	Significant difference
Archie[40]	1987	200	15	5	0	Yes
Hertzer et al.[29]	1987	917	21	31	9	Yes
Katz et al.[53]	1987	89	24	19	2.4	Yes
Rosenthal et al.[54]	1990	1000	33	4	4	No
Moore et al.[55]	1998	720	31	16	4.6	Yes

patch, the cost of the longer operative time required for patch closure, the cost of antibiotic coverage, and, in the case of saphenous vein patches, the cost of procuring the patch and closing the wounds. While each of these elements is relatively small, on an aggregate scale they would represent a significant addition to the cost of care.

Several large studies have compared the results of patch angioplasty and primary closure with regard to postoperative neurological events as well as the incidence of restenosis (Table 22.3). In a series of 200 consecutive patients, Archie[52] noted four recurrent stenoses and one occlusion in patients who underwent primary closure. This contrasted with no such events in the patch closure group. Katz et al.[53] reported a series of 47 primary closures and 42 patch closures following CEA. The primary closure group developed restenosis in 19% of closures and the patched group developed restenosis in 2.4%.

Hertzer et al.[29] compared patch closure with primary closure in a series of 917 endarterectomies performed at Cleveland Clinic between 1983 and 1985. An increased incidence of perioperative carotid occlusion was observed in the primary closure group (total of 15 events), while the patch group suffered only two such events.

In 1990, Rosenthal et al.[54] reviewed 1000 consecutive endarterectomies and compared four groups: primary closure, PTFE patch closure, Dacron patch closure, and vein patch closure. The incidence of early postoperative neurological events was similar in all groups. Furthermore, they discovered no significant difference in the incidence of restenosis between any groups. They concluded that the method of carotid closure did not appear to affect the occurrence of ipsilateral stroke or restenosis.

A recent review of data collected for the ACAS trial by Moore et al. noted that recurrent carotid stenosis occurred with greater frequency in those without patch closure.[55] The authors noted that the cumulative rates of recurrent stenosis were 16.9% for primary closure and 4.5% for patch closure of the endarterectomy. Since some hyperplastic lesions will regress over time, the incidence of recurrence was 2.8% for primary closure and 0.6% for patch closure after 18 months.

PROSPECTIVE RANDOMIZED STUDIES

A survey of the English literature indicates that there are 10 prospective randomized studies which deal with the question of recurrent carotid stenosis. Of these, one compares two different patches, one is a pharmacologic study, one reports immediate postoperative results, and three report results with only 1 year of follow-up data. Given the natural history of recurrent stenosis, it is clear that a longer follow-up period is required. Thus, four prospective randomized studies comparing patch closure with primary closure are available for evaluation (Table 22.4).

Clagett et al.[28] randomized patients between vein patch angioplasty and primary closure. Recurrent stenosis was defined as any evident lesion, including those causing < 50% diameter reduction. Recurrent lesions were identified in 1.7% of the primary closure group and 12.9% of the vein patch group. Most of the recurrent lesions resulted in less than 30% stenosis. The authors also noted that patch

Table 22.4
Prospective randomized studies of impact of surgical technique on carotid restenosis: primary closure vs patch closure

Author	Year	n	Mean follow-up (months)	Primary (%)	Patch (%)	Significance (P)
Clagett et al.[28]	1989	152	22	1.7	12.9	<0.01
De Letter et al.[27]	1994	129	60	27	12	<0.01
Myers et al.[57]	1994	163	59	7.8	14.3	NS
Katz et al.[56]	1994	100	36	3.9	0	NS

closure resulted in a significant increase in the operative time and did not result in a reduction of perioperative or late postoperative neurological events.

De Letter et al.[27] divided 129 endarterectomies into two groups: saphenous vein patch closure and primary closure. The immediate postoperative stroke and death rate was similar in the two groups (6.4% primary closure, 4.5% patch closure). Long-term follow-up (5 years) indicated a 27% incidence of recurrent stenosis (> 50%) in the primary closure group and 12% in the patch group. Subgroup analysis among the women in the study revealed a dramatic difference between the primary closure group and the patch group (70% vs 5.5%). No such difference was noted in the men. Unfortunately, the authors were not able to explain the reason for the dramatic incidence of restenosis among the women undergoing primary closure.

The last two prospective randomized studies appeared in 1994. Katz et al.[56] reported 100 patients followed closely with serial duplex scans over a 36-month follow-up period. The authors noted no significant differences between the groups with respect to perioperative neurological events (4% primary vs 2% patch), or recurrent stenosis (4% primary vs 0 patch). One patient required reoperation for infection of a PTFE patch. The authors concluded that both primary closure and patch closure result in acceptably low rates of restenosis.

Myers et al.[57] reported a series of 163 endarterectomies randomized over a 46-month period. Early postoperative results recorded three strokes: one in the primary closure group, and two in the obligatory vein patch group. On long-term follow-up recurrent stenoses were identified: primary closure

7.8%, vein patch 14.3%. The authors concluded that the use of vein patch did not yield a superior result and had no impact on the durability of CEA.

When examined as a group, the prospective randomized studies do not support the routine use of patch angioplasty in CEA. While there may be some reason to use patch angioplasty in selected groups of high-risk patients, there appears to be no rationale for routine patch closure. Careful attention to detail in performing the endarterectomy and primary closure appear to be as effective as patch closure in both perioperative and long-term results.

CONCLUSIONS

Primary closure of CEA is a safe and simple technique which economizes in time and resources. Of particular importance is the appropriate application of this technique. When used properly it is not associated with an increase in occlusion, stroke, or recurrent stenosis. It further avoids the potential complications associated with patch closure: infection, aneurysm, embolization, and arterial disruption.

Patch angioplasty closure of a CEA is advised in selected instances. Patients who are at an increased risk of developing hemodynamically significant problems with primary closure should undergo patch angioplasty. Thus, patients with very small arteries (<0.5cm) or those whose arterial closure appears to compromise the carotid lumen may merit patch angioplasty. Use of patch angioplasty for patients with risk factors known to be associated with an increased risk for restenosis, such as female gender, smoking, hyperlipidemia, and diabetes, seems to be reasonable. Stronger data are needed before routine patch closure should be generally accepted.

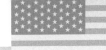

REFERENCES

21 Asymptomatic Carotid Atherosclerosis Study Group. Endarterectomy for asymptomatic carotid artery stenosis. *Journal of the American Medical Association* 1995; **273**: 1421–1427.

22 CASANOVA Study Group. Carotid surgery versus medical therapy in asymptomatic carotid stenosis. *Stroke* 1991; **22**: 1229–1235.

23 NASCET Collaborators. Beneficial effect of carotid endarterectomy in symptomatic patients with high grade carotid stenosis. *New England Journal of Medicine* 1991; **325**: 445–453.

24 Mayberg MR, Wilson SE, Yatsu F *et al*. Carotid endarterectomy and prevention of cerebral ischemia in symptomatic carotid stenosis. *Journal of the American Medical Association* 1991; **266**: 3289–3294.

25 Hobson R, Weiss D, Fields W *et al*. Efficacy of carotid endarterectomy for asymptomatic carotid stenosis. *New England Journal of Medicine* 1993; **328**: 221–227.

26 Das M, Hertzer N, Ratliff N, O'Hara P, Beven E. Recurrent stenosis. A five year series of 65 reoperations. *Annals of Surgery* 1985; **202**: 28–35.

27 De Letter JA, Moll FL, Welten RJ *et al*. Benefits of carotid patching: a prospective randomized study with long-term follow-up. *Annals of Vascular Surgery* 1994; **8**: 54–58.

28 Clagett GP, Patterson CB, Fisher D Jr *et al*. Vein patch versus primary closure for carotid endarterectomy. A randomized prospective study in a selected group of patients. *Journal of Vascular Surgery* 1989; **9**: 213–223.

29 Hertzer NR, Beven EG, O'Hara PJ, Krajewski LP. A prospective study of vein patch angioplasty during carotid endarterectomy. Three-year results for 801 patients and 917 operations. *Annals of Surgery* 1987; **206**: 628–635.

30 Ricotta J, O'Brien M, DeWeese J. Natural history of recurrent and residual stenosis after carotid endarterectomy: implications for postoperative surveillance and surgical management. *Surgery* 1992; **112**: 656–663.

31 Sanders EA, Hoeneveld H, Eikelboom BC, Ludwig JW, Vermeulen FE, Ackerstaff RG. Residual lesions and early recurrent stenosis after carotid endarterectomy. A serial follow-up study with duplex scanning and intravenous digital subtraction angiography. *Journal of Vascular Surgery* 1987; **5**: 731–737.

32 Bandyk D, Kabenick H, Adams M, Towne J. Turbulence occurring after carotid bifurcation endarterectomy: a harbinger of residual and recurrent carotid stenosis. *Journal of Vascular Surgery* 1988; **7**: 261–274.

33 Sawchuck A, Flanigan D, Machi J, Schuler J, Siegel B. The fate of unrepaired minor technical defects detected by intraoperative ultrasonography during carotid endarterectomy. *Journal of Vascular Surgery* 1989; **9**: 671–676.

34 Reilly LM, Okuhn SP, Rapp JH *et al*. Recurrent carotid stenosis: a consequence of local or systemic factors? The influence of unrepaired technical defects. *Journal of Vascular Surgery* 1990; **11**: 448–459.

35 Clagett G, Rich N, McDonald P *et al*. Etiologic factors for recurrent carotid artery stenosis. *Surgery* 1983; **93**: 313–318.

36 Nicholls S, Phillips D, Bergelin R, Beach K, Primozich J, Strandness D. Carotid endarterectomy. Relationship of outcome to early restenosis. *Journal of Vascular Surgery* 1985; **2**: 375–381.

37 Eikelboom BC, Ackerstaff RG, Hoeneveld H *et al*. Benefits of carotid patching: a randomized study. *Journal of Vascular Surgery* 1988; **7**: 240–247.

38 Salenius JP, Haapanen A, Harju E, Jokela H, Riekkinen H. Late carotid restenosis: aetiologic factors for recurrent carotid artery stenosis during long-term follow-up. *European Journal of Vascular Surgery* 1989; **3**: 271–277.

39 Atnip RG, Wenrovitz M, Gifford RR, Neumyer MM, Thiele BL. A rational approach to recurrent carotid stenosis. *Journal of Vascular Surgery* 1990; **11**: 511–516.

40 Archie J. The geometry and mechanics of saphenous vein patch angioplasty after carotid endarterectomy. *Texas Heart Journal* 1987; **14**: 395–400.

41 Archie J, Green J. Saphenous vein rupture pressure, rupture stress, and carotid endarterectomy vein patch reconstruction. *Surgery* 1990; **107**: 89–96.

42 Donovan D, Schmidt S, Townshend S, Njus G, Sharp W. Material and structural characterization of human saphenous vein. *Journal of Vascular Surgery* 1990; **112**: 531–537.

43 Smith JW. Delayed postoperative bleeding from polytetrafluoroethylene carotid artery patches. *Journal of Vascular Surgery* 1992; **16**: 663.

44 Riles TS, Lamparello PJ, Giangola G, Imparato AM. Rupture of the vein patch: a rare complication of carotid endarterectomy. *Surgery* 1990; **107**: 10–20.

45 O'Hara PJ, Hertzer NR, Krajewski LP, Beven EG. Saphenous vein patch rupture after carotid endarterectomy. *Journal of Vascular Surgery* 1992; **15**: 504–509.

46 Scott EW, Dolson L, Day AL, Seeger JM. Carotid endarterectomy complicated by vein patch rupture. *Neurosurgery* 1992; **31**: 373–376.

47 Spetzler RF. Carotid endarterectomy complicated by vein patch rupture. *Neurosurgery* 1993; **32**: 151–152.

48 Tawes R Jr, Treiman RL. Vein patch rupture after carotid endarterectomy: a survey of the Western Vascular Society members. *Annals of Vascular Surgery* 1991; **5**: 71–73.

49 Van Damme H, Grenade T, Creemers E, Limet R. Blowout of carotid venous patch angioplasty. *Annals of Vascular Surgery* 1991; **5**: 542–545.

50 Motte S, Wautrecht JC, Bellens B, Vincent G, Dereume JP, Delcour C. Infected false aneurysm following carotid endarterectomy with vein patch angioplasty. *Journal of Cardiovascular Surgery* 1987; **28**: 734–736.

51 Mattes M, van Bemmelen P, Barkmeire L, Hodgson K, Ramsey D, Sumner D. Routine surveillance after carotid endarterectomy: does it affect clinical management? *Journal of Vascular Surgery* 1993; **17**: 819–831.

52 Archie J Jr. Prevention of early restenosis and thrombosis-occlusion after carotid endarterectomy by saphenous vein patch angioplasty. *Stroke* 1986; **17**: 901–905.

53 Katz MM, Jones GT, Degenhardt J, Gunn B, Wilson J, Katz S. The use of patch angioplasty to alter the incidence of carotid restenosis following thromboendarterectomy. *Journal of Cardiovascular Surgery* 1987; **28**: 2–8.

54 Rosenthal D, Archie J Jr, Garcia-Rinaldi R *et al*. Carotid

patch angioplasty: immediate and long-term results. *Journal of Vascular Surgery* 1990; **12**: 326–333.

55 Moore W, Kempczenski R, Nelson J, Toole J. Recurrent carotid stenosis. *Stroke* 1998; **29**: 2018–2025.

56 Katz D, Snyder SO, Gandhi RH *et al*. Long-term follow-up for recurrent stenosis: a prospective randomized study of expanded polytetrafluoroethylene patch angioplasty versus primary closure after carotid endarterectomy. *Journal of Vascular Surgery* 1994; **19**: 198–203.

57 Myers SI, Valentine RJ, Chervu A, Bowers BL, Clagett GP. Saphenous vein patch versus primary closure for carotid endarterectomy: long-term assessment of a randomized prospective study. *Journal of Vascular Surgery* 1994; **19**: 15–22.

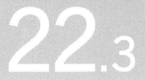

22.₃ Editorial Comment

KEY POINTS

1 Meta-analyses suggest that a policy of routine patching is preferable to routine primary closure.
2 There have been no randomized trials comparing routine with selective patching.
3 There is no evidence that either vein or prosthetic patches are superior.
4 The risk of vein patch rupture is similar to the risk of prosthetic patch infection.

The role of patching has been one of the most enduring controversies in carotid surgery. Surgeons usually fall into three camps, advocating routine patching, selective patching, or routine primary closure. Excellent results have been published by each group.

There have been a number of randomized trials to address this issue. Although accurate interpretation of the subsequent meta-analyses is potentially confounded by certain methodological problems (method of randomization, losses to follow-up, bilateral procedures), the available evidence suggests that routine primary closure is associated with a threefold increase in stroke or thrombosis within 30 days of surgery and a threefold risk of stroke or recurrent stenosis long-term. However, because of the relatively low number of end-points and the methodological problems highlighted above, to the purists the results may not be considered statistically robust. The latter conclusion is based on the highly improbable scenario that, if all patched patients lost to follow-up or duplex assessment are assumed to have suffered a stroke or occlusion, whilst all primarily closed patients who are lost to follow-up are not, then all statistical benefit favoring patching is lost. This seems a rather extreme method of interpretation. In practice, there appears to be more evidence supporting a policy of selective or routine patching as opposed to routine primary closure – an observation also borne out in the long-term follow-up data from ACAS.

For those who prefer to adopt a policy of selective patching, the available evidence suggests that patching is preferentially indicated in: first, those patients with an internal carotid artery diameter < 5mm; second, females; and third, those situations where the arteriotomy extends > 2cm beyond the carotid bifurcation.

There is no evidence, to date, that either vein or prosthetic patches are superior. The advantages of vein include ease of insertion, the presence of endothelial cells, and resistance to infection. The principal disadvantages include rupture (hence the need to harvest the saphenous vein in the groin), groin wound complications, and using up a valuable source of vein for the future. The advantages of prosthetic patches include instant availability and preservation of vein for further use while the principal disadvantage is the risk of infection. In practice, the incidence and associated morbidity/mortality risk of vein patch rupture are about the same as those of prosthetic patch infection.

When should I abandon a planned endarterectomy?

Nicholas JM London (Europe)

INTRODUCTION

The simple answer to the question posed in this title is, rarely. Although the frequent abandonment of a carotid endarterectomy (CEA) implies inadequate patient assessment, it is important that the occasional decision to abandon a planned endarterectomy is not perceived as a failure. The surgeon should, therefore, always carefully assess the risk/benefit ratio in any one particular situation and ensure that surgical machismo does not get the better of common sense!

The following discussion is based on the not unreasonable assumption that most patients in the surgeon's practice undergo colour duplex scanning as the principal preoperative imaging technique, that the procedure is performed under general anaesthesia, that transcranial Doppler (TCD) is used to monitor middle cerebral artery (MCA) blood flow velocity intraoperatively and that the surgeon routinely inserts a carotid shunt. It is accepted that in many situations there are no evidence-based data to support some of these strategies, but in order to focus the discussion on the subject in question, it is necessary to make certain assumptions concerning the nature of the operative procedure.

WHEN MIGHT I HAVE TO ABANDON THE PROCEDURE?

Broadly speaking, there are five occasions when a surgeon may need to consider abandoning a CEA:

1   The disease process in the internal carotid artery (ICA) may extend unexpectedly high/low.
2   There may be an unsuspected hypoplastic ICA instead of an underfilled but patent ICA.
3   There may be uncontrollable bleeding.
4   The patient may have a 'hostile neck'.
5   The anaesthetist may decide that it is not safe to continue because of anaesthetic problems.

This last instance is an anaesthetic decision that will not be discussed further.

With respect to the 'hostile neck', the surgeon should first have discussed the concept of a trial dissection with the patient preoperatively and if at operation the carotid artery is firmly adherent to adjacent structures, then the operation may have to be abandoned. It is only in the context of a hostile neck that the properly trained carotid surgeon should encounter uncontrollable bleeding. In day-to-day carotid practice, it is the first two scenarios – disease extending unexpectedly high/low or an unsuspected hypoplastic ICA – that may ultimately lead to a decision to abandon the procedure.

PREOPERATIVE IMAGING

All patients for CEA should have a repeat carotid duplex scan in the 24h preceding the operation. This is because a small number of patients will suffer an asymptomatic ICA occlusion whilst awaiting surgery and, of course, these patients do not then require CEA. It is therefore vitally important that the surgeon establishes a good working relationship with the technologists who perform the duplex scans on his or her patients. In particular, they should be asked to warn the surgeon if they think that the carotid bifurcation is very high, if they cannot see the upper border of the disease process in the ICA, or if the disease process in the common carotid artery (CCA) extends particularly low. Additionally, the vascular technologist should warn the surgeon if it is thought that the ICA is very small or if there is a subtotal occlusion.

If the proximal or distal extent of the disease process cannot be delineated or if the CCA waveform is damped, then this is an indication for preoperative carotid arteriography. In our own experience of 494 CEAs performed between 1992 and 1996 with colour duplex as the primary imaging procedure and arteriograms performed selectively using the above criteria,[1] arteriograms were required on only 13 (2.6%) occasions in order to define the extent of proximal or distal disease.

DISTAL CAROTID DISEASE EXTENSION

Despite the preoperative work-up, the surgeon will occasionally encounter unexpected distal disease extension, usually in the form of a posterior tongue of plaque. There are a number of operative manoeuvres that can help to deal with disease extending high up in the ICA and these have been highlighted elsewhere. However, as a matter of routine, the surgeon should gently palpate the ICA prior to clamping the vessels and performing an arteriotomy. If the upper extent of the disease cannot be felt, then ICA exposure should continue higher up into the neck. If at this point the carotid artery is still diseased, then at least the carotid artery has not been clamped and opened and the surgeon still has the option of abandoning the endarterectomy if necessary.

It is at this stage that the surgeon has to decide whether to continue or not. This decision is, essentially, a risk/benefit ratio analysis in much the same way as the original decision to operate. The difference now is that the risk of the operation is considerably higher than had been originally discussed with the patient! The surgeon must, therefore, carefully consider the indication for surgery.

If the carotid lesion was asymptomatic and the patient has a patent contralateral ICA, then the procedure should probably be abandoned. Although the Asymptomatic Carotid Atherosclerosis Study (ACAS) showed that CEA conferred a 5% absolute risk reduction over best medical therapy alone,[2] this trial did not routinely include patients with disease extending very high. Moreover, as the risk reduction

was only 1% per annum and did not prevent disabling stroke, discretion may occasionally be the better part of valour!

If, however, the ipsilateral lesion was asymptomatic, and the contralateral carotid was occluded, then the surgeon should try to predict the effect of ipsilateral ICA occlusion on cerebral perfusion. This can be done by sequentially clamping or compressing the ICA and external carotid artery (ECA) and observing the changes on TCD. If the MCA velocities did not change significantly (< 50% fall in velocity or a mean clamp velocity > 20cm/s) I would abandon the procedure and subsequently warfarinize the patient.

However, if there was no significant change in MCA velocity with ICA clamping but there was a fall when the ECA was clamped, this would suggest that the ECA was an important source of collateral flow to the brain. In that situation, I would leave the ICA alone but endarterectomize and/or patch the ECA as appropriate and thereafter warfarinize the patient.

If, however, compression of the ipsilateral ICA caused a significant drop in MCA velocity I would once again confirm that I could not expose the distal extent of the ICA disease process. If this proved to be the case, and in the light of recent reports concerning the lack of compelling evidence for CEA in asymptomatic patients,[3] I would abandon the procedure and subsequently warfarinize the patient. As the artery has not, as yet, been opened this decision is much easier to make.

The principles underlying the decision-making process in the symptomatic patient are essentially the same as described above for the asymptomatic patient. The difference, of course, is that the risks of abandoning the procedure are much higher. This again reinforces the importance of knowing preoperatively whether the surgeon is likely to encounter distal disease.

If faced with disease going right up to the skull base and if, despite all manoeuvres to improve access, it is not possible to get above it then the surgeon has no choice but to abandon the procedure. If it is thought possible to perform an endarterectomy, but at an increased risk, the surgeon must again balance this increased risk against the risk of abandoning the procedure. My own view is that if the patient's only symptoms were amaurosis fugax or if the patient has had a single transient ischaemic attack (TIA) or has been symptom-free for 6 months then I would be inclined to abandon the procedure.[4] However, if the patient had frequent or crescendo TIAs then I would have to proceed with the endarterectomy.

PROXIMAL CAROTID DISEASE EXTENSION

Preoperative duplex scanning should have identified any areas in the CCA that were causing a significant narrowing (damped inflow signal or a peak velocity ratio increase of > 2.0 across a stenosis). Thus, generally speaking, if the preoperative duplex scan has not shown a significant narrowing in the CCA and yet at operation it seems rather diseased, I would not continue the endarterectomy down the CCA, but instead finish the endarterectomy and patch in the normal way. However, if I was seriously concerned that the duplex might be incorrect and that the CCA might contain significant disease extending down towards the aortic arch, I would test the CCA inflow by releasing the CCA clamp momentarily. If the flow appeared abnormally low I would organize an intraoperative arteriogram. If arteriography shows significant inflow disease, the treatment will depend on its anatomical distribution. In general terms, localized stenoses of the CCA or innominate artery can be dealt with by intraoperative retrograde balloon angioplasty.[5] Diffuse disease of the CCA/innominate artery will require some form of bypass (e.g. subclavian-carotid or carotico-carotid). In practice, the surgeon should never encounter problems such as these if the preoperative evaluation has been done properly.

In the rare patient in whom it is necessary to dissect quite far proximally down the CCA, the surgeon should remain aware that, if the shunt accidentally slips out, it can occasionally be very difficult to replace it rapidly. This is particularly the case if the dissection extends to the level of the sternoclavicular joint. To prevent this from happening, the Pruitt–Inahara shunt balloon is held in place with a sling whilst proximal dissection continues (Fig. 23.1). Once a healthier segment of proximal CCA has been identified, a fresh sling is

placed around the CCA and the shunt balloon is carefully manipulated below the second sling.

CAROTID SUBOCCLUSION

As discussed above, the vascular technologist should already have alerted the carotid surgeon to the possibility of an ICA subocclusion and the decision process will then vary from one surgeon to another. This is because, to my knowledge, there are no randomized studies to guide management in this situation.

My own thoughts are as follows. If the ipsilateral symptomatic ICA appears suboccluded on colour duplex or angiography, this can result from either a truly hypoplastic ICA (Fig. 23.2) or a severe stenosis and extremely low distal flow in a normal-calibre artery (Fig. 23.3). In the former situation, because the flow is so low within the ICA, I consider that it no longer poses a significant embolic risk and, similarly, it does not contribute significantly to circle of Willis blood flow. In this situation, if the ICA occludes, it can no longer pose an embolic risk and it is unlikely to cause a haemodynamic stroke.

However, post-mortem studies in patients with ICA occlusion have shown that, in 33% of cases, the thrombus extends beyond the ICA bifurcation and that the presence or absence of a normal anterior segment of the circle of Willis had no influence on whether the thrombus extended into the MCA.[6] In addition, these patients often have recent emboli in the MCA. In other words, roughly one-third of patients who suffer ICA occlusion will have thrombus extending across into the MCA and/or embolism distally.

For this reason, although it is possible to use transcranial colour duplex to ascertain the completeness of the circle of Willis, it is not possible to predict which patients will propagate thrombus or embolize into their MCA in the event of ICA occlusion. I do not therefore request transcranial colour duplex of the circle of Willis because, although it might help to predict haemodynamic stroke in the event of ICA occlusion, it cannot predict the likelihood of thrombus propagation or embolization into the MCA. Instead I would favour warfarinizing patients in whom a diagnosis of ICA subocclusion

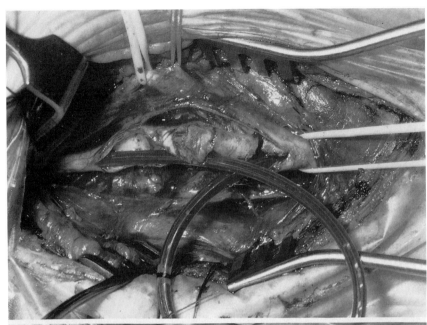

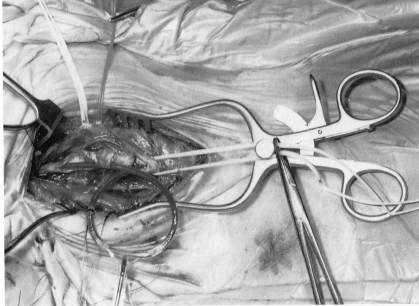

Fig. 23.1
The proximal balloon of the Pruitt–Inahara shunt is secured by passing a sling around the common carotid artery and then round the hub of the West retractor, where it is secured with an artery clip. If further proximal dissection is necessary, a second sling is placed more proximally and the shunt balloon is gently manipulated below the second sling.

had been made preoperatively, in the expectation that their ICA will thrombose in due course and that warfarinization will hopefully minimize the risk of clot propagation or embolization into the MCA. However, should duplex or angiography indicate a normal-calibre artery beyond the symptomatic stenosis (Fig. 23.3), reconstruction is still indicated.

The difficult question arises, however, as to what one should do if one encounters a true hypoplastic carotid artery at operation. As discussed above, a hypoplastic ICA discovered at operation could result

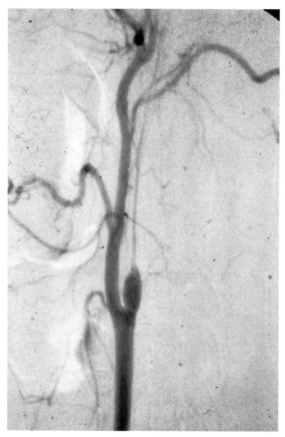

Fig. 23.2
Digital subtraction angiogram demonstrating a tiny residual lumen extending up to the skull base. This is not suitable for reconstruction.

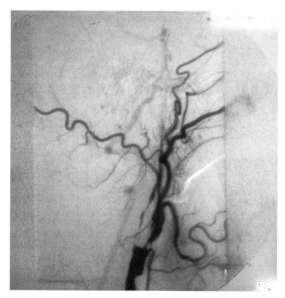

Fig. 23.3
Severe stenosis at the origin of the internal carotid artery. The stenosis extends quite far distally but opens out into a normal-calibre lumen. This is suitable for reconstruction.

from either a subocclusion with distal vessel wall collapse or genuine hypoplasia and it is not always possible to distinguish between these two situations, even at operation.

In practice, the surgeon is usually faced with a tiny ICA that disappears into the distal reaches of the neck (Fig. 23.2). The less commonly encountered scenario is where there is a short narrowed segment of ICA at its origin with a larger, normal-looking ICA higher up (Fig. 23.3). The difference between the two situations is, of course, that in the former it is not possible safely to reconstruct the ICA, whereas in the latter it is.

If only a short segment of the ICA origin is hypoplastic, I would perform some form of

reconstruction – usually a short reversed vein graft – because I would be concerned about the hypoplastic ICA origin acting as a source of embolism or propagated thrombus. If all the visible length of the ICA were hypoplastic, I would consider this inoperable and then the only remaining surgical issue is whether the ipsilateral ECA is a significant contributor to cerebral perfusion. I would evaluate this using TCD in the manner described earlier. If the procedure is abandoned, I would warfarinize the patient.

UNCONTROLLED HAEMORRHAGE
The first issue is to ascertain whether the bleeding is venous or arterial. It is usually straightforward to tell this from the colour of the blood and whether the blood is welling up or spurting. In practice the bleeding is predominantly venous and usually arises from small veins around the occipital artery or behind the digastric muscle. In this situation the bleeding can always be controlled by careful packing with a small gauze swab and by placing the patient

a little more head-up. The assistant should be discouraged from prodding the wound with swabs as, on occasion, this may dislodge emboli. Unless the bleeding is major, I would then continue with another part of the operation for 5–10min, gently remove the pack and stop the bleeding using a 5–0 or 6–0 Prolene suture.

As stated above, the experienced (or properly supervised) carotid surgeon should not encounter serious arterial bleeding during a standard CEA. However, in the context of a hostile neck, carotid aneurysm or carotid body tumour, profuse bleeding from the distal ICA may occur. A particular problem may also arise in patients in whom dissection has extended very high and overall access is poor. Initial control of the bleeding can be obtained by clamping the ICA proximally and applying finger pressure distally. The surgeon should then slowly withdraw the compressing finger whilst using suction to visualize the bleeding point. If the bleeding is from a small tear or hole, then it may be possible to repair the defect using 6–0 or 7–0 Prolene sutures. If this is possible and the surgeon is certain that the ICA has not been narrowed, nothing further need be done. If there is any concern that the ICA lumen has been compromised by the repair, an intraoperative arteriogram should be performed. Any narrowing of significance will then require patch repair at some stage during the procedure.

If the bleeding cannot be controlled by finger pressure, I would carefully pass a number 2 Fogarty balloon catheter into the distal ICA and gently inflate the balloon cranial to the bleeding point. Provided that a three-way tap has been fitted to the catheter hub, haemostatic control can then be maintained whilst further treatment continues. If the TCD suggests that MCA velocity is satisfactory (i.e. > 15cm/s), I would then repair the artery under direct vision. If, however, the MCA velocities are less than 15cm/s, I would insert a Pruitt–Inahara shunt.

This carries a potential risk of further tearing the artery at the site of the original tear. However, the patient is otherwise at high risk of suffering a stroke and cerebral blood flow must be maintained. If it proves impossible to control the distal ICA bleeding or if, having controlled the bleeding and trying to repair the ICA, the repair starts to 'fall apart' then the surgeon has to make the difficult decision as to whether to ligate the proximal ICA and oversew the distal ICA.

The risk of suffering a TIA or stroke after carotid occlusion or ligation ranges from 25% to 30% with roughly half of these patients dying.[7-9] Interestingly, a proportion of patients will develop a hemiplegia some days *after* surgery, presumably due to propagated thrombus. Thus, if faced with no other alternative, I would proceed to carotid ligation if the ipsilateral MCA velocity was >15 cm/s during carotid clamping but would prefer a velocity > 20cm/s.

The vascular audit at Leicester Royal Infirmary shows that only one CEA in 800 since 1992 has had to be abandoned because of distal haemorrhage. This arose in a young male with a severe symptomatic stenosis in association with a distal aneurysm. Despite the patient having had the benefit of preoperative angiography, the aneurysm extended almost to the skull base and was very inflammatory. During the course of a difficult dissection, the arterial lumen was breached and a Fogarty catheter had to be inserted to control the bleeding. The arterial wall proved to be very friable and could not be repaired as the sutures kept tearing out. TCD, however, indicated that the MCA velocity was 26cm/s during clamping and the distal ICA was ultimately overseen and the patient systemically heparinized then warferinized. Postoperatively, the patient recovered from anaesthesia with no neurological deficit and has since remained asymptomatic.

However, if MCA velocities are < 15cm/s I would then have to review the possibility of operation and do my utmost to effect an ICA repair and restore cerebral perfusion. Certainly, it would be with a heavy heart that I would take the decision to ligate the ICA in the presence of an ipsilateral MCA velocity of < 15cm/s.

REFERENCES

1 Loftus IM, McCarthy MJ, Pau H *et al*. Carotid endarterectomy without angiography does not compromise operative outcome. *European Journal of Vascular and Endovascular Surgery* 1998; **16**: 489–493.

2 Executive Committee for the Asymptomatic Carotid Atherosclerosis Study. Endarterectomy for asymptomatic carotid artery stenosis. *Journal of the American Medical Association* 1995; **273**: 1421–1428.

3 Benavente O, Moher D, Pham B. Carotid endarterectomy for asymptomatic carotid stenosis; a meta-analysis. *British Medical Journal* 1998; **327**: 1477–1480.

4 Streifler JY, Benavente OR, Harbison JW *et al*. Prognostic implications of retinal versus hemispheric TIA in patients with high grade carotid stenosis. Observations from NASCET. *Stroke* 1992; **23**: 159 (abstract).

5 Levien LJ, Benn C-A, Veller MG, Fritz VU. Retrograde balloon angioplasty of brachiocephalic or common carotid artery stenoses at the time of carotid endarterectomy. *European Journal of Vascular and Endovascular Surgery* 1998; **15**: 521–527.

6 Castaigne P, Lhermitte F, Gautier J-C, Escourolle R, Derouesne C. Internal carotid artery occlusion. A study of 61 instances in 50 patients with post-mortem data. *Brain* 1970; **93**: 231–258.

7 Shanik GD, Moore DJ, Leahy A, Grouden MC, Colgan M-P. Asymptomatic carotid stenosis; a benign lesion? *European Journal of Vascular and Endovascular Surgery* 1992; **6**: 10–15.

8 Klop RBJ, Taks ACJM, Welten RJ Th, Eikelboom BC. Outcome of progression from carotid stenosis to occlusion. *European Journal of Vascular and Endovascular Surgery* 1992; **6**: 263–268.

9 Brackett CE Jr. The complications of carotid artery ligation in the neck. *Journal of Neurosurgery* 1953; **10**: 91–106.

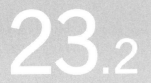

23.2

When should I abandon a planned endarterectomy?
Jonathan P Gertler (USA)

INTRODUCTION

Despite advances in CEA over the last decade, the final arbiters of success or failure of this procedure are the judgment and technical skill exercised by the surgeon. Preoperative cardiac risk stratification has significantly improved patient selection and the safety of endarterectomy. Improved preoperative imaging has further refined patient selection by allowing precise correlation of symptoms with lesions and precise determination of degree of stenosis and plaque morphology in asymptomatic patients. None the less, under certain circumstances imaging data may force the surgeon to abandon plans for CEA or may mislead the surgeon into attempting an endarterectomy which must be abandoned intraoperatively. This chapter will review radiologic findings which militate against successful endarterectomy and intraoperative experience which has led to abandonment or modification of the procedure.

The precise evaluation of cardiac comorbidity is described in Chapter 14 and will not be reviewed here. It is incumbent on the carotid surgeon in all elective circumstances to insure that perioperative morbidity and mortality risk is within acceptable range and that anticipated longevity is sufficient to insure accrual of benefit. Except in emergency cases where imminent threat of major stroke outweighs longer-term concerns, endarterectomy should not be carried out, especially in asymptomatic patients, if comorbid conditions (e.g. unreconstructable coronary disease with severe ventricular dysfunction, incurable cancer) strictly limit survival potential. Furthermore, certain specific anatomic conditions (extensive head and neck cancer, extensive previous radiation therapy, local infection, tracheostomy) may disqualify patients from consideration for endarterectomy.

PREOPERATIVE IMAGING AND INOPERABILITY

The purpose of preoperative imaging is threefold: to provide documentation of the source of carotid territory symptoms, to stratify the degree of stenosis and overall severity of disease, and to demonstrate operability. Generally accepted criteria for operability are listed below:

1 lesion consistent with symptoms or severe enough to warrant intervention in an asymptomatic patient;
2 absence of total occlusion;
3 bifurcation accessible from cervical incision with or without adjunctive mandibular maneuvers;
4 accessible end-point to plaque;
5 absence of secondary critical arch or intracranial lesions which might obviate benefit from CEA or mandate additional procedures.

Obviously, a planned CEA should be canceled if the lesion is not severe enough to explain the patient's symptoms or to warrant repair in the asymptomatic setting.

With very rare exceptions, total occlusion of the internal carotid mandates abandonment of plans for CEA. Internal carotid occlusions can occur asymptomatically with a residual bruit from an external carotid lesion resulting in imaging devaluation. Occlusion is more commonly associated with hemispheric or ocular TIA or stroke. Duplex criteria which are highly sensitive and specific for internal carotid occlusion include absent visualization of ICA flow, echodense material filling the internal carotid lumen, and a 'thump' at the bifurcation and ICA orifice with reflected waves emanating backwards from the obstructed lumen. With these findings, unless there are ongoing TIAs or a fluctuating neurologic status, no further imaging studies are warranted and the diagnosis of an occluded and, therefore inoperable, carotid is virtually certain. If there are ongoing TIAs or neurologic fluctuation, implying either ongoing embolization or hemodynamic insufficiency, further investigation is appropriate. In this setting, either formal contrast angiography including 'trickle' studies or spiral computed tomography (CT) with three-dimensional reconstruction is needed to assess definitively the internal and external carotids and identify the source of the patient's symptoms.[10,16,17,18] Magnetic resonance angiography (MRA) has been disappointing in this setting, since it is another flow-dependent imaging modality which might miss a patent ICA in the presence of sluggish flow, and which lacks the resolution to identify with reliability potential sources of emboli in the ECA or ICA stump.[12] It should be stressed, however, that the vast majority of patients with ICA occlusion will be neurologically stable and will not require extensive invasive evaluation.

Significant difficulty can be encountered in the evaluation of patients with very high grade carotid stenosis causing pseudo-occlusion.[19] String sign, slim sign, and hypoplasia are alternative terms used to describe an underfilled carotid in which sluggish flow results in layering of contrast (or no contrast filling at all), lack of continuity in the CT angiogram image, and a long flow void on MRA. Distinguishing which of these lesions are operable and which inoperable is difficult and sometimes impossible, even with extensive non-invasive and invasive imaging evaluation. The possible causes of a radiologic string sign or pseudo-occlusion include:

1 tight stenosis with poor filling secondary to very slow flow or contrast layering;
2 layered fresh thrombus distal to critical stenosis;
3 chronic layered thrombus distal to critical stenosis;
4 severe diffuse atheromatous disease with distal extension;

5 distal arterial fibrosis secondary to old thrombus related to flow stagnation from a critical proximal stenosis;
6 arterial atrophy secondary to a critical proximal stenosis with poor flow and low pressure.

Even with the use of multiple imaging modalities it may be impossible to distinguish among these entities, The detection of a patent distal lumen of reasonable diameter on any imaging modality is reassuring; however, the absence of this finding does not always preclude successful endarterectomy. Careful review of all available imaging data, correlation of these data with the patient's clinical presentation, and risk–benefit analysis of surgical exploration should be carried out on a case-by-case basis when deciding which patients with a string sign should undergo operation.

INTRAOPERATIVE FINDINGS PRECLUDING ENDARTERECTOMY

Findings at surgery which preclude safe completion of a planned endarterectomy are usually, but not always, detectable on preoperative evaluation. Rarely, a carotid will thrombose in the interval between imaging evaluation and surgery. More commonly, however, the necessity to abandon endarterectomy intraoperatively represents a failure of preoperative imaging or a failure of the surgeon to recognize the significance of preoperative imaging findings. A variety of intraoperative findings that might lead to abandonment and their appropriate management are discussed below.

Tightly Stenotic Proximal Internal Carotid with Underfilling Secondary to Low Flow

Exploration of the carotid bifurcation in this setting reveals severe bifurcation disease with a normal, though sometimes quite small, pliable distal ICA with no external evidence of disease.[11] Maneuvers should include Doppler insonation of the distal ICA as well as high circumferential dissection. If Doppler flow in the ICA above the plaque is present and the artery appears free of disease at the distal extent of exposure, the artery should be opened and the arteriotomy extended above the plaque end-point. If the artery probes normally for a few centimeters above this, the endarterectomy can be completed in standard fashion and closed with a patch. If the artery does not probe easily, or if the lumen is of small caliber, pre-reconstruction on-table angiography can be carried out to confirm distal patency and vessel quality. With small distal arteries, vein patching may be preferable to minimize thrombogenic potential in the early postoperative period.

Layering Fresh Thrombus Distal to a Critical Stenosis

This finding is often encountered in emergent or urgent clinical settings, crescendo TIAs or stroke in evolution. Rarely, the surgeon may encounter this in an elective endarterectomy in which the interval between diagnosis of a critical stenosis and surgery has been prolonged.

The arbiters of whether to proceed with or abort the endarterectomy in this setting are whether the thrombus can be removed safely and completely and whether the underlying arterial wall is sufficiently healthy to permit restoration of antegrade flow across a reasonably thromboresistant surface. Re-establishing flow, only to have a postoperative thrombosis with the attendant risk of embolization, may well result in a poorer outcome than would have occurred if the artery had been left alone or ligated and the patient treated with anticoagulants.

In the setting of an acutely thrombosed artery or in the setting of apparent non-occlusive soft thrombus, distal clamps should not be applied. Rather, common and external carotid clamps should be applied as per routine, the artery opened, and the arteriotomy extended up the ICA. Clot should be gently extracted. If a clear end-point of clot is reached with resultant vigorous back-bleeding, and the distal artery is soft and palpably free of disease and residual clot, the CEA should proceed with patch closure. In this setting, a completion arteriogram or duplex study seems advisable.

If there is no back-bleeding, or scant back-bleeding, a thrombectomy catheter may be passed gently for a short distance ($\leq$ 8cm), but if strong back-bleeding is not re-established, the procedure should be abandoned. Overvigorous attempts at thrombectomy can result in catastrophic distal

arterial rupture or carotid cavernous fistula. If reasonable back-bleeding is established, a pre-reconstruction arteriogram is wise to rule out retained non-occlusive thrombus, but in the absence of good back-bleeding, such an arteriogram is unwise, since distal clot is likely to be dislodged.

Chronic Layered Thrombus Distal to a Critical Stenosis or Fibrosis of the Artery Secondary to Recanalized Old Thrombus Distal to a Critical Stenosis

This situation is similar to that described above for more acute thrombus, but the fibrosis of the vessel wall should lead the surgeon away from standard ICA endarterectomy. Attempts to remove chronic adherent thrombus and fibrotic intima, especially in the more distal carotid, may be hazardous and are unlikely to result in re-establishment of a satisfactory lumen and flow surface. Except in the rare circumstance where the chronic thrombus and fibrosis are quite focal and the more distal artery appears normal, abandonment of the procedure is by far the wisest course.

Diffuse Atheromatous Disease[15]

The presence of a diffusely and extensively diseased ICA mandates several maneuvers to maximize the chances for a good outcome. Hopefully, the presence of diffuse plaque extending high into the ICA will be noted on preoperative duplex and lead to arteriography for optimal visualization. With confirmation of the presence of extensive distal disease, plans can be made for maneuvers (such as mandibular subluxation, see Chapter 18) to enhance distal exposure. Alternatively, if the disease extends prohibitively high, the procedure can be canceled and the patient offered medical management. If the need for high exposure is not recognized preoperatively, the surgeon may try several maneuvers such as digastric division and cranial nerve mobilization (described in detail in Chapter 18). Alternatively, the neck can be closed temporarily and intraoperative oral surgery consultation for mandibular subluxation requested.

The artery should be opened, as always, beyond the point of significant disease. There is great danger, if inadequate length of artery remains between the arteriotomy and the base of the skull, for distal control, end-point establishment (with or without tacking sutures), shunt placement if required, or ligation of the artery should this be necessary. Loss of control of the distal carotid near the skull base is usually catastrophic.

The decision as to whether or not to proceed with endarterectomy in the setting of extensive distal disease is based on whether or not a safe, adequate end-point can be established. Although a ridge of thickened intima held down by a row of 7–0 tacking sutures is less appealing than a finely feathered end-point, it will usually result in a satisfactory outcome. Medial calcinosis, although not esthetically pleasing to the surgeon, should have little impact on luminal diameter and therefore little impact on surgical outcome. However, leaving significant plaque with an elevated ridge at the distal end-point poses the threat of thrombosis and/or embolization with perioperative stroke. Therefore, if a satisfactory distal end-point cannot be achieved because of severe distal disease with shelf-like plaque remnants, the artery should be ligated. Intraoperative monitoring with electroencephalogram, TCD, or regional anesthesia can facilitate this decision by demonstrating the adequacy of collateral flow in most patients.

THE ABANDONED ENDARTERECTOMY

Once the decision is made to abandon attempts at standard carotid endarterectomy, several steps are necessary to optimize outcome:

1   The remaining plaque in the CCA and ECA must be removed.
2   The arteriotomy should be redirected so that the ECA can be included in the patch closure and kept in continuity with common carotid flow, insuring the maintenance of this critical collateral pathway.
3   The internal carotid must be divided from the CCA and the area oversewn to eliminate any possible cul-de-sac and provide a smooth common carotid surface.
4   The distal internal carotid must be securely ligated.
5   Perform perioperative anticoagulation with heparin and conversion to coumadin for 3–6 months, much as is done after spontaneous carotid occlusion – this is usually appropriate.

CONCLUSION

Abandonment of a CEA is appropriate under specific circumstances to prevent potential medical or surgical catastrophes. Prohibitive medical risk, limited life expectancy, and unreconstructable anatomy are the most frequent reasons for abandonment. When it is necessary to abandon a planned endarterectomy intraoperatively, several maneuvers, including carotid ligation, external CEA with patch angioplasty, and anticoagulation can help to optimize outcome in what is often a frustrating and potentially dangerous operative setting.

REFERENCES

10   Ammar AD, Turrentine NM, Farha SJ. The importance of arteriographic interpretation in occlusion or pseudo-occlusion of the carotid artery. *Surgery, Gynecology and Obstetrics* 1988; **167**: 119–123.
11   Archie JP. Carotid endarterectomy when the distal internal carotid artery is small or poorly visualized. *Journal of Vascular Surgery* 1994; **19**: 23–31.
12   Barnett HJM, Peerless SJ, Kaufman JCE. Stump of the internal carotid: a source of further cerebral embolic ischemia. *Stroke* 1978; **9**: 448–456.
13   Clark OH, Moore WS, Hall AD. Radiographically occluded anatomically patent carotid arteries. *Archives of Surgery* 1971; **102**: 604–606.
14   Gertler J, Blankensteijn J, Brewster D *et al.* Carotid endarterectomy for unstable and compelling neurologic conditions: do results justify an aggressive approach? *Journal of Vascular Surgery* 1994; **19**: 32–42.

15   Hertzer NS. Management of totally and nearly occluded extracranial internal carotid arteries. In: Ernst CB, Stanley JC (eds) *Current Therapy in Vascular Surgery*, (2nd edn.) London: Mosby 1991; 70–76.
16   Lippman BH, Sundt TM, Holman CB. The poststenotic string sign: spurious internal carotid hypoplasia. *Mayo Clinic Proceedings* 1970; **45**: 762–767.
17   Mehigan JT, Olcott C. The carotid string sign: differential diagnosis and management. *American Journal of Surgery* 1980; **140**: 137–143.
18   Newton TH, Couch RSC. Possible errors in the arteriographic diagnosis of internal carotid occlusion. *Radiology* 1960; **75**: 776–783.
19   Yonas H, Meyer J. Extreme pseudo-occlusion of internal carotid artery. *Neurosurgery* 1982; **11**: 681–686.

Editorial Comment

In short, plans to abandon CEA should be considered whenever the perceived risk of the procedure exceeds the probable long-term benefit. For example, the patient with prohibitive medical comorbidity or with a short life expectancy is unlikely to benefit from the stroke prevention afforded by successful surgery. Similarly, the hostile neck (extensive cancer, radiation therapy) significantly increases the risks of the procedure to the point where they might outweigh any potential benefit. The other remaining preoperative indication for abandonment is when the duplex scan indicates that the ICA has now undergone asymptomatic occlusion. There is no indication for CEA in this situation, as attempts to unblock the artery can be hazardous.

Intraoperative abandonment of a CEA suggests a failure of preoperative imaging to define adequately the extent or severity of disease or failure by the surgeon to appreciate the significance of the imaging findings in the context of his or her ability to complete the procedure. Thus, in the situation of a surgeon unexpectedly finding him- or herself having to consider a high distal exposure in a patient with unilateral asymptomatic disease, the risks are now much higher than were discussed with the patient preoperatively and abandonment may be the most judicious strategy.

When confronted, otherwise, with potentially inoperable carotid disease in the operating room, the surgeon has to make several critical decisions. If a hypoplastic artery has not been opened, it can either be left intact or ligated. The authors are divided on this issue and there is no good evidence to guide the surgeon in this situation. Clearly, ligation should not be performed if this will render the ipsilateral hemisphere ischemic (based on TCD or awake testing EEG findings) but, in practice, there is so little flow going up a hypoplastic ICA that this is rarely a problem. If the consensus is that the hypoplastic ICA is a continuing source of embolism, it should probably be ligated. If not, it may well be best to leave it alone. Either way, the patient should be anticoagulated immediately following the procedure to minimize the risks of embolization into the circle of Willis. Ideally, warfarinization should continue for 6 months thereafter. If a long hypoplastic artery has been opened already, it should be ligated distally and the patient anticoagulated. It is important, of course, to consider reconstruction of the ECA in this situation as it may be a vital source of collateral flow to the brain via reversed flow in the ophthalmic artery. Similarly, if the surgeon opens the carotid bifurcation to find that it is occluded and the thrombus extends beyond surgical accessibility, the procedure should be abandoned. Attempts at thrombectomy may restore back-bleeding but retained mural thrombus or intimal damage may result in catastrophic secondary embolization or thrombosis. If thrombectomy is carried out, completion angiography would be prudent to exclude retained thrombus or underlying plaque.

Is there any evidence that perioperative monitoring and quality control assessment alter clinical outcome?
A Ross Naylor (Europe)

Despite a plethora of published literature on the role of monitoring during carotid endarterectomy (CEA), no randomized trial has ever been performed and, consequently, no consensus exists amongst vascular surgeons as to whether it confers any overall benefit. However, before simply dismissing the concept of monitoring as a waste of time or resources, it is important to review some of the principles upon which it should be based.

WHY HAS MONITORING NOT MADE A DIFFERENCE?

The reason why monitoring has significantly failed to reduce the risk of operation-related stroke is probably a simple failure to ask the right questions.[1] For example, most monitoring methods have been used to develop criteria for guiding selective shunt deployment, despite the fact that haemodynamic failure remains a relatively rare cause of intraoperative stroke.[2] Virtually none has been developed and thereafter applied to identify and prevent thromboembolism, which continues to be the principal cause of operative stroke.[3]

Moreover, despite the fact that the largest single predisposing cause for perioperative thromboembolism is inadvertent technical error,[3] most vascular surgeons rarely include some form of quality control assessment in their operative protocol. There also remains the flawed assumption that one monitoring method is superior to all others and that, by using it routinely, one can prevent all operation-related strokes. For example, is it reasonable to blame the electroencephalogram (EEG) for not having prevented an intraoperative stroke due to embolization of luminal thrombus at the time of restoration of flow if no attempt was made to identify this and remove it beforehand?

Operation-related stroke is a multifactorial problem and, despite protestations to the contrary, surprisingly few reliable audit data are available concerning the exact aetiology, timing and combination of circumstances that predispose towards its evolution. Accordingly, it should come as no surprise that surgeons frequently prefer to condemn monitoring to the role of scapegoat (should any complication arise) rather than focus attention on why such complications occur and how monitoring may be used to help prevent them in the future.[1]

IS THERE AN UNDERLYING PROBLEM?

The European Carotid Surgery Trial (ECST) and the North American Symptomatic Carotid Endarterectomy Trial (NASCET) have shown that, in selected patients, CEA confers a 50% reduction in the long-term risk of stroke as compared with best medical therapy alone.[4,5] However, the benefits of CEA are inextricably linked to the initial operative risk and surgeons must accept that these results may not be instantly generalizable to routine clinical practice. All of the international randomized trials to date have used experienced surgeons with proven records and a significant proportion of trial applicants were rejected because their complication rate was considered too high.[6]

Following publication of the trials, the number of CEAs performed annually has increased dramatically throughout the world and there is now evidence that the current risk of operative stroke or death may be significantly higher than that pertaining to by the original trial centres.[7–11] For example, more than 90% of CEAs in the US are currently performed in non-NASCET centres with an operative mortality rate that is both higher than that of the NASCET centres and directly proportional to the annual operative workload.[10] This therefore suggests that there may be an underlying problem to be addressed and now is an excellent opportunity to review many of our current attitudes and, in particular, the complementary role of perioperative monitoring.

PRINCIPLES UNDERLYING THE ROLE OF MONITORING

The principal causes of operation-related stroke are detailed in Table 24.1. For the purposes of rationalizing the role of monitoring, it is useful to subdivide such stroke into intraoperative stroke (i.e. apparent upon recovery from anaesthesia) and postoperative stroke (occurring after normal recovery from anaesthesia).

The initiating factor in most patients is thromboembolism, which is followed, in sequence, by a variable period of focal or global hypoperfusion, loss of cerebral electrical activity and finally neuronal death. The rate of progression through each phase is controlled by external factors, including the state of the collateral circulation, the anatomical severity of the insult (major vessel or branch occlusion) and the presence or absence of spontaneous embolic fragmentation, which will also be influenced to some degree by the underlying cerebral perfusion pressure. Thus, when considering whether monitoring might be clinically useful, it is important to determine which monitoring modality detects which phase in the sequence (Table 24.2).

The most important end-point is the onset of a neurological deficit. However, unless the operation is performed under regional anaesthesia, this is clearly not possible to detect. Moreover, although awake testing will be of practical value in detecting critical

---

Table 24.1
Aetiology of stroke following carotid endarterectomy

Intraoperative stroke*	Postoperative stroke[†]
Embolism	*Embolism*
Spontaneous embolization (unstable plaque)	Particulate emboli from endarterectomy zone
Particulate emboli during carotid dissection	Particulate emboli following external carotid artery thrombosis
Particulate emboli dislodged by shunt	
Major air embolism through shunt malfunction	
Particulate embolization from endarterectomy zone	
Thrombosis	*Thrombosis*
Peri-shunt thrombosis	Secondary to technical error
On-table carotid thrombosis	Secondary to hypotension
	Secondary to syphon disease
	Secondary to coagulation disorder
Miscellaneous	*Miscellaneous*
Haemodynamic failure (no shunt used)	Hypertensive encephalopathy
Haemodynamic failure (shunt malfunction)	Primary intracerebral haemorrhage
	Haemorrhagic transformation of infarct
	Hyperperfusion syndrome

*Intraoperative stroke, patient recovers from anaesthetic with a new neurological deficit.
[†]Postoperative stroke, patient suffers a stroke some time after a normal recovery from anaesthetic.

Table 24.2
The role of monitoring methods in the detection of cerebral ischaemia

Detection of thromboembolism	Detection of reduced cerebral perfusion	Detection of loss of electrical activity	Detection of neuronal injury
TCD	Reduced stump pressure Reduced back flow Near infra-red spectroscopy Jugular venous oxygen saturation Xenon CBF measurement TCD	EEG SSEP	Awake testing

TCD, transcranial Doppler; CBF, cerebral blood flow; EEG, electroencephalogram; SSEP, somatosensory evoked potential.

ischaemia during carotid clamping (thereby enabling shunt insertion), it provides no benefit in terms of detecting and preventing intra- or postoperative embolization other than documenting that it happened.

Similarly, because the perfusion threshold for suffering neuronal cell injury and thus the onset of neurological signs (10ml/100g brain per min) is significantly less than the corresponding threshold for the loss of cerebral electrical activity (12–15ml/100g brain per min), monitoring modalities such as EEG and somatosensory evoked potential (SSEP) will already have registered a loss of normal cerebral electrical activity.[12] In summary, just because the EEG or SSEP is abnormal, it does not necessarily follow that neuronal injury is inevitable. Thus, although EEG- or SSEP-detected abnormalities can also guide selective shunt deployment, they are of little clinical value in the event of embolization other than indicating that something has happened.

The phase immediately preceding loss of cerebral electrical activity is focal or global hypoperfusion. Monitoring modalities such as transcranial Doppler (TCD), near infra-red spectroscopy, jugular venous oxygen saturation measurements, xenon-based cerebral blood flow studies and stump pressure can be used to monitor crudely the overall adequacy of cerebral perfusion but they frequently do not provide clinically useful information regarding *why* the insult occurred. Many are also limited in their ability to provide subtle resolution regarding focal ischaemia, particularly in patients who present with a pre-existing cerebral infarct and a vulnerable ischaemic penumbra.

Finally, TCD remains the only monitoring method capable of providing an on-line diagnosis of embolization because the back-scattered signal from an embolus is significantly greater than that of flowing blood.[13,14] However, there has always been considerable scepticism amongst surgeons as to the relevance of these TCD-diagnosed emboli or so-called high-intensity transients. This is largely because they can occur in relatively large numbers during CEA (often with little morbidity), and represent a variety of artefacts, and gaseous and particulate elements.

However, recent evidence suggests that artefacts can be readily excluded,[15] while gaseous emboli appear to have little clinical relevance.[16,17] More attention is therefore being directed towards those phases in the operation when the emboli have to be particulate, as there does appear to be an increased risk of stroke, cognitive impairment and ischaemic change on magnetic resonance imaging (MRI).[14,16–18]

WHAT IS THE ROLE OF QUALITY CONTROL ASSESSMENT?

TCD will therefore detect an embolus entering the cerebral circulation, methods capable of monitoring cerebral perfusion may register either global or, less likely, focal hypoperfusion, EEG and SSEP will document any subsequent loss of cerebral electrical activity and awake testing will record the onset of any neurological deficit. Unfortunately, however, because most of these methods will only act once the primary insult has occurred, they can hardly be expected to *prevent* the initial thromboembolic event!

In a comprehensive review of complications following CEA, Riles *et al.* showed that inadvertent technical error was present in most cases.[3] Yet, despite the fact that few surgeons would undertake a femorodistal bypass without completion angiography, the same principle of quality control assessment is rarely applied following CEA. However, as with the basic monitoring methods described above, there are also a number of quality control techniques and, unless they are considered in the context of what they can and cannot detect (Table 24.3), it will still be difficult to plan a rational strategy for evaluation.

The principal roles for quality control assessment are the diagnosis of particulate embolization, the detection of unexpected phenomena, the monitoring of shunt integrity, the detection of luminal thrombus and intimal flaps and the diagnosis of a residual stenosis.

Embolization

Spontaneous particulate embolization during initial carotid dissection warns the surgeon of an unstable plaque with overlying thrombus[19] and its detection permits either a gentler dissection technique or prompts the surgeon to clamp the ICA as soon as possible. Spontaneous embolization is significantly more likely in patients with recent symptoms, particularly crescendo transient ischaemic attacks (TIAs) and, in our experience, the routine use of TCD has been associated with a 50% drop in the number of especial emboli (Table 24.4) detected during the procedure.[20] Although this has been of especial benefit in the training of obsessional surgical technique to younger colleagues,[21] even the more senior surgeon can occasionally learn a thing or two!

Gaseous embolization is relatively common after shunt insertion and following restoration of flow but is probably of little clinical relevance.[14,16,17] There are, however, three other important phases of particulate embolization that require careful monitoring.

Immediately following restoration of flow, particulate emboli can also be released into the cerebral circulation. The principal source of these emboli appears to be bleeding from the vasa vasorum during the endarterect or closure phase with thrombus formation on the highly thrombogenic endarterectomized surface. Because TCD will only document its passage through the brain, some other form of quality control assessment is required to prevent this from causing a stroke (see section on detection of luminal thrombus, below).

The other critical phases in the operation regarding embolization are the period of neck closure (on-table thrombosis) and early postoperative thrombosis. As early as 1967, Blaisdell *et al.* reported that up to 2% of patients suffered an on-table carotid thrombosis during CEA.[22] Evidence now shows that, despite the high rate of blood flow through the carotid artery, platelets will begin to

Table 24.3
Role of quality control methods during carotid endarterectomy

Embolization	Shunt malfunction	Luminal thrombus	Intimal flap	Distal stenosis
TCD	TCD	Angioscopy Angiography Duplex CW Doppler	Angioscopy Angiography Duplex	Angioscopy Angiography Duplex CW Doppler

TCD, transcranial Doppler, CW, continuous-wave.

Table 24.4
Reduction in median number (95% confidence intervals) of emboli detected during carotid surgery

Operative phase	Group 1 (1992/1993) ($n = 75$)	Group 2 (1995) ($n = 75$)	P
Carotid dissection	10 (4–14)	2 (1–5)	0.0193
Shunt opening	7 (5–9)	4 (3–5)	0.0032
During shunting	7 (4–11)	4 (2–7)	0.1378
ECA flow restoration	8 (5–12)	4 (3–7)	0.0782
ICA flow restoration	19 (14–27)	16 (12–21)	0.7508
Total particulate emboli	21 (16–29)	9 (7–14)	0.0008
Total air emboli	18 (14–24)	15 (11–19)	0.1303
Total emboli	43 (33–55)	25 (19–31)	0.0023

ECA, external carotid artery; ICA, internal carotid artery. Adapted from Smith et al.[20] with permission.

adhere to the endarterectomy zone within 2min of flow restoration.[23] However, until the advent of TCD, it was not possible to diagnose and monitor the evolution of this process.

The diagnosis of incipient on-table carotid thrombosis can now be made by the detection of increasing numbers of embolic signals in the middle carotid artery (MCA) after about 5min have elapsed following flow restoration.[24] Unless steps are thereafter taken to intervene, the carotid artery will thrombose. This can be recognized by MCA velocities falling to levels observed during initial clamping. In our experience this is a rare phenomenon (affecting 2 patients in the last 800 CEAs: 0.25%) but only TCD allows one to recognize immediately its evolution and implement steps to prevent it from progressing to complete occlusion.

Similarly, postoperative carotid thrombosis has remained hitherto an unpreventable condition with devastating consequences. It affects up to 3% of patients, usually in the first 6 postoperative hours. It had previously been assumed that carotid thrombosis was primarily due to some underlying technical error but evidence now suggests that, as with on-table carotid thrombosis, it follows enhanced platelet aggregation within the endarterectomy zone. There are now studies from three continents that have shown that increasing rates of asymptomatic embolization (often for 1–2h) precede the onset of thrombotic stroke.[14,18,24–26] This has been an

important breakthrough because, for the first time, TCD can be used to identify the at-risk patient and thereafter guide surgical or therapeutic intervention. At the Leicester Royal Infirmary, we routinely monitor all patients for 3h after surgery with TCD. Those patients with sustained embolization (> 25 emboli in any 10-min period, or large emboli distorting the MCA waveform) are commenced on an incremental dose of intravenous dextran. Since implementing this strategy, only 5% of patients have received adjuvant dextran therapy and no patient in the last 500 has progressed on to thrombotic stroke.[27] This protocol is discussed more fully in Chapter 26.

Ensuring Shunt Integrity
There is a tendency to assume that, once a shunt is inserted, nothing further need be done. In fact, up to 3% of shunts malfunction to some degree during CEA[28] and it seems illogical to take the trouble to insert a shunt and not ensure that it is functioning optimally. TCD fulfils the role very effectively.

The most common problems include inadvertent kinking (which is usually transient and clinically irrelevant), but the shunt lumen can occasionally impinge on the vessel wall and occlude distal flow. The latter follows overinflation of the shunt balloon or, more commonly, impaction of the shunt tip against a distal carotid artery loop or kink (Fig. 24.1; see plate section). We have also observed 2 patients in our last 500 CEAs in whom we had preferentially to shunt the external carotid artery in order to obtain satisfactory MCA flow. We aim to maintain mean blood flow velocity in the MCA > 15cm/s, which is equivalent to the threshold for loss of cerebral electrical activity.[29] If, following shunt insertion, MCA velocity was less than this, we would first partially deflate the proximal and/or distal shunt balloons, followed by repositioning of the distal shunt tip. Special care is taken to ensure that a distal carotid loop is not occluding flow. In a prospective study in 550 patients (unpublished data), only 2% of patients have had an MCA velocity < 15cm/s after repositioning and checking the shunt. In each case, however, velocities increased to > 15cm/s following therapeutic elevation of blood pressure.

Luminal Thrombus and Intimal Flaps

While it is well recognized that distal intimal flaps can predispose towards postoperative stroke, the fact that thrombus can form undetected within the endarterectomy zone and subsequently embolize with flow restoration has been treated with scepticism. In a preliminary pilot study, however, Gaunt *et al.* showed that luminal thrombi (> 3mm) remained undetected and adherent to the endarterectomy zone in 4% of their patients despite flushing with heparinized saline.[25] The source of the thrombus was subsequently found to be bleeding from the vasa vasorum on to the highly thrombogenic endarterectomized surface.[30]

There are a number of methods for detecting these thrombi (Table 24.3). We currently prefer to use completion angioscopy (Figs 24.2 and 24.3) because it is performed *before* flow restoration (Fig. 24.4; see plate section), thereby enabling immediate detection and removal of thrombus (Figs 24.5; see plate section and 24.6; see plate section). With angiography and duplex, there is the ever-present risk that embolization might occur with flow restoration. All three methods are effective at detecting intimal flaps. In practice, we have only had to revise < 4% of distal anastomoses following angioscopy but 4% will have thrombus removed prior to restoration of flow. In practice, it is not necessary to take down the anastomosis in order to remove thrombus, as this can easily be done with repeated irrigation and direct suction. Since

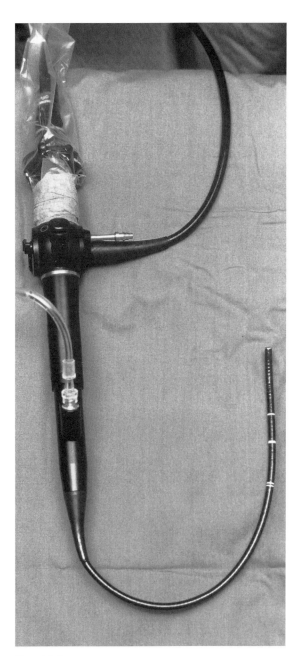

Fig. 24.2
A flexible hysteroscope with irrigation channel is used to inspect the lumen of the endarterectomy zone prior to restoration of flow. We previously used a multifibre angioscope, but the light fibres tended to break.

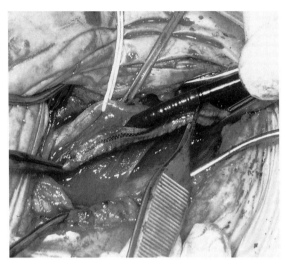

Fig. 24.3
The hysteroscope is introduced through a 5mm
defect in the patch closure, usually adjacent to the
origin of the external carotid artery.

introducing our programme of completion
angioscopy and intraoperative TCD, the rate of
intraoperative stroke (i.e. apparent upon
recovery from anaesthesia) has fallen from 4% to
0.3%.[30]

Residual Stenoses

This comprises two forms. The detection of
significant residual disease sufficient to cause a
detectable stenosis (i.e. due to the original
atheromatous process) should not occur because it
implies that the endarterectomy was not
performed properly. Although it may
occasionally be preferable to leave distal mural
plaques, the need to leave significant residual
disease implies either inexperience (i.e. reluctance
to proceed to a high dissection) or poor
preoperative work-up.

The second type of stenosis occurs during
arteriotomy closure and is commoner with
primarily as opposed to patch-closed
arteriotomies.[31] Clinically important stenoses (i.e.
> 30%) can be detected by angiography, duplex
and continuous-wave Doppler (angioscopy is
probably less effective in this situation) and the
distal anastomosis revised accordingly. In our
hands, we have had more problems with intimal
flaps and luminal thrombus than distal stenoses,
possibly because our routine use of a shunt acted
as a stent for closure.

CONCLUSIONS

If one adopts the fatalistic approach – perioperative
strokes are either not preventable or prevention is not
worth the effort – patients as a whole will not receive
the true benefit from the operation. It is a salutary
fact that, despite its long-term effectiveness, more
than 100 000 patients worldwide will have suffered
an operation-related stroke since the introduction of
CEA in 1953.

Although the international trials have
demonstrated a role for CEA, it is incumbent upon
surgeons everywhere to quote their *own* results
when discussing risks with their patients. Each unit
must therefore regularly review its outcomes and
ask itself whether they remain within accepted
limits (preferably < 5% for death and/or any stroke
rate), and whether they might be improved.

The Leicester monitoring protocol has evolved
over the last 7 years (> 800 CEAs) and is based on
the following observations. First, although there is a
plethora of causes of operation-related stroke,
thromboembolism predominates. Second, although
it may be a hard concept for surgeons to accept,
inadvertent technical error remains an important
predisposing factor. Third, it is always easier to
prevent a stroke rather than treat it. Fourth, no single
monitoring or quality control technique is infallible
and thus the final choice must reflect a compromise
between idealism and reality. Finally, surgeons must
stop using the ongoing controversies regarding
patches, shunts and monitoring methods as a
scapegoat for complications should they arise.
Monitoring and quality control assessment will only
help the surgeon if the right questions are asked!

Our choice of monitoring therefore reflects a
desire to identify and prevent problems before they
arise, rather than taking action once trouble has
started. We therefore use intraoperative TCD, where
possible, in order to detect spontaneous
embolization, to ensure optimal shunt function and
to identify the small number of patients at risk of

suffering an on-table carotid thrombosis. Completion angioscopy is primarily used to identify residual mural thrombus but large intimal flaps (> 3mm) are repaired. TCD monitoring is restarted in the recovery room and/or high-dependency unit for 3h following restoration of flow in order to identify those at risk of thrombosis.

Since this combined protocol was implemented in 1995, 500 patients have undergone CEA. The rate of intraoperative stroke has fallen from 4% to 0.2%, while the incidence of postoperative thrombotic stroke has fallen from 3% to 0%. Overall, there has been a 60% decrease in the 30-day risk of stroke or death, from 6% to 2.25%,[27] despite the fact that more than 50% of the operations were performed by trainees under supervision. It is our firm belief that a carefully planned strategy of monitoring and quality control assessment has contributed towards this sustained improvement.

REFERENCES

1 Naylor AR. Prevention of operation related stroke: are we asking the right questions? *Cardiovascular Surgery* 1999; **7**: 155–157.

2 Krul JM, van Gijn J, Ackerstaff RG, Eikelboom BC, Theodorides T, Vermeulen FE. Site and pathogenesis of infarcts associated with carotid endarterectomy. *Stroke* 1989; **20**: 324–328.

3 Riles TS, Imparato AM, Jacobowitz GR et al. The cause of peri-operative stroke after carotid endarterectomy. *Journal of Vascular Surgery* 1994; **19**: 206–214.

4 European Carotid Surgery Trialists' Collaborative Group. Randomised trial of endarterectomy for recently symptomatic carotid stenosis: final results of the MRC European Carotid Surgery Trial (ECST). *Lancet* 1998; **351**: 1379–1387.

5 Barnett HJM, Taylor DW, Eliasziw M et al. Benefit of carotid endarterectomy in patients with symptomatic moderate or severe stenosis. *New England Journal of Medicine* 1998; **339**: 1415–1425.

6 Moore WS, Young B, Baker WH et al. Surgical results: a justification of the surgeon selection process for the ACAS Trial. The ACAS investigators. *Journal of Vascular Surgery* 1996; **23**: 323–328.

7 Hsai DC, Krushat WM, Moscoe LM. Epidemiology of carotid endarterectomy among Medicare beneficiaries. *Journal of Vascular Surgery* 1992; **16**: 201–208.

8 Hsai DC, Krushat WM, Moscoe LM. Epidemiology of carotid endarterectomy among Medicare beneficiaries: 1985–1996 update. *Stroke* 1998; **29**: 346–350.

9 CAVATAS Investigators. Results of the Carotid and Vertebral Artery Transluminal Angioplasty Study (CAVATAS). Proceedings of the Annual Vascular Society Meeting of Great Britain and Ireland (Hull, November 1998).

10 Wennberg DE, Lucas FL, Birkmeyer JD, Bredenberg CE, Fisher ES. Variation in carotid endarterectomy mortality in the Medicare population. *Journal of the American Medical Association* 1998; **279**: 1278–1281.

11 Karp HR, Flanders D, Shipp CC, Taylor B, Martin D. Carotid endarterectomy among Medicare beneficiaries: a statewide evaluation of appropriateness and outcome. *Stroke* 1998; **29**: 46–52.

12 Astrup J, Siesjo BK, Symon L. Thresholds in cerebral ischaemia: the ischaemic penumbra. *Stroke* 1981; **12**: 723–725.

13 Smith JL, Evans D, Fan L et al. Interpretation of embolic phenomena during carotid endarterectomy. *Stroke* 1995; **26**: 2281–2284.

14 Spencer MP. Transcranial Doppler monitoring and causes of stroke from carotid endarterectomy. *Stroke* 1997; **28**: 685–691.

15 Smith JL, Evans DH, Naylor AR. Differentiation between emboli and artefacts using dual gated transcranial Doppler ultrasound. *Ultrasound Medicine and Biology* 1996; **22**: 1031–1036.

16 Gaunt ME, Martin PJ, Smith JL et al. The clinical relevance of intra-operative embolisation detected by transcranial Doppler monitoring during carotid endarterectomy: a prospective study in 100 patients. *British Journal of Surgery* 1994; **81**: 1435–1439.

17 Ackerstaff RG, Jansen C, Moll FL, Vermeulen FE, Hamerlijnck RP, Mauser HW. The significance of microemboli detection by means of transcranial Doppler ultrasonography monitoring in carotid endarterectomy. *Journal of Vascular Surgery* 1995; **21**: 963–969.

18 Cantelmo NL, Babikian VL, Samaraweera RN, Gordon JK, Pochay VE, Winter MR. Cerebral microembolism and ischaemia changes associated with carotid endarterectomy. *Journal of Vascular Surgery* 1998; **27**: 1024–1030.

19 Gaunt ME, Brown L, Hartshorne T, Thrush A, Bell PRF, Naylor AR. Unstable carotid plaques: preoperative identification and association with intra-operative embolisation detected by transcranial Doppler. *European Journal of Vascular and Endovascular Surgery* 1996; **11**: 78–82.

20 Smith JL, Goodall S, Evans D, London NJM, Bell PRF, Naylor AR. Experience with transcranial Doppler reduces the incidence of embolisation during carotid endarterectomy. *British Journal of Surgery* 1998; **85**: 56–59.

21 Naylor AR, Thompson MM, Varty K, Sayers RD, London NJM, Bell PRF. Provision of training in carotid surgery does not compromise patient safety. *British Journal of Surgery* 1998; **85**: 939–942.

22 Blaisdell FW, Lim R, Hall AD. Technical result of carotid endarterectomy: arteriographic assessment. *American Journal of Surgery* 1967; **114**: 239–245.

23 Stratton JR, Zierler ZE, Kazmers A. Platelet deposition at carotid endarterectomy sites in humans. *Stroke* 1987; **18**: 722–727.

24 Gaunt ME, Smith J, Martin PJ, Ratliff DA, Bell PRF, Naylor AR. On-table diagnosis of incipient carotid artery thrombosis during carotid endarterectomy using transcranial Doppler sonography. *Journal of Vascular Surgery* 1994; **20**: 104–107.

25 Gaunt ME, Smith JL, Martin PJ, Ratliff DA, Bell PRF, Naylor AR. A comparison of quality control methods applied to carotid endarterectomy. *European Journal of Vascular and Endovascular Surgery* 1996; **11**: 4–11.

26 Levi CR, O'Malley HM, Fell G *et al.* Transcranial Doppler detected cerebral embolism following carotid endarterectomy: high microembolic signal loads predict post-operative cerebral ischaemia. *Brain* 1997; **120**: 621–629.

27 Naylor AR, Hayes PD, Allroggen H *et al.* Reducing the risk of carotid surgery: a seven year audit of the role of monitoring and quality control assessment. *Journal of Vascular Surgery* (in press).

28 Ghali R, Palazzo EG, Rodriguez DI *et al.* Transcranial Doppler intra-operative monitoring during carotid endarterectomy: experience with regional or general anaesthesia, with and without shunting. *Annals of Vascular Surgery* 1997; **11**: 9–13.

29 Halsey JH, McDowell HA, Gelmon S, Morawetz RB. Blood flow velocity in the middle cerebral artery and regional cerebral blood flow during carotid endarterectomy. *Stroke* 1989; **20**: 53–58.

30 Lennard N, Smith JL, Gaunt ME *et al.* A policy of quality control assessment reduces the risk of intra-operative stroke during carotid endarterectomy. *European Journal of Vascular and Endovascular Surgery* 1999; **17**: 234–240.

31 Counsell C, Salinas R, Naylor AR, Warlow CP. A systematic review of the randomised trials of carotid patch angioplasty in carotid endarterectomy. *European Journal of Vascular and Endovascular Surgery* 1997; **13**: 345–354.

Is there any evidence that perioperative monitoring and quality control assessment alter clinical outcome?
D Preston Flanigan (USA)

INTRODUCTION

Ever since the first elective CEA was performed, vascular surgeons have been striving to perfect the procedure. This striving for perfection has included the selection of appropriate patients for the procedure and the quest for technical excellence. The selection of appropriate patients as it relates to operative complications is mostly resolved for elective CEA. It is now generally accepted that the totally occluded carotid artery should not be operated upon and most would agree that patients with acute stroke older than 2h with significant neurologic deficits should be managed non-operatively. With the recent conduction of the many prospective randomized trials, many of the questions regarding patient selection relative to percent stenosis have been significantly addressed, although some unanswered questions remain.[32–34] These remaining questions will hopefully be answered satisfactorily when all arms of the studies are completed. Once patient selection is perfected, the main remaining obstacle to a complication-free procedure will be technical misadventure.

The significant complications of CEA include cranial nerve injury, stroke, and death. Deaths as a result of the procedure are most commonly from stroke, cardiac complications, or operative complications such as neck hematomas. Diligent preoperative cardiac evaluation coupled with modern techniques of perioperative cardiac monitoring has probably reduced cardiac mortality from the procedure. Neck hematomas and cranial nerve injuries are primarily technical errors and can be reduced by meticulous operative technique. Stroke is primarily caused by technical errors at the time of

surgery. If technical errors during the procedure can be eliminated, then the incidence of stroke and death associated with the procedure should plummet.

Technical errors are of several types and are thought to include excessive manipulation of the artery during dissection with resultant embolization; inadequate cerebral circulation because of failure to provide cerebral protection through shunting; malfunctioning shunts; embolization at the time of shunt insertion or removal; and embolization from inadequate flushing and improper sequence of flow restoration. Thrombosis and embolization may also occur in the intraoperative and postoperative periods as a result of retained thrombi, strictures, or intimal flaps. It is these latter technical defects that may be found and corrected using intraoperative assessment.

Although many technical points of the operative procedure remain controversial, this author believes that the bulk of the available evidence indicates that the elements providing for the safest operation include performing minimal manipulation of the artery during dissection; clamping the internal carotid artery first, making sure the arteriotomy extends proximal and distal to all plaque whenever possible; routinely using a T-type indwelling shunt to provide cerebral protection and to allow adequate flushing to prevent embolization; performing a meticulous endarterectomy without the need for tacking sutures unless absolutely necessary; routine patching of the artery, except possibly in males with very large internal carotid arteries; using meticulous flushing before and after shunt removal; and re-establishing flow to the ECA first. These technical standards have evolved over the roughly 45 years that the procedure has been performed and are, for the most part, agreed upon by most vascular surgeons, except for some minor disagreements regarding patching, shunting, and the optimal type of anesthesia. Nevertheless, despite the widespread application of these evolved standards, stroke rates continue to be reported at alarmingly high rates.[35] These higher than desired stroke rates have driven vascular surgeons to find additional ways to improve on the technical results of CEA.

HISTORY OF INTRAOPERATIVE ASSESSMENT

In 1967 Blaisdell et al. reported on the use of completion intraoperative arteriography to assess the technical results of CEA. In this report the incidence of technical error was 26%.[36] Although many of these errors resulted in only strictures, the report pointed out the inability of clinical examination reliably to detect technical errors in many patients. Despite this report, completion arteriography for CEA did not become widely utilized. Although other reports substantiated Blaisdell's report, there were also reports of complications from intraoperative arteriography which may have, in part, discouraged the utilization of the technique.[37,38]

In an effort to discover safer and more easily applied methods of intraoperative assessment, attention turned toward the use of intraoperative ultrasound. Initially, continuous-wave Doppler was employed. This technique allowed the detection of flow disturbances but was not a good tool for quantification of the abnormality or for identifying the type of defect present. Objective criteria were never established.

In 1984 Zierler et al.[39] reported on the use of combined pulsed Doppler and spectral analysis to identify technical defects. This method was sensitive in the detection of defects but had the shortcoming of the inability to identify the type of defect, thus limiting the role of the technique in the decision process regarding criteria for re-exploration. Nevertheless, this report provided a big step forward

in the ability to detect, non-invasively, technical errors occurring during CEA.

In 1986, Flanigan et al.[40] reported on 155 CEAs assessed by intraoperative imaging ultrasound. Technical defects were detected in 27.7% of the procedures and included intimal flaps (73%), strictures (18%), and arterial kinks, residual plaque, and intraluminal thrombi (9% collectively). This incidence of technical error was similar to that found by Blaisdell et al. using intraoperative arteriography 19 years earlier.[36]

Like many other studies, these answered questions and created new questions. It seemed inappropriate to repair all lesions detected since many were minor and probably insignificant. Reopening the artery would be expected to increase the chance of stroke and should not be performed unnecessarily. The decision on which defects to correct was empirical. In the study of Flanigan et al.[40] 7% of the arteries (26% of those with defects) were re-entered and defects were found and corrected. The incidence of stroke in this group was similar to that found in patients who had normal intraoperative ultrasound results (3.3% vs 3.8% respectively). No patient thought to have a significant technical defect was left unrepaired for comparison purposes.

At this time it would probably be unethical to conduct a study in which some defects are randomly left unrepaired for the purpose of determining which defects require repair. In Flanigan's study, data analysis suggested that intimal flaps ˝ 1mm in the internal carotid artery, 1–3mm intimal flaps in the common and external carotid arteries, and strictures less than 30% can be safely left uncorrected.

The decision to correct a defect should not only consider the immediate effect as regards the risk of stroke but also the long-term effects as regards restenosis of the artery. Using the criteria previously described by Flanigan, Sawchuk et al.[41] followed 80 carotid endarterectomies, of which 21 had unrepaired defects, with serial postoperative duplex ultrasound scans for 1–96 months. Seventeen of 19 intimal flaps healed and 2 of 2 strictures resolved. One 1-mm internal carotid flap was associated with a stable 30% stenosis and a 2-mm external carotid flap was associated with occlusion of the external carotid artery. These data suggested that the criteria empirically decided upon in Flanigan's study for correction of defects to prevent perioperative stroke were also applicable to the prevention of restenosis, although the criteria were far from proven.

In 1988, Schwartz et al.[42] reported on the use of intraoperative duplex ultrasound during CEA. They found defects in 22% of the arteries studied and defects were repaired in 11% of cases. These results were similar to results reported previously for arteriography, pulsed Doppler, and B-mode ultrasound.

For over 10 years now, this author has used intraoperative duplex scanning as the preferred method of intraoperative assessment not only for CEA but also for most vascular reconstructions. The technique has improved over the years as new probe design and higher-resolution equipment have become available. Specific to CEA, the hockey-stick design of the intraoperative probe has nearly eliminated the previous problem of not being able to insonate the most distal part of the reconstruction because of spatial limitations. With imaging ultrasound there was a problem with poor echogenicity of fresh clot. The application of newer duplex technology has compensated for this short-coming of older imaging ultrasound. The author has had experience with 3 patients now in whom the B-mode image was unremarkable but color flow Doppler and velocity measurements detected significant defects.

TECHNIQUE OF INTRAOPERATIVE DUPLEX SCANNING

The technique of intraoperative duplex scanning is easily learned and takes only a few minutes of operating time. The ultrasound technologist places a non-sterile 10MHz probe into a sterile condom into which sterile or non-sterile acoustic gel has been placed. The probe should be placed so that no air bubbles are present as they will generate artifacts in the image. The patient is positioned so that saline will remain in the neck wound. The common,

internal, and external carotid arteries are then imaged in B mode looking for any defects. Color flow is then employed to look at the same areas. Velocity measurements are then measured in all three vessels at an angle as close to 60° as possible. Particular attention is paid to the velocity just past the distal end-point of the endarterectomy. Criteria for analysis are discussed below. If a defect is seen that is judged to warrant repair, repair is performed, after which the ultrasound exam is repeated. If the velocity measurements are abnormal but no defect is visualized, an intraoperative arteriogram is obtained. If a patch closure is used, it is important to consider the patch material if duplex scanning is to be employed. Good images can be obtained through patches of vein or bovine pericardium. Satisfactory images can usually be obtained through patches of thin-walled polytetrafluoroethylene (PTFE) or Dacron. Scans are often unsatisfactory when insonating through regular-wall PTFE or Dacron.

Strict criteria for interpreting intraoperative velocity data obtained from duplex scans are lacking. From available data, however, it appears that the same criteria used for transcutaneous measurements of carotid velocities are applicable to intraoperative studies.[43] Values in excess of 120cm/s are considered abnormal. When abnormal-velocity data are obtained in the face of a normal B-mode image, arteriography is probably indicated. The other indication for intraoperative arteriography is technical problems leading to an incomplete or suboptimal duplex scan.

CLINICAL OUTCOMES

Numerous reports have documented the incidence of technical imperfection during the performance of CEA (Table 24.5). It is striking to note that the incidence (average = 25%) has changed little since the report by Blaisdell et al. in 1967[36] (26%). Despite this overwhelming evidence that vascular surgeons make numerous technical errors in performing this procedure, questions still remain as to whether or not intraoperative quality assurance makes any difference to the outcome of the procedure.

Table 24.5
Incidence of total intraoperative defects found and defects repaired

Author	Technique	Defects found	Defects repaired
Baker et al.[44]	Duplex	62/316 (19.6%)	9/316 (3%)
Dorffner et al.[45]	Duplex	19/50 (38%)	9/50 (18%)
Flanigan et al.[40]	B-mode	43/155 (27.7%)	11/155 (7%)
Hoff et al.[46]	Duplex	6/16 (37.5%)	NA
Papanicolaou et al.[43]	Duplex	10/78 (11%)	10/78 (11%)
Sawchuk et al.[41]	B-mode	18/80 (22.5%)	NA
Schwartz et al.[42]	Duplex	17/84 (22%)	8/84 (11%)
Scott et al.[48]	Arteriography	56/170 (52%)	12/107 (11%)
Walker et al.[47]	Duplex	21/50 (42%)	3/50 (6%)

There are numerous reasons why the effectiveness of intraoperative assessment of technical results is unlikely to be proven conclusively. Probably the most significant reason is the already low stroke rate associated with CEA. Because of this low stroke rate, the number of patients included in such a study would need to be quite large. Also, in order to answer the question of which defects should be corrected, there would need to be a group of patients in whom defects detected by intraoperative duplex scanning would be left uncorrected. This fact would raise ethical questions that would most likely preclude such a study from being performed.

Despite these limitations, there is evidence, both direct and indirect, that intraoperative assessment does decrease the incidence of perioperative stroke in patients having CEA. Scott et al.[48] evaluated two consecutive groups of patients having CEA. In the first group of 146 procedures, the perioperative stroke rate was 6.8% and the mortality rate was 4.8%. In a second group of 107 procedures, intraoperative arteriography was performed. Fifty-two percent of the arteriograms showed defects. In this latter group of 107 procedures, the incidence of stroke was 3.6% and the mortality was 1.5%. The difference was attributed to 12 patients in whom significant defects were detected and corrected in the internal carotid artery. Repeat intraoperative arteriograms in these patients were all normal. The differences were not significantly different, but this could have been due to an insufficient number of patients.

Roon[49] compared 157 procedures performed without intraoperative arteriography to 535 procedures using intraoperative carotid arteriography. The group having intraoperative arteriography had a significantly lower stroke rate than the group not having ($P < 0.01$). Also there was a statistically significant difference in the incidence of reoperations for recurrent stenosis in favor of the group having intraoperative arteriography ($P < 0.01$).

Baker et al.[44] found that patients having intraoperative minor defects which were left uncorrected had a significantly higher incidence of restenosis (> 75%) than those in whom defects detected by intraoperative ultrasound were repaired ($P < 0.001$, 17% vs 4.3%).

Dykes et al.[50] reported a statistically significant reduction in residual stenosis following CEA in patients having intraoperative duplex scanning ($P < 0.05$). These authors also reported a lower stroke rate for the group undergoing intraoperative duplex scanning, but the difference was not significant.

Kinney et al.[51] found an increase in the postoperative incidence of internal carotid stenosis or occlusion in patients with uncorrected residual flow abnormality or no intraoperative study compared to those in whom defects were corrected or having a

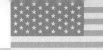

normal study ($P < 0.007$). Also, patients with normal intraoperative studies had a lower incidence of late ipsilateral stroke compared to the remaining patient cohort.

Courbier et al.[52] reduced the incidence of perioperative stroke from 1.9% to 1% through the use of intraoperative arteriography, in a study comparing 206 patients not undergoing intraoperative arteriography to 100 patients subjected to this procedure. A lower incidence of restenosis was demonstrated in patients with no or minimal residual defects when arteriograms were performed 1 year later.

CONCLUSIONS

These contemporary studies show rather conclusively that intraoperative assessment decreases the incidence of residual and recurrent stenosis. They also strongly suggest a lowering of the perioperative stroke rate. From a deductive reasoning standpoint, it seems more than reasonable to assume that, if the incidence of significant unrepaired technical defects can be reduced – which it clearly can be through the application of intraoperative duplex scanning or arteriography – then a decrease in the incidence of perioperative stroke would follow.

Intraoperative quality assurance for CEA does, indeed, alter clinical outcome.

REFERENCES

32 North American Symptomatic Carotid Endarterectomy Trial Collaborators. Beneficial effect of carotid endarterectomy in symptomatic patients with high-grade carotid stenosis. *New England Journal of Medicine* 1991; **325**: 445–453.

33 Executive Committee for the Asymptomatic Carotid Atherosclerosis Study. Endarterectomy for asymptomatic carotid artery stenosis. *Journal of the American Medical Association* 1971; **273**: 1421–1428.

34 European Carotid Surgery Trialists' Collaborative Group. MRC European carotid surgery trial: interim results for symptomatic patients with severe (70–99%) or with mild (0–29%) carotid stenosis. *Lancet* 1985; **337**: 1235–1243.

35 Moore WS. Extracranial cerebrovascular disease: the carotid artery. In: Moore WS (ed.) *Vascular Surgery: A Comprehensive Review*, 5th edn, pp. 555–597. Philadelphia: WB Saunders, 1998.

36 Blaisdell FW, Lim R, Hall AD. Technical result of carotid endarterectomy. *American Journal of Surgery* 1967; **114**: 239–245.

37 Anderson CA, Collins GJ, Rich NM. Routine operative arteriography during carotid endarterectomy: a reassessment. *Surgery* 1978; **83**: 67–71.

38 Ansell G. Adverse reactions to contrast agents: scope of the problem. *Investigative Radiology* 1970; **5**: 373–384.

39 Zierler RE, Bandyk DF, Thiele BL. Intraoperative assessment of carotid endarterectomy. *Journal of Vascular Surgery* 1984; **1**: 73–83.

40 Flanigan DP, Douglas DJ, Machi J et al. Intraoperative ultrasonic imaging of the carotid artery during carotid endarterectomy. *Surgery* 1986; **100**: 893–898.

41 Sawchuk AP, Flanigan DP, Machi J et al. The fate of unrepaired minor technical defects by intraoperative ultrasonography during carotid endarterectomy. *Journal of Vascular Surgery* 1989; **9**: 671–679.

42 Schwartz RA, Peterson GJ, Noland KA et al. Intraoperative duplex scanning after carotid artery reconstruction: a valuable tool. *Journal of Vascular Surgery* 1988; **7**: 620–628.

43 Papanicolaou G, Toms C, Yellin AE et al. Relationship between intraoperative color-flow duplex findings and early restenosis after carotid endarterectomy: a preliminary report. *Journal of Vascular Surgery* 1996; **24**: 588–595.

44 Baker WH, Koustas G, Littooy FN et al. Intraoperative duplex scanning and late carotid artery stenosis. *Journal of Vascular Surgery* 1994; **19**: 829–832.

45 Dorffner R, Metz VM, Tratting S et al. Intraoperative and early postoperative colour Doppler sonography after carotid artery reconstruction: follow-up of technical defects. *Neuroradiology* 1997; **39**: 117–121.

46 Hoff C, de Gier P, Buth J. Intraoperative duplex monitoring of the carotid bifurcation for the detection of technical defects. *European Journal of Vascular Surgery* 1994; **8**: 441–447.

47 Walker RA, Fox AD, Magee TR et al. Intraoperative duplex scanning as a means of quality control during carotid endarterectomy. *European Journal of Vascular Surgery* 1996; **11**: 364–367.

48 Scott SM, Sethi GK, Bridgeman AH. Perioperative stroke during carotid endarterectomy: the value of intraoperative angiography. *Journal of Cardiovascular Surgery* 1982; **23**: 353–358.

49 Roon AJ, Hoogerwerf D. Intraoperative arteriography and carotid surgery. *Journal of Vascular Surgery* 1992; **16**: 239–243.

50 Dykes JR 2nd, Bergamini TM, Lipski DA et al. Intraoperative duplex scanning reduces both residual stenosis and postoperative morbidity of carotid

endarterectomy. *American Surgeon* 1997; **63**: 50–54.

51 Kinney EV, Seabrook GR, Kinny LY *et al*. The importance of intraoperative detection of residual flow abnormalities after carotid artery endarterectomy. *Journal of Vascular Surgery* 1993; **17**: 912–923.

52 Courbier R, Jausseran J, Reggi M *et al*. Routine intraoperative carotid angiography: its impact on operative morbidity and carotid restenosis. *Journal of Vascular Surgery* 1986; **3**: 343–350.

Editorial Comment

KEY POINTS

1 There is no randomized trial evidence that a policy of quality control or intraoperative monitoring alters outcome.
2 Each surgeon should, however, be aware of his or her own operative stroke risk. If it is too high, monitoring or quality control assessment may improve outcomes.
3 No single monitoring or quality control technique is infallible.
4 Surgeons should stop blaming the shunt, patch, or monitoring modality for perioperative strokes. Each provides specific information or benefit, but none will prevent a stroke due to undiagnosed technical error.

A number of centers have reported excellent CEA results without using any form of monitoring and, somewhat predictably, this has been used by others as an argument against its use. However, a 1–2% operative risk is not the overall norm in Europe and North America and evidence suggests that outcomes may be significantly worse than those reported in the randomized trials. This should not come as a surprise, as > 90% of CEAs are now performed in non-trial hospitals. Thus, if we are to reduce the operative risk to levels at or below those observed in the randomized trials, it is important to consider all reasonable options, including the concept of intraoperative monitoring and quality control assessment.

Both authors make strong arguments for the adoption of monitoring and quality control protocols to reduce the incidence of perioperative stroke. Flanigan advocates routine use of intraoperative duplex assessment, while Naylor advocates completion angioscopy. Clearly, there is no evidence to indicate that one is superior to the other, but the advantage of angioscopy is that it is performed before restoration of flow so intraluminal thrombus can be identified and removed. It is important to note that some technical defects detected by either modality might be insignificant. However, the fact that intraoperative stroke rates were significantly reduced using either of these methods proves their utility. More clearly defined criteria are required in the future so as to avoid unnecessary re-exploration.

Until recently, duplex probes were too cumbersome for use in the limited space afforded by the standard carotid incision, although this has now been improved by L-shaped probes. In addition, synthetic patches significantly interfere with the ability of duplex ultrasound to image for small defects and some centers will find it difficult to arrange for the duplex technologist and equipment to be brought to the operating room whenever required. Few hospitals today can afford to have a state-of-the-art duplex unit dedicated solely to operating room use. Transcranial Doppler monitoring involves a significant learning curve but is otherwise an easy monitoring method to use and interpret. Its main intraoperative use is in warning of spontaneous embolization and for monitoring shunt function. However, its ability to predict those at risk of suffering a postoperative carotid thrombosis and thereafter guide therapy or surgery is probably its most important potential role. While routine postoperative TCD monitoring is unlikely to become universally accepted, it may be possible to use it in

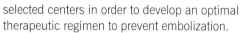

selected centers in order to develop an optimal therapeutic regimen to prevent embolization.

What then is the ideal quality control and monitoring protocol? The answer is that any one of several is justified, as long as it is strictly followed and results in a minimal perioperative stroke rate. Every surgeon performing CEA must look critically at his or her own results. In centers where the operative risk is $< 4\%$ in symptomatic patients and $< 2\%$ in asymptomatic patients, changes in practice are unnecessary. For surgeons with higher complication rates, merely to dismiss the concept of monitoring and quality control assessment because others can achieve stroke rates of $1-2\%$ without using them is not acceptable.

25.1

Is there a role for carotid angioplasty or stenting?
Jonathan D Beard (Europe)

INTRODUCTION

Randomized trials have demonstrated a clear benefit for carotid endarterectomy (CEA) in symptomatic patients with a severe stenosis while asymptomatic patients may reap a small benefit. Neurologists now question whether endovascular intervention can produce the same benefit, based on their philosophy that 'medicine aims to avoid surgery'. Percutaneous transluminal balloon angioplasty has become a well-established procedure for the treatment of peripheral arterial disease. However, using it to treat a carotid artery stenosis has come about only recently. Technically, angioplasty of a short stenosis in a relatively large high-flow carotid vessel should produce good results, as the situation seems analogous to the iliac vessels (Fig. 25.1).

Interventional radiologists and cardiologists, especially in North America, have also embraced angioplasty and stenting enthusiastically for financial reasons. However, speciality partisanship seems a poor basis for recommending a new treatment. A world of difference may exist between the endovascular treatment of a lesion which causes morbidity due to emboli, and that of the majority of other arterial stenoses that produce symptoms by limiting flow.

POTENTIAL ADVANTAGES

Patients will naturally prefer an endovascular intervention to an operation that requires an incision. However, patient preference will depend on reassurance that the endovascular procedure is very safe and efficacious. They need to know that carotid angioplasty has yet to achieve full validity regarding safety and efficacy in order to avoid a future backlash from the press and patients' associations,

as occurred after the unchecked introduction of laparoscopic interventions.

The standard transfemoral approach increases the technical difficulty of the procedure due to the distance from the carotid artery. Direct puncture of the common carotid artery aids guidewire and catheter manipulation, but risks embolization and neck haematoma.[1] The carotid occlusion time is short, as most radiologists only inflate the angioplasty balloon for 1 min or less, but no evidence exists to suggest that this results in a lower incidence of intraoperative haemodynamic stroke.

Neurologists frequently quote cranial nerve injuries as a reason for avoiding surgery. Up to 50% of patients may suffer some degree of cranial nerve injury,[2] but most such injuries seem transitory and resolve within a few days. The area of cutaneous numbness anterior to the scar also diminishes with time and does not usually cause long-term problems.

The other quoted advantages of carotid angioplasty include a shorter recovery time and lower cost. This may be true for major vascular procedures such as coronary bypass or aortobifemoral bypass, but probably not for CEA, which represents a relatively safe and inexpensive procedure. Indeed, a recent comparative study found no difference between balloon angioplasty and stenting versus CEA in terms of the length of hospitalization or total costs.[3]

POTENTIAL HAZARDS

The risk of embolization following angioplasty remains the principal concern of any surgeon who has seen the soft 'porridge-like' plaques inside carotid arteries. Cerebral emboli, detected by transcranial Doppler (TCD) during conventional CEA,

315

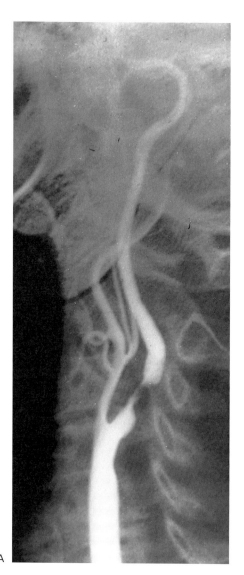 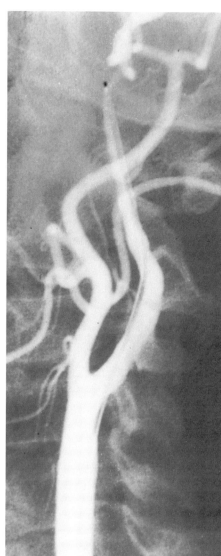

A

B

Fig. 25.1
Tight stenosis of the internal carotid artery successfully treated by balloon dilatation (A) without the need for stenting (B).

can cause stroke[4] as well as cognitive impairment. In Sheffield, all carotid angioplasties and endarterectomies undergo monitoring with TCD. Cerebral emboli always occur during angioplasty and in far greater numbers than associated with CEA (Fig. 25.2). This probably accounts for the 6% incidence of transient ischaemic attacks (TIAs) that we have observed during angioplasty. Plaque characterization may help identify those stenoses that have a low risk of embolization[5] but the techniques, as yet, remain unvalidated.

Two techniques might reduce the risk of cerebral embolization: use of protective balloons and stents respectively. Theron et al.[6] reported a series of 259 carotid angioplasties performed since 1984. A total of 174 patients received treatment for an atherosclerotic stenosis of the carotid bifurcation or internal carotid artery. The first 38 angioplasties without cerebral protection resulted in a dissection rate of 5% and an embolic complication rate of 8%. In 1987 they introduced a cerebral protection system, where a balloon is mounted on the end of a

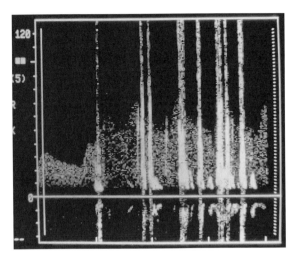

Fig. 25.2
Transcranial Doppler signal from the middle cerebral artery demonstrating multiple emboli on deflation of the angioplasty balloon.

guiding catheter and positioned beyond the stenosis via a triple-lumen catheter. This balloon is then inflated prior to angioplasty. After withdrawing the angioplasty balloon, any debris is aspirated and the artery is flushed with saline before deflating the distal protection balloon. Since introducing this revised technique, Theron et al. have reported a 5% dissection rate but no embolic complications. Since 1990, this group has also used stents in 65 out of 93 cases when the result appeared suboptimal after angioplasty alone. This resulted in no dissections and a 2% rate of embolic complications. Kachel[7] has also reported a low risk of embolic complications using a similar cerebral protection system (2 strokes and 1 TIA in 60 cases of internal carotid angioplasty without the use of stents).

The Theron protection balloon passes across the stenosis without a guidewire. This increases the risk of dissection and embolization before inflation of the protective balloon. Development of guidewires with integral low-profile balloons or filters continues but some have described stroke caused by a dissection of a high-grade stenosis by the guidewire alone.[8] Use of a protective balloon increases the carotid occlusion time and the risk of cerebral ischaemia.[9] Cerebral embolization can occur via the external

carotid collaterals, even with the balloon inflated.

Primary stenting may reduce embolization by trapping the atheroma against the wall of the artery but, conversely, passage of a stent across the stenosis may increase the risk of embolization. Furthermore, the use of a stent increases the cost of the procedure and balloon expandable stents can become crushed by pressure on the neck. Roubin et al. have reported stent deformation in 8 of 69 Palmaz stents[10] and the same problem has occurred with Strecker stents.[11] If a stent becomes necessary because of a suboptimal result after angioplasty, it seems sensible to use a self-expanding stent such as the Memotherm or Wallstent.

Although the early results of endovascular carotid intervention have received widespread attention, the incidence of restenosis due to myointimal hyperplasia seems less well documented but appears to be higher than that reported after CEA. Gil-Peralta et al.[12] reported a 25% restenosis rate at 12 months after angioplasty alone. Stents may lower the short-term restenosis rate and Yadav et al.[13] described a 5% restenosis rate at 6 months using stents routinely. Similarly, Theron et al.[6] reported a higher restenosis rate of 16% in patients treated by angioplasty, as compared to only 4% once stents were introduced. However, in Sheffield we have found little difference in the longer-term restenosis rates between angioplasty and stenting. The Carotid And Vertebral Artery Transluminal Angioplasty Study (CAVATAS) has also found no difference in the rate of restenosis at 1 year following either surgery or angioplasty.[14]

The higher restenosis rates after endovascular treatment may not matter as the vast majority of carotid restenoses remain asymptomatic. Repeated dilatation remains the best treatment of symptomatic restenosis after angioplasty, but restenosis within stents does not respond at all well. Atherectomy would probably carry a high risk of cerebral embolization and so endarterectomy of the entire atheroma/ stent/hyperplasia complex may be the best option.[11]

EVIDENCE FOR ANGIOPLASTY AND STENTING?

The first reports of carotid angioplasty appeared in 1980.[15] The best represent prospective series of consecutive patients compared with a similar group of patients undergoing conventional endarterectomy at the same institution, with complete long-term follow-up. Unfortunately, the majority represent uncontrolled studies of small numbers of selected patients with ill-defined indications and inadequate follow-up, performed by doctors with little previous experience of managing patients with carotid disease.[16,17]

Dietrich et al. claimed that a stroke rate of 6.4% after carotid stenting bore comparison to the outcomes reported in the European Carotid Surgery Trial (ECST) and North American Symptomatic Carotid Endarterectomy Trial (NASCET).[18] However, another 4.5% of the 110 patents developed TIAs and the inclusion of asymptomatic stenoses accounted for a large proportion of procedures. Direct comparisons with the randomized trials can therefore mislead as they only included symptomatic patients and neurologists performed the follow-up. Many neurological deficits may go undiagnosed in the absence of neurological evaluation.[19] In this respect, it is interesting to observe that Yadav et al. reported a higher stroke and death rate of 10.8% after carotid stenting for 74 symptomatic patients where neurologists performed the evaluation.[13] We have treated 182 patients with 189 symptomatic atherosclerotic stenoses (50–99%) by angioplasty and stenting. We achieved a 30-day death and disabling stroke rate of 6.9%, as assessed by a neurologist, and this compares favourably with the results of the ECST and NASCET trials.

Even when comparing results within the same institution, analytical bias can arise. A recent presentation to the American Heart Association compared carotid stenting and CEA in patients over the age of 80.[20] One major stroke, three minor strokes and one death occurred in the 30 patients who underwent stenting compared to no strokes or deaths and three temporary cranial nerve palsies in the endarterectomy group. The authors concluded that: 'even though the stented patients had higher co-morbidity, the non-neurological complications were lower and the hospital stay was shorter'; a triumph of optimism over experience!

CAVATAS represents the only large randomized controlled trial of endovascular therapy for carotid disease, funded by the UK Medical Research Council.[21] Thirteen centres from around the world recruited 504 patients fit for carotid surgery between 1992 and 1997. Patients with symptomatic carotid stenoses > 50% underwent randomization to carotid endarterectomy (n = 253) or angioplasty/stenting (n = 251), according to the uncertainty principle used in the ECST trial.

The groups match well in terms of the indication for treatment and the severity of stenosis. On an intention-to-treat analysis, the 30-day death and any stroke rate showed no difference between the two groups (9.9% for surgery and 10% for endovascular treatment). Some have criticized these high complication rates, but almost half of the events took place after randomization and before treatment. This emphasizes the need to avoid delay between randomization and treatment in future trials. The lack of a record of eligible patients who did not enter the trial, and the reasons why, represents a more serious criticism, as selection bias might have occurred in some centres. Furthermore, 20 patients randomized to angioplasty crossed over to surgery or medical treatment due to treatment failure, and more than half of the 504 patients received treatment in just two centres. The preliminary data also suggest no difference in stroke-free survival at 3 years, despite a higher restenosis rate for angioplasty.

FUTURE TRIALS?

We have now entered an era of industry-sponsored trials of carotid stents. Although these trials seem carefully organized, with independent monitoring committees, they aim to produce a commercial product. For this reason they ignore the fact that no good evidence exists to support the need for primary stenting. In 1997, the American National Institutes of Health (NIH) received two proposals for randomized trials to compare CEA and carotid stenting: the Carotid Revascularization Endarterectomy versus Stent Trial (CREST) and the Carotid Artery Stenting versus Endarterectomy Trial (CASET). Funding for the CREST trial has now been approved, but why use stents when angioplasty alone would be less expensive, especially as cost will be a major end-point?

Table 25.1
Current indications for carotid angioplasty

Primary, symptomatic carotid stenoses where surgical access seems difficult or hazardous (Fig. 25.3)
Symptomatic restenosis after conventional carotid endarterectomy
Patients unfit for carotid endarterectomy
In trial centres, where the requisite teams and experience have already developed, to maintain expertise and evaluate new technology.

In the UK, the Medical Research Council and the UK Stroke Association have agreed to fund CAVATAS II, which aims to extend the original trial, but again stents will now be used routinely without good evidence. The success of any trial will require the enrolment of an adequate number of patients, and follow-up for a minimum of 2 years to allow a comparison with adequate statistical power. To demonstrate equivalence within 2% – assuming a disabling stroke/death rate after surgery of 5% – requires 5000 patients, i.e. more than NASCET and ECST combined. This implies that we should only have one trial which should include all major centres in North America, Europe and elsewhere. Alternatively, the organizers of the two funded trials

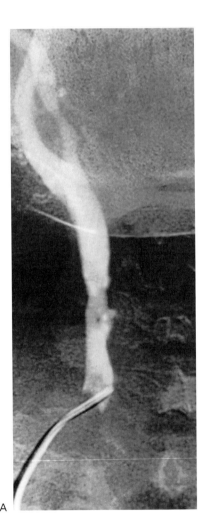

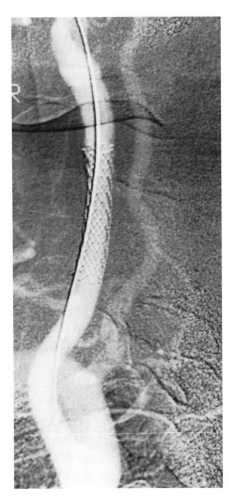

Fig. 25.3
Symptomatic, irregular stenosis of the common carotid artery following radiotherapy for laryngeal carcinoma (A), successfully treated by stenting (B).

A

B

319

must agree on common criteria to permit subsequent aggregation of data.

Such a trial will require the establishment of teams (neurologist, vascular surgeon or neurosurgeon and interventional radiologist or cardiologist) that will develop experience to avoid the problems associated with learning curves. Such experience would need careful monitoring by registries such as that proposed by the American Heart Association Science Advisory and Co-ordinating Committee[21] and the Joint Working Party of the Vascular Surgical Society of Great Britain and Ireland and the British Society of Interventional Radiologists. A trial will also need to determine the situations in which clinical equipoise permits ethical randomization of patients and also allow for the future inclusion of any technological advances.

In the absence of such a randomized trial, the following situations seem appropriate for carotid angioplasty or stenting (see also Table 25.1).

The first category includes stenoses at the origin of the common carotid or brachiocephalic artery as endovascular treatment gives good results and surgical access requires a median sternotomy.[22] Post-radiotherapy stenoses of the common carotid artery (Fig. 25.3)[23] and distal stenoses of the internal carotid artery[24] represent other indications.[25] Surgery for restenosis after CEA can be technically difficult and may be associated with a higher morbidity and mortality. Yadav et al.[26] have reported good results after treating 25 carotid restenoses by stenting. All procedures appeared

successful on angiogram with one minor stroke and no restenosis > 50% at 6 months, although follow-up seemed incomplete.

As has been discussed elsewhere, there remains no consensus as to the optimal treatment of patients with combined cardiac and coronary artery disease. Most surgeons prefer a synchronous operation but angioplasty before coronary artery bypass graft (CABG) represents a reasonable alternative in these high-risk cases. We have successfully performed 11 carotid angioplasties in patients with such stenoses prior to CABG.

CONCLUSIONS

In summary, carotid angioplasty results in significantly more cerebral emboli and probably more TIAs than CEA. Little evidence exists that cerebral protection balloons or stents reduce the risk of cerebral embolism, nor has a reliable method of selecting 'safe' stenoses for endovascular treatment emerged. Endovascular treatment avoids the risk of cranial nerve damage but demonstrates few other clinical or economic advantages. Stenting might reduce the high incidence of restenosis after carotid angioplasty but, as with surgery, most restenoses cause no symptoms. The only randomized trial of endovascular treatment versus surgery (CAVATAS) has shown no short-term difference in terms of stroke or death but could not prove equivalence. There are few current indications for carotid angioplasty or stenting unless performed as part of a randomized controlled trial.

REFERENCES

1 Bergeron P. Carotid angioplasty and stenting: is endovascular treatment for cerebrovascular disease justified? Journal of Endovascular Surgery 1996; 3: 129–131.
2 Forrsell C, Bergqvist D, Bergenz SE. Peripheral nerve injuries in carotid artery surgery In: Greenhalgh RM, Hollier LH (eds) Surgery for Stroke, pp. 217–234. London: WB Saunders, 1993.
3 Jordan WD, Roye GD, Fisher WS, Reddon D, McDowell HA. A cost comparison of balloon angioplasty and stenting versus endarterectomy for the treatment of carotid artery stenosis. Journal of Vascular Surgery 1998; 27: 16–22.
4 Ackerstaff RGA, Janson C, Moll FL. The significance of microemboli detection by means of transcranial Doppler

ultrasonography monitoring in carotid endarterectomy. Journal of Vascular Surgery 1995; 21: 963–970.
5 Biasi GM, Mingazzi PM. Should the type of carotid plaque determine the carotid procedure: a conventional or endovascular? In: Greenhalgh RM (ed.) Indications in Vascular and Endovascular Surgery, pp. 73–79 London: WB Saunders, 1998.
6 Theron JG, Payelle GG, Coskum O, Hoet HF, Guimaraems L. Carotid artery stenosis: treatment with protected balloon angioplasty and stent placement. Radiology 1996; 201: 627–636.
7 Kachel R. Results of balloon angioplasty in the carotid arteries. Journal of Endovascular Surgery 1996; 3: 22–30.
8 Tsai F, Higashida R, Meoli C. Percutaneous transluminal

angioplasty of extracranial and intracranial arterial stenosis of the head and neck. *Neuroimaging Clinics of North America* 1992; **3**: 371–384.

9 Brockenheimer S, Mathias K. Percutaneous transluminal angioplasty in arteriosclerotic internal carotid artery stenosis. *American Journal of Neuroradiology* 1983; **4**: 791–792.

10 Roubin GS, Yadav S, Iyer SS, Vitek J. Carotid stent-supported angioplasty: a neurovascular intervention to prevent stroke. *American Journal of Cardiology* 1996; **78**: 8–12.

11 Calvey TAJ, Gough MJ. A late complication of internal carotid artery stenting. *Journal of Vascular Surgery* 1998; **27**: 753–755.

12 Gil-Peralta A, Mayol A, Gonzalez Marcos JR *et al*. Percutaneous transluminal angioplasty of the symptomatic atherosclerotic carotid arteries. *Stroke* 1996; **27**: 2271–2273.

13 Yadav JS, Roubin GS, Iyer S *et al*. Elective stenting of the extracranial carotid arteries. *Circulation* 1997; **95**: 376–381.

14 Brown MM *et al*. The carotid and vertebral artery transluminal angioplasty study. *Lancet* 1999 (in press).

15 Mullan S, Duda E, Petronas N. Some examples of balloon technology in neurosurgery. *Journal of Neurosurgery* 1980; **52**: 321–329.

16 Brown MM, Clifton A, Taylor RS. Concern about safety of carotid angioplasty. *Stroke* 1996; **27**: 1435–1436.

17 Hurst RW. Carotid angioplasty. *Radiology* 1996; **201**: 613–616.

18 Dietrich EB, Mohamadon N, Reid DB. Stenting the carotid artery: initial experience in 110 patients. *Journal of Endovascular Surgery* 1996; **3**: 42–62.

19 Rothwell P, Slattery J, Warlow C. A systematic review of the risks of stroke and death due to endarterectomy for symptomatic carotid stenosis. *Stroke* 1996; **27**: 260–265.

20 Chastain HD, Roubin GS, Iyer SS, Mathew A, Gomez CR, Vitek JJ. Carotid stenting versus carotid endarterectomy in octogenarians. *Circulation* 1997; **96**: (Suppl 8): I–441.

21 Bettmann MA, Katzen BT, Whisnant J *et al*. Carotid stenting and angioplasty. A statement for healthcare professionals from the Councils on Cardiovascular Radiology, Stroke, Cardiothoracic and Vascular Surgery, Epidemiology and Prevention and Clinical Cardiology, American Heart Association. *Circulation* 1998; **97**: 121–123.

22 Whitbread T, Cleveland TJ, Beard JD, Gaines PA. A combined approach to the treatment of proximal arterial occlusions of the upper limb with endovascur stents. *European Journal of Vascular and Endovascular Surgery* 1998; **15**: 29–35.

23 Yadav JS, Roubin GS, King P, Iyer S, Vitek J. Angioplasty and stenting for restenosis after carotid endarterectomy. *Stroke* 1996; **27**: 2075–2079.

24 Callahan AS 3rd, Berger BL. Balloon angioplasty of intracranial vessels for stroke prevention. *Journal of Neuroimaging* 1997; **7**: 232–235.

25 Criado FJ, Wellons E, Clark NS. Evolving indications for and early results of carotid artery stenting. *American Journal of Surgery* 1997; **174**: 111–114.

26 Yadav JS, Roubin GS, King P, Iyer S, Vitek J. Angioplasty and stenting for restenosis after carotid endarterectomy. *Stroke* 1996; **27**: 2075–2079.

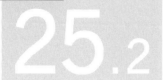

25.2

Is there a role for carotid angioplasty or stenting?
Robert W Hobson II (USA)

INTRODUCTION
CEA has become the preferred method for treatment of symptomatic[27–29] and asymptomatic[30,31] patients with high-grade carotid stenosis, displacing optimal medical management alone. However, during the last several years, the performance of carotid angioplasty–stenting (CAS) has been recommended by some clinicians as an alternative to CEA for patients who have symptomatic extracranial carotid occlusive disease. Emergence of a position of clinical equipoise[32,33] in the assessment of the value of these alternatives has resulted in the initiation of two randomized clinical trials[34,35] and in NIH funding for a large-scale multicentered North American trial, CREST.[36]

CEA, performed with a low periprocedural complication rate, is the only form of mechanical cerebral revascularization for which definitive evidence of clinical effectiveness has been reported. In the NASCET data,[27] life-table estimates of the cumulative risk of stroke at 2 years were 26% in the medical group vs 9% in the surgical group (absolute risk reduction ($\pm$SE): 17$\pm$3.5%, $P < 0.001$). The corresponding estimates for major or fatal ipsilateral stroke were 13.1% vs 2.5% (absolute risk reduction ($\pm$SE): 10.6$\pm$2.6%, $P < 0.001$) and for any stroke or death were 32% vs 16% (absolute risk reduction: 16.5$\pm$4.2%, $P < 0.001$). Complementary findings were reported in the ECST[28] and the Veterans' Administration symptomatic endarterectomy trial.[29] Although recent presentation of data by the NASCET investigators on patients with symptomatic disease[37] has also confirmed efficacy of CEA in male patients with 50–69% stenosis, the benefit was not confirmed in women with the same degree of stenosis. In ACAS,[31] after a median follow-up of

2.7 years, the aggregate risk over 5 years for ipsilateral stroke and any periprocedural stroke or death was estimated to be 5.1% for surgical patients and 11% for patients treated medically (aggregate risk reduction: 53%, 95% confidence interval (CI) 22–72%). Results from these trials have provided the basis for current indications for CEA throughout this country and abroad.

Although CAS has been proposed as an alternative to CEA, the safety and clinical effectiveness of CAS have not been established and no prospective comparisons of CAS and CEA have been conducted in the US. Furthermore, a recently published Science Advisory from the American Heart Association[38] concluded that: 'with few exceptions, use of carotid stenting should be limited to well-designed, well-controlled randomized studies with careful dispassionate oversight.'

CAROTID ANGIOPLASTY AND ANGIOPLASTY–STENTING
Morris et al.[39] reported the first balloon dilatation of a carotid artery in 1968; it was performed for fibromuscular dysplasia. However, Kerber and colleagues[40] performed the first human carotid artery dilatation for an atherosclerotic lesion in 1980, and demonstrated that atherosclerotic lesions of the carotid artery could be dilated without necessarily provoking symptomatic atherothromboembolism.

Numerous case reports and clinical series have been published since then.[41–65] The first report of a multicenter prospective protocol-based study of CAS, the North American Percutaneous Transluminal Angioplasty Register (NACPTAR),[66,67] was published in 1993. Interim results were reported on 165 angioplasties in 147 symptomatic non-surgical patients. The average stenosis pre-angioplasty was 84% (range 70–99%). The average stenosis immediately post-angioplasty was 37% ($P < 0.01$). This corresponded to an immediate success rate of 83% (95% CI, 76–88%). Death from all causes occurred in 3% of procedures, and stroke in an additional 6%. The 30-day combined rate of death and stroke from all causes was 9% (95% CI, 5–51%). Data concerning the rate of restenosis in 44 lesions with angiographic follow-up at a mean of 260 days have also been reported.[68] The definition of restenosis was angiographic documentation of stenosis exceeding 70%. Of the 37 lesions that were " 70% after the initial dilatation, restenosis occurred in 8 (22%; 95% CI, 10–38%). Of the patients who had restenosis, 5/8 (63%) were symptomatic at the time of follow-up. Cox proportional hazards modeling demonstrated that symptoms and the degree of stenosis pre-angioplasty were independent predictors of angiographic restenosis in follow-up. These data suggested that restenosis after angioplasty alone would be a significant problem and stimulated clinicians to perform stenting after angioplasty as a routine practice.

In 1996, Dietrich et al.[64] reported results of CAS in 110 symptomatic patients with ≥ 70% stenoses from a single institution. One procedure failed (0.9%) for technical reasons and was converted to CEA. Two deaths (1.8%) were observed (1 from stroke and 1 due to a cardiac event). Seven strokes (2 major (1.8%) and 5 minor (4.5%)) and 5 transient neurological events (4.5%) occurred. Based on this early experience, the authors concluded that the incidence of periprocedural neurological complications was excessive. In an accompanying editorial, Dietrich[65] suggested that CAS should be restricted to cases of carotid restenosis after prior CEA, instances in which the internal carotid stenosis was anatomically higher than readily treated by CEA, and radiation-induced stenosis.

A larger prospective protocol-based study of CAS in 204 patients was reported by Roubin and colleagues.[69] Ages ranged from 36 to 86 years, 75% had significant coronary artery disease, and 70% of the patients had medical comorbidities that would have made them ineligible for the NASCET study. Of these 238 arteries treated (204 patients), 145 arteries (61%) presented in patients with ipsilateral symptoms (60 strokes, 85 TIAs), while 93 arteries were treated in asymptomatic patients. Nine percent of the patients had an occluded contralateral carotid artery and 15% had restenosis following prior CEA. Eighteen percent of patients had complex lesions with ulcerated plaques. Technical success was achieved in 99% of patients. In 2 patients, the carotid could not be accessed via the transfemoral approach. In 1 patient, the procedure was aborted after initial angiography was complicated by an air embolism. Of the 204 patients, there was 1 death (0.5%) and 2 major (0.98%; NIH stroke scale > 4 with residual disability > 30 days) strokes. One was due to the single episode of stent thrombosis and the second to a cardiogenic embolus causing a contralateral stroke on the second post-procedural day. Minor strokes (NIH stroke scale < 3 and resolution within 30 days) were observed in 15 patients (7.4%). During follow-up, 1 minor ischemic stroke occurred in these 204 patients. Three patients suffered TIAs with no evidence of stent restenosis. Four patients died during follow-up (congestive heart failure (1), pneumonia (1), intracranial hemorrhage (1) (patient not on anticoagulation), renal failure (1)). Repeat carotid imaging (angiography or ultrasound) has been performed in 75% of patients reaching 6 months of follow-up. Restenosis (> 70% diameter reduction) has been documented in 5 of 104 (5%) patients re-studied. Stent deformation occurred in 14% of balloon-expandable stents deployed. Consequently, only self-expanding stents have been employed by the authors thereafter. As a result of these data, a self-expandable stent has been recommended for use by CREST investigators.

Recently, Mathur and colleagues[70] updated their previous report.[69] These data included 271 procedures in 231 patients (139 symptomatic: 60%). Of the arteries treated, 214 (79%) were excluded by NASCET and Asymptomatic Carotid Atherosclerosis Study (ACAS) criteria. Major strokes occurred in 2 patients (0.9%) and minor strokes were observed in 17 patients (7.4%); however, among NASCET–ACAS eligible patients, only

1 minor stroke (1.8%) was reported. Predictors of stroke in the overall clinical update included advanced age, lesion severity, and long/multiple lesions. In a recent update on 40 NASCET-eligible patients, Gomez and coauthors[71] reported 1 transient (2.5%) neurological event and no deaths, major strokes, or myocardial infarctions. These investigators suggested a comparability of complications between CAS and CEA.

Currently, two randomized clinical trials comparing the efficacy of CAS and CEA are ongoing. In Europe, CAVATAS is comparing surgical intervention and angioplasty for treatment of carotid and vertebral occlusive lesions.[34] Dr Martin Brown, Principal Investigator, CAVATAS, presented the results from phase I of his multicentered trial during the American Heart Association's international stroke meeting in Nashville, TN, in February 1999. Among 504 patients randomized primarily to angioplasty alone and considered suitable candidates for CEA, 30-day stroke and death rates were comparable: 6.3% for CEA and 6.4% for the CAS group. Phase II will be initiated later in 1999 and will utilize angioplasty–stenting in all symptomatic carotid cases. These are the only data available on cases randomized to CEA or CAS; however, their influence may be blunted by the somewhat higher than expected complication rate in the CEA group.

Alberts and coauthors[35] described the methodology of the other randomized clinical trial comparing carotid stenting versus endarterectomy in symptomatic patients as sponsored by the Schneider Corporation (now Boston Scientific Vascular, manufacturers of the Wallstent endoprosthesis). Patients with symptomatic stenoses (50–99%) are randomized. A sample size of 700 is anticipated. The goal is to determine whether or not carotid stenting is equivalent to CEA in the prevention of any ipsilateral stroke, periprocedural death (within 30 days), or vascular death within 1 year of treatment. To date, only about 200 patients have been randomized, from 22 centers (personal communication, M. Schollmeyer, DVM, Boston Scientific Vascular) during the last 24 months. The study's monitoring committee has not invoked any actions to curtail the trial's recruitment of patients, suggesting that no differences have occurred

between treatment groups in this early phase of the trial. However, the trial's future is being reviewed because of the low recruitment rates of symptomatic patients at clinical sites.

Conclusions regarding the results of these clinical trials await future review. However, it appears that, in selected patients, CAS can produce a significant decrease or eliminate the extracranial carotid stenosis in NASCET-eligible patients with periprocedural complications which may be comparable to those reported for CEA.

CURRENT PRACTICE AND TECHNICAL CONSIDERATIONS

Current practice suggests consideration for CAS in several areas: anatomically high internal carotid stenoses, carotid restenosis following prior CEA, radiation-induced carotid stenosis, and occasional high-risk patients with severe medical comorbidity. While these are not universally accepted indications for CAS, this represents a reasonable approach in view of the American Heart Association's position against use of CAS for initially symptomatic carotid stenosis in the absence of a clinical trial.

We have restricted our use of CAS primarily to carotid restenosis after CEA within the previous 3 years.[72] Symptomatic or asymptomatic carotid restenosis after CEA is relatively uncommon and is generally attributed to myointimal hyperplasia during the early postoperative period (within 36 months) or recurrent atherosclerosis thereafter.[73–77] Surgical management of carotid restenosis is controversial for two major reasons. First, indications for operative management in the asymptomatic patient with high-grade (≥ 80%) restenosis remain controversial due to the low risk of stroke or progression to total occlusion.[73,78,79] Second, reoperation is associated with a marginally increased risk of perioperative neurological events and cranial nerve palsies.[75,80,81] Because of these issues, some authors[82–86] recommend CAS as an alternative to operative management.

We prospectively collected data and intervened using endovascular techniques on patients with symptomatic and asymptomatic (≥ 80%) carotid restenosis due to myointimal hyperplasia for the purpose of defining technical feasibility and

Table 25.2
Protocol for carotid angioplasty–stent (CAS) procedure

- Transfemoral 8 F introducer sheath; open carotid cannulation considered in presence of severe aortoiliac disease; preprocedural aspirin and Ticlid or Plavix
- 0.035 in J-guidewire with moveable core to aortic arch; heparinization to ACT of 225–250
- NH-2 Vitek catheter for cannulation of aortic arch branches
- 0.035 in coated Terumo long exchange guidewire to external carotid artery. Occasional use of the 0.035 in Amplatz stiff guidewire is recommended to advance the NH-2 catheter or the 8 F guide sheath
- 8 F (internal diameter) guide sheath (100cm length) to common carotid artery proximal to lesion
- 0.018in. guidewire to cross common internal carotid stenosis
- 4mm low-profile balloon for pre-stent dilatation
- Deployment of 8×20mm or 10×20mm Wallstent over 0.018in. wire
- Post-stent dilatation using 5 or 6mm balloons
- Intermittent hand-injection angiography during procedure; utilize bony landmarks for balloon and stent placements
- Remove sheath once ACT < 150; continue aspirin, while Ticlid or Plavix is discontinued 3 weeks after CAS

Modified from Hobson et al.[72] with permission.

periprocedural outcomes. Technical considerations in the performance of CAS are outlined in Table 25.2. Examples of pre- and post-procedural arteriograms (Figs 25.4 and 25.5) are presented and demonstrate placement of an 8 or 10mm $\times$ 20mm Wallstent (Boston Scientific Vascular, Natick, MA). In each case, 4mm low-profile balloons were used initially to dilate the lesions, followed by placement of appropriately sized stents with post-stent balloon dilatation to obtain the final result. Intravascular ultrasound was utilized to insure adequate apposition of the stent to the arterial wall. In these cases and all but one other case, stents were placed across the carotid bifurcation. Serial duplex ultrasonography has demonstrated patency of all external and internal carotid arteries.

Our carotid restenosis series has now been expanded to 24 patients (25 procedures). Immediate post-procedural hypotension and bradycardia were observed in 2 patients (8%), which responded to pharmacologic intervention without further complications. All patients were discharged on the morning following the procedure and no periprocedural strokes have been observed. One recently treated 78-year-old woman with severe coexisting coronary artery disease had undergone CAS during the week before a right CAS procedure. The patient was alone at home and died suddenly 10 days after CAS. Presumed to be due to an acute myocardial infarction or cardiac arrhythmia, she represents the only mortality in our series of now 31 cases (3.2%).

CREST ORGANIZATIONAL PLAN

Based on our experience with this subset of restenosis patients and the other data presented above, clinical equipoise between CEA and CAS is at hand. These data suggest a substantial enough improvement in the technology of CAS as to allow performance of a clinical trial. The CREST investigators have recommended that a trial be initiated using Wallstent technology, but anticipate use of run-in phase data and high-risk registry cases to introduce new stents as well as cerebral protection devices during the conduct of the trial.

CREST will compare the efficacy of CEA and CAS in symptomatic patients with high-grade ($\geq 70\%$) stenoses. Recently, discussions have been completed to reduce the threshold lesion to $\geq 50\%$. Recognizing that CAS is a relatively new procedure, each participating center will be required to complete a credentialing phase to reassure clinicians that the safety of these procedures has been reviewed and established before proceeding with the randomized phase of the trial.

Assuming that a credentialing phase which requires performance of up to 15 interventional

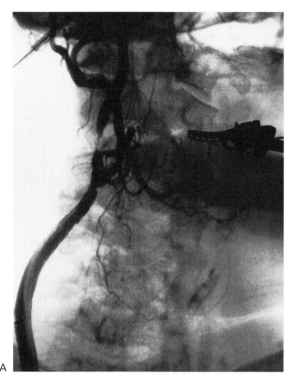

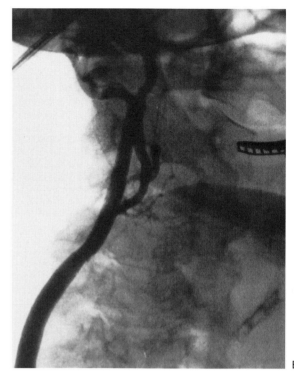

A

B

Fig. 25.4
Example of (A) pre-procedural arteriogram and (B) post-procedural arteriogram.

procedures at each of 50 or more participating
centers is completed to the satisfaction of the study's
interventional management committee,
randomization of patients between the two
treatments will then proceed. The primary outcome
events for this clinical trial will include any stroke,
myocardial infarction, or death during the 30-day
perioperative or periprocedural period, or ipsilateral
stroke after 30 days. End-points will be reviewed by
an adjudication committee blinded to the assigned
treatment. Stroke will be determined by a positive
TIA/stroke questionnaire confirmed by neurologist
evaluation. Myocardial infarction will be determined
by electrocardiogram and enzyme abnormalities.
Secondary goals include:

1 Describe differential efficacy of the two
  treatments in men and women.
2 Contrast perioperative procedural (30-day)

morbidity and post-procedural (after 30 days)
mortality for CEA and CAS.
3 Estimate and contrast the restenosis rates for the
  two procedures.
4 Identify subgroups of participants at differential
  risk for the two procedures.
5 Evaluate differences in health-related quality of
  life and cost-effectiveness issues.

Differential efficacy assessment of CEA and CAS
based on gender is a secondary goal for CREST. In
patients with high-grade asymptomatic stenosis
reported by ACAS, CEA offered a 66% reduction in
events over a 5-year period for men, but only a 17%
reduction for women.[31] In NASCET, while no
differential gender effects were reported among
symptomatic patients with stenosis greater than
70%, male patients demonstrated greater benefit after
CEA than did women for stenoses of 50–69%.[37]

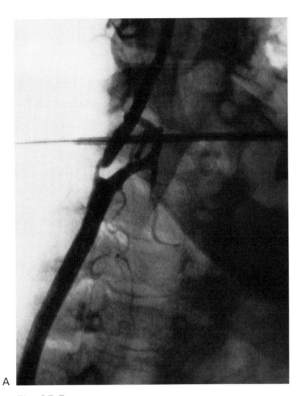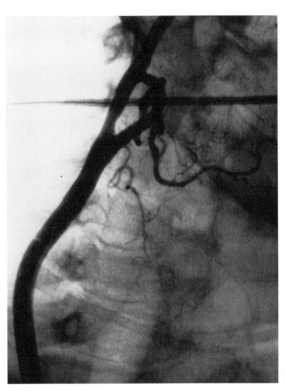

A   B

Fig. 25.5
Example of (A) pre-procedural arteriogram and (B) post-procedural arteriogram.

While the causes for these examples of differential efficacy between genders are not well understood, the effect may be attributed to a higher complication rate for CEA in women, possibly caused by their reported smaller arterial sizes and a greater surgical morbidity. Unfortunately, neither ACAS nor NASCET suspected the possibility of a differential gender effect, and as such could not be reasonably expected to provide design parameters to evaluate definitively the possibility of a differential gender effect. However, given the results of these two randomized clinical trials, a requirement for *a priori* plans to evaluate the possibility of a differential gender effect has become an important component of CREST. Centers are being selected with a goal as high as 50% women in the randomized sample of patients and a minimum of 40% women.

Patients will be evaluated at baseline, 24h post-procedure, 30 days, and 6 months, and thereafter at 6-month intervals. Baseline procedures will include a brief medical history and physical examination, a risk factor evaluation, performance of neurological status questionnaires, a neurological examination, electrocardiogram, and a baseline carotid duplex scan. The 30-day follow-up will include evaluation of the neurological status through questionnaires, electrocardiogram, and a follow-up carotid duplex scan. All 6-month follow-up visits will include a brief physical, completion of the neurological questionnaire, risk factor evaluation, and carotid duplex scan. All patients with a positive neurological status questionnaire will be evaluated by a neurologist. The sample size for the study is approximately 2500 symptomatic patients, which will be sufficient to detect a relative difference of 25–30% between treatment groups. Lesser differences would be considered sufficiently small to declare the treatments equivalent.

CONCLUSIONS

Current clinical practice dictates that CAS be considered in limited subsets of patients, as outlined. Conduct of clinical trials (CREST and others) will provide level I evidence from which solid clinical recommendations can be established. Until these data are available during the next several years, performance of CAS should be limited to randomized clinical trials and defined unique subsets of high-risk patients. CEA continues to be recommended for the management of most patients with symptomatic and asymptomatic extracranial carotid occlusive disease.

REFERENCES

27 North American Symptomatic Carotid Endarterectomy Trial Collaborators. Beneficial effect of carotid endarterectomy in symptomatic patients with high-grade carotid stenosis. *New England Journal of Medicine* 1991; **325**: 445–453.

28 European Carotid Surgery Trialists' Collaborative Group. MCR European Carotid Surgery Trial: interim results for symptomatic patients with severe (70–99%) or with mild (0–29%) carotid stenosis. *Lancet* 1991; **337**: 1235–1243.

29 Mayberg MR, Wilson SE, Yatsu F and the VA Symptomatic Carotid Stenosis Group. Carotid endarterectomy and prevention of cerebral ischemia in symptomatic carotid stenosis. *Journal of the American Medical Association* 1991; **266**: 3289–3294.

30 Hobson RW, Weiss DG, Fields WS *et al*. Efficacy of carotid endarterectomy for asymptomatic carotid stenosis. *New England Journal of Medicine* 1993; **328**: 221–227.

31 Executive Committee for the Asymptomatic Carotid Atherosclerosis Study. Endarterectomy for asymptomatic carotid stenosis. *Journal of the American Medical Association* 1995; **273**: 1421–1428.

32 Freedman B. Equipoise and the ethics of clinical research. *New England Journal of Medicine* 1987; **317**: 141–145.

33 Brown M. Balloon angioplasty for cerebrovascular disease. *Neurological Research* 1992; **14**(Suppl): 159–163.

34 Major ongoing stroke trials: carotid and vertebral artery transluminal angioplasty study (CAVATAS). *Stroke* 1996; **27**: 358.

35 Alberts MJ, McCann R, Smith TP *et al*. A randomized trial: carotid stenting versus endarterectomy in patients with symptomatic carotid stenosis, study designs. *Journal of Neurovascular Disease* 1997; **6**: 228–234.

36 Hobson RW, Brott T, Ferguson R *et al*. Letter to the editor, regarding 'statement regarding carotid angioplasty and stenting'. *Journal of Vascular Surgery* 1997; **25**: 1117.

37 Barnett HJM, Taylor DW, Eliasziw M *et al*. Benefit of carotid endarterectomy in patients with symptomatic moderate or severe stenosis. *New England Journal of Medicine* 1998; **339**: 1415–1425.

38 Bettmann MA, Katzen BT, Whisnant J *et al*. Carotid stenting and angioplasty. A statement from the Councils on Cardiovascular Radiology, Stroke, Cardio-thoracic and Vascular Surgery, Epidemiology and Prevention, and Clinical Cardiology, American Heart Association. *Stroke* 1998; **29**: 336–346.

39 Morris GC, Lechter A, DeBakey ME. Surgical treatment of fibromuscular disease of the carotid artery. *Archives of Surgery* 1968; **96**: 636–643.

40 Kerber CW, Cromwell LD, Leohden OL. Catheter dilatation of proximal stenosis during distal bifurcation endarterectomy. *American Journal of Neuroradiology* 1980; **1**: 348–349.

41 Namaguchi Y, Puyau FA, Provenza LJ, Richardson DE. Percutaneous transluminal angioplasty of the carotid artery: its application to post surgical stenosis. *Neuroradiology* 1984; **26**: 527–530.

42 Tsia FY, Matovich V, Hieshima G *et al*. Percutaneous angioplasty of the carotid artery. *American Journal of Neuroradiology* 1986; **7**: 349–358.

43 Becker G, Katzen B, Dake M. Noncoronary angioplasty. *Radiology* 1989; **170**: 921–940.

44 Theron J, Raymond J, Casasco A, Courtheoux F. Percutaneous angioplasty of atherosclerotic and postsurgical stenosis of carotid arteries. *American Journal of Neuroradiology* 1987; **8**: 495–500.

45 Theron J. Angioplasty of brachiocephalic vessels. In: Vinuela F, Halbach VV, Dion JE (eds) *Interventional Neuroradiology: Endovascular Therapy of the Central Nervous System*, pp. 167–180. New York: Raven Press, 1992.

46 Munari LM, Belloni G, Perretti A, Ghia HF, Moschini L, Porta M. Carotid percutaneous angioplasty. *Neurological Research* 1992; **14**(Suppl): 156–158.

47 Freitag G, Freitag J, Koch RD, Wagemann W. Percutaneous angioplasty of carotid artery stenoses. *Neuroradiology* 1986; **28**: 126–127.

48 Freitag G, Freitag J, Koch RD *et al*. Transluminal angioplasty for the treatment of carotid artery stenosis. *VASA* 1987; **16**: 67–71.

49 Higashida RT, Hieshima GB, Tsai FY, Halbach W, Norman D, Newton TH. Transluminal angioplasty of the vertebral and basilar artery. *American Journal of Neuroradiology* 1987; **8**: 745–749.

50 Kachel R, Endert G, Basche S, Grossman K, Glaser FH. Percutaneous transluminal angioplasty (dilatation) of carotid, vertebral, and innominate artery stenoses. *Cardiovascular and Interventional Radiology* 1987; **10**: 142–146.

51 Higashida RT, Tsai FY, Halbach W *et al*. Transluminal angioplasty for atherosclerotic disease of the vertebral and basilar arteries. *Journal of Neurosurgery* 1993; **78**: 192–198.

52 Kachel R, Basche ST, Heerklotz I, Grossman K, Endler S. Percutaneous transluminal angioplasty (PTA) of supra-aortic arteries especially the internal carotid artery. *Neuroradiology* 1991; **33**: 191–194.

53 Theron J, Courtheoux P, Alachkar F, Maiza D. New triple

coaxial catheter system for carotid angioplasty with cerebral protection. *American Journal of Neuroradiology* 1990; **11**: 869–874.

54 Rostomily RC, Mayberg MR, Eskridge JM, Goodkin R, Winn HR. Resolution of petrous internal carotid artery stenosis after transluminal angioplasty. *Journal of Neurosurgery* 1992; **76**: 520–523.

55 Dietrich EB, Rodriguez-Lopez J, Lopez-Garcia L. Stents for vascular reconstruction in the carotid arteries. *Circulation* 1995; **92**(Suppl 8): I–383.

56 Yamamura A, Oyama H, Matsuno F, Ishiguro M, Nakagawa T, Hashi K. Percutaneous transluminal angioplasty for cervical carotid artery stenosis. *No Shinkei Geka* 1995; **23**: 117–123.

57 Chen CC, Lirng JF, Chou YH *et al*. Percutaneous transluminal angioplasty of neck vessels. *Chung Hua I Hsueh Tsa Chih* 1994; **54**: 251–258.

58 Motarjeme A. Percutaneous transluminal angioplasty of supra-aortic vessels. *Journal of Endovascular Surgery* 1996; **3**: 171–181.

59 Bergeron P, Chambran P, Hartung O, Bianca S. Cervical carotid artery stenosis. *Journal of Cardiovascular Surgery* 1996; **37**(Suppl 1–5): 73–75.

60 Shawl FA, Efstratiou A, Hoff S, Dougherty K. Combined percutaneous carotid stenting and coronary angioplasty during acute ischemic neurologic and coronary syndromes. *American Journal of Cardiology* 1996; **77**: 1109–1112.

61 Eckert B, Zanella FE, Thie A, Steinmetz J, Zeumer H. Angioplasty of the internal carotid artery: results, complications and follow-up in 61 cases. *Cerebrovascular Disease* 1996; **6**: 97–105.

62 Babatasi G, Theron J, Masetti M, Payelle G, Rossi A, Khayat A. Intérêt de l'angioplastic carotidienne percutanée avant chirugie cardiaque. *Annales de Cardiologie et d'Angeiologie (Paris)* 1996; **45**: 24–29.

63 Karnik R, Ammerer HP, Valentin A, Slany J, Brenner H. Intraoperative transluminal angioplasty of the supra-aortic vessels. *Acta Neurochirurgica (Wien)* 1993; **121**: 53–57.

64 Dietrich EB, Ndiye M, Reid DB. Stenting in the carotid artery: initial experience in 110 patients. *Journal of Endovascular Surgery* 1996; **3**: 42–62.

65 Dietrich EB. Indications for carotid artery stenting: a preview of the potential derived from early clinical experience. *Journal of Endovascular Surgery* 1996; **3**: 132–139.

66 Ferguson R, Ferguson J, Schwarten D *et al*. Immediate angiographic results and in-hospital central nervous system complications of cerebral percutaneous transluminal angioplasty. *Circulation* 1993; **88**(Suppl 4): I–393.

67 The NACPTAR investigators. Update of the immediate angiographic results and in-hospital central nervous system complications of cerebral percutaneous transluminal angioplasty. *Circulation* 1995; **92**: I–383.

68 NACPTAR Investigators. Restenosis following cerebral percutaneous transluminal angioplasty. *Stroke* 1995; **26**: 186.

69 Roubin GS, Yadav S, Iyer SS *et al*. Carotid stent-supported angioplasty: a neurovascular intervention to prevent stroke. *American Journal of Cardiology* 1996; **78**: 8–12.

70 Mathur A, Roubin GS, Piamsomboom C, Liu MW, Gomez CR, Iyer SS. Predictors of stroke following carotid stenting: univariate and multivariate analysis. *Circulation* 1997; **96**: A1710.

71 Gomez CR, Roubin GS, Vitsk JJ *et al*. Safety of carotid artery stenting in NASCET-comparable patients. *Neurology* 1998; **50**: 76A.

72 Hobson RW II, Goldstein JE, Jamil Z *et al*. Carotid restenosis: operative and endovascular management. *Journal of Vascular Surgery* 1999; **29**: 228–238.

73 Lattimer CR, Burnand KG. Recurrent carotid stenosis after carotid endarterectomy. *British Journal of Surgery* 1997; **84**: 1206–1219.

74 Stoney RJ, String ST. Recurrent carotid stenosis. *Surgery* 1976; **80**: 705–710.

75 Bartlett FF, Rapp JH, Goldstone J, Ehrenfeld WK, Stoney RJ. Recurrent carotid stenosis: operative strategy and late results. *Journal of Vascular Surgery* 1987; **5**: 452–456.

76 Atnip RG, Wengrovitz M, Gifford RRM, Neumyer MM, Thiele BL. A rational approach to recurrent carotid stenosis. *Journal of Vascular Surgery* 1990; **11**: 511–516.

77 Sterpetti AV, Schultz RD, Feldhaus RJ *et al*. Natural history of recurrent carotid artery disease. *Surgery, Gynecology and Obstetrics* 1989; **168**: 217–223.

78 Healy DA, Zierler RE, Nicholls SC *et al*. Long-term follow-up and clinical outcome of carotid restenosis. *Journal of Vascular Surgery* 1989; **10**: 662–669.

79 Washburn WK, Mackey WC, Belkin M, O'Donnell TF. Late stroke after carotid endarterectomy: the role of recurrent stenosis. *Journal of Vascular Surgery* 1992; **15**: 1032–1037.

80 Treiman GS, Jenkins JM, Edwards WH *et al*. The evolving surgical management of recurrent carotid stenosis. *Journal of Vascular Surgery* 1992; **16**: 354–363.

81 Das MD, Hertzer NR, Ratliff NB, O'Hara PJ, Beven EG. Recurrent carotid stenosis: a five-year series of 65 operations. *Annals of Surgery* 1985; **202**: 28–35.

82 Roubin GS, Yadav S, Iyer SS, Vitek J. Carotid stent-supported angioplasty: a neurovascular intervention to prevent stroke. *American Journal of Cardiology* 1996; **78**(Suppl. 3A): 8–12.

83 Bergeron P, Chambran P, Benichou H, Alessandri C. Recurrent carotid disease: will stents be an alternative to surgery? *Journal of Endovascular Surgery* 1996; **3**: 76–79.

84 Yadav JS, Roubin GS, King P, Iyer S, Vitek J. Angioplasty and stenting for restenosis after carotid endarterectomy. Initial experience. *Stroke* 1996; **27**: 2075–2079.

85 Theron J, Raymond J, Casasco A, Courtheoux F. Percutaneous angioplasty of atherosclerotic and postsurgical stenosis of carotid arteries. *American Journal of Neuroradiology* 1987; **8**: 495–500.

86 Yadav JS, Roubin GS, Iyer S *et al*. Elective stenting of the extracranial carotid arteries. *Circulation* 1997; **95**: 376–381.

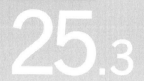

25.3 Editorial Comment

KEY POINTS

1 Carotid angioplasty is clearly technically feasible and has been associated with good outcomes in selected case series. However, no randomized trial has shown to date that angioplasty confers any consistent benefit over CEA.
2 The CAVATAS trial suggests that, following a successful angioplasty, the risk of late stroke is similar to that of surgery.
3 Carotid angioplasty involves a learning curve and this must be taken into account for the results of future randomized trials to be generalizable.
4 Although future developments in catheter technology are inevitable, future randomized trials must not be deferred on the basis that 'now is not the time'.

Vascular surgeons were equally vocal in their fears about peripheral angioplasty in the 1970s but, for the most part, these fears have proved to be unfounded. Ironically, although the current debate relates to the respective roles of angioplasty and CEA, similar criticisms were levelled at surgeons about their reluctance in the 1980s to participate in randomized trials comparing CEA with best medical therapy. It seems intuitive that angioplasty will have some role in the future. It is essential, therefore, that future indications are based on science rather than being driven by industry and the media.

The importance of the so-called learning curve will continue to dominate debate regarding the generalizability of angioplasty into routine clinical practice. There is currently a tendency to dismiss adverse published results following angioplasty as being simply secondary to the learning-curve experience. However, were angioplasty to become accepted practice in the future, this learning curve will apply to current interventionists and all future trainees just as it currently applies to carotid surgeons. Moreover, it seems that, on reviewing the literature, the original pioneers of angioplasty did not encounter any learning curve at all and simply developed a technique that was immediately safer than diagnostic carotid angiography alone. However, just as the interventionists face a potential credibility issue regarding some of the published results, vascular surgeons must also accept that current outcomes following CEA may not be as good as were published in the randomized trials in 1991. The role of angioplasty must be evaluated properly in well-designed randomized trials that are generalizable and applicable to all patients, all radiologists, and all surgeons.

Part Four Postoperative Management

26.1

How should I manage the patient who suffers a perioperative neurological deficit?

A Ross Naylor (Europe)

INTRODUCTION

In order to plan a strategy for managing the patient who suffers a stroke after carotid endarterectomy (CEA), it is helpful first to consider the likeliest causes (Table 26.1). In an earlier chapter, perioperative stroke was classified as intraoperative if the patient recovered from anaesthesia with a new neurological deficit and postoperative if the deficit

occurred some time after an uneventful recovery from anaesthesia. This simple classification allows the clinician to prioritize investigation and management strategies, which is extremely important as too much delay can be as dangerous as too much haste.

The immediate management of perioperative stroke is largely governed by the clinician's access to

Table 26.1
Aetiology of stroke following carotid endarterectomy

Intraoperative stroke*	Postoperative stroke[†]
Embolism	*Embolism*
Spontaneous embolization (unstable plaque)	Particulate emboli from endarterectomy zone
Particulate emboli during carotid dissection	Particulate emboli following external carotid artery thrombosis
Particulate emboli dislodged by shunt	
Major air embolism through shunt malfunction	
Particulate embolization from endarterectomy zone	
Thrombosis	*Thrombosis*
Peri-shunt thrombosis	Secondary to technical error
On-table carotid thrombosis	Secondary to hypotension
	Secondary to syphon disease
	Secondary to coagulation disorder
Miscellaneous	*Miscellaneous*
Haemodynamic failure (no shunt used)	Hypertensive encephalopathy
Haemodynamic failure (shunt malfunction)	Primary intracerebral haemorrhage
	Haemorrhagic transformation of infarct
	Hyperperfusion syndrome

*Intraoperative stroke, patient recovers from anaesthetic with a new neurological deficit.
[†]Postoperative stroke, patient suffers a stroke some time after a normal recovery from anaesthetic.

333

monitoring equipment. Because this varies between units, this chapter will summarize management strategies based upon whether the surgeon has rapid access to duplex ultrasound or transcranial Doppler (TCD) ultrasound.

THE CONVENTIONAL APPROACH TO MANAGEMENT

The Intraoperative Stroke

The first evidence that something has gone wrong is usually a delay in the patient recovering from anaesthesia. The immediate priority is to identify those patients who have suffered an on-table carotid thrombosis because they have most to gain from immediate re-exploration. If the patient makes a slow recovery from anaesthesia and exhibits the triad of hemiplegia, homonymous hemianopia and higher cortical dysfunction (aphasia/visuospatial neglect) then it is highly likely that either the internal carotid artery (ICA) or the mainstem of the middle cerebral artery (MCA) is occluded.[1,2] Unfortunately, without access to TCD the two cannot be differentiated on clinical grounds alone.

Thus, for surgeons with no access to duplex or TCD, any patient who recovers from anaesthesia with a new neurological deficit should be assumed to have suffered an on-table thrombosis and immediately re-explored. This will inevitably mean that some patients with focal embolism and haemodynamic stroke are subjected to an unnecessary re-exploration, but currently this cannot be avoided. If the decision is taken to re-explore the patient, it should be performed as soon as possible as any delay beyond 1h reduces the chances of a good functional outcome.[3]

It is our current practice to administer 8mg of intravenous dexamethasone and further antibiotics at the time of re-exploration in order to reduce cerebral oedema. However, there is no randomized trial evidence to support this practice. Great care must be taken to avoid unnecessary neck movements whilst positioning the patient on the operating table as this may dislodge friable thrombus contained within the endarterectomy zone.

The neck wound is carefully reopened; the practice of simply palpating the carotid artery for a

reassuring pulse avoided as it is both insensitive and potentially dangerous.[4] The patient should be systemically heparinized, the vessels cross-clamped and the arteriotomy reopened. In most cases, the thrombus is localized to the carotid bifurcation with surprisingly little distal extension. If good back-bleeding occurs following thrombectomy it is probably safe to insert a shunt. If back-bleeding is poor or non-existent then careful passage of a number 2/3 Fogarty catheter may be the only option to improve outflow. In the future, however, there may be a role for catheter-guided thrombolysis in this difficult situation.

Prior to arteriotomy closure, any underlying technical error should be corrected. If a primary closure was performed at the original procedure, a patch should now be inserted. It is our practice to perform a completion angiogram following re-exploration in order to ensure a technically satisfactory result, particularly in the distal ICA. The patient is then electively ventilated overnight in the intensive care unit to minimize the risks of laryngeal oedema. Two further doses of intravenous dexamethasone and antibiotic are administered postoperatively.

If at re-exploration there is no evidence of carotid thrombosis the surgeon will have to assume that the stroke was due to either focal embolism or haemodynamic failure. In either situation, the immediate management is conservative and it would be reasonable to administer two further bolus doses of dexamethasone.

The Postoperative Stroke

The early postoperative period remains a potentially dangerous time for the patient, not least because it often coincides with evening when the surgeon may be at home. As with the intraoperative stroke, should the patient develop a new neurological deficit the surgeon has the continuing dilemma of having to decide whether or not to re-explore the patient. As a general rule, should a stroke occur in the first 6–12h following surgery it will almost certainly be thrombo-embolic and, in the absence of any monitoring to guide the surgeon, the patient should return to theatre for re-exploration. For those wishing a simple but more discriminating clinical guide to the likely pathogenesis, patients with the complete triad of hemiplegia, homonymous hemianopia and higher cortical dysfunction (e.g. dysphasia) are highly likely to have suffered a major vessel occlusion,[1,2] and warrant urgent re-exploration. Patients with an isolated monoparesis have usually suffered branch occlusion(s) of the MCA[1,2] and have a good prognosis and probably have less to gain from re-exploration. Unfortunately, the surgeon has no way of knowing whether there is any underlying technical error or ongoing embolization in these less severely disabled patients and may have to proceed to re-exploration on the grounds of uncertainty. In practice, we would not request an urgent computed tomography (CT) scan if the stroke occurred within 12h of surgery. Time is of the essence in this situation and the chances of having suffered an intracranial haemorrhage are extremely remote.

It has been our experience that strokes occurring after 3–5 days have elapsed are less likely (though not impossible) to be due to thromboembolism. In our last 500 audited CEAs, 1 patient (0.12%) suffered an embolic stroke on the fifth postoperative day.[5] As a general rule, after 3 days have elapsed one is concerned about intracranial haemorrhage and, less commonly, stroke secondary to hyperperfusion. It would therefore be useful to undertake an urgent CT scan in any patient who develops a neurological deficit during this period. Intracranial haemorrhage (ICH) complicates 1–2% of all endarterectomies and, while a number of aetiological factors have been implicated (poorly controlled hypertension, hyperperfusion syndrome, undiagnosed intracranial aneurysms), there are currently no means of predicting those at highest risk.

Unfortunately there is currently no active treatment available for ICH and the patient should be managed conservatively. Isolated cases may be considered for emergency neurosurgical intervention, although there is currently no consensus on the role of craniotomy in this situation. If this were to be considered, the carotid surgeon should take steps to discuss this possible therapeutic option in advance with neurosurgical colleagues. Otherwise, particular care must be taken to regulate the blood pressure. If the blood pressure is too high it can precipitate further bleeding whilst precipitous lowering can cause a critical reduction in perfusion pressure and secondary ischaemic injury.

The so-called hyperperfusion syndrome is an increasingly quoted diagnosis that is poorly understood, badly defined and engenders considerable scepticism. Evidence suggests that most patients undergoing CEA will have a transient increase in cerebral blood flow following CEA but fewer than 2% overall will progress on to the syndrome comprising seizure, irritability and confusion, while ischaemic stroke and/or ICH is rare. Patients at risk of suffering the hyperperfusion syndrome share similar characteristics to those at risk of ICH. These include severe, bilateral extracranial occlusive disease, treated hypertension, poor collateralization via the circle of Willis and impaired cerebral autoregulation.

The prevailing viewpoint is that impaired autoregulation takes some days to reset after CEA, during which time the brain is subjected to massively increased flow through the chronically vasodilated cerebral arterioles.[6] To date, however, we have only encountered two definite cases of hyperperfusion syndrome in 800 audited CEAs (0.25%). This indicates that, although the condition is interesting, it is not as important as thromboembolism or ICH. In keeping with the experience of others, our two patients presented on days 5 and 7 with seizures and confusion and, in 1 case, a transient hemiparesis. Both had high MCA blood flow velocities and both had grossly elevated blood pressures (260/150mmHg in one patient!).

The mainstay of management is control of the seizures. As an emergency first-line treatment we use titrated intravenous diazepam and thereafter ask our neurology colleagues to advise immediately on appropriate pharmacotherapy. It is vital to control the seizures as the patient is at some risk of asphyxiation and the grossly elevated central venous pressures can precipitate bleeding into either the brain or neck. The next priority is control of blood pressure. Jorgensen and Schroeder have shown that, although the interrelationship between blood pressure and cerebral blood flow is complex, careful administration of antihypertensive agents can reduce the elevated blood pressure and cerebral blood flow accordingly.[7] Our policy is to use a titrated labetalol infusion but there is no clear evidence that one agent is preferable to another.

Following stabilization, we would then arrange for a CT scan to be performed as soon as possible. This normally shows varying degrees of cerebral oedema (sometimes surprisingly little) but it is useful to exclude secondary haemorrhage. Evidence suggests that most patients will make a good recovery once the blood pressure and seizures are brought under control.

'PREVENTIVE' MANAGEMENT OF OPERATIVE STROKE

As will have been noted, most of the management decisions described above tend to be retrospective, i.e. something has to be done once the event has occurred. It would clearly be preferable to prevent the stroke from happening in the first place. The next section summarizes the current management strategy at Leicester Royal Infirmary. It is based on observations during a 7-year prospective audit of complications following 800 CEAs, during which time there has been a routine policy of intraoperative TCD and completion angioscopy and, latterly, postoperative TCD monitoring.[4,5,8–12] The practical aspects of the protocol are summarized in Tables 26.2–26.4.

The Intraoperative Stroke

One of the advantages of TCD is that it is an easy means of monitoring the patient throughout the procedure and can be of particular help in differentiating between a stroke due to on-table thrombosis, focal embolism or haemodynamic failure. At this difficult time, the key decision is to identify those patients with on-table carotid thrombosis who require immediate re-exploration.

In the author's experience, TCD remains the optimal method for differentiating between ICA thrombosis and MCA occlusion. The pathognomonic feature of on-table carotid thrombosis is a fall in ipsilateral MCA velocity to levels observed during carotid clamping (Table 26.2) and this is invariably associated with increasing rates of embolization.[4,8,10] Flow reversal in the ipsilateral

anterior cerebral artery (ACA), i.e. indicating that flow is derived from the contralateral hemisphere, is a corroborative but not necessarily exclusive feature.[13] With mainstem MCA occlusion, no MCA signal is detectable where one was present intraoperatively and there may be increased flow velocity in the ipsilateral ACA.[13]

On-table carotid thrombosis

Since 1992, 800 patients undergoing CEA in our institution have been monitored intraoperatively by continuous TCD (provided there is an accessible cranial window) and completion angioscopy. As described in Chapter 24, the main aim of angioscopy is to identify the 3–4% of patients with residual luminal thrombus and thereafter remove this before flow is restored.[9]

Only 2 patients (0.25%) recovered after suffering an anaesthesia-related stroke. In both cases, this followed on-table carotid thrombosis. On average, 3–4% of patients throughout the 7-year period of study underwent removal of small fragments of thrombus before restoration of flow (diagnosed by angioscopy) and we suspect that prior to our using angioscopy, embolization of retained luminal thrombus was the principal reason for our original 4% rate of intraoperative stroke.[8,9] The first case of on-table thrombosis was correctly diagnosed using TCD[4] but there was considerable scepticism on the part of the operating surgeon about reopening an otherwise normal-looking artery. The second occurred 5 years later and involved a patient with a vein bypass to the base of the skull. He had no collateral flow on TCD, and in the absence of TCD providing an immediate warning of impending trouble, he would almost certainly have suffered a major (fatal) stroke. We were therefore aware of a problem while he was still unconscious and were able to revise his vein graft.[5] After 9h of surgery, he recovered from anaesthesia with a dysphasic stroke which had almost recovered by day 30. In practice, therefore, on-table carotid thrombosis is extremely rare but it can be immediately diagnosed using TCD. This enables the surgeon to take pre-emptive steps to correct the underlying problem rather than waiting for the patient to recover from anaesthesia.

Table 26.2
Protocol for managing the patient who recovers from anaesthesia with a new neurological deficit

Clinical	Duplex	Transcranial Doppler	Likely diagnosis	Immediate treatment
Slow to awaken Hemiparesis* Monoparesis*	Normal	Normal MCA velocity No embolization Low intraoperative MCA flow	Haemodynamic	Conservative management 8mg intravenous dexamethasone CT scan at 3–5 days
Slow to awaken Hemiplegia Homonymous hemianopia Aphasia	No ICA flow	MCA flow same as during carotid clamping ACA flow reversed*	Carotid thrombosis	Urgent thrombectomy 8mg intravenous dexamethasone (× 3) Ventilate postoperatively CT scan at 3–5 days
Slow to awaken Hemiplegia Homonymous hemianopia Aphasia	Damped ICA flow Exclude luminal irregularity	MCA signal not detectable ACA flow increased	MCA mainstem occlusion	Conservative management 8mg intravenous dexamethasone (× 3) Re-explore if evidence of luminal thrombus CT scan at 3–5 days
Slow to awaken Hemiparesis* Monoparesis*	Normal ICA flow Exclude luminal irregularity	Will be normal if < 3 MCA branches are occluded but > 30% asymmetry suggests > 3 branches occluded	MCA branch occlusion	Conservative management 8mg intravenous dexamethasone Re-explore if embolizing Re-explore if evidence of luminal thrombus CT scan at 3–5 days

ICA, internal carotid artery; MCA, middle cerebral artery; ACA, anterior cerebral artery
*Findings may vary.

Focal cerebral embolism

As discussed above, the clinical features of a patient recovering from anaesthesia with a stroke secondary to MCA mainstem occlusion are indistinguishable from those of ICA thrombosis. Using TCD, any patient who suddenly loses their MCA signal following restoration of flow can be assumed to have suffered an MCA mainstem occlusion. At present there is relatively little that one can do about this, although catheter-guided thrombolysis might be of value in the future. In our experience, the use of completion angioscopy to identify luminal thrombus (prior to restoration of flow) has abolished this problem and we have not had any patient recover from anaesthesia in the last 500 patients with a focal embolic stroke.[5]

In contrast to the hemiplegic patient who is slow to recover following MCA mainstem occlusion, the patient who awakens relatively quickly and who is found to have a monoparesis or dysphasia is highly

Table 26.3
Protocol for postoperative transcranial Doppler monitoring and selective dextran therapy

No evidence of sustained embolization during 3h of monitoring
Normal postoperative care

> 25 emboli detected in any 10-min period or emboli which distort the middle cerebral artery waveform
20ml bolus of intravenous dextran 40, infusion rate started at 20ml/h
If rate of embolization reduces, continue dextran for 12h
If rate of embolization does not reduce, increase dextran dose every 10min to maximum of 40ml/h
If neurological deficit occurs whilst patient is on dextran, proceed to immediate re-exploration

unlikely to have suffered a major vessel occlusion. Patients with focal embolism and MCA branch occlusion (recognized by the development of significant (> 30%) interhemispheric MCA velocity asymmetry[14] are treated conservatively provided that there is no evidence of ongoing embolization on TCD. If there was evidence of ongoing embolization we would currently re-explore these patients, although this has not been necessary since introducing our intraoperative monitoring protocol. Patients with stroke secondary to branch occlusion of the MCA have a good prognosis[1,2] and treatment, in the absence of ongoing embolization, is directed at supportive therapy, which includes careful control of blood pressure and intravenous dexamethasone.

Haemodynamic stroke

This is an easy diagnosis to make, largely because it is difficult to disprove! If, however, the patient recovers from anaesthesia with a new neurological deficit and there has been a documented period of sustained hypoperfusion on TCD (usually < 10 cm/s[15]) in conjunction with no other duplex or TCD abnormality, then this diagnosis can be made with greater confidence. If there is no evidence of ongoing embolization, this diagnosis can be made

with even greater certainty. If a haemodynamic stroke is suspected, a CT scan performed 4–5 days postoperatively should show boundary zone infarction. Although this is useful information regarding personal audit and future prevention, the management of patients with stroke due to haemodynamic failure is conservative. Thus, if we were faced with a patient who recovered rapidly from anaesthesia with a new neurological deficit and who had a normal MCA velocity (but low flow at some stage in the procedure) and no evidence of ongoing embolization, we would treat him or her conservatively.

Postoperative Stroke

With the exception of prevention of thrombotic stroke, our management strategy is the same as that for the conventional approach to management.

Postoperative thrombotic stroke

Most of the decisions regarding the management of postoperative thromboembolic stroke tend to be implemented once the event has occurred. It would clearly be preferable to prevent the phase of platelet accumulation and embolism and subsequent progression on to thrombosis in the first place. In the past, the general viewpoint has been that postoperative carotid thrombosis was invariably due to some underlying technical error. However, several studies have enabled us to review many aspects of the pathophysiology of postoperative thromboembolism.

First, evidence suggests that, while implementation of an intraoperative quality control programme reduces the incidence of intraoperative stroke, it has little or no effect on the incidence of postoperative thrombotic stroke.[8,9] Second, provided intraoperative technical error has been excluded by a quality control programme, patients suffering a postoperative carotid thrombosis will not usually be found to have an underlying technical error at re-exploration.[8] Instead, these patients are found to have platelet-rich thrombus adherent to the endarterectomy zone.[8] Third, there is now evidence from three continents that patients destined to suffer a postoperative carotid thrombosis have a 1–2h phase of increasing embolization before any neurological deficit develops.[4,8,16–18]

Table 26.4
Protocol for managing the patient with a new neurological deficit in the late postoperative period

Results of investigations	Likely diagnosis	Management
Absent ICA flow on duplex MCA velocity same as during carotid clamping Reversed flow in ipsilateral ACA*	Carotid thrombosis	Immediate thrombectomy 8mg intravenous dexamethasone CT scan should not delay surgery
Damped ICA flow on duplex Absent MCA signal Increased ipsilateral ACA flow*	MCA mainstem occlusion	Re-explore if luminal irregularity suspected on duplex, otherwise treat conservatively 8mg intravenous dexamethasone Exclude cardiac source if necessary
Normal duplex examination Normal or slightly asymmetric MCA velocity	MCA branch embolism	*No ongoing embolization* Conservative management Exclude cardiac source *Embolizing + deficit resolving* Dextran 40 infusion Re-explore if deficit worsens *Embolizing + deficit persisting* Urgent re-exploration CT scan should not delay surgery
Intracranial haemorrhage on CT scan TCD mainstem may be deviated Normal duplex scan	Intracranial haemorrhage	Conservative management Careful blood pressure control
Increased ICA flow and MCA flow CT scan may show oedema Seizures may be present	Hyperperfusion syndrome	Conservative management 8mg intravenous dexamethasone Control of seizures, reduce blood pressure, maintain airway

ICA, internal carotid artery; MCA, middle cerebral artery; ACA, anterior cerebral artery; CT, computed tomography; TCD, transcranial Doppler
*Findings may vary
All patients undergo clinical, duplex and TCD assessment plus emergency CT scan.

Thus, recognition of this premonitory phase of embolization enables clinicians, for the first time, to intervene early and so prevent progression on to complete thrombosis. As a consequence, we have now revised our perioperative monitoring protocol to include routine TCD monitoring in all patients for 3h postoperatively. Evidence suggests that at least 50% of patients undergoing CEA will have one or more emboli detected postoperatively[5,11,12] but only 5% will develop the sustained pattern of embolization (> 25 emboli detected in any 10-min period or those with large emboli that distort the MCA waveform) that is associated with an increased risk of stroke. Evidence suggests that 50–60% of patients with this pattern of embolisation will suffer a thrombotic stroke.[8,16,17]

Accordingly, in our unit any patient with sustained postoperative embolization is considered high-risk for thromboembolic stroke and treated with a 20ml bolus of intravenous dextran followed by infusion of dextran 40 (Table 26.3). Dextran is initially started at a rate of 20ml/h and increased every 10min thereafter to a maximum of 40ml/h if there is no reduction in the rate of embolization.[11,12] If this fails to abolish the embolization or if the patient develops a neurological deficit whilst on dextran therapy, our protocol requires us to urgently re-explore the carotid artery, although we have not had to do this in our last 500 patients.[5] Prior to implementing this protocol, our incidence of postoperative thrombotic stroke was 2.7%.[8,9]

It might be argued that all patients should receive dextran in the early postoperative period. At first sight this has an attractive logic but our experience shows that the dextran dose has to be increased in 36% of patients in order to control the high rates of embolization in the small number of high-risk patients.[5] Moreover, caution must be exercised in those with a history of cardiac failure or renal impairment. When we did adopt a policy of routine postoperative dextran therapy in early 1995, we encountered no ICA thromboses but 1 patient died as a consequence of dextran-mediated multiorgan failure and the incidence of neck haematomas and clinical cardiac failure increased significantly.[11]

Delayed postoperative embolic stroke

The patient who develops a new neurological deficit in the postoperative period, particularly if several days have elapsed, must undergo a CT scan to exclude haemorrhage (Table 26.4). If, however, the CT scan is normal and TCD/duplex suggests a likely embolic aetiology, we would advocate immediate re-exploration if there was TCD evidence of ongoing embolization and no early improvement in the severity of the deficit in order to exclude an underlying source of embolism in the endarterectomized ICA. Conversely, if the deficit had started to improve, we would be more likely to treat the patient with intravenous dextran therapy but re-explore the patient if there was any evidence of clinical deterioration. In practice, only 1 patient in

the last 500 CEAs suffered a documented embolic stroke after the first 3 postoperative hours had elapsed. This patient suffered a monoparesis on day 5 and was found to have profuse embolization. His original operation involved a high carotid dissection and, in view of the fact that thrombus dislodgement was a potential problem (notwithstanding the inevitable neck oedema) and he was starting to recover, we chose to treat him with dextran. The embolization ceased with dextran therapy and he went on to make a near complete recovery with no recurrence of symptoms thereafter.[5]

CONCLUSIONS

In the absence of monitoring, management decisions are extremely difficult and the inevitable result is that most patients with a new neurological deficit will need to be re-explored. The strategy of management at Leicester Royal Infirmary has evolved from an integrated audit and clinical research programme which has systematically tried to prevent avoidable morbidity and mortality. In our experience, intraoperative TCD and completion angioscopy have reduced the risk of intraoperative stroke from 4% to 0.2%. Those few cases that do occur have exclusively arisen from on-table carotid thrombosis. Although this can be difficult to treat, the only means of diagnosing it is TCD.

Postoperatively, a 3h period of TCD monitoring with selective use of dextran has reduced our postoperative thrombotic stroke rate from 2.7% to 0% in the last 500 CEAs.[5] Of most practical importance has been the observation that no patient who had no evidence of postoperative embolization suffered a thromboembolic stroke in the postoperative period. During the last 500 CEAs, when the full monitoring protocol has been employed (continuous TCD, completion angioscopy and 3h of postoperative TCD with selective dextran therapy), our 30-day death and/or any stroke rate has fallen by 60% to 2.25%,[5] with the principal source of operative morbidity and mortality now being cardiac pathology and intracranial haemorrhage.

REFERENCES

1 Bamford J, Sandercock PAG, Dennis M *et al*. The clinical features and natural history of the four major subtypes of cerebral infarction. *Lancet* 1991; **337**: 1521–1526.

2 Naylor AR, Sandercock PAG, Sellar RJ, Warlow CP. Patterns of vascular pathology in acute, first-ever cerebral infarction. *Scottish Medical Journal* 1993; **38**: 41–44.

3 Takolander R, Bergentz SE, Bergqvist D *et al*. Management of early neurologic deficits after carotid thromboendarterectomy. *European Journal of Vascular Surgery* 1987; **1**: 67–71.

4 Gaunt ME, Smith J, Martin PJ, Ratliff DA, Bell PRF, Naylor AR. On-table diagnosis of incipient carotid artery thrombosis during carotid endarterectomy using transcranial Doppler sonography. *Journal of Vascular Surgery* 1994; **20**: 104–107.

5 Naylor AR, Hayes PD, Allroggen H *et al*. Reducing the risk of carotid surgery: a seven year audit of the role of monitoring and quality control assessment. *Journal of Vascular Surgery* (in press).

6 Naylor AR, Ruckley CV. The post-carotid endarterectomy hyperperfusion syndrome. *European Journal of Vascular and Endovascular Surgery* 1995; **9**: 365–367.

7 Jorgensen L, Schroeder TV. Defective cerebrovascular autoregulation after carotid endarterectomy. *European Journal of Vascular Surgery* 1993; **7**: 370–379.

8 Gaunt ME, Smith JL, Martin PJ, Ratliff DA, Bell PRF, Naylor AR. A comparison of quality control methods applied to carotid endarterectomy. *European Journal of Vascular and Endovascular Surgery* 1996; **11**: 4–11

9 Lennard N, Smith JL, Gaunt ME *et al*. A policy of quality control assessment reduces the risk of intra-operative stroke during carotid endarterectomy. *European Journal of Vascular and Endovascular Surgery* 1999; **17**: 234–240.

10 Gaunt ME, Martin PJ, Smith JL *et al*. The clinical relevance of intra-operative embolisation detected by transcranial Doppler monitoring during carotid endarterectomy: a prospective study in 100 patients. *British Journal of Surgery* 1994; **81**: 1435–1439.

11 Lennard N, Smith JL, Dumville J *et al*. Prevention of post-operative thrombotic stroke after carotid endarterectomy: the role of transcranial Doppler ultrasound. *Journal of Vascular Surgery* 1997; **26**: 579–584.

12 Lennard N, Smith JL, Hayes P *et al*. Transcranial Doppler directed dextran therapy in the prevention of carotid thrombosis: 3 hours monitoring is as effective as 6 hours. *European Journal of Vascular and Endovascular Surgery* 1999; **17**: 301–305.

13 Naylor AR, Ruckley CV. Complications after carotid surgery. In: Campbell B (ed.) *Complications in Arterial Surgery*, pp. 73–88. Oxford: Butterworth-Heinemann, 1996.

14 Zannette EM, Fieschi C, Bozzao I *et al*. Comparison of cerebral angiography and transcranial Doppler sonography in acute stroke. *Stroke* 1989; **20**: 899–903.

15 Halsey JH, McDowell HA, Gelmon S *et al*. Blood flow velocity in the middle cerebral artery and regional blood flow during carotid endarterectomy. *Stroke* 1989; **20**: 53–58.

16 Levi CR, O'Malley HM, Fell G *et al*. Transcranial Doppler detected cerebral embolism following carotid endarterectomy: high microembolic signal loads predict post-operative cerebral ischaemia. *Brain* 1997; **120**: 621–629.

17 Cantelmo NL, Babikian VL, Samaraweera RN, Gordon JK, Pochay VE, Winter MR. Cerebral microembolism and ischaemia changes associated with carotid endarterectomy. *Journal of Vascular Surgery* 1998; **27**: 1024–1030.

18 Spencer MP. Transcranial Doppler monitoring and causes of stroke from carotid endarterectomy. *Stroke* 1997; **28**: 685–691.

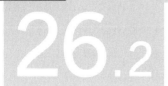

How should I manage the patient who suffers a perioperative neurological deficit?
David Rosenthal (USA)

INTRODUCTION

After more than four decades of carotid artery surgery, the pathogenesis and management of postoperative neurologic deficits remain controversial. Several reports[19-21] attribute temporary cerebral ischemia during carotid occlusion to the pathogenesis of postoperative deficits, while others[22-24] suggest that reperfusion injury or technical error resulting in thromboembolic events is the cause. It is often difficult to determine the exact cause of a postoperative deficit, but all these factors may play some role. The purpose of this chapter is first, to investigate the pathogenesis of neurologic deficits after CEA and second, to evaluate the best means of managing such patients in order to minimize permanent neurologic impairment.[25]

CLINICAL EXPERIENCE

Our protocol for managing postoperative neurologic deficits is based on our experience in 1033 CEAs performed from 1980 through 1996. The indications for these operations were: hemispheric transient ischemic attacks (TIAs: $n = 477$), symptoms of vertebrobasilar insufficiency ($n = 214$), reversible ischemic neurologic deficit (RIND) or stroke ($n = 149$), prophylactic CEA prior to major abdominal or cardiovascular reconstruction ($n = 95$), amaurosis fugax ($n = 79$), and stroke in evolution ($n = 19$).

Postoperative neurologic deficits were classified into three categories:

1 A focal episode of neurologic dysfunction which resolved within 24h was defined as a TIA.
2 A neurologic deficit which lasted more than 24h, yet resolved completely within 3 weeks, was designated a RIND.
3 A fixed non-progressive neurologic deficit that lasted longer than 24h and was due to cerebral infarction was characterized as a stroke.

The incidence of postoperative neurologic deficits (Table 26.5) was not significantly different in patients with routine shunting, routine non-shunting, and selective shunting based on electroencephalogram (EEG) criteria. In the routine shunt patients ($n = 408$), transient deficits occurred in 2.9% and permanent deficits in 1.9%. In the no-shunt group ($n = 274$), transient deficits occurred in 2.9% of patients, while permanent deficits occurred in 2.2%. Similarly, in patients shunted selectively

Table 26.5
Postoperative neurologic deficits

Carotid endarterectomy ($n = 1033$)		Transient ($n = 29$)	Permanent ($n = 21$)
Shunt	($n = 408$)	2.9% (12)	1.9% (8)
No shunt	($n = 274$)	2.9% (8)	2.2% (6)
Electroencephalogram	($n = 351$)	2.5% (9)	1.9% (7)

Table 26.6
Postoperative deficits and indication for operation

Indications		Transient	Permanent
Transient ischemic attack	(n = 477)	2.0% (10)	1.8% (9)
Vertebrobasilar insufficiency	(n = 214)	2.8% (6)	2.3% (5)
Prophylactic	(n = 95)	1.0% (1)	1.0% (1)
Amaurosis fugax	(n = 79)	2.5% (2)	(0)
Stroke in evolution (no shunt)	(n = 19)	16.0% (3)	5.3% (1)
Post RIND/CVA (no shunt)	(n = 63)	7.9% (5)	6.3% (4)
Post RIND/CVA (shunt)	(n = 86)	2.3% (2)	1.2% (1)

RIND, reversible ischemic neurologic deficit; CVA, cerebrovascular accident.

based on EEG criteria (n = 351), transient deficits were noted in 2.5% and permanent deficits in 1.9%. Overall, 29 patients experienced transient postoperative deficits and 21, permanent deficits. There was no significant statistical difference in the incidence of postoperative neurologic deficits when the three methods of cerebral monitoring/protection were compared (P > 0.25).

The incidence of postoperative neurologic complications was evaluated on the basis of indication for operation (Table 26.6). The incidence of both transient and permanent neurologic deficits was lower in patients with stable neurologic status (TIA, amaurosis, vertebrobasilar, or prophylactic) than in those with stroke in evolution or prior established stroke. This difference was especially noteworthy when no shunt was utilized in this group. When the RIND/stroke patients underwent CEA with a temporary indwelling shunt, the incidence of postoperative neurologic complications was reduced almost to the level for the patients without prior stroke.

The preoperative arteriograms of all patients experiencing postoperative neurologic deficits were reviewed. Of 29 patients experiencing postoperative transient deficits, 20 (69%) had ulcerated plaques. Of the 21 patients with permanent deficits, 10 (48%) had ulcerated plaques. This suggests that

intraoperative embolization from the ulcer may have played a role in the pathogenesis of the event. Contralateral stenosis (> 75%) or occlusion was noted in only 3 (6%) of the 50 patients with deficits. On the other hand, intracranial lesions were noted in 52% of these patients.

In the immediate postoperative period (< 6h), 29 patients experienced transient neurologic deficits: 8 occurred in the CEA/no-shunt group, 12 in the CEA/shunt group, and 9 in the CEA/EEG group. Fourteen patients experienced minor focal deficits which resolved rapidly and uneventfully. Fifteen patients experienced more pronounced deficits such as contralateral sensory and motor changes of the face and extremities upon awakening from anesthesia. Thirteen were re-anesthetized and had immediate operative arteriography. Carotid re-exploration was necessary in 3 patients, while the others had normal arteriograms. All 15 patients with more pronounced deficits had 72-h interval CT brain scans which were normal, and all regained normal neurologic function within 1 month of operation. By definition, these were classified as postoperative RINDs.

Twenty-one patients with immediate profound postoperative deficits required emergency operation. Nineteen deficits were identified upon awakening from anesthesia and 2 occurred in the recovery room within 1 h of operation. A patent CEA site was identified in 9 patients, and a thrombosed carotid artery in 12. Of the first 9 patients, arteriography verified an intracranial embolic shower in 6, while 3 arteriograms were normal. After the second operation, 7 patients improved gradually and 2 died. Of the 12 patients with thrombosed CEA sites, 4 had thrombectomy of platelet–fibrin aggregates or 'white clot.' Despite arteriography, the cause of the thromboses could not be identified. The other thromboses were caused by technical error, where an intimal flap in 5 and a lateral tear repair site in 3 were demonstrated. At reoperation, 10 patients had placement of a patch graft (2 autogenous vein, and 8 prosthetic material) and 2 had replacement of the carotid bifurcation with saphenous vein interposition graft. Three patients had immediate return of neurologic function, 2 improved slowly, 6 were unchanged, and 2 died of stroke-related causes.

Four late (> 12h) postoperative strokes occurred, all due to thrombosis of the CEA site. Three of these strokes were related to cardiac causes. Two patients suffered a postoperative myocardial infarction and the other had an episode of ventricular tachycardia resulting in prolonged hypotension. After resuscitation, the patients were hemiplegic and emergent reoperation demonstrated thrombosis of the CEA sites. Re-exploration and thrombectomy re-established carotid flow, but only minimal neurologic function was regained in these patients, despite successful thrombectomy verified by arteriography. The fourth patient aspirated and developed hemiplegia 40h after CEA. He progressed to coma and died 4 days later.

LESSONS LEARNED FROM OUR CLINICAL EXPERIENCE

Neurologic deficits after CEA occur infrequently (transient 2.8% and permanent 2.0% in our experience). Both the etiology of these deficits and their management remain ill-defined. The goal of this chapter is to elucidate the causes of these deficits and discuss their safest and most expeditious management.

It is noteworthy that asymptomatic and TIA patients had a lower incidence of transient and permanent deficits than did patients with prior stroke or acute stroke (Table 26.6). This has been observed by others.[26,27] After a RIND/stroke event or during a stroke in evolution, a zone of ischemic brain tissue is present which may be more vulnerable to diminished perfusion during carotid cross-clamp than normal brain tissue.[28,29] This ischemic zone is supplied by highly resistant collateral vessels and a drop in perfusion pressure during carotid cross-clamp may cause further ischemia. The risk of postoperative neurologic problems in these patients can be diminished by shunting.

Assessment of the preoperative arteriograms suggested two findings of interest. First, most complications (27/29 transient, 10/21 permanent deficits) occurred in patients who had ulcerative plaque disease identified at arteriography. It seems likely that patients with ulcerated plaque disease are more prone to an embolic event during carotid artery mobilization, where intraluminal cellular debris is not adherent within the ulcer bed, than patients with calcific high-grade obstructive lesions. Second, of the 50 patients who suffered a postoperative deficit, 26 had intracranial occlusive disease (stenoses at the siphon or stenoses within the circle of Willis). Severe intracranial disease has been previously demonstrated to place patients at high risk for postoperative neurologic complications.[30] In the absence of intraoperative EEG monitoring in the patient with severe intracranial occlusive disease, shunting seems most appropriate.

Since most surgeons, thankfully, have little experience with neurologic deficits after endarterectomy, a clear protocol for management is necessary (Fig. 26.1). When a minor focal deficit occurs which resolves within minutes, supportive non-operative treatment is most appropriate. Urgent carotid color flow duplex ultrasonography, however, should be performed to evaluate the operative site. All patients with minor deficits in this series resolved their deficits uneventfully. If, however, there is progression of the deficit, the symptoms wax and wane, the surgeon is unsure, or an abnormal ultrasound examination is found, the safest and most expeditious means of managing the patient is prompt return to the operating room for arteriography. Arteriography was performed on 13 patients with more severe postoperative deficits

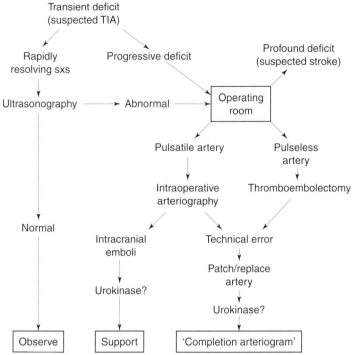

Fig. 26.1
Protocol for management of postoperative neurologic deficit. TIA, transient ischemic attack.

to identify possible intimal flaps, intraluminal thrombi, clamp injuries, or other technical problems which might serve as an embolic foci; in 10 patients no technical problem was found and all regained normal neurologic function within a month of operation.

If intracranial emboli are demonstrated by arteriography, recent reports indicate that local intra-arterial thrombolysis may be beneficial.[31,32] The thrombotic agent may be administered by a microcatheter placed via the ICA into the intracranial vessels or via an indwelling shunt. These reports offer encouraging results; however, it must be remembered that perioperative neurologic deficits caused by an 'embolic shower' are most often due to cholesterol and platelet–fibrin aggregates and thrombolysis may have little benefit in this setting. Further investigation is, however, warranted in this area.

When the patient awakens from anesthesia with a neurologic deficit, he or she is immediately re-anesthetized and the wound reopened for assessment of the endarterectomy site. The surgeon should never leave the operating theater until satisfied that the patient is neurologically intact. If the deficit occurs in the recovery room the patient should immediately be returned to the operating room. If a pulsatile vessel is found at reoperation, an arteriogram is obtained through a common carotid puncture proximal to the endarterectomy site. In this manner, the previous common carotid clamp site as well as the extra- and intracranial ICA may be visualized. When a pulseless, thrombosed endarterectomy site or some other obvious defect is found, the common and external carotid arteries are cross-clamped, the endarterectomy site is opened, and the ICA is allowed freely to back-bleed in the hope of removing any thromboembolic material. If no back-bleeding occurs, gentle thromboembolectomy with a Fogarty catheter is mandatory. Once back-bleeding is established, a temporary shunt is inserted to insure restoration of cerebral blood flow. In this setting, thrombolysis may be an excellent adjunct as thrombus may have propagated to the intracranial vasculature. Technical errors should be corrected, but unfortunately these may not always be found. The arteriotomy should be closed with a patch graft or the artery replaced with saphenous vein depending on the condition of the artery and the nature of the technical defect. A completion arteriogram or ultrasound examination is then mandatory.

Of the 4 late postoperative strokes (> 12h) which occurred, 3 patients had permanent hemiplegia and the other died. Uniformly poor results are reported with these late-occurring deficits, but if a mechanical problem is the cause, prompt return to the operating room affords the only opportunity to correct the problem and hopefully avert a neurologic catastrophe.[33,34]

Four endarterectomy sites were thrombosed by white clot composed of platelet–fibrin aggregates. There were no obvious reasons for the thromboses and the pathogenesis of this phenomenon remains obscure. It may, however, be due either to a heparin-dependent platelet membrane antibody which will induce platelet aggregation in the presence of heparin or to a disequilibrium in the balance of the prostaglandin systems (thromboxane A_2 and prostacyclin), where platelet proaggregation and disaggregation activity is affected.[35,36] It was of interest to note that, of the patients experiencing either a transient (29) or permanent (21) postoperative deficit, 23 had been on a regimen of aspirin and/or dipyridamole until the day of operation. In the patient with arterial disease severe enough to warrant CEA, platelet inhibition by aspirin and/or dipyridamole may not be sufficient to prevent a white clot thrombosis after endarterectomy. The newer antiplatelet agents, clopidogrel and ticlopidine, may play a role in preventing such events. Low-molecular-weight dextran, given systemically or topically over the endarterectomized surface, may also help to prevent platelet adherence and aggregation.

The incidence of the postoperative neurologic deficits in our experience was not significantly influenced by the method of monitoring and cerebral protection in the group as a whole (Table 26.5). The concept of inadequate cerebral collateral flow during CEA could not, therefore, be indicted as the cause of the postoperative neurologic complications. It must be emphasized that technical errors which cause carotid thrombosis or cerebral emboli, and not inadequate collateral cerebral flow, account for most neurologic deficits after CEA.

As patient selection, assessment of neurologic stability, intraoperative monitoring, and surgical technique become more sophisticated and standardized, the incidence of post-endarterectomy neurologic deficits will continue to decrease. If a perioperative neurologic deficit does occur, the most appropriate management of the patient is immediate return to the operating room where all diagnostic and therapeutic resources are available to the surgeon. A few selected patients with minimal focal postoperative neurologic deficits will improve without surgical reintervention, but these patients must be monitored closely and their endarterectomy site proven normal by duplex.

REFERENCES

19 Frawley JE, Hicks RG, Reardon M, Woodey R. Hemodynamic ischemic stroke during carotid endarterectomy: an appraisal of risk and cerebral prootection. *Journal of Vascular Surgery* 1997; **25**: 611–619.

20 Archie JP. Technique and clinical results of carotid stump back-pressure to determine selective shunting during carotid endarterectomy. *Journal of Vascular Surgery* 1991; **13**: 319–327.

21 Owens MC, Wilson SE. Prevention of neurologic complications of carotid endarterctomy. *Archives of Surgery* 1982; **117**: 551–555.

22 Riles TS, Imparato AM, Jacobowitz GR *et al*. The cause of perioperative stroke after carotid endarterectomy. *Journal of Vascular Surgery* 1994; **19**: 201–206.

23 Rosenthal D, Zeichner WD, Pano LA, Stanton PE. Neurologic deficit after carotid endarterectomy: pathogenesis and management. *Surgery* 1983; **94**: 776–780.

24 Hertzer NR, Beven EG, Greenstreet RL, Humphries AW. Internal carotid artery back pressure, intraoperative shunting, ulcerated atheromata, and the incidence of stroke during carotid endarterectomy. *Surgery* 1978; **83**: 306–312.

25 Moore WS, Barnett HJM, Beebe HG *et al*. Guidelines for carotid endarterectomy: a multidisciplinary consensus statement from the Ad Hoc Committee, American Heart Association. *Stroke* 1995; **26**: 188–201.

26 Whittemore AD, Ruby ST, Couch NP *et al*. Early carotid endarterectomy in patients with small fixed neurologic deficits. *Journal of Vascular Surgery* 1984; **1**: 795–799.

27 Giordano JM, Trout HH, Kozloff L, DePalma RG. Timing carotid arterial endarterectomy surgery after stroke. *Journal of Vascular Surgery* 1985; **2**: 250–255.

28 Pomposelli FB, Lamparello PJ, Riles TS *et al*. Intracranial hemorrhage after carotid endarterectomy. *Journal of Vascular Surgery* 1988; **7**: 240–247.

29 Rothwell PM, Slattery J, Warlow CP. A systematic comparison of the risks of stroke and death due to carotid endarterectomy for symptomatic and asymptomatic stenosis. *Stroke* 1996; **27**: 266–269.

30 Thompson JE, Talkington CM. Carotid endarterectomy. *Advances in Surgery* 1993; **26**: 99–131.

31 Castol N, Moschinil FT, Camerlingo M *et al*. Local intraarterial thrombolysis for acute stroke in the carotid territories. *Acta Neurologica Scandinavica* 1992; **86**: 308–311.

32 Barr JD, Harowitz MB, Mathis JM *et al*. Intraoperative urokinase infusion for embolic stroke during carotid endarterectomy. *Neurosurgery* 1995; **36**: 606–611.

33 Perdue GI. Management of postendarterectomy neurologic deficits. *Archives of Surgery* 1982; **117**: 1079–1081.

34 Treiman RL *et al*. Management of postoperative stroke after carotid endarterectomy. *American Journal of Surgery* 1981; **142**: 236–238.

35 Kapsch D, Silver D. Heparin induced thrombocytopenia and hemorrhage. *Archives of Surgery* 1981; **116**: 1423–1429.

36 Adams JG, Humphrey LJ, Zhang X, Silver D. Do patients with heparin-induced thrombocytopenia syndrome have heparin specific antibodies? *Journal of Vascular Surgery* 1995; **21**: 247–254.

26.3 Editorial Comment

KEY POINTS

1 Patients who awaken from anesthesia with a new neurologic deficit, or who develop one in the early postoperative period, will almost certainly have a thromboembolic cause. In order definitively to exclude carotid thrombosis or an underlying technical error, the patient should be immediately re-explored.
2 Patients with acute carotid thrombosis have most to gain from re-exploration, which should be performed as soon as possible.
3 Further refinement in the indications for immediate re-exploration may, in the future, be made by those with access to TCD and/or emergency duplex ultrasound.
4 TCD may be used to identify patients at high risk for progression on to carotid thrombosis and thereafter guide therapeutic or surgical intervention as appropriate.

The fundamental priority in the management of patients with an early postoperative neurological deficit is the identification of carotid thrombosis and elimination of the potential for further embolization.

In most centers, this will require immediate return to the operating theater as any delay beyond 1h can adversely affect outcome. The chances of having suffered an intracranial hemorrhage within 6–12h of operation are remote and an emergency CT scan is therefore unnecessary and may delay emergency re-exploration. Because it is not possible to exclude carotid thrombus in the absence of monitoring, such a policy will mean that some patients will undergo an unnecessary and possibly dangerous re-exploration. Unfortunately, however, a carotid thrombosis and an MCA mainstem occlusion cannot be differentiated on clinical grounds alone.

Carotid re-exploration should be done with great care so as not to dislodge friable thrombus into the brain. Palpation for a reassuring pulsation should be avoided for the same reason. The patch or arteriotomy should be reopened and the thrombus removed. If there is good back-flow, a shunt can be inserted. Any underlying defect should be repaired. If no defect is found and a white friable thrombus is encountered, it may be appropriate to start a dextran infusion. If the vessel had been closed primarily, a vein patch should now be inserted and a completion angiogram performed.

There is, however, growing evidence that patients destined to suffer a postoperative thrombosis will have a 1–2h phase of increasing embolization before developing any neurological signs. By using TCD to detect this warning phase, antiplatelet or antithrombotic agents can be administered to prevent progression on to thrombosis. In those centers with access to this facility, evidence suggests that few patients require emergency re-exploration.

All patients developing a stroke after 12–24h have elapsed should undergo an urgent CT scan to exclude hemorrhage unless TCD or duplex findings can make a confident diagnosis of acute ICA or MCA occlusion. If there is any doubt, a definitive decision regarding management should await the CT scan. Patients with intracranial hemorrhage should be treated conservatively, with special care directed at avoiding extremes of blood pressure. These patients

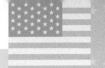

are best managed with the input of specialist stroke physicians wherever possible. A diagnosis of hyperperfusion stroke should be suspected in any patient suffering a neurologic deficit in association with seizures, headaches, hypertension, and evidence of high MCA velocities on TCD. The mainstay of management is control of seizures and reduction in blood pressure.

27.1

How can I balance patient safety and cost-effectiveness in planning early postoperative care and hospital discharge?
Peter R Taylor (Europe)

INTRODUCTION

The safety of the patient is paramount in any form of surgery and nothing should ever be done which will compromise that. However, there are certain traditions which continue to be regularly adhered to in patients undergoing carotid endarterectomy (CEA) for which there is no supporting rationale.

The fundamental reason for looking closely at current practice is the limited amount of money available for health care together with the increasing demand for resources. It is therefore important that all stages of the patient's progress through the system are closely monitored to identify where savings can safely be made. For example, one of the many traditions in carotid surgery is the reliance on angiography for preoperative imaging. In Chapter 8 the replacement of angiography by duplex scan has been discussed and Strandness has calculated that this could amount to a saving of $712 million annually in the US.[1]

The Operation

The most important factor in ensuring the safety of the patient, and thus an early and safe discharge, is to make sure that the operation is performed with technical excellence. Early work has shown that some form of intraoperative quality control assessment can identify abnormalities and that this can predict the risk of late restenosis.[2,3] The development of small transducer heads with high-resolution imaging has enabled improved visualization of the endarterectomized segment. Some progress has been made to identify which duplex-detected abnormalities should be corrected in order to improve patency rates.[4] Defects which are present at the end of the operation can progress or resolve when the artery is assessed by transcutaneous duplex at 6 weeks. Lesions at the proximal endarterectomy site seem to resolve, but lesions at the distal site are usually still present and may progress. This is probably important in determining outcome, as there is evidence that patients with normal intraoperative findings have a significantly lower rate of late ipsilateral stroke compared with patients with abnormal results.[5] Other methods have been recommended for quality control, such as angiography and angioscopy.[6]

The Early Postoperative Period

The next most important period is the immediate postoperative phase. The risk of stroke appears to be highest intraoperatively and seems to decrease exponentially thereafter. It was previously traditional (particularly in the US) for all patients undergoing CEA to be admitted to the intensive care unit (ICU) for overnight observation. However, in a retrospective review of 129 patients, 31 were deemed not to require intensive care[7] and the authors thereafter recommended that 8h should elapse before it was safe for the patient to return to the ward and then only if no intervention was required.

However, pressure on intensive care beds from other disciplines and the expense of keeping a patient overnight in such a unit have encouraged a reappraisal of this strategy. In a further study of 331 patients, only 12 (3.6%) were considered appropriate for admission to the ICU: 9 for cardiorespiratory problems and 3 for control of blood pressure.[8]

In a further prospective study, 79% of 185 patients were admitted to the recovery area for 3h and thereafter transferred to the ward when haemodynamically and neurologically stable.[9] Thirty-nine (21%) required admission to the ICU for the treatment of hypertension ($n = 14$), hypotension ($n = 14$), possible myocardial infarction ($n = 3$), neurological deficit ($n = 3$), arrhythmias ($n = 2$), wound haematomas ($n = 2$) and reintubation ($n = 1$). This latter group of patients spent an average of 20h on the ICU with a further 32h in hospital.

Many will, no doubt, observe that the ICU was not necessarily the appropriate place to treat all these patients. The development of a high-dependency unit (HDU) would further increase cost-effectiveness by avoiding the high cost of ICU whilst maintaining an increased level of nursing and medical supervision. If such a unit had been used, about 72% of Morasch's patients could, in theory, have avoided ICU care.

In our centre, the HDU has fulfilled the important role of nursing high-risk patients and monitoring the haemodynamic and neurological status of the patient. Patients should be nursed sitting upright as this tends to decrease the incidence of neck haematoma formation. If a haematoma is developing, great care should be taken to monitor the patient's saturation, and if he or she develops stridor, the patient should be taken back to theatre for exploration of the neck and evacuation of the haematoma. The most senior anaesthetist available should be present as reintubation may be difficult and hazardous. Patients dying through loss of the airway following haemorrhage into the wound are unfortunately still being reported. Under these circumstances it is safer to look and see rather than wait and see.

The control of blood pressure is crucial at this time, and all patients should have an arterial line for continuous monitoring. Most patients have a decrease in blood pressure compared with their preoperative measurements. This may be a physiological response to the removal of the tight carotid stenosis, or may be a reflection of postoperative analgesia and sedation.

Hypotension should be actively treated if the systolic pressure falls below 100mmHg. The first line of therapy in our unit is to increase the rate of infusion of intravenous fluids, usually with colloid. This is sufficient to bring most patients above the threshold for intervention but, in refractory patients, ephedrine may be necessary. On very rare occasions, the patient may require treatment with more potent inotropes and these cases should be transferred to the ICU.

Hypertension should also be actively treated: the threshold for intervention in our centre is any systolic pressure 10% above the patient's preoperative level. Initial measures include adequate analgesia and sedation, but some patients require hypotensive medications such as sublingual nifedipine or infusions of glyceryl trinitrate. Long-acting drugs and those prone to cause rapid and profound hypotension should be avoided as these may precipitate a stroke.

Careful attention is also paid to the patient's neurological status during the early postoperative phase. Neurological observations should be performed every 5min for the first 30min, after which the frequency can be lengthened if the patient is stable. The protocol for managing the patient with a new neurological deficit is discussed elsewhere.

Hospital stay

One further tradition which has recently been questioned is the length of postoperative stay. In the US, this has been driven by the medical insurance companies. In the UK, patients have traditionally been kept in hospital for 5–7 days following surgery. However, studies have shown that patients can safely be discharged home on the first postoperative day,[10] and there is little evidence that keeping patients longer results in any better outcome.

In a prospective study of 72 patients having CEA under general anaesthesia who were admitted on the day of surgery following outpatient work-up, 88% were discharged home the following day. There were no strokes or deaths, and only 2 patients suffered a transient ischaemic attack.[11]

Other centres have developed similar clinical pathways following elective CEA. Collier used outpatient angiograms on selected patients, same-day admission, regional anaesthesia, selective use of the ICU, and discharge on day 1 wherever possible.[12] Of the 186 patients entered into the study, 3 (1.6%) had neurological complications and 18 (10%) required admission to the ICU. Most CEA patients (84%) were discharged on the first postoperative day and the average length of stay for all patients was 1.27 days. There was 1 death on the 28th day from cardiac causes. No patient was subsequently readmitted. The use of this clinical pathway resulted in an average saving of $3000 per patient. Neurological complications, admission to the ICU and length of stay all decreased the overall cost-effectiveness of CEA. However, the type of anaesthesia and the use of a shunt or a patch did not affect cost.

Other studies have confirmed these findings and have forced surgeons at least to question their practice. In a retrospective review of 331 patients, admission to the ICU was deemed necessary in only 12 patients.[8] Hospital stay was reduced by an average of 2.1 days and the overall costs of CEA were reduced by 29%, which equated to an average reduction of nearly $2000 per case. In common with other studies, this was not achieved at the cost of increase in morbidity and mortality. The overall stroke rate was 0.78% and the death rate 0.26%.

For any centre wishing to implement some of these changes, it is clear that in addition to changing physician attitudes, it is vitally important to involve and reassure the patient and to brief the family doctor. Clear patient information is essential and written instructions covering the operation, length of stay and potential complications are helpful. Subcuticular absorbable sutures negate visits to have clips or non-absorbable sutures removed by medical or nursing staff. Patients should also be told of the likelihood of wound swelling, which usually increases until the third or fourth postoperative day. The patient should have an information sheet which details the symptoms or signs that require reporting to the hospital and there should also be a list of emergency phone numbers so that the patient can always contact the unit should any problem arise.

It is also important that the patient and family are informed from the outset that it is the current policy to discharge patients on the first postoperative day. This alters attitudes and enables the family to plan to be with the relative in the early postoperative period.

We recently instituted such a policy in my institution. In common with other series, most patients were discharged on the first postoperative day and 82% felt that this length of hospital stay was satisfactory. Only 12% had seen their general practitioner within the 4-week period after discharge. The operative risk – (3.8% (8/211)) was not adversely affected by this change in protocol.

Only 1 patient has required readmission, having suffered a stroke on the second postoperative day, which was thought to be due to cardiogenic embolism. In practical terms, the cost saving achieved per case has been about £2550. This study confirms the findings of many others that valuable savings can be achieved by reducing the preoperative investigations, reducing the requirement for intensive care and by early discharge from hospital, and that these changes do not result in a decrease in patient safety.

CONCLUSIONS

There is relatively little scientific evidence to support the previously held viewpoint that patients should remain in hospital for 5–7 days following carotid surgery. In the UK, there has always been a natural reluctance routinely to admit CEA patients to the ICU after surgery. In practice, the HDU can fulfil this role, with few patients meriting admission thereafter to the ICU. Provided arrangements and information have been communicated to the family doctor, most patients can be discharged on day 1 after CEA without adversely affecting outcome. Evidence suggests that most patients approve of the concept of early discharge. The reappraisal of many of the aspects of how we investigate and treat patients with carotid artery disease could lead to significant cost benefits.

REFERENCES

1 Strandness DE Jr. Extracranial arterial disease. In: Strandness DE Jr (ed.) *Duplex Scanning in Vascular Disorders*, 2nd edn, pp. 113–158. New York: Raven Press, 1993.

2 Flanigan DP, Douglas DJ, Machi J *et al*. Intraoperative ultrasonic imaging of the carotid artery during carotid endarterectomy. *Surgery* 1986; **100**: 893–898.

3 Bandyk DF, Kaebnick HW, Adams MB *et al*. Turbulence

occurring after carotid bifurcation endarterectomy: a harbinger of residual and recurrent stenosis. *Journal of Vascular Surgery* 1988; **10**: 261–274.

4 Padayachee TS, Brooks MD, Modaresi KB, Arnold AJ, Self GW, Taylor PR. Intraoperative high resolution duplex imaging during carotid endarterectomy: which abnormalities require surgical correction? *European Journal of Vascular and Endovascular Surgery* 1998; **15**: 387–393.

5 Kinney EV, Seabrook GR, Kinney LY *et al*. The importance of intraoperative detection of residual flow abnormalities after carotid artery endarterectomy. *Journal of Vascular Surgery* 1993; **17**: 912–922.

6 Gaunt ME, Smith JL, Martin PJ, Ratliff DA, Bell PRF, Naylor AR. A comparison of quality control methods applied to carotid endarterectomy. *European Journal of Vascular and Endovascular Surgery* 1996; **11**: 4–11.

7 Lipsett PA, Tierney S, Gordon TA, Perler BA. Carotid endarterectomy – is intensive care unit care necessary? *Journal of Vascular Surgery* 1994; **20**: 403–409.

8 Hoyle RM, Jenkins JM, Edwards WH Sr, Edwards WH Jr, Martin RS 3rd, Mulherin JL Jr. Case management in cerebral revascularisation. *Journal of Vascular Surgery* 1994; **20**: 396–401.

9 Morasch MD, Hirko MK, Hirasa T *et al*. Intensive care after carotid endarterectomy: a prospective evaluation. *Journal of the American College of Surgeons* 1996; **183**: 387–392.

10 Taylor PR, Panayiotopoulos YP, Edmondson RA, Sandison AJP. Strengths of carotid endarterectomy were understated. *British Medical Journal* 1995; **311**: 1575.

11 Friedman SG, Tortolani AJ. Reduced length of stay following carotid endarterectomy under general anaesthesia. *American Journal of Surgery* 1995; **170**: 235–236.

12 Collier PE. Are one-day admissions for carotid endarterectomy feasible? *American Journal of Surgery* 1995; **170**: 140–143.

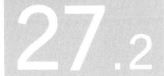

27.2

How can I balance patient safety and cost-effectiveness in planning early postoperative care and hospital discharge?
Paul E Collier (USA)

INTRODUCTION

Spiraling medical costs have been consuming an increasing percentage of the budgets of both the federal government and big businesses. Economists and regulators have focused attention on bringing these expenses under control. The introduction of the diagnosis-related group (DRG) system by the US government challenged hospitals and physicians to maximize cost-effectiveness in clinical practice. Business turned to managed care and self-insurance plans to decrease insurance costs. In an effort to economize while maintaining high standards of patient care, physicians have increasingly turned to a business model. Quality has been defined as the 'conformance to requirements or the norm.'[13] Only those products that fall outside the norm receive extra attention. When analyzed from this perspective, most patients who underwent elective CEA were demonstrated to follow a well-defined and predictable course, which called into question traditional norms such as routine preoperative contrast angiography, routine postoperative ICU care, and 4–7 days of postoperative inpatient care.[14,15]

The institution of total quality management business principles allowed us to question the validity of each step in the process of performing a CEA at our institution. A clinical pathway was developed and instituted with five major components:

1 duplex scanning as the sole diagnostic study;
2 admission on the morning of operation;
3 use of regional anesthesia whenever possible;
4 use of a short recovery room stay to select those patients who require the ICU;
5 discharge on the first postoperative morning.

Although many other important considerations are involved, these are the key steps in the clinical pathway that facilitate the performance of safe, cost-efficient CEAs.

Because preoperative imaging protocols are covered in detail in Chapters 8–11, our protocol of using duplex alone as the routine preoperative imaging modality and using angiography only in highly selected cases (approximately 7%) will not be discussed further. It has been clearly demonstrated that, for the vast majority of patients, duplex when performed by experienced technicians, interpreted in the context of the patient's history and physical findings by an experienced clinician, and supplemented when necessary by other imaging studies, gives sufficient preoperative information to allow safe endarterectomy.[17,18]

This chapter focuses on our methods for streamlining hospital care by admission on the day of surgery, routine use of regional anesthesia to improve the likelihood of early discharge, selective use of the critical care unit, and early postoperative discharge. Experience has proven that in both the community hospital and in the academic medical center environment, CEA can be carried out safely with limited resource utilization and a short, efficient hospital stay. Strict adherence to an established clinical pathway with built-in flexibility when clinical circumstances and patient safety concerns dictate a longer, more closely monitored course is the key to maintenance of excellent clinical outcomes and patient satisfaction in a short-stay program.

SAME-DAY ADMISSION

In a modern carotid surgery practice, most elective patients can be admitted on the morning of operation. Preoperative education regarding the pre-, intra-, and postoperative management protocols is essential to insure that patients are comfortable with the routines involved in their management. Patients with cardiac problems should be fully evaluated and prepared for operation before admission. Diabetics should be operated upon early in the day to avoid problems with hypoglycemia. Patients with renal failure should receive their outpatient dialysis on the day before surgery. It is essential that patients with hypertension be well controlled before operation and ordinarily they should take their normal medications on the morning of surgery.[19] Over the last 6 years all patients scheduled for elective CEA who were not already in hospital for another reason were admitted on the day of surgery.[16] This has also been achieved in tertiary care and teaching institutions.[15,20]

OPERATION UNDER REGIONAL ANESTHESIA

No single operative protocol has been demonstrated to optimize adherence to the clinical pathway. CEA can be performed in a safe, cost-efficient manner using either general or regional anesthesia.[15,16] In our practice regional anesthesia is preferred because of the ease of neurologic monitoring and the reported shorter length of postoperative hypertension.[19] Allen et al. concluded that cervical block anesthesia is safer and results in a more efficient use of hospital resources than general anesthesia in the treatment of patients undergoing CEA.[20] Hirko et al. safely discharged 73% of their endarterectomy patients on the first postoperative day using general anesthesia.[15] Similarly, Kaufman et al.[21] discharged 80% of their patients within 2 days using general anesthesia. General anesthesia is used only 15% of the time in my practice. At my institution, the average length of stay was 1.1 days for elective CEA performed using cervical block techniques, and 1.32 days when general anesthesia was used. When we compared general with regional anesthesia, we found that there was a threefold increase in the number of patients who stayed longer than 1 day in the hospital. The debate over optimal anesthetic technique is covered in detail in Chapter 16.

SHORT RECOVERY ROOM STAY TO SELECT ONLY THOSE PATIENTS IN NEED OF THE INTENSIVE CARE UNIT

An essential step in optimizing resource utilization in CEA patients is to limit ICU utilization to those situations where it is essential. One day in the ICU has been shown to increase the charges for CEA by 12.5% on average.[22] Before 1990, all my patients undergoing CEA went to the ICU postoperatively. In 1990, we began keeping patients in the recovery room for 4h in order to select only those patients who required acute care in the ICU. This recovery room stay was found to be much less expensive than a day in the ICU. Recovery room stay has since been decreased to 3h. There are two reasons for this duration of recovery room observation. First, all of the perioperative strokes at my institution occurred within 3h of reaching the recovery room, and second, 95% of the patients who developed hypertension normalized within 3h.

Patients are transferred to the vascular floor if they are unchanged neurologically, have no new cardiac problems, have no hematomas that may compromise their airway, and maintain a systolic blood pressure less than 180mmHg without new medication. Between 6% and 14% of patients per year required the ICU at our institution.[23] The reasons for ICU admission in my practice are outlined in Table 27.1. The most frequent cause for ICU admission is persistent hypertension. Although our policy has been a 3-h recovery room stay, we now keep a hypertensive patient in the recovery room longer if he or she is normalizing blood pressure. This has been shown at our institution to be more cost-efficient than a day in the ICU. The safety of highly selective use of the ICU has been demonstrated by other authors.[24]

Initially, we were concerned about hypotension. Patients with persistent asymptomatic hypotension went to the ICU. After review, we found that these patients all gradually normalized their blood pressure. Now, if patients have persistent systolic hypotension above 90mmHg with no adverse neurologic or cardiac problems, they are transferred to the vascular floor. This has resulted in no adverse consequences.

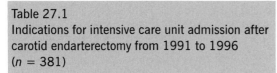

Table 27.1
Indications for intensive care unit admission after carotid endarterectomy from 1991 to 1996 (n = 381)

Indication	Number
Blood pressure control	
Refractory hypertension	17
Hypotension	6
Neurologic complications	
Transient	3
Permanent	7
Cardiac	
Premature ventricular contractions	3
Ventricular tachycardia	1
Angina pectoris	1
Asystole (protamine reaction)	1
Subendocardial myocardial infarction	1
Hematomas	3

Over the last 7 years, only 1 patient was transferred to the ICU after originally going to the floor. This patient developed severe sustained hypertension, which was later found to be secondary to urinary retention. Only 1 patient required readmission to the ICU after being transferred out. She developed an intracerebral hemorrhage on the second postoperative day.

DISCHARGE ON THE FIRST POSTOPERATIVE DAY

Discharge is scheduled for the morning after operation if certain criteria are met. It has even been possible to discharge patients from the ICU if their admitting problem has resolved itself. The patient must be neurologically intact or at neurologic baseline. He or she must be afebrile and have normal vital signs. The blood pressure must be within an acceptable range and the patient must not have a significant headache. The wound must be dry and without excessive swelling. The patient must be able to eat, void, and ambulate. Just as importantly, the patient must be willing to be discharged, have transportation home, and have

someone with him or her for a least the next 2 days. It is essential that this aspect of the care be discussed preoperatively so that the support systems are in place before discharge.

In my practice over the last 5 years, 85–95% of patients per year are discharged on the first postoperative day.[16] Persistent hypertension, cardiac issues, and neurologic complications were the main reasons for lengths of stay greater than 1 day in decreasing order of frequency. Hospital charges averaged over $2000 less than the DRG reimbursement for the last 6 years. A linear progression in patient charges occurred with each extra day spent in the hospital. Follow-up quality surveys have demonstrated that patients were happy to go home when they did and did not feel pushed out of the hospital.[25]

Table 27.2
Process changes and results

Key actions	Results
Duplex-only routine imaging study	Cost reduction Improved patient satisfaction Enhanced safety
Same-day admission	Cost reduction
Regional anesthesia	Improved monitoring Less postoperative hypertension
Selective use of the intensive care unit	Cost reduction
Discharge on the first postoperative day	Greater patient satisfaction Decreased length of stay Cost savings

CONCLUSIONS

Streamlining the care of patients undergoing CEA has been shown to be feasible in both community and university hospitals. Though not essential, a formal clinical pathway is helpful in establishing and monitoring a short-stay program. These changes have been clearly demonstrated to result in cost savings and decreased length of stay without jeopardizing patient outcome and safety. The actions taken to establish our short-stay program and the results of these actions are summarized in Table 27.2. At no point has patient safety been compromised. Essential components of a short-stay program are adequate patient education and preparation, an experienced care team guided by well-established protocols, and experienced carotid surgeons who are completely comfortable with the program.

ACKNOWLEDGEMENTS
Special thanks to Loretta Thomas and Nancy Collier, RN, for their technical and editorial assistance, and the staff at Sewickley Valley Hospital for their help in making this program work successfully.

REFERENCES

13 Crosby PB. *Quality is Free: The Art of Making Quality Certain*. New York: McGraw-Hill, 1979.

14 Collier PE. Carotid endarterectomy: a safe cost-efficient approach. *Journal of Vascular Surgery* 1992; **16**: 926–933.

15 Hirko MK, Morasch MD, Burke K, Greisler HP, Littooy FN, Baker WH. The changing face of carotid endarterectomy. *Journal of Vascular Surgery* 1996; **23**: 622–627.

16 Collier PE. Are one-day admissions for carotid endarterectomy feasible? *American Journal of Surgery* 1995; **70**: 140–143.

17 Nicholas GG, Osborne MA, Jaffe JW, Reed JF. Carotid artery stenosis: preoperative noninvasive evaluation in a community hospital. *Journal of Vascular Surgery* 1995; **22**: 9–16.

18 Kuntz KM, Skillman JJ, Whittemore AD, Kent KC. Carotid endarterectomy in asymptomatic patients – is contrast angiography necessary? A morbidity analysis. *Journal of Vascular Surgery* 1995; **22**: 706–716.

19 Corson JD, Chang BB, Leopold PW et al. Perioperative hypertension in patients undergoing carotid endarterectomy: shorter duration under regional block anesthesia. *Circulation* 1986; **74** (Suppl 1): 1–4.

20 Allen BT, Anderson CB, Rubin BG et al. The influence of anesthetic technique on perioperative complications after carotid endarterectomy. *Journal of Vascular Surgery* 1994; **19**: 834–843.

21 Kaufman JL, Frank D, Rhee SW, Berman JA, Friedmann P. Feasibility and safety of one-day postoperative hospitalization for carotid endarterectomy. *Archives of Surgery* 1996; **131**: 751–755.

22 O'Brien MS, Ricotta JJ. Conserving resources after carotid endarterectomy: selective use of the intensive care unit. *Journal of Vascular Surgery* 1991; **14**: 796–802.

23 Collier PE. How essential is the intensive care unit after carotid endarterectomy? *Vascular Surgery* 1997; **31**: 563–566.

24 McConnell DB, Yeager RA, Moneta GL, Edwards JM, Deveney CW. "Just in time" decision making for ICU care after carotid endarterectomy. *American Journal of Surgery* 1996; **171**: 502–504.

25 Collier PE, Friend S, Gentile C, Ruckert D, Vescio L, Collier NA. Carotid endarterectomy clinical pathway: an innovative approach. *American Journal of Quality in Medicine* 1995; **10**: 18–27.

27.3 Editorial Comment

KEY POINTS

1 There is no scientific evidence to support the previously held viewpoint that patients should remain in hospital for 5–7 days following CEA. Many centers have now demonstrated the safety and cost savings associated with discharge on day 1 or 2 after CEA.
2 There is no rationale for using routine ICU admission post-CEA. Most monitoring requirements are possible in a post-anesthesia care unit or recovery area of theater prior to discharge to the ward. Occasionally patients may require overnight stay in an intermediate-care unit or HDU.
3 The key to implementing a policy of early post-endarterectomy discharge is to develop practice guidelines (critical pathways) which fundamentally change expectations regarding length of hospital stay without compromising patient safety and professional standards.
4 The commonest reasons for delayed discharge include blood pressure management, social issues, wound complications, and cardiac problems.

Since there is no doubt that discharge on day 1 or 2 can be achieved in most patients without compromising outcome, it is important to consider what steps need to be taken to implement this.

First, the hospital has to have a sufficient volume of CEAs in order that the procedure for admission, operation, and discharge is made routine. Second, all professional staff must accept the concept of early discharge as being safe and appropriate. Third, patient expectations with regard to the length of stay, postoperative pain and disability, and post-discharge care must be established at the outpatient consultation when the risks and rationales of the procedure are discussed and informed consent is obtained. This is facilitated by the provision of written information concerning arrangements for postoperative care (see below). Fourth, social issues such as transportation and home care (e.g., living alone) must be anticipated and planned for in advance. In the New England Medical Center, this is facilitated by having a full-time outpatient clinic nurse who works in close concert with a discharge planning nurse.

In practice, there are two types of patient who cannot be discharged early after CEA. The first group are predictable preoperatively and include:

1 those with significant comorbidity (e.g. severe airway disease);
2 patients living alone and who have been unable to arrange for a friend or relative to stay with them for the first 48h;
3 patients with stable stroke but a residual neurologic deficit which may limit the capability for self-care.

The second group are those whose postoperative course requires unanticipated changes to planned inpatient care. These include:

1 perioperative neurological deficit;
2 blood pressure control;
3 cardiac problems;
4 local wound complications such as neck edema or hematoma.

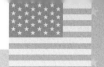

Early discharge protocols, when combined with other changes in resource management, can result in significant institutional cost savings (30% reduction at the New England Medical Center) without compromising outcome or patient satisfaction.

NEW ENGLAND MEDICAL CENTER PATIENT GUIDANCE REGARDING POSTOPERATIVE CARE AFTER CAROTID ENDARTERECTOMY

Patient's Understanding of Diagnosis and Hospital Course

Surgery is required to remove a plaque from the carotid artery, widen the blood vessel and decrease the risk of a fragment breaking free and causing a stroke.

Instructions for care at home

Treatments/special instructions

1 Steristrips remain in place until they begin to curl up and peel off.
2 Do not irritate incision line with tight or restrictive clothing.
3 Incision is to be left open to air unless otherwise instructed.
4 Men should be careful when shaving due to temporary numbness around the jaw. Electric razors are preferable.
5 *No smoking!*

Activity

1 Refrain from all heavy work, lifting, and physical exercise until your doctor has given approval.
2 Walking and light activity are beneficial.
3 Do not drive for 7 days or until after the follow-up appointment with your doctor.

4 A shower is discouraged for the first week following surgery because of the risk of dizziness. Bathing is allowed: do not immerse the neck, but gentle washing is encouraged after the 5th day of surgery.

Normal activity

1 Numbness and discomfort around the incision site, ear, and jaw are common on the side of the wound.
2 Slight voice hoarseness may occur.
3 There may be slight headache or dizziness (bend slowly at the knees if picking up an object; sudden changes in position may lead to dizziness and fainting).

Reasons to notify surgeon or clinic

1 Intense or worsening headache or pain not relieved by Acetaminophen (Tylenol®).
2 Chest pain.
3 Difficulty breathing or swallowing.
4 Numbness: tingling, weakness or paralysis of arms or legs.
5 Enlarged neck mass or drainage from incision site.
6 Slurred voice.
7 Visual changes.
8 Wound separation.
9 Fevers greater than 101°F.

For questions and concerns

1 In case of emergency call:
2 Surgical ward telephone number:
3 Surgical outpatient clinic telephone number:
4 Surgeon's telephone number:

28.1

Does serial postoperative clinical or duplex surveillance reduce the long-term stroke risk?

Jonathan D Beard (Europe)

INTRODUCTION

The rationale underlying an effective programme of postoperative surveillance is that:

1 there must be a clinically important end-point, i.e. stroke;
2 the risk of stroke is high enough to justify surveillance;
3 there must be a definite association between the risk of stroke and the development of either a restenosis or contralateral disease progression;
4 there must be an effective and safe intervention.[1]

In practice, no one would dispute that stroke is an important end-point to prevent, nor that carotid endarterectomy (CEA) is an effective and safe intervention. However, the evidence supporting the position that the risk of late stroke is high enough to justify surveillance and that there is a definite association between restenosis or contralateral disease progression and late stroke is the subject of critical debate.

WHAT IS THE RISK OF LATE STROKE AFTER CAROTID SURGERY?

The evidence from the international trials suggests that, following a successful CEA, the risk of ipsilateral late stroke is about 1–2% per annum.[2,3] Similarly, evidence suggests that the risk of stroke in the contralateral non-operated hemisphere is also about 1–2% per annum.[4] Thus, from the outset, one is faced with the situation that, unless there is a good correlation between disease progression/restenosis and late stroke, any programme of clinical or ultrasound-based surveillance is unlikely to be either clinically or cost-effective.

RESTENOSIS

Definition of Restenosis?

The term restenosis implies the recurrence of a stenosis after treatment and yet some authors have also included residual disease, adjacent stenoses and technical defects after surgery in this category. Purists demand intraoperative or early post-operative imaging to provide a baseline that allows identification of subsequent changes and excludes any residual abnormalities.[5] Methods used to assess the technical success of CEA include completion angiography,[5] intraoperative duplex scanning[6] and angioscopy.[7] The list of identifiable residual lesions includes residual plaques, intimal flaps, adherent thrombi, suture stenoses and kinks.

The reported incidence of these abnormalities varies from 5% to 65%[8,9] and generates much debate as to which of them justify correction, especially the small intimal flaps and fronds often seen on duplex scanning. Although some authors have advised re-exploration and revision,[10] no study has shown any significant improvement in outcome as a result of such a policy.

Traditionally, primary carotid stenosis measurements have relied on angiographic criteria using the European Carotid Surgery Trial (ECST), North American Symptomatic Carotid Endarterectomy Trial (NASCET) or (CCA) methods.[11] However, using angiography for routine surveillance is unjustifiable and duplex scanning has become the most common method used for follow-up. Most centres would currently define restenosis as the development of a recurrent stenosis causing a greater than 50% diameter (75% area) reduction based on Strandness' criteria of a systolic peak velocity greater than 1.25m/s (4 kHz) with marked spectral broadening.[12]

Incidence

The reported incidence of restenosis after CEA varies widely because of differences in the definition of restenosis, method of detection, length of follow-up and method of analysis.[13] Latimer and Burnand have performed an extensive literature review[14] and found the incidence of restenosis to range from 1% to 37%, but only 0–8% of patients had symptoms related to restenosis. Unsurprisingly, studies based solely on the presence of symptoms or a bruit[15] had the lowest incidence, whereas those with the highest rates used duplex assessment with a long follow-up.[16,17]

Fredriks et al. recently performed a systematic review of the Medline database using standard meta-analytical techniques.[18] They identified 20 publications that met all of their requirements, which included long-term follow-up of more than 100 patients subjected to regular non-invasive assessment. These showed a risk of restenosis of 10% in the first year, 3% in the second year and 2% in the third year. The longer-term risk was about 1% per annum. The reported relative risk of stroke in patients with restenosis, compared to those without a stenosis, showed considerable heterogeneity and ranged from 0.1 to 10. The heterogeneity meant that it was difficult to calculate an overall estimate of the relative risk.

Aetiology

Many reports on follow-up after CEA have examined the influence of sex, age, hypertension, diabetes, smoking and hyperlipidaemia on the development of restenosis. Unfortunately, many authors have investigated these possible aetiological factors by retrospectively comparing patients with restenosis to those without.[19] Such case control studies have intrinsic flaws since they only include survivors and tend to overrepresent women. Continued smoking has an association with a threefold increase in the relative risk of restenosis.[20] Several case control studies have reported hypercholesterolaemia as a risk factor and some have proposed trials of lipid-lowering therapy after CEA.[21] However, other studies based on life-table analysis have not shown

hypercholesterolaemia as an independent risk factor, especially as women undergoing carotid surgery have higher cholesterol levels than men.[20] The smaller size of the female carotid artery could also explain the increased incidence of restenosis observed in women in a number of series.

Ouriel and Green[22] found that small internal carotid arteries (< 4mm diameter) had a significantly increased risk of restenosis compared to those of diameter $\geq$ 4mm (37% vs 12%). Some have suggested that abnormalities left uncorrected at the end of the CEA may contribute to restenosis, although small intimal flaps probably do not matter.[23] Sawchuk et al.[24] observed that 16 out of 19 small intimal flaps detected by intraoperative duplex scanning in 80 patients undergoing CEA had completely resolved before the first postoperative scan. Kinks and stenoses of between 25% and 50% that cause turbulent flow, probably have an association with the development of restenosis. Bandyk et al.[25] found that 17% of carotid arteries that contained such defects had a greater than 75% area stenosis at follow-up (mean 21.6 months) as compared to only 4.3% of endarterectomized arteries that were deemed satisfactory. Other studies have also confirmed this finding.[26]

Conversely, serial angiography[27] has demonstrated regression of postoperative carotid stenosis. It therefore seems likely that an early stenosis has the potential to improve, stabilize or deteriorate. Subsequent studies using duplex scanning have reported regression rates varying from 1.4%[28] to 27%.[29] Healy et al.[16] have estimated a 30% cumulative incidence of restenosis at 7 years with a 10% cumulative incidence of regression. Regression may be caused by remodelling, i.e. an adaptive response of the arterial wall to new haemodynamic conditions or a reduction of the intimal mass due to the organization and resolution of intimal thrombus (see below).

Pathophysiology

Carotid arteries respond to a surgical insult in much the same way as arteries and vein grafts elsewhere. Residual disease or technical defects cause immediate stenoses, myointimal hyperplasia causes early stenoses (less than 2 years) and recurrence or progression of atherosclerosis causes later lesions.[30] On the basis of these findings, some would consider the pathogenesis of carotid restenosis to be a dynamic process of early myointimal hyperplasia and later atherosclerotic degeneration.[31] Other suggested causes of carotid restenosis include clamp injury, shunt trauma and the use of distal tacking sutures.[32]

Thrombus formation can occur at any time, but especially in the immediate postoperative period, and is responsible for most neurological deficits occurring at this time.[33] Resolution of thrombus may explain why some early stenoses regress but it may also play an important part in the restenotic process. However, while several histological studies have demonstrated a high incidence of surface and intraplaque thrombus in carotid restenoses,[34] others have not found that thrombosis plays a major part in the development of restenosis.[35]

CONTRALATERAL DISEASE PROGRESSION

It has also been suggested that one of the reasons for undertaking serial postoperative surveillance imaging is to prevent stroke in the non-operated hemisphere. This is based on the premise that contralateral disease progression is associated with a high risk of stroke. This is supported by the observation that, when a patient presents with a stroke or transient ischaemic attack (TIA) in the non-operated hemisphere, there may be a severe stenosis present in the ipsilateral carotid artery.[36] However, evidence is increasingly showing that the onset of symptoms usually *precedes* recognition that disease progression has occurred, i.e. the patient may now have a severe stenosis but if one reviews the last surveillance scan before onset of symptoms, the stenosis may well be of only moderate severity. Subsequent to this, some form of acute intraplaque change occurs (e.g. fissuring or haemorrhage) with secondary thrombosis which then causes the stenosis to progress rapidly to a more severe form.[36] In practice, the incidence of stroke in the contralateral hemisphere is only about 2% per annum and in many cases there is no severe stenosis present.[4]

POSTOPERATIVE SURVEILLANCE

Many centres in North America routinely follow up CEA patients with duplex ultrasound in order to detect restenosis and contralateral disease progression.[37,38] This is not the case in much of Europe, which adopts a more conservative policy.

The Operated Carotid Artery

The results of any operative procedure must be judged in the context of its long-term durability, especially when performed prophylactically. Therefore it is understandable that surgeons may wish to audit their results. However, audit of long-term outcome is expensive and, once it has been established that results are satisfactory, routine audit of *process* is all that is required.

The vast majority of patients with restenosis are asymptomatic, and the justification for surveillance programmes has therefore been based on the results of the asymptomatic carotid surgery trials. Symptom-free patients with a primary carotid stenosis greater than 75% have an annual ipsilateral ischaemic stroke rate of only 2.5–3% and a 4–8% annual chance of cardiac death.[38] Thus, prophylactic carotid surgery in these individuals has to have a combined stroke and death rate of less than 2% to be justifiable and the cost of preventing one stroke is high.

Reoperation in patients with restenosis is even harder to justify as the annual risk of ipsilateral stroke is lower (see section on aetiology, above) and the perioperative stroke and death rate is higher (4.9% and 1% respectively).[14] In addition, the cost of identifying and repairing these lesions has been calculated at $133 000 per stroke saved, at 1995 prices.[37]

Most restenoses are due to neointimal hyperplasia. These smooth stenoses rarely embolize, which is why they behave differently from primary atheromatous disease. However, when symptoms do occur, the cause is usually embolism rather than reduced blood flow.[39] Fortunately most patients present with TIAs or amaurosis fugax,[40] which means that any investigation and treatment is only required for those with recurrent symptoms (Figs 28.1 and 28.2). The possibility that a high-grade asymptomatic restenosis may progress to

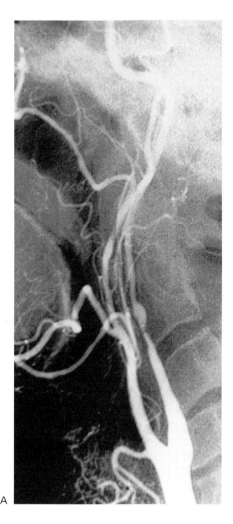
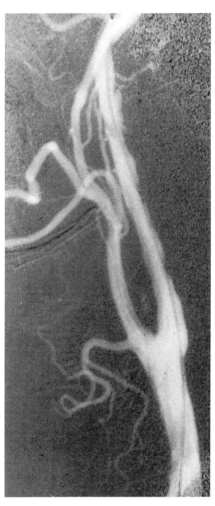

Fig. 28.1
Severe, symptomatic restenosis of the internal carotid artery at the distal end of an endarterectomy performed 2 years previously (A). This was successfully treated by balloon angioplasty (B).

A

B

occlusion and stroke does exist, but it is an extremely rare event.

Thus, if serial imaging is to have any impact in the future, it must address the issue of what precipitates acute changes within the restenosis, such as fissuring, ulceration and thrombus formation. Two surveillance scans are perhaps the most that can possibly be justified: one in the early postoperative period (to serve as a baseline) and the other at 1 year, as the incidence of a significant stenosis developing after this time is only 1% per annum. There may, however, be an argument for more frequent scans in carotid bypass grafts and after angioplasty/stenting, because the risk of restenosis is higher (25% at 1 year).[41]

An increasing number of studies are now showing that serial duplex surveillance does not alter outcome relative to the operated artery.[1,42,43] If non-invasive surveillance is unjustified, then invasive imaging by arteriography certainly cannot be. Clinical follow-up, once the patient has recovered from surgery, is also pointless as there is little correlation between bruits and the presence of a stenosis. Symptoms, if they do occur, will tend to develop in the intervals between appointments. Patients should therefore be seen once postoperatively, to ensure that there are no wound or neurological problems, and then discharged if none is found. However, they should be encouraged to reattend the clinic without delay if neurological symptoms referable to either carotid

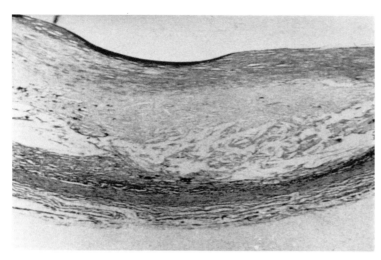

Fig. 28.2
Photomicrograph of internal carotid artery wall 6 months after carotid angioplasty (patient died of myocardial infarction). Although atheroma is still present, the luminal surface is smooth due to myointimal hyperplasia and remodelling.

territory develop. Patient information leaflets or alert cards may help in this respect.

The Non-operated Carotid Artery

The same principles also apply to surveillance of the non-operated carotid artery, largely because the annual rate of stroke is only about 2%.[4] In essence, therefore, it means that if you do not advocate operating upon patients with an asymptomatic, unilateral carotid artery stenosis in excess of 70% (which is the policy in most European centres), then the indications for serially surveying the non-operated carotid artery almost disappear. The object of any surveillance programme is to prevent unheralded stroke. It has no role in preventing TIA or amaurosis fugax as these patients would thereafter be suitable for surgery if they have a severe stenosis. Evidence suggests that, however attractive the logic, few strokes will be prevented by adopting a policy of prophylactic CEA in patients with asymptomatic disease in the non-operated carotid artery. More often than not, many of the strokes that do occur will do so in the absence of a severe stenosis.[4]

CONCLUSIONS

In summary, the risk of carotid restenosis (diameter loss > 50%) is 10% in the first year, 3% in the second and 2% in the third. The longer-term risk is about 1% per annum. The cumulative risk of developing a stenosis > 70% or occlusion over a 12-month period is only 1–2%. The reported relative risk of stroke in patients with restenosis, compared to those without, ranges from 0.1 to 10. However, in most cases the onset of symptoms precedes recognition of the development of a severe restenosis or disease progression. Risk factors for the development of restenosis within the operated artery include a carotid artery < 4mm in diameter, technical defects causing turbulence and continued smoking. Restenosis is usually due to myointimal hyperplasia which, being smooth, rarely causes cerebral embolization. Serial duplex surveillance does not alter patient outcome, as reoperation for what is asymptomatic restenosis cannot be justified in terms of clinical effectiveness or cost benefit. Similarly, evidence suggests that the risk of stroke in the non-operated carotid artery with a severe (unilateral) asymptomatic stenosis, over a 12-month period, is low. Patients should be encouraged to return to the clinic without delay if they develop ipsilateral or contralateral carotid territory symptoms.

REFERENCES

1 Naylor AR, John T, Howlett J, Gillespie I, Allan P, Ruckley CV. Serial surveillance imaging does not alter clinical outcome following carotid endarterectomy. *British Journal of Surgery* 1996; **83**: 522–526.

2 European Carotid Surgery Trialists' Collaborative Group. MRC European Carotid Surgery Trial: interim results for symptomatic patients with severe (70–99%) or with mild (0–29%) carotid stenosis. *Lancet* 1991; **337**: 1235–1243.

3 North American Symptomatic Carotid Endarterectomy Trial Collaborators. Beneficial effect of carotid endarterectomy in symptomatic patients with high grade carotid stenosis. *New England Journal of Medicine* 1991; **325**: 445–453.

4 Naylor AR, John T, Howlett J, Gillespie I, Allan P, Ruckley CV. Fate of the non-operated carotid artery after contralateral endarterectomy. *British Journal of Surgery* 1995; **82**: 44–48.

5 Moore WS. Recurrent carotid stenosis. In: Bernstein EF, Callow AD, Nicolaides AN, Shifrin EG (eds) *Cerebral Revascularization*, vol. 26, pp. 327–332. New York: Med Orion, 1993.

6 Schwartz RA, Peterson GJ, Noland KA, Hower JF Jr, Narnheim KS. Intraoperative duplex scanning after carotid artery reconstruction: a valuable tool. *Journal of Vascular Surgery* 1988; **5**: 620–624.

7 Raithel D, Kasprzak P. Angioscopy after carotid endarterectomy. In: Greenhalgh RM (ed.) *Vascular Imaging for Surgeons*, pp. 141–146. London: WB Saunders, 1995.

8 Courbier R, Jansseran JM, Reggi M, Bergeron P, Formichi M, Ferdani M. Routine intraoperative angiography: its impact on operative morbidity and carotid restenosis. *Journal of Vascular Surgery* 1986; **3**: 343–350.

9 Anderson CA, Collins GJ Jr, Rich NM. Routine operative arteriography during carotid endarterectomy: a reassessment. *Surgery* 1978; **83**: 67–71.

10 Kinney EV, Seabrook GR, Kinney LY, Bandy KDF, Towne JB. The importance of intraoperative detection of residual flow abnormalities after carotid endarterectomy. *Journal of Vascular Surgery* 1993; **17**: 912–923.

11 Naylor AR, Beard JD, Gaines PA. Extracranial carotid disease. In: Beard JD, Gaines PA (eds) *Vascular and Endovascular Surgery*, vol. 13, pp. 317–350. London: WB Saunders, 1998.

12 Jacobs NM, Grant EG, Schellinger D, Byrd MC, Richardson JD, Cohan SL. Duplex carotid sonography: criteria for stenosis accuracy and pitfalls. *Radiology* 1985; **154**: 385–391.

13 Civil ID, O'Hara PJ, Hertzer NR, Krajewski LP, Beven EG. Late patency of the carotid artery after endarterectomy. Problems of definition, following methodology and data analysis. *Journal of Vascular Surgery* 1988; **8**: 79–85.

14 Latimer CR, Burnand KG. Recurrent carotid stenosis after carotid endarterectomy. *British Journal of Surgery* 1997; **84**: 1206–1219.

15 Hertzer NR, Martinez BD, Benjamin SP, Beven EG. Recurrent stenosis after carotid endarterectomy. *Surgery, Gynecology and Obstetrics* 1979; **149**: 360–364.

16 Healy DA, Zierler RE, Nicholls SC. Long-term follow-up and clinical outcome of carotid restenosis. *Journal of Vascular Surgery* 1989; **10**: 662–669.

17 Sterpetti AV, Shultz RD, Fieldhaus RJ. Natural history of recurrent carotid artery disease. *Surgery, Gynecology and Obstetrics* 1989; **168**: 217–223.

18 Fredriks H, Kievit J, van Baalen JM, van Bockel JH. Carotid recurrent stenosis and risk of ipsilateral stroke. A systematic review of the literature. *Stroke* 1998; **29**: 244–250.

19 Clagett GP, Rich NM, McDonald PT. Etiologic factors for recurrent carotid artery stenosis. *Surgery* 1983; **93**: 313–318.

20 Powell JT, Cuming R, Greenhalgh RM. In: Greenhalgh RM, Hollier LH (eds) *Surgery for Stroke*, pp. 45–41. London: WB Saunders, 1993.

21 Rapp JH, Qvarfordt P, Krupski WC, Ehrenfeld WK, Stoney RJ. Hypercholesterolaemia and early restenosis after carotid endarterectomy. *Surgery* 1987; **101**: 277–282.

22 Ouriel K, Green RM. Clinical and technical factors influencing recurrent carotid stenosis and occlusion after endarterectomy. *Journal of Vascular Surgery* 1987; **5**: 702–706.

23 Dorffner R, Metz VM, Trattnig S. Intraoperative and early postoperative colour Doppler sonography after carotid artery reconstruction: follow-up of technical defects. *Neuroradiology* 1997; **39**: 117–121.

24 Sawchuk AP, Flanigan DI, Machi J, Schuler JJ, Sigel B. The fate of unimpaired minor technical defects detected by intraoperative ultrasonography during carotid endarterectomy. *Journal of Vascular Surgery* 1989; **4**: 671–676.

25 Bandyk DF, Kaebrick HW, Adams JB, Towne JB. Turbulence occurring after carotid bifurcation endarterectomy: a harbinger of residual and recurrent carotid stenosis. *Journal of Vascular Surgery* 1988; **7**: 261–274.

26 Golledge J, Cuming R, Ellis M, Davies AH, Greenhalgh RM. Duplex imaging findings predict stenosis after carotid endarterectomy. *Journal of Vascular Surgery* 26: 43–48.

27 Diaz FG, Patel S, Boulos R, Mehta B, Ausman JI. Early angiographic changes following carotid endarterectomy. *Neurosurgery* 1982; **10**: 151–161.

28 Bernstein EF, Toren S, Dilley RB. Does carotid restenosis predict an increased risk of late symptoms, stroke or death? *Annals of Surgery* 1990; **212**: 629–636.

29 Atnip RG, Wengrovitz M, Gifford RRM, Neumeyer MM, Thiele BL. A rational approach to recurrent carotid stenosis. *Journal of Vascular Surgery* 1990; **6**: 511–516.

30 Storey RJ, String ST. Recurrent carotid stenosis. *Surgery* 1976; **80**: 705–710.

31 Callow AD. Recurrent stenosis after carotid endarterectomy. *Archives of Surgery* 1982; **117**: 1082–1085.

32 Aukland A, Hurlow BA. Carotid restenosis due to clamp injury. *British Medical Journal* 1981; **282**: 2013.

33 Takolander R, Bergentz SE, Bergqvist D, Persson NH. Management of early neurologic defects after carotid thromboendarterectomy. *European Journal of Vascular Surgery* 1987; **1**: 67–72.

34 Clagett GP, Robinowitz M, Youkey JR. Morphogenesis and

clinicopathologic characteristics of recurrent carotid disease. *Journal of Vascular Surgery* 1986; **3**: 10–23.

35 Schwartz TH, Yates GN, Ghobrial M, Baker WH, Pathologic characteristics of recurrent carotid artery stenosis. *Journal of Vascular Surgery* 1987; **5**: 280–288.

36 Bock RW, Gray-Weale AC, Mock PA. The natural history of asymptomatic carotid artery disease. *Journal of Vascular Surgery* 1987; **17**: 160–171.

37 Ricotta JR, DeWeese JA. Is routine carotid ultrasound surveillance after carotid endarterectomy worthwhile? *American Journal of Surgery* 1996; **172**: 140–143.

38 Ouriel K, Green RM. Appropriate frequency of carotid duplex testing following carotid endarterectomy. *American Journal of Surgery* 1995; **170**: 144–147.

39 Norris JW, Zhu CZ, Bornstein NM, Chambers BR. Vascular risks of asymptomatic carotid stenosis. *Stroke* 1991; **22**: 1485–1490.

40 Hunter BC, Palmaz JC, Hayashi HH, Raviola CA, Vogt PJ, Guernsey JM. The aetiology of symptoms in patients with recurrent carotid stenosis. *Archives of Surgery* 1987; **122**: 311–315.

41 Cook JM, Thompson BW, Barnes RW. Is routine duplex examination after carotid endarterectomy justified? *Journal of Vascular Surgery* 1990; **12**: 334–340.

42 Mattos MA, van Benmelen PS, Barakmeier LC, Hodgson KJ, Ramsey DE, Sumnar DS. Routine surveillance after carotid endarterectomy: does it affect clinical management? *Journal of Vascular Surgery* 1993; **17**: 819–831.

43 Golledge J, Cuming R, Ellis M, Beattie DK, Davies AH, Greenhalgh RM. Clinical follow-up rather than duplex surveillance after carotid endarterectomy. *Journal of Vascular Surgery* 1997; **25**: 55–63.

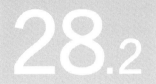

28.2 Does serial post-operative clinical or duplex surveillance reduce the long-term stroke risk?

William C Mackey (USA)

The rationale for serial clinical and duplex follow-up examinations following CEA rests on four premises:

1. Carotid restenosis occurs frequently.
2. Carotid restenosis is a potential cause of neurologic morbidity.
3. Timely reoperation in patients with restenosis results in better neurologic outcomes than conservative follow-up.
4. Detection and treatment of progressive contralateral carotid disease prevent neurologic morbidity.

The incidence of significant (≥ 50%) recurrent carotid stenosis is well known. The results of our original post-endarterectomy duplex surveillance program are seen in Table 28.1. As shown, 16.2% of our patients developed ≥ 50% restenosis or occlusion at some time following endarterectomy.[44] This incidence of significant recurrence is consistent with some reports citing incidences of 18–22%[45,46] although some more recent reports have noted a lower (6.5–8%) incidence.[47,48] With more liberal use of patching, the incidence of significant restenosis should decline.

The morbidity associated with recurrent carotid stenosis has also been well described. The clinical outcomes in 55 of the patients in our original surveillance program found to have developed ≥ 50% recurrent carotid stenosis are shown in Table 28.2. More than half of our ≥ 50% restenoses remained asymptomatic without intervention and did not progress to carotid occlusion over a mean follow-up period of 52.6 months.[44] Of note, however, is the fact that there were 2 unheralded strokes related to sudden carotid occlusion and 8 carotid occlusions not resulting in permanent neurologic deficits in this group. Ten (18.2%) of our 55 patients with ≥ 50% restenosis suffered an adverse outcome.[44]

Table 28.1
Incidence of restenosis following carotid endarterectomy

Normal	205/348	58.9%
30–49% Restenosis	87/348	25.0%
50–74% Restenosis	26/348	7.5%
75–99% Restenosis	19/348	5.5%
Occlusion	11/348	3.2%

Table 28.2
Clinical outcome in patients with a recurrent stenosis after CEA

Asymptomatic, no occlusion, no reoperation	29/55	52.8%
Occlusion with no neurologic residua	8/55	14.5%
Reoperation for transient ischemic attack	8/55	14.5%
Reoperation for asymptomatic restenosis	8/55	14.5%
Unheralded stroke	2/55	3.6%

Review of our CEA follow-up databank gives further evidence that recurrent stenosis can lead to stroke. In 688 patients with a mean follow-up of approximately 5 years, the incidence of late stroke was 35/688 (5.1%).[49] Of these 35 late strokes,

11 (31.4% or 1.6% of the total group) were clearly related to recurrent stenosis. Only 3 of 20 (15%) strokes occurring within 36 months of endarterectomy were related to recurrent stenosis, while 8 of 15 (53.3%) strokes occurring after 36 months from the endarterectomy were related to restenosis. It is likely, therefore, that early restenoses related to neointimal fibrous hyperplasia are less likely to result in stroke than later restenoses related to atherosclerotic degeneration of the endarterectomized segment.[49] Neointimal hyperplastic lesions are of smooth uniform fibrous consistency, while recurrent atherosclerotic lesions are more likely to have irregular ulcerated surfaces lined by thrombus and pultaceous debris. This difference in plaque morphology may explain the possible difference in clinical behavior of the early and late restenoses.[50]

Intervention for carotid restenosis appears beneficial in selected cases. Most neurologists and vascular surgeons agree that patients with symptoms related to a high-grade (75–99%) recurrent stenosis should undergo redo endarterectomy, although no prospective randomized trials support this approach. More debatable is the role of re-do endarterectomy in the management of asymptomatic recurrences. It must be kept in mind that the favorable results in the surgical groups in both NASCET and ACAS were dependent on maintenance of low perioperative mortality and stroke morbidity rates. Because the risks of re-do endarterectomy (especially the risk of local anatomic complications such as cranial nerve injury) are somewhat higher than the risks of primary endarterectomy the results of NASCET and ACAS cannot be extrapolated to patients with recurrent disease.

In the absence of randomized controlled trials for the management of patients with recurrent disease, justification for operative intervention must be based on a comparison of the natural history of conservatively followed recurrent stenosis with the outcome of surgical intervention. In our most recent series of 48 re-do CEAs, there was 1 operative mortality (2.1%) related to myocardial ischemia, and 1 stroke (2.1%).[51]

Some of our most recent patients with asymptomatic restenoses are followed conservatively because of advanced age or significant comorbidity.

In these patients there was a 33% neurologic event (2 strokes and 1 TIA) rate in 9 patients.[51] In addition, 3 of 10 (30%) patients whose recurrent stenosis progressed to occlusion suffered a stroke. In contrast, in 21 patients with 50–75% restenosis there was only 1 (4.7%) TIA, and no strokes.[51] Comparison of these natural history data with our surgical results (2.1% mortality and stroke rates) suggests that our aggressive approach to reoperation for asymptomatic critical lesions is appropriate.

The late results of reoperative carotid surgery offer further justification for its use in managing restenoses. Life-table stroke-free rates (92% 1-year and 83.3% 5-year) following re-do endarterectomy in our series are acceptable and only slightly lower than those following primary operation (96.7% 1-year and 90.9% 5-year).[52] Comparison of stroke-free rates from the time of primary operation in our patients who did and did not develop restenosis requiring reoperation revealed no statistically significant difference.[52]

Duplex follow-up post-endarterectomy is also useful for the detection of disease progression in the contralateral artery. Since the ACAS data prove that intervention for asymptomatic lesions exceeding 60% prevents strokes, it is most likely that detection of such lesions in the contralateral artery will be beneficial. Still, most carotid surgeons reserve surgery for higher-grade asymptomatic lesions (> 75% or > 80%). In our experience, with duplex follow-up in 324 patients, the contralateral artery progressed to ≥75% stenosis over 5 years in 28% of patients.[53] Using multivariate analysis, age > 65 or initial stenosis > 50% contributed to the likelihood of disease progression. Patients > 65 had a 34% likelihood of disease progression, and those with > 50% stenosis at initial duplex had a 39% likelihood of progression. In patients aged > 65 with > 50% stenosis at initial scan there was a 49% risk of progression, while in those < 65 with initial stenosis < 50%, the risk of progression was only 15% ($P < 0.0001$).[53] Thus, at least in patients > 65, or in those with > 50% stenosis at initial duplex, surveillance of the contralateral artery is reasonable, especially in light of the results of ACAS.

In summary, carotid restenosis is common, although the incidence may decrease with more liberal use of carotid patching. Significant restenosis,

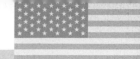

especially ≥80% restenosis, may result in unheralded stroke or progression to carotid occlusion. Overall, approximately one-third of late post-endarterectomy strokes are related to recurrent stenosis. Reoperation for recurrent stenosis is associated with acceptable mortality and neurologic morbidity rates and with long-term outcomes similar to those of patients without restenosis. Duplex surveillance over 5 years will detect progression of contralateral disease to > 75% in about

28% of all endarterectomy patients and in about 49% of patients over 65 with > 50% contralateral stenosis at initial presentation. Data from the ACAS trial prove that detection and treatment of these progressive lesions will prevent strokes. Although the optimal protocol for clinical and duplex surveillance has not yet been defined, these facts strongly suggest that post-endarterectomy surveillance will reduce long-term stroke risk.

REFERENCES

44 Mackey WC, Belkin M, Sindhi R, Welch H, O'Donnell TF. Routine postendarterectomy duplex surveillance: does it prevent late stroke? *Journal of Vascular Surgery* 1992; **16**: 934–940.

45 Cook JM, Thompson BW, Barnes RW. Is routine duplex examination after carotid endarterectomy justified? *Journal of Vascular Surgery* 1990; **12**: 334–339.

46 Nichols SC, Phillips DJ, Bergelin RO, Beach KW, Primozich JF, Strandness DE. Carotid endarterectomy: relationship of outcome to early restenosis. *Journal of Vascular Surgery* 1985; **2**: 375–381.

47 Gelabert HA, El Massry S, Moore WS. Carotid endarterectomy with primary closure does not adversely affect the rate of recurrent stenosis. *Archives of Surgery* 1994; **129**: 648–654.

48 Carballo RE, Towne JB, Seabrook GR, Freischlag JA, Cambria RA. An outcome analysis of carotid endarterectomy: the incidence and natural history of recurrent stenosis. *Journal of Vascular Surgery* 1996; **23**: 749–754.

49 Washburn WK, Mackey WC, Belkin M, O'Donnell TF. Late stroke after carotid endarterectomy: the role of recurrent stenosis. *Journal of Vascular Surgery* 1992; **15**: 1032–1037.

50 O'Donnell TF, Callow AD, Scott G, Shepard AD, Heggerick P, Mackey WC. Ultrasound characteristics of recurrent carotid disease: hypothesis explaining the low incidence of symptomatic recurrence. *Journal of Vascular Surgery* 1985; **2**: 26–41.

51 O'Donnell TF, Rodriguez A, Fortunato J, Welch HJ, Mackey WC. The management of recurrent carotid stenosis: should asymptomatic lesions be treated surgically? *Journal of Vascular Surgery* 1996; **24**: 207–212.

52 Nitzberg RS, Mackey WC, Prendiville E *et al*. Long-term follow-up of patients operated on for recurrent carotid stenosis. *Journal of Vascular Surgery* 1991; **13**: 121–127.

53 Iafrati MD, Mackey WC, Salamipou H, Young C, O'Donnell TF. Surveillance of the contralateral carotid artery: who needs it? *American Journal of Surgery* 1996; **172**: 136–139.

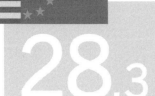

28.3 Editorial Comment

KEY POINTS

1 No randomized controlled trials either support or refute the value of routine post-endarterectomy duplex surveillance.
2 Those who practice postoperative surveillance are those who believe in the value of re-do CEA for asymptomatic carotid restenosis and/or believe that the natural history of contralateral disease warrants systematic follow-up.
3 Current models suggest that, because of the low incidence of severe recurrent stenosis and neurologic events related to either recurrent stenosis or contralateral disease, routine surveillance is not cost-effective ($130 000 per stroke prevented).
4 For research and quality control purposes, selected centers should systematically follow post-endarterectomy patients, if only to establish guidelines for optimal cost-effective follow-up in the future.

In an ideal world, routine post-endarterectomy duplex surveillance would be generally accepted, since it will detect virulent restenosis or rapid contralateral disease progression. Although it would not prevent all instances of post-endarterectomy strokes, a surveillance program would contribute to the prevention of some. Because duplex surveillance is costly, detects significant restenosis or progressive contralateral stenosis in relatively few patients, and because the natural history of recurrent stenosis and contralateral disease is benign in most patients, the value of routine surveillance has been questioned. Accordingly, most European centers no longer practice any routine long-term surgical follow-up.

The approach to post-endarterectomy follow-up will inevitably reflect ease of access to and cost of duplex and attitudes towards re-do CEA for asymptomatic restenosis or endarterectomy for progressive asymptomatic contralateral disease. Those who aggressively operate for asymptomatic recurrent lesions or progressive contralateral disease will have to adopt some form of surveillance to identify patients at high risk, while those who reserve operation for symptomatic restenoses or contralateral disease will find no role at all for surveillance.

Because more frequent patching is being performed, there may be a decreased incidence in the future of significant restenosis (both symptomatic and asymptomatic). Even ardent advocates of surveillance may need to reassess their position.

In those centers with research interests in neointimal hyperplasia and progression of the atherosclerotic process, surveillance is unavoidable and should serve to elucidate more aspects of the natural history and clinical significance of these two disease processes.

29.1 When should I reoperate for recurrent carotid stenosis?
Michael Horrocks (Europe)

INCIDENCE OF RESTENOSIS

The incidence of recurrent stenosis following carotid endarterectomy depends largely on the definition used.[1-3] Intraoperative quality monitoring may demonstrate that, following reconstruction there is an incidence of technical error of up to 10% which, if unrecognized, might be termed a recurrent stenosis when the patient is subsequently followed up.[4] Techniques for identifying residual stenosis at the time of operation include completion angiography, intraoperative duplex scanning and angioscopy. After residual lesions have been excluded, restenosis is usually defined as a > 50% diameter (75% area) reduction based on duplex criteria of a systolic peak velocity > 1.25m/s (4 kHz), with spectral broadening.[5]

Two recent overviews have examined the incidence and clinical significance of recurrent carotid stenosis.[6,7] Overall, the incidence of restenosis ranges from 1% to 37%,[6] but these figures will inevitably be distorted by the duration of follow-up, the number of patients studied and the method for diagnosing restenosis. Thus, when Latimer and Burnand's overviews are reanalysed to take this into account, the incidence of recurrent restenosis following carotid endarterectomy is found to be 6–14%, which equates to an average annual restenosis or occlusion rate of 1.5–4.5%. However, the rate of restenosis may not be linear throughout the period of follow-up and the overview of Frericks et al.[7] suggests that the risk of restenosis is approximately 10% in the first year of follow-up, 3% in the second year and 2% in the third year. The risk thereafter of developing a significant recurrent stenosis is probably about 1% per annum.

CAUSES OF EARLY AND LATE RESTENOSIS

Once intraoperative technical errors and residual disease have been excluded, a true restenosis can be defined as the development of a further stenosis following operation. Early restenosis is defined as a restenosis occurring within the first year and almost invariably follows neointimal hyperplasia. This hyperplastic stenosis often occurs in the first 6 months following operation, and is seen as a diffuse generalized narrowing, usually in relation to the upper half of the carotid endarterectomy site (Fig. 29.1).

Late restenosis can be defined as stenosis which occurs after more than 1 year has elapsed following successful carotid endarterectomy, with no evidence of restenosis in the first year. This secondary form tends to be slow and progressive and appears to be related to recurrent atherosclerosis rather than intimal hyperplasia.[1]

Factors which are thought to influence the development of neointimal hyperplasia include surgical injury during the operation (e.g. clamp damage), trauma following insertion of an indwelling shunt and the use of distal tacking sutures. This last phenomenon may reflect the presence of residual disease or because turbulent flow predisposes towards neointimal hyperplasia.[8] Similarly, restenosis appears to be more common in patients with small carotid arteries (< 4 mm in diameter) and in those who continue to smoke. There is no evidence that either antiplatelet agents or anticoagulant therapy reduce the incidence of restenosis.

WHY OPERATE ON A RECURRENT STENOSIS?

Surgeons assume that the secondary lesions of intimal

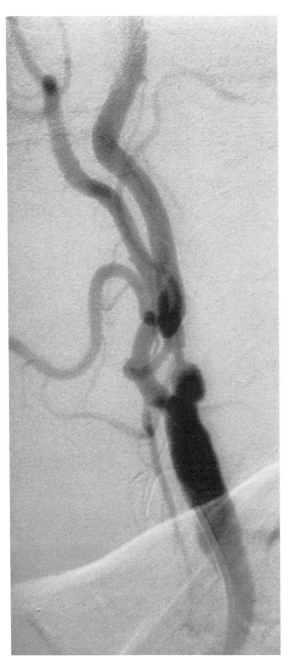

Fig. 29.1
Typical appearance of restenosis following carotid
endarterectomy.

hyperplasia and recurrent atherosclerosis carry the
same increased risk of obstructive and thromboembolic
ischaemia as primary obstructive and atherosclerotic
lesions. Until more reliable data are available, Frericks
has concluded that this reasoning by analogy is
probably safe way to follow.[7]

To date, there have been no randomized controlled
trials to evaluate the role of re-do carotid
endarterectomy in the management of patients with
a recurrent stenosis. Thus, although Frerick's
rationale is superficially attractive, it remains
unproven. The question is, therefore, not whether
recurrent stenoses are a common phenomenon
following carotid endarterectomy (which clearly they
are), but first whether they significantly increase the
risk of late ipsilateral stroke and second, whether the
risks of reoperation outweigh the natural history risk
of late stroke.

It is difficult to determine the true risk of ipsilateral
stroke in patients with a recurrent carotid stenosis
because many are subjected to a prophylactic re-do
operation during the course of follow-up. However,
in the overview of Frericks et al.,[7] there are
10 published series where the risks of stroke were
examined relative to whether the patient had a
recurrent stenosis or not. Having corrected for the
confounding effects of differing lengths of follow-up
and study size, a reanalysis of this data suggests that
the incidence of ipsilateral stroke in patients with a
recurrent stenosis > 50% is approximately 5.5%
over 3 years (i.e. about 2% per annum). For those
with no evidence of a recurrent stenosis, the risk of
ipsilateral stroke is 3.3% over 3 years (i.e. incidence
about 1% per annum). These figures also correlate
closely with the follow-up data reported in the
international trials.[9,10]

Thus, even if a policy of operating upon every
patient with a recurrent carotid stenosis was
associated with a zero early and late stroke risk, re-do
carotid endarterectomy could only ever realistically
confer a 2–3% absolute risk reduction over 3 years
(i.e. an absolute risk reduction of about 1% per
annum). However, as we all know, re-do carotid
surgery is not without risk. Fifteen recently published
series have detailed the risks and outcomes of re-do
carotid endarterectomy in the management of 995

patients with recurrent carotid stenosis.[11-25] Overall, the 30-day mortality rate was 1.29% while the stroke rate was 3.8%, giving an overall death/any stroke rate of approximately 5%. Thus, given that the 3-year risk of ipsilateral stroke in patients with a significant recurrent stenosis is probably only about 5.5%, most, if not all, long-term benefit will be lost through the early risks of re-do surgery. Moreover, because evidence suggests that 11-22% will develop a second recurrent stenosis following re-do endarterectomy,[15,23,25] the potential attractions of re-do surgery increasingly diminish.

In view of this, there seems to be little evidence to advocate reoperating on any patient with recurrent carotid stenosis in the absence of symptoms. Thus, as is the practice in most north European centres, re-do carotid endarterectomy is reserved in my practice for patients with recurrent carotid territory symptoms. The only exception might be the patient who has had a saphenous vein graft bypass of the carotid artery. As with lower-limb vein grafts, these patients have a high incidence of focal, hyperplastic restenosis (up to 30% within 18-24 months) and far greater a risk of progressing on to occlusion.

HOW BEST TO TREAT RECURRENT CAROTID DISEASE?

Few surgeons have extensive experience of re-do carotid surgery and clearly any such procedure should not be undertaken lightly. The patient should be warned that the procedure carries an increased risk of stroke and/or cranial nerve injury as compared with the original procedure. In my experience, performing the operation under local anaesthesia has many benefits, not least the fact that infiltration with Marcain and adrenaline allows easier dissection through the scar tissues. Great care must be taken to identify the cranial nerves. The procedure may take considerably longer than a primary operation, and planning should take this into account.

It is advisable to dissect the common carotid artery lower than normal in the neck and the internal carotid artery right up to and behind the posterior belly of digastric. Once the artery has been isolated, the nerves identified and the vessels controlled, the operation will proceed as for a primary endarterectomy. In my experience it is much easier to close these recurrent endarterectomies with a long patch, extending this up into normal internal carotid artery above the previous endarterectomy site to allow easy suturing of the patch at the top end.

A more recent alternative to surgery is balloon angioplasty. Treatment by angioplasty has been advocated by many as the preferred treatment for recurrent stenosis in that it obviates the necessity for dissection of the carotid artery, thus reducing any possible cranial nerve injury. Four studies have recently described their experience in angioplasty on 85 patients with a recurrent carotid stenosis,[26-29] with an overall procedural stroke rate of 3.5%. However, up to 12% will develop a second recurrence,[29] which is similar to that observed following re-do carotid surgery. Although these patients were inevitably highly selected, should there ever be a proven role for reintervention in patients with recurrent stenoses, it may be that angioplasty will become the preferred option. In those patients who have had a vein graft implanted, then it is perfectly feasible to dilate the stenoses that may complicate these vein grafts, with similar results to those who have stenoses in femoropopliteal bypass grafts.

REFERENCES

1 Stoney RJ, String ST. Recurrent carotid stenosis. *Surgery* 1976; **80**: 705-710.

2 Cossman D, Callow AD, Stein A, Matsumoto G. Early restenosis after carotid endarterectomy. *Archives of Surgery* 1978; **113**: 275-278.

3 Colgan MP, Kingston V, Shanik G. Stenosis following carotid endarterectomy. Its implication in management of asymptomatic carotid stenosis. *Archives of Surgery* 1984; **119**: 1033-1035.

4 Barnes RW, Nix ML, Wingo JP, Nichols BT. Recurrent versus residual carotid stenosis. Incidence detected by Doppler ultrasound. *Annals of Surgery* 1986; **203**: 652-660.

5 Eikelboom BC, Ackerstaff RGA, Heonveld H *et al*. Benefits of carotid patching: a randomized study. *Journal of Vascular Surgery* 1988; **7**: 240-247.

6 Latimer CR, Burnand KG. Recurrent carotid stenosis after carotid endarterectomy. *British Journal of Surgery* 1997; **84**: 1206-1219.

7 Frericks H, Kievit J, van Baalen JM, van Bockel JH. Carotid recurrent stenosis and risk of ipsilateral stroke. A

systematic review of the literature. *Stroke* 1998; **29**: 244–250.

8 Bandyk DF, Kaebnick HW, Adams MB, Towne JB. Turbulence occurring after carotid bifurcation endarterectomy: a harbinger of residual and recurrent stenosis. *Journal of Vascular Surgery* 1988; **7**: 261–274.

9 European Carotid Surgery Trialists' Collaborative Group. Randomised trial of endarterectomy for recently symptomatic carotid stenosis: final results of the MRC European Carotid Surgery Trial (ECST). *Lancet* 1998; **351**: 1379–1387.

10 Barnett HJM, Taylor DW, Eliasziw M *et al*. Benefit of carotid endarterectomy in patients with symptomatic moderate or severe stenosis. *New England Journal of Medicine* 1998; **339**: 1415–1425.

11 Clagett GP, Rich NM, McDonald PT *et al*. Aetiological factors for recurrent carotid artery stenosis. *Surgery* 1983; **93**: 313–318.

12 Bartlett FF, Rapp JH, Goldstone J, Ehrenfeld WK, Stoney RJ. Recurrent carotid stenosis: Operative strategy and late results. *Journal of Vascular Surgery* 1987; **5**: 452–456.

13 Kazmers A, Zierler RE, Huang TW, Pulliam CW, Radke HM. Reoperative carotid surgery. *American Journal of Surgery* 1988; **156**: 346–352.

14 Bernstein EF, Torem S, Dilley RB. Does carotid restenosis predict an increased risk of late symptoms, stroke or death? *Annals of Surgery* 1990; **212**: 629–636.

15 Trieman GS, Jenkins JM, Edwards WH *et al*. The evolving surgical management of recurrent carotid stenosis. *Journal of Vascular Surgery* 1992; **16**: 354–363.

16 AbuRahma AF, Snodgrass KR, Robinson PA, Wood DJ, Meek RB, Patton DJ. Safety and durability of redo carotid endarterectomy for recurrent carotid artery stenosis. *American Journal of Surgery* 1994; **168**: 175–178.

17 Lattimer CR, Lockhart S, Irvine A, Browse NL, Burnand KG. Surgery for carotid restenosis: a 13 year review. *British Journal of Surgery* 1996; **83** (Suppl): 16.

18 Coyle KA, Smith RB, Gray BC *et al*. Treatment of recurrent cerebrovascular disease: review of a 10 year experience. *Annals of Surgery* 1995; **221**: 517–521.

19 Meyer FB, Piepgras DG, Fode NC. Surgical treatment of recurrent carotid artery stenosis. *Journal of Neurosurgery* 1994; **80**: 781–787.

20 O'Donnell TF, Rodriguez AA, Fortunato JE, Welch HJ, Mackey WC. Management of recurrent carotid stenosis: should asymptomatic lesions be treated surgically? *Journal of Vascular Surgery* 1996; **24**: 207–212.

21 Hertzer NR, O'Hara PJ, Mascha EJ, Krajewski LP, Sullivan TM, Beven EG. Early outcome assessment for 2228 consecutive carotid endarterectomy procedures: the Cleveland Clinic experience from 1989 to 1995. *Journal of Vascular Surgery* 1997; **26**: 1–10.

22 Ballinger BA, Money SR, Chatman DM, Bowen JC, Ochsner JL. Sites of recurrence and long term results of redo surgery. *Annals of Surgery* 1997; **225**: 512–515.

23 Mansour MA, Kang SS, Baker WH *et al*. Carotid endarterectomy for recurrent stenosis. *Journal of Vascular Surgery* 1997; **25**: 877–883.

24 Hobson RW, Goldstein JE, Jamil Z *et al*. Carotid restenosis: operative and endovascular management. *Journal of Vascular Surgery* 1999; **29**: 228–235.

25 Rockman CB, Riles TS, Landis R *et al*. Redo carotid surgery: an analysis of materials and configurations used in carotid reoperations and their influence on peri-operative stroke and subsequent recurrent stenosis. *Journal of Vascular Surgery* 1999; **29**: 72–80.

26 Bergeron P, Chambran P, Benichou H, Alessandri C. Recurrent carotid disease: will stents be an alternative to surgery? *Journal of Endovascular Surgery* 1996; **3**: 76–79.

27 Lorenzi G, Domanin M, Costantini A, Rolli A, Agrifoglio G. Intra-operative transluminal angioplasty of recurrent carotid stenosis. *Journal of Cardiovascular Surgery (Torino)* 1993; **34**: 163–165.

28 Yadav JS, Roubin GS, King P, Iyer S, Vitek J. Angioplasty and stenting for restenosis after carotid endarterectomy: initial experience. *Stroke* 1996; **27**: 2075–2079.

29 Lanzino G, Mericle RA, Lopes DK, Wakhloo AK, Guterman LR, Hopkins LN. Percutaneous transluminal angioplasty and stent placement for recurrent carotid artery stenosis. *Journal of Neurosurgery* 1999; **90**: 688–694.

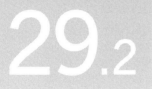

29.2

When should I reoperate for recurrent carotid stenosis?

G Patrick Clagett (USA)

INTRODUCTION

The answer to the question posed in the chapter title is straightforward. I recommend reoperative endarterectomy in good-risk patients with anticipated significant longevity using the same indications as in patients with primary carotid stenosis. These indications include focal neurologic symptoms ipsilateral to a hemodynamically significant stenosis (≥ 50% linear stenosis measured angiographically[30]) and, in the absence of focal symptoms, an advanced or progressive (≥ 70–80%) stenosis. However, appropriate application of these indications to patients with carotid restenosis requires careful consideration of the incidence, natural history, and pathology of recurrent carotid disease, its risk factors, the technical features of reoperation necessary to minimize morbidity, and the results of reintervention.

INCIDENCE AND NATURAL HISTORY

Recurrent stenosis is infrequent but not rare. A recent systematic overview documented the risk to be about 10% in the first year after primary endarterectomy, 3% in the second, and 2% in the third[31] (Fig. 29.2). Long-term risk was estimated to be about 1% per year. The risk of ipsilateral stroke varies widely according to published series in which patients with recurrence are compared retrospectively to patients with no recurrence.[32–41] The data are extremely heterogeneous, reflecting the retrospective nature of most of these studies, selection bias, lack of consistent follow-up of all patients at risk, varying lengths of follow-up, and inconsistent definitions of events. Despite the short-comings in available data, the overview by Frericks et al. concluded that the risk of stroke with recurrence was moderately increased (relative risk 2.0).[31]

Stroke and other neurologic events from recurrent stenoses appear more likely to occur several years after original endarterectomy and are less likely in the first 2–3 years after the primary procedure.[42–44] This may be related to the underlying pathology of

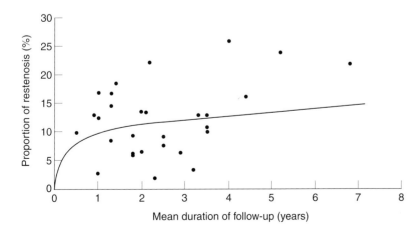

Fig. 29.2
Cumulative incidence of recurrent carotid stenosis plotted against average follow-up period. Modified from Frericks et al.[31] with permission.

recurrent lesions relative to the time interval from primary operation to lesion diagnosis. The pathology of carotid restenosis is discussed below.

The risk of recurrent stenosis may be decreasing. Pooled data from 24 published studies that assessed the incidence of recurrent stenosis by duplex ultrasonography yield a crude recurrence rate of 14 ± 12% (mean ± SD) with a wide range (0–49%).[39,41,42,44–62] If one plots study year against recurrence rate in individual studies (Fig. 29.3), the incidence has clearly decreased in more recent studies. When life-table methods are used to calculate recurrence risk over time, older data suggest that the cumulative risk of hemodynamically significant lesions developing 5 years after endarterectomy is 25%.[63] More contemporary data suggest that this figure is much lower: 5–10%.[55,56] In North American Symptomatic Carotid Endarterectomy Trial (NASCET) surgical patients, the need for reoperation at 2–5 years after carotid endarterectomy was less than 1% (HJM Barnett, personal communication). Explanations for a decreasing incidence of recurrent stenosis remain speculative but probably include recognition and control of multiple systemic and local risk factors, wider use of intraoperative surveillance techniques leading to correction of reconstruction site abnormalities, wider use of patch angioplasty closure in small arteries and in women, and, perhaps, better training.

Despite a possible decrease in risk for recurrent stenosis, the number of reoperative carotid endarterectomies in major centers may increase because of renewed enthusiasm for carotid endarterectomy generated by positive results from major multicenter trials.[30,64–67] Large-scale epidemiologic studies have already documented a marked increase in the number of endarterectomies being performed for asymptomatic disease.[68,69] With the announcement of the second phase of NASCET documenting the beneficial effects of endarterectomy in symptomatic patients with moderate stenoses (50–69%), as well as the durable stroke-free survival after operation in those with advanced stenoses (≥ 70%),[30] the performance of carotid endarterectomy will increase further.

PATHOLOGY AND RISK FACTORS

In assessing the risk of neurologic events stemming from recurrent lesions, several factors bear consideration. Many authors have documented that recurrences in the first 2–3 years after primary endarterectomy are relatively benign and infrequently cause symptoms.[42–44] Later recurrences – those occurring more than 3 years after endarterectomy – appear much more likely to be associated with neurologic events.[44,70] This temporal relationship is most likely due to the underlying pathologic features of early and late recurrences. Some studies have documented partial regression of early lesions within the first year after primary procedure.[35] This waxing and waning of lesions suggests some remodeling at the endarterectomy site, but the precise nature of the remodeling process

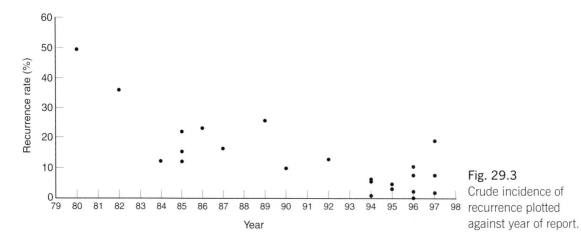

Fig. 29.3 Crude incidence of recurrence plotted against year of report.

is unknown. In our histopathologic studies, we noted adherent, organized thrombus lining the surface of hypercellular early recurrences with cellular material infiltrating thrombus. It is tempting to speculate that the remodeling process may be related to thrombus growth, dissolution by lytic processes, and organization.

Early lesions (recurrence less than 2–3 years) are predominantly neointimal fibromuscular hyperplasia consisting of smooth-muscle cells surrounded by proteoglycans. Late recurrent lesions (recurrence interval greater than 2–3 years) tend to have elements of atherosclerosis (foam cells, cholesterol clefts, abundant collagen, and calcium). However, the histopathologic differentiation between early and late lesions is indistinct because focal areas of neointimal fibromuscular hyperplasia can frequently be found in late recurrences.[71] It seems most likely that these histologic differences account in large part for the distinct natural histories of early and late recurrent lesions.

In considering which patients might be likely to develop recurrent stenosis, it is important to consider risk factors. These can be broadly categorized into local or systemic risk factors. One of the more important local determinants is residual defects at the endareterectomy site.[72–74] In assessing recurrence of disease, it is necessary to consider residual stenosis. Several series using angiography have studied the presence of disease in the early postoperative period;[72–79] residual disease is present in $12 \pm 12\%$ of patients with a range of 0–29%. This is important because residual stenosis may progress to significant recurrent disease. The most significant risk factor for this appears to be the degree of residual plaque left at the time of original carotid endarterectomy.[79] Flaps and other technical defects may also be important.[50–52] Several studies have documented that technical defects leading to turbulence and hemodynamic abnormalities as detected by intraoperative duplex scanning are more likely to progress to recurrent stenosis, in comparison to endarterectomy sites free of defects with normal, luminal flow.[64,83–88] These data suggest that some sort of intraoperative assessment at the completion of carotid reconstruction is important and that detection of abnormalities mandates immediate correction.

Systemic factors that have been associated with development of recurrent disease include female gender, continued smoking after endarterectomy, hypercholesterolemia, diabetes mellitus, hypertension, young age at original endarterectomy, and associated severe atherosclerotic disease.[37,41,52,60,83,84] Female gender is one of the most consistently reported risk factors for recurrence of disease.[83,85–87] The high incidence of recurrence in females may be related to the smaller vessel size in these patients.[51] We first reported continued smoking after primary endarterectomy to be a potent risk factor for recurrence.[83] This has been confirmed in subsequent studies of our own,[84] as well as those of others.[44,53,57,80,86] Patients with premature atherosclerosis appear to have a particularly virulent form of the disease and are at especially high risk for restenosis.[88,89]

All local and many systemic factors associated with restenosis are subject to modification to prevent restenosis. A technically precise primary operation and liberal use of patching in patients at highest risk for restenosis are critical to minimize local factors leading to restenosis. Careful management of hypercholesterolemia, hypertension, and diabetes, as well as smoking cessation, are essential to minimize the systemic factors.

REOPERATIVE TECHNIQUE

Precise technique is required in reoperative carotid surgery to minimize risk and insure benefit. The operation for recurrent disease is markedly different from that for primary disease. Because these operations take much longer, we employ general anesthesia and use a shunt without electroencephalogram or other monitoring techniques. During the initial dissection, dense fibrosis usually obscures the planes of the carotid sheath. This is much more pronounced with early recurrent lesions, for which reoperative surgery is performed within 1 year of the primary carotid endarterectomy. Sharp (scalpel) dissection is the optimum technique to use. The key point in the initial dissection is exposure of the common carotid artery well below the bifurcation. Once the vessel is identified, the periadventitial plan is found and dissection along and around the vessel is continued *close* to the vessel wall. Frequently, the vagus nerve is adherent to the wall more anteriorly than anticipated and cannot be readily distinguished from the vessel wall and surrounding fibrous tissue. Therefore, dissection of the common carotid artery is best begun medially. By staying close to the wall with scalpel dissection, the vagus nerve can be atraumatically dissected free.

Once the common carotid artery is isolated circumferentially, the dissection is continued upward along the anterior lateral aspect of the bulb and the internal carotid artery. The 'no-touch' technique of avoiding dissection of the disease-bearing carotid bifurcation by first isolating the common, internal, and external carotid arteries is advocated for primary carotid endarterectomy. However, for reoperative endarterectomy, this is frequently impossible because one cannot separately identify the internal carotid artery in the fibrous reaction and dissect it free. Therefore, it is necessary to proceed cautiously from caudad to cephalad along the bulb and origin of the internal carotid artery. Identification of the old suture line, which serves as a road map, is helpful. Once an adequate length of internal carotid artery is exposed (beyond the end of old suture line or extent of recurrent disease) on its anterior lateral borders, it is mobilized circumferentially. During this portion of the dissection, one should be wary of the possibility of a low-lying hypoglossal nerve. Again, scalpel dissection close to the vessel wall would help prevent injury to this nerve. Dissection must always be gentle, methodical, and precise. Recurrent lesions (especially later ones) frequently have associated thrombus and loose pultaceous debris that can easily be dislodged. Because the 'no-touch' technique cannot be used, 'gentle-touch' technique is mandatory. Although we almost always circumferentially mobilize the external carotid artery before primary endarterectomy, we rarely do so for recurrent disease. Dissection of enough of the circumference to allow control with a small angled vascular clamp is all that is necessary.

Frequently, high carotid exposure is necessary for recurrent carotid disease. This may be due to the initial disease extending above the C_2 level or, on occasion, because the fibrotic reaction surrounding the internal carotid is so dense that exposure of the vessel in an area above the previous dissection (virgin territory) is desirable. We have found mandibular subluxation for carotid exposure helpful in such cases.[90]

The ease of endarterectomy for recurrent carotid disease is closely tied to the pathological characteristics of recurrent lesions. Early recurrences are usually pale, white, rubbery lesions that are densely adherent to the vascular wall. The cells comprising these lesions stem from smooth-muscle cells in the adherent media left from the original endarterectomy; therefore, recurrent lesions are also adherent. This presents technical challenges in that the re-endarterectomy plane is uneven and frequently obscured. Because of this, some authors have advocated reconstruction with venous patch angioplasty alone without endarterectomy. However, with careful technique, we are almost always able to remove most of the hyperplastic recurrent lesion by establishing a subadventitial plane. Often, early recurrences must be removed piecemeal. In cases where the subadventitial plane is obscured, one must not persist in trying to remove the entire lesion for fear of destroying the carotid wall. Resection of the bulk of the lesion, coupled with vein patch closure, is effective. Despite the fear of leaving hyperplastic media which may further proliferate and cause recurrence, this is rare and is not borne out by clinical experience.

Late recurrences are more typically atherosclerotic and are easier to endarterectomize. Even though late recurrences stem from neointimal fibromuscular hyperplastic lesions that have undergone time-dependent atheroscleortic change, the subadventitial endarterectomy plane is much easier to find. This may be because atherosclerotic change has also progressed in the adherent media left after initial endarterectomy, thus allowing this media, along with the recurrent lesion, to separate easily from the outer wall. Despite this, the subadventitial planes often remain somewhat obscured distally and proximally and end-point feathering is difficult. The same caveats with regard to trying to be too compulsive and complete in removing all grossly visible diseases are appropriate. It is far better to leave some diseased intima and media and to protect the reconstruction with a vein patch closure than to risk

Table 29.1
Recurrent carotid disease: results of reoperation

Series	Year	Number of patients	Stroke	Death	Cranial nerve injury
Bartlett et al.[96]	1987	116	1(1.5%)	2(3.1%)	7(11%)
Nitzberg et al.[91]	1991	29	1(3.4%)	0	5(17%)
Treiman et al.[91]	1992	57(vein graft)	2(3.5%)	1(1.8%)	
		105(re-do CEA)	2(1.9%)	1(1.0%)	
Gagne et al.[92]	1993	41	0	0	2(5%)
AbuRahma et al.[93]	1994	46	3(7%)	0	3(7%)
Coyle et al.[98]	1995	69	1(1.4%)	2(2.9%)	0
Rosenthal et al.[86]	1996	31*	0	0	3(10%)
O'Donnell et al.[70]	1996	48	1(2.1%)	1(2.1%)	9(18.9%)
Ballinger et al.[94]	1997	70	1(1.4%)	1(1.4%)	11(15.7%)
Mansour et al.[95]	1997	69	4(5.8%)	0	6(8.7%)

*Tertiary operations.
CEA, carotid endarterectomy.

getting into too deep a dissection plane and destroying the integrity of the wall.

Patch angioplasty is necessary with most reoperations for recurrent carotid artery disease. On rare occasions, we have performed a primary closure in a patient with a pliable, large carotid artery in which a complete re-endarterectomy was possible for a late recurrent lesion. Although we have used a prosthetic material patch in the past, we now use saphenous vein because of the theoretical advantages of non-thrombogenicity and enhanced endothelial coverage of the endarterectomy site. In patients with extensive, long-segment recurrent disease or patients with recurrence a second or third time, resection and replacement of the carotid artery is advocated. For replacement of the carotid artery, we prefer to use the greater saphenous vein and, if this is not available, we have successfully used superficial femoral vein.

RESULTS OF REOPERATION
The final factor bearing on the decision to reoperate for recurrent stenosis is the expected outcome. The

results of reoperation for recurrent carotid disease from several major series are shown in Table 29.1.[70,86,91–98] The overall incidence of major morbidity and mortality is approximately that of primary endarterectomy, except for the incidence of cranial nerve injury. In general, the mean risk of stroke with reoperation is approximately 3%, with a death rate of approximately 1% and a cranial nerve injury rate of approximately 10%. Many recent series document excellent results from reoperative carotid endarterectomy, with overall low morbidity and mortality indistinguishable from those of primary endarterectomy.[91–98]

CONCLUSIONS AND RECOMMENDATIONS
The overall incidence of recurrent carotid stenosis may be decreasing, but the total number of cases will probably increase because more carotid endarterectomies are being performed. Although our knowledge of the natural history of recurrent stenosis is imperfect, the risk of stroke with recurrence is increased, particularly with late lesions. Because of the increased risk of stroke and the excellent results of reoperation when performed appropriately, I favor

an aggressive approach and recommend reoperation for all patients with symptomatic recurrence who have an ipsilateral hemodynamically significant stenosis and in asymptomatic patients with an advanced or progressive (≥ 70–80%) stenosis.

Because patients with early (< 3 years) restenosis appear to be at somewhat lower risk than those with late restenosis, I am more conservative with stable asymptomatic early lesions, which usually remain asymptomatic and may even regress.

REFERENCES

30 North American Symptomatic Carotid Endarterectomy Trial Collaborators. The benefit of carotid endarterectomy in symptomatic patients with moderate and severe stenosis. *New England Journal of Medicine* (in press).

31 Frericks H, Kievit J, van Baalen JM, van Bockel JH. Carotid recurrent stenosis and risk of ipsilateral stroke. A systematic review of the literature. *Stroke* 1998; **29**: 244–250.

32 Civil ID, O'Hara PJ, Hertzer NR, Krajewski LP, Beven EG. Late patency of the carotid artery after endarterectomy; problems of definition, follow-up methodology, and data analysis. *Journal of Vascular Surgery* 1988; **8**: 79–85.

33 Cuming R, Worrell P, Woolcock NE, Franks PJ, Greenhalgh RM, Powell JT. The influence of smoking and lipids on restenosis after carotid endarterectomy. *European Journal of Vascular Surgery* 1993; **7**: 572–576.

34 Hansen F, Lindblad B, Persson NH, Bergqvist D. Can recurrent stenosis after carotid endarterectomy be prevented by low-dose acetylsalicylic acid? A double-blind, randomised and placebo-controlled study. *European Journal of Vascular Surgery* 1993; **7**: 380–385.

35 Healy DA, Zierler RE, Nichols SC *et al*. Long-term follow-up and clinical outcome of carotid restenosis. *Journal of Vascular Surgery* 1989; **10**: 662–669.

36 Kinney EV, Seabrook GR, Kinney LY, Bandyk DF, Towne JB. The importance of intraoperative detection of residual flow abnormalities after carotid artery endarterectomy. *Journal of Vascular Surgery* 1993; **17**: 912–923.

37 Mackey WC, Belkin M, Sindhi R, Welch H, O'Donnell TF Jr. Routine postendarterectomy duplex surveillance; does it prevent late stroke? *Journal of Vascular Surgery* 1992; **16**: 934–940.

38 Mattos MA, van Bemmelen PS, Barkmeier LD, Hodgson KJ, Ramsey DE, Sumner DS. Routine surveillance after carotid endarterectomy: does it affect clinical management? *Journal of Vascular Surgery* 1993; **17**: 819–831.

39 Ouriel K, Green RM. Clinical and technical factors influencing recurrent carotid stenosis and occlusion after endarterectomy. *Journal of Vascular Surgery* 1987; **5**: 702–706.

40 Rosenthal D, Archie JP Jr, Garcia-Rinaldi R *et al*. Carotid patch angioplasty: immediate and long-term results. *Journal of Vascular Surgery* 1990; **12**: 326–333.

41 Zbornikova V, Elfstrom J, Lassvik C, Johansson I, Olsson JE, Bjornlert U. Restenosis and occlusion after carotid surgery assessed by duplex scanning and digital subtraction angiography. *Stroke* 1986; **17**: 1137–1142.

42 O'Donnell TF Jr, Callow AD, Scott G, Shepard AD, Heggerick P, Mackey WC. Ultrasound characteristics of recurrent carotid disease: hypothesis explaining the low incidence of symptomatic recurrence. *Journal of Vascular Surgery* 1985; **2**: 26–41.

43 Washburn WK, Mackey WC, Belkin M, O'Donnell TF Jr. Late stroke after carotid endarterectomy: the role of recurrent stenosis. *Journal of Vascular Surgery* 1992; **15**: 1032–1037.

44 Ricotta JJ, O'Brien-Irr MS. Conservative management of residual and recurrent lesions after carotid endarterectomy: long-term results. *Journal of Vascular Surgery* 1997; **26**: 963–972.

45 Bodily KC, Zeirler RE, Marinelli MR *et al*. Flow disturbances following carotid endarterectomy. *Surgery, Gynecology and Obstetrics* 1980; **151**: 77–80.

46 Zierler RE, Bandyk DF, Thiele BL *et al*. Carotid artery stenosis following endarterectomy. *Archives of Surgery* 1982; **117**: 1408–1415.

47 Colgan MP, Kingston V, Shanik G. Stenosis following carotid endarterectomy. Its implication in management of asymptomatic carotid stenosis. *Journal of Cardiovascular Surgery* 1985; **26**: 300–302.

48 Nichols SC, Phillips DJ, Bergelin RO *et al*. Carotid endarterectomy: relationship of outcome to early restenosis. *Journal of Vascular Surgery* 1985; **2**: 375–381.

49 Glover JL, Bendick PJ, Dilley RS *et al*. Restenosis following carotid endarterectomy. Evaluation by duplex ultrasonography. *Archives of Surgery* 1985; **120**: 678–684.

50 Keagy BA, Erdington RD, Pool MA *et al*. Incidence of recurrent or residual carotid stenosis after carotid endarterectomy. *American Journal of Surgery* 1985; **149**: 722–725.

51 Healy DA, Clowes AW, Zierler RE *et al*. Immediate and long-term results of carotid endarterectomy. *Stroke* 1989; **20**: 1138–1142.

52 Bernstein EF, Torem S, Dilley B. Does carotid restenosis predict an increased risk of late symptoms, stroke, or death? *Annals of Surgery* 1990; **212**: 629–636.

53 Ladowski JS, Shinabery LM, Peterson D, Peterson AC, Deschner WP. Factors contributing to recurrent carotid disease following carotid endarterectomy. *American Journal of Surgery* 1997; **174**: 118–120.

54 Carballo RE, Towne JB, Seabrook GR, Freischlag JA, Cambria RA. An outcome analysis of carotid endarterectomy: the incidence and natural history of recurrent stenosis. *Journal of Vascular Surgery* 1996; **23**: 749–754.

55 Gelabert HA, El-Massry S, Moore WS. Carotid endarterectomy with primary closure does not adversely affect the rate of recurrent stenosis. *Archives of Surgery* 1994; **129**: 648–654.

56 Myers SI, Valentine RJ, Chervu A, Bowers BL, Clagett GP. Saphenous vein patch versus primary closure for carotid endarterectomy: long-term assessment of a randomized prospective study. *Journal of Vascular Surgery* 1994; **19**: 15–22.

57 Dempsey RJ, Moore RW, Cordero S. Factors leading to early recurrence of carotid plaque after carotid endarterectomy. *Surgical Neurology* 1995; **42**: 278–283.

58 Mattos MA, Hodgson KJ, Londrey GL et al. Carotid endarterectomy: operative risks, recurrent stenosis, and long-term stroke rates in a modern series. *Journal of Cardiovascular Surgery* 1992; **33**: 387–400.

59 Golledge J, Cuming R, Davies AH, Greenhalgh RM. Outcome of selective patching following carotid endarterectomy. *European Journal of Vascular and Endovascular Surgery* 1996; **11**: 458–463.

60 Perler BA, Ursin F, Shanks U, Williams GM. Carotid Dacron patch angioplasty; immediate and long-term results of a prospective series. *Cardiovascular Surgery* 1995; **3**: 631–636.

61 Johnson BL, Gupta AK, Bandyk DF, Shulman C, Jackson M. Anatomic patterns of carotid endarterectomy healing. *American Journal of Surgery* 1996; **172**: 188–190.

62 Baker WH, Koustas G, Burke K et al. Intraoperative duplex scanning and later carotid artery stenosis. *Journal of Vascular Surgery* 1994; **19**: 829–833.

63 DeGroote RD, Lynch TG, Jamil Z, Hobson RW II. Carotid restenosis: long-term noninvasive follow-up after carotid endarterectomy. *Stroke* 1987; **18**: 1031–1036.

64 North American Symptomatic Carotid Endarterectomy Trial Collaborators. Beneficial effect of carotid endarterectomy in symptomatic patients with high-grade stenosis. *New England Journal of Medicine* 1991; **325**: 445–453.

65 European Carotid Surgery Trialists' Collaborative Group. Endarterectomy for moderate symptomatic carotid stenosis: interim results from the MRC European Carotid Surgery Trial. *Lancet* 1996; **347**: 1591–1593.

66 Mayberg MR, Wilson SE, Yatsu F et al. Carotid endarterectomy and prevention of cerebral ischemia in symptomatic carotid stenosis. *Journal of the American Medical Association* 1991; **266**: 3289–3294.

67 Asymptomatic Carotid Atherosclerosis Study Group. Carotid endarterectomy for patients with asymptomatic internal carotid artery stenosis. *Journal of the American Medical Association* 1995; **273**: 1421–1428.

68 Huber TS, Wheeler KG, Cuddeback JK, Dame DA, Flynn TC, Seeger JM. Effect of the Asymptomatic Carotid Atherosclerosis Study on carotid endarterectomy in Florida. *Stroke* 1998; **29**: 1099–1105.

69 Kozak LJ, Owings MF. Ambulatory and inpatient procedures in the United States, 1995. National Center for Health Statistics. *Vital Health Statistics* 1998; **135**: 1–116.

70 O'Donnell TF Jr, Rodriguez AA, Fortunato JE, Welch HJ, Mackey WC. Management of recurrent carotid stenosis: should asymptomatic lesions be treated surgically? *Journal of Vascular Surgery* 1996; **24**: 207–212.

71 Clagett GP, Robinowitz M, Youkey JR et al. Morphogenesis and clinicopathologic characteristics of recurrent carotid disease. *Journal of Vascular Surgery* 1986; **3**: 10–23.

72 Blaisdell FW, Lim R Jr, Hall AD. Technical result of carotid endarterectomy. *American Journal of Surgery* 1967; **114**: 239–246.

73 Shutz H, Flemming JF, Awerbuck B. Arteriographic assessment after carotid endarterectomy. *Annals of Surgery* 1970; **171**: 509–521.

74 Sundt TM Jr, Houser OW, Fode NC et al. Correlation of postoperative and two-year follow-up angiography with neurological function in 99 carotid endarterectomies in 86 consecutive patients. *Annals of Surgery* 1986; **203**: 90–100.

75 Hans SS. Late follow-up of carotid endarterectomy with venous patch angioplasty. *American Journal of Surgery* 1991; **162**: 50–54.

76 Diaz FG, Patel S, Boulos R et al. Early angiographic changes after endarterectomy. *Stroke* 1980; **11**: 135.

77 Holder J, Binet EF, Flanigan S et al. Arteriography after carotid endarterectomy. *American Journal of Roentgenology* 1981; **137**: 483–487.

78 Hertzer NR, Beven EG, Modic MT et al. Early patency of the carotid artery after endarterectomy: digital subtraction angiography after 262 operations. *Surgery* 1982; **92**: 1049–1057.

79 Archie JP Jr. Early and late geometric changes after carotid endarterectomy patch reconstruction. *Journal of Vascular Surgery* 1991; **14**: 258–266.

80 Reilly LM, Okuhn SP, Rapp JH et al. Recurrent carotid stenosis: a consequence of local or systemic factors? The influence of unrepaired technical defects. *Journal of Vascular Surgery* 1990; **11**: 448–460.

81 Golledge J, Cuming R, Ellis M, Davies AH, Greenhalgh RM. Duplex imaging findings predict stenosis after carotid endarterectomy. *Journal of Vascular Surgery* 1997; **26**: 43–48.

82 Jackson MR, D'Addio VJ, Gillespie DL, O'Donnell SD. The fate of residual defects following carotid endarterectomy detected by early postoperative duplex ultrasound. *American Journal of Surgery* 1996; **172**: 184–187.

83 Clagett GP, Rich NM, McDonald PT et al. Etiological factors for recurrent carotid artery stenosis. *Surgery* 1983; **93**: 313–318.

84 Clagett GP, Patterson CB, Fisher DF et al. Vein patch versus primary closure for carotid endarterectomy. *Journal of Vascular Surgery* 1989; **9**: 213–223.

85 Eikelboom BC, Ackerstaff RGA, Hoeneveld H et al. Benefits of carotid patching: a randomized study. *Journal of Vascular Surgery* 1988; **7**: 240–247.

86 Rosenthal D, Archie JP, Avila MH et al. Secondary recurrent carotid stenosis. *Journal of Vascular Surgery* 1996; **24**: 424–449.

87 AbuRahma AF, Robinson PA, Saiedy S, Khan JH, Boland JP. Prospective randomized trial of carotid endarterectomy with primary closure and patch angioplasty with saphenous vein, jugular vein, and polytetrafluoroethylene: long-term follow-up. *Journal of Vascular Surgery* 1998; **27**: 222–234.

88 Valentine RJ. Premature peripheral atherosclerosis. *Cardiovascular Surgery* 1993; **1**: 473–480.

89 Valentine RJ, Myers SI, Hagino RY, Clagett GP. Late outcome of patients with premature carotid atherosclerosis after carotid endarterectomy. *Stroke* 1996; **27**: 1502–1506.

90 Fisher DF, Clagett GP, Parker JL et al. Mandibular subluxation for high carotid exposure. *Journal of Vascular Surgery* 1984; **1**: 727–733.

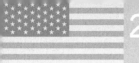

91 Nitzberg RS, Mackey WC, Prendiville E *et al.* Long-term follow-up of patients operated on for recurrent carotid stenosis. *Journal of Vascular Surgery* 1991; **13**: 121–126.

92 Gagne PJ, Riles TS, Jacobowitz GR *et al.* Long-term follow-up of patients undergoing reoperation for recurrent carotid artery disease. *Journal of Vascular Surgery* 1993; **18**: 991–1001.

93 AbuRahma AF, Snodgrass KR, Robinson PA, Wood DJ, Meek RB, Patton DJ. Safety and durability of redo carotid endarterectomy for recurrent carotid artery stenosis. *American Journal of Surgery* 1994; **168**: 175–178.

94 Ballinger BA, Money SR, Chatman DM, Bowen JC, Ochsner JL. Sites of recurrence and long-term results of redo surgery. *Annals of Surgery* 1997; **225**: 512–517.

95 Mansour MA, Kang SS, Baker WH *et al.* Carotid endarterectomy for recurrent stenosis. *Journal of Vascular Surgery* 1997; **25**: 877–883

96 Bartlett FF, Rapp JH, Goldstone J *et al.* Recurrent carotid stenosis: operative strategy and late results. *Journal of Vascular Surgery* 1987; **5**: 452–456.

97 Treiman GS, Jenkins JM, Edwards WH Sr *et al.* The evolving surgical management of recurrent carotid stenosis. *Journal of Vascular Surgery* 1992; **16**: 354–362.

98 Coyle KA, Smith RB III, Gray BC *et al.* Treatment of recurrent cerebrovascular disease. Review of a 10-year experience. *Annals of Surgery* 1995; **211**: 517–524.

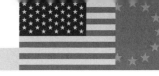

29.3 Editorial Comment

In the previous chapter, it was clear that the surgeon's policy regarding the role of surveillance was primarily dictated by attitude to the role of carotid endarterectomy (CEA) in asymptomatic disease. The same dilemma (and conclusions), not surprisingly, confronts surgeons in the management of recurrent carotid stenosis. Recurrent stenosis is relatively common following CEA; however, surprisingly few patients will develop symptoms. There is a clear consensus amongst the authors that patients presenting with recurrent symptoms should be considered for re-do endarterectomy or carotid bypass. Whether or not angioplasty will have a role in the future remains to be seen. Symptomatic patients undergoing re-do CEA should be counseled as to the increased risks of death, stroke, and cranial nerve injury, as compared with their first CEA, and should be warned that up to 20% may develop second or even third restenoses.

There is no consensus on the role of re-do surgery in the management of patients with an asymptomatic recurrent stenosis. Supporters of re-do CEA will quote the twofold excess risk of ipsilateral stroke in patients with a recurrent stenosis but what is rarely quoted is the fact that the onset of symptoms usually precedes recognition of a severe recurrent stenosis, i.e. if one reviewed the preceding surveillance study prior to stroke onset it is likely that no severe recurrent stenosis was present. Thus, in the absence of any evidence-based data, surgeons considering re-do surgery in asymptomatic (rather than symptomatic) patients must ensure that the initial operative risk does not exceed 6%, as otherwise evidence suggests that any benefit in terms of long-term stroke prevention is negated by the initial operative stroke rate.

How should I manage a patient with an infected prosthetic patch?

Peter RF Bell (Europe)

INTRODUCTION

The question as to whether or not one should patch the endarterectomy zone after carotid endarterectomy (CEA) remains unanswered. Thus, the simplest answer to this question would be not to put any prosthetic patches into anyone! However, a number of randomized controlled studies have shown that patching reduces the incidence of stroke and it is an easy technique for surgeons to learn.[1,2] Meta-analyses[3] also suggest that patching is superior in terms of a reduced incidence of restenosis. Thus, despite the various methodological problems that are inherent when trying to interpret the results of meta-analyses, I have concluded that routine patching is probably the right strategy to adopt. The question is, which patch to use?

Vein patches are certainly more user-friendly, but unless they are harvested from the upper end of the long saphenous vein, patch rupture is likely.[4] Moreover, if this is done, the vein cannot thereafter be used for other purposes such as coronary artery bypass surgery or distal bypass. The obvious alternative is some form of prosthetic patch and this can either be expanded polytetrafluoroethylene (PTFE) or Dacron. PTFE has been used by a number of authors[5] but, in my experience, the main problem with its use has been prolonged bleeding from the suture holes. Apart from the time it takes for this to stop, there is always the risk that any secondary wound haematoma can become infected. The principal alternative is Dacron. The newer patches are now much thinner and, because they are impregnated with albumin or collagen, they do not leak.

PROSTHETIC PATCH INFECTION

The problem with any prosthetic patch is, of course, that they can get infected. Although the infection rate

is extremely low (0.6% in our institution) infection of a patch can be a desperate situation. Moreover, as with many other rare but life-threatening problems, consensus as to the best way of managing it is absent.

Initial management

The patient usually presents with an obvious abscess or sinus related to the wound or with haemorrhage. Patients presenting with the former usually have a 'window of opportunity' with regard to operative planning and this should be exploited. One absolute rule is that *no one* should incise any abscess related to a carotid endarterectomy wound before referral to an experienced vascular surgeon. A bacteriological swab should be taken as soon as possible, as this might provide valuable information from an immediate Gram stain as to the likely underlying organism. My next choice of investigation would be a duplex scan which will, on occasion, demonstrate a small false aneurysm (Fig. 30.1; see plate section). This presence of a false aneurysm related to the carotid patch should not be ignored as it will inevitably rupture and it will warn the surgeon of the extent of the underlying inflammatory reaction. As a general rule, I do not require any further investigations and would plan for urgent surgery. The patient should be warned about the increased risks of such a procedure, particularly with regard to stroke, death and cranial nerve injury. In practice, there should be as little delay as possible in taking the patient to theatre but, unless there was any evidence of incipient haemorrhage, I would probably add the patient to one of the elective vascular lists the next day. The benefit of having vascular anaesthetists and trained nursing staff experienced in dealing with complex vascular cases is obvious.

On a practical note, I would counsel that this is definitely not an operation for the occasional carotid surgeon and, wherever possibly, the patient should immediately be transferred to a regional centre.

The second form of presentation is acute profuse haemorrhage which may have been preceded by a small herald bleed. In this situation, there is usually little time to transfer patients elsewhere and the local vascular surgeon will have no alternative but to deal with it. In practice, firm pressure should be applied to the wound to staunch any bleeding, but care must be taken to avoid complete occlusion of the artery.

Operative procedure

This can be a difficult procedure and usually requires complete removal of the patch and insertion of a vein patch or interposition vein graft. Wherever possible, this should be harvested from the long saphenous vein in the groin. Prophylactic antibiotics (usually a cephalosporin and metronidazole) should be administered with induction of anaesthesia with the intention of modifying this regimen once definitive cultures are available postoperatively. If there is any question of the underlying infection being methicillin-resistant *Staphylococcus aureus*, intravenous vancomycin should be given.

It would be my preference to have transcranial Doppler (TCD) monitoring available. This enables every phase of what is otherwise a stressful procedure to be monitored and it will guide the surgeon on the immediacy and urgency of shunt insertion if the carotid artery has to be clamped before the bifurcation is exposed. As a general rule,

provided the middle cerebral artery blood flow velocity is greater than 15–20cm/s, haemodynamic failure is unlikely.

The best way to approach an infected carotid patch is to incise the neck well below the previous incision and access the proximal common carotid artery to gain control before doing anything else (Fig. 30.2). This vessel should be controlled with a sling and the incision lengthened distally, thereby opening up the old wound. As likely as not, a sudden rush of blood will occur as the friable infected tissues disrupt and the patch comes away from the artery. At this point, the common carotid artery should be clamped and a Pruitt–Inahara shunt inserted through the dehiscence in the patch (Fig. 30.3). If the patch is not immediately visible in the depths of the wound, the TCD will alert the surgeon as to the urgency of dissection to expose it.

Once the shunt has been inserted the patch can be removed by grasping it with a pair of forceps at the free edge and continuing with dissection of the carotid artery in a distal direction. This usually has to be done with a scalpel because of severe fibrosis around the area. Sufficient dissection is done to remove the patch only and allow its replacement with a piece of saphenous vein. Too much dissection should be discouraged, as this will inevitably lead to an increased risk of cranial nerve injury.

If this approach shows that the edges of the artery are not suitable for suture then it may be necessary to insert a reversed vein graft. In practice, this can be difficult and is not to be recommended as the first-line approach. Minimal dissection is what is necessary. The wound should be thoroughly irrigated

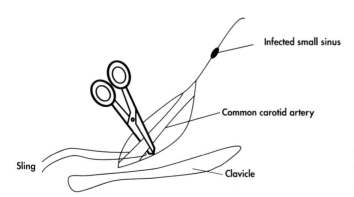

Infected small sinus

Common carotid artery

Sling

Clavicle

Fig. 30.2
The common carotid artery should be clamped well below the original patch.

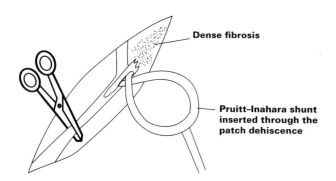

Dense fibrosis

Pruitt–Inahara shunt inserted through the patch dehiscence

Fig. 30.3
The shunt should be inserted into the dehisced area of the patch. Bleeding from the orifice of the external carotid artery can be controlled using a balloon occlusion catheter and a three-way tap.

and a vein patch inserted after debridement of the artery and adjacent tissues. It is also useful to wrap the reconstructed artery with a gentamicin-impregnated sponge, which delivers high local doses of the antibiotic and little risk of systemic toxicity. The wound should then be closed over a suction drain and the patient given antibiotics for at least 6 weeks thereafter.

What If the Reconstruction Appears to be Impossible?

If the above strategy proves impossible and the situation becomes desperate because of complete breakdown of the artery, it may then be possible to take other options. The key is to have the shunt in place to buy time and minimize the risk of ischaemia and the trauma that can be associated with injudicious haste. If there was truly little prospect of achieving a safe reconstruction, I would next clamp the shunt and assess the overall change in middle cerebral artery blood flow. If the middle cerebral artery blood flow velocities exceed 20cm/s, the prospects of inducing a haemodynamic stroke are lessened. The shunt can then be removed and the artery oversewn. If this is done, I recommend that the patient should be systemically heparinized and formally anticoagulated to reduce the risks of thrombus propagation or embolism from the distal internal carotid artery into the circle of Willis. It would be my practice to maintain the patient on warfarin for 6 months (possibly even long-term), although there is little evidence-based literature to support this.

A second option is to expose the carotid artery higher up, exposing the facial nerve with or without mandibular subluxation to gain access to a segment of uninfected carotid artery. In practice, this is a daunting prospect for the inexperienced surgeon and it may be worth seeing if a vascular surgeon from the regional unit is available to help. Provided the shunt is in place, the patient is at greater risk if the surgeon proceeds with dissection in unfamiliar territory. If this is done, it might be possible to place a vein patch even higher, although the glossopharyngeal and facial nerves are at severe risk of damage. In practice, however, it is not usually possible to perform a mandibular subluxation once the operation has started. This should have been planned for preoperatively wherever possible.

CONCLUSIONS

Prosthetic patch infection is rare but associated with a high risk of death and stroke. A vascular surgeon should always be involved in the management of any patient suspected of having an infected prosthetic patch. The absolute rule is never to incise a carotid wound abscess without having made arrangements for what is likely to be a complex reconstruction. Wherever possible, patients with infected prosthetic patches should be transferred to a regional vascular centre.

In order to avoid catastrophic haemorrhage, never expose the carotid vessels through the original wound. The proximal common carotid artery should always be exposed first. Access to TCD monitoring is invaluable, particularly if there is any question of having to ligate the carotid artery. The optimal treatment is to replace the prosthetic patch with autologous vein. Carotid bypass should be viewed as a secondary but important option. If a vein bypass is inserted, it will require long-term surveillance.

REFERENCES

1 Eikelboom BC, Ackerstaff RGA, Hoenveldt H *et al.* Benefits of carotid patching and randomised study. *Journal of Vascular Surgery* 1988; **7**: 240–247.

2 Ranaboldo CT, Barros D'Sa ABB, Bell PRF *et al.* Randomised controlled trial of patch angioplasty for carotid endarterectomy. *British Journal of Surgery* 1993; **80**: 1528–1530.

3 Counsell CE, Salinas R, Naylor R *et al.* A systematic review of the randomised trials of carotid patch angioplasty in carotid endarterectomy. *European Journal of Vascular and Endovascular Surgery* 1997; **13**: 345–355.

4 Murie JA, John TG, Morris PJ. Carotid endarterectomy in Great Britain and Ireland. Practice between 1984 and 1992. *British Journal of Surgery* 1994; **81**: 827–831.

5 Abu Rahma A, Khan J, Robinson P *et al.* Prospective randomised trial of carotid endarterectomy with primary closure and patch angioplasty with saphenous vein jugular vein and polytetrafluoroethylene. Perioperative [30 days] results. *Journal of Vascular Surgery* 1996; **24**: 998–1007.

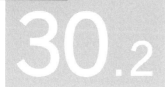

30.2

How should I manage a patient with an infected prosthetic patch?

Bruce A Perler (USA)

Since its introduction in the 1950s, CEA has rapidly become the most frequently performed peripheral vascular operation in the US, with more than 100 000 procedures now carried out annually. The demonstrated safety and efficacy of the operation in multicenter randomized prospective clinical trials, and the dramatic expansion of the older segment of our population in whom cerebrovascular disease predominates, suggest the potential for continued substantial growth in the performance of this operation in the years ahead.

It is axiomatic that the superiority of CEA when compared to the medical management of patients with significant carotid bifurcation disease is intimately dependent upon a low incidence of perioperative complications as well as the long-term durability of the procedure. This last concern has been the focus of intense and increasing attention over the last two decades. While recurrent symptomatic disease has been noted infrequently, the incidence of asymptomatic recurrent carotid stenoses has been reported in from 9% to 19% of patients. Although not universally accepted, in the view of this writer the preponderance of evidence today indicates that the routine, or selective, repair of the carotid arteriotomy as a patch angioplasty has significantly reduced the incidence of recurrent stenoses.[6–10] The controversy over primary versus patch arteriotomy closure is covered in detail in Chapter 22. The current chapter outlines a logical algorithm for dealing with the serious and potentially devastating complication of prosthetic patch infection.

INCIDENCE

Infection is an extremely uncommon complication of carotid surgery. In a review of his personal series of 1140 CEAs performed upon 903 patients, for example, Thompson reported 1 (0.09%) wound infection.[11] The true incidence of carotid prosthetic patch infection is unknown, but must be exceedingly low. Several recent series of patients undergoing Dacron patch angioplasty have failed to identify a single case of patch infection.[7,8,10,12] In a review of the literature, 57 patients were identified with carotid pseudoaneurysms, and in 40 cases they were associated with patch grafting. However, only 4 (10%) were proven to be secondary to infection.[13] Nevertheless, in view of the anticipated increased performance of CEA in general, and the greater acceptance of carotid patch angioplasty in particular, it can be assumed that this complication of CEA will be encountered in the occasional patient in the future, and therefore the busy carotid surgeon should be prepared for its management.

PREVENTION

The frequency with which carotid patch infection has been encountered is so low that the fundamental principles of management must be surmised from our unfortunately larger experience with prosthetic graft infection in other anatomic sites. Since it is axiomatic that in most cases prevention of complications is far easier on the patient and the surgeon than their treatment, I feel compelled to express some personal prejudices with respect to the prevention of carotid prosthetic patch infection. Although infection of synthetic material implanted within the vascular system may not become apparent from months to years post-operatively, there is convincing evidence that most episodes of bacterial seeding of prosthetic material occur at the original operation. While the risk of bacterial

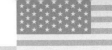

inoculation of a prosthetic patch placed through a clean, extremely well vascularized neck incision is theoretically far less than that of a prosthetic graft placed in the groin, for example, the principles of infection prophylaxis are the same.

Two specific issues merit comment. First, there is substantial evidence that perioperative antibiotics reduce the incidence of wound and more serious graft infection in the vascular surgical patient population. Although the benefit of perioperative antibiotics has not been demonstrated specifically in the setting of CEA, and although this is a typically brief and clean procedure, I nevertheless favor the administration of a broad-spectrum antibiotic perioperatively. Since *Staphylococcus* has been the most common species identified in carotid patch infections, a cephalosporin is most appropriate.[14]

This dogma has not been universally accepted, however.[15,16] It has been argued that if primary arterial suture line repair is anticipated, thus obviating the use of prosthetic material, antibiotics are superfluous.[14] However, since the decision to employ a patch may not be made until the artery has been explored, or the endarterectomy completed, and since the value of prophylactic antibiotics is dependent upon their circulation prior to skin incision, it is logical to administer prophylactic antibiotics in all cases. While reflecting purely anecdotal experience, it is nevertheless interesting to note that, in two recently published cases of carotid prosthetic patch infection[16] and an infected carotid wound hematoma,[15] respectively, prophylactic antibiotics had not been administered. In a recent review of 8 patients who presented with infected carotid pseudoaneurysms, prophylactic antibiotics had been administered in no cases.[17] I also routinely employ topical irrigation of the wound with an antibiotic solution prior to wound closure, both for its antibiotic as well as its mechanical role in removing devitalized tissue from the operative site. Furthermore, in view of the role of transient bacteremia in seeding prosthetic vascular materials, I favor continuing antibiotic administration postoperatively until invasive vascular lines and/or urinary drainage catheters, if used, are removed.

A second point upon which there is a lack of a consensus is the use of a drain postoperatively.

There is no question that the development of a hematoma is an important factor predisposing to postoperative wound infection. Since I begin my patients on aspirin preoperatively, administer heparin intraoperatively, and do not reverse it at the completion of the procedure, and infuse low-molecular-weight dextran for the first postoperative day, I routinely drain my carotid incisions. Although others have challenged this policy,[15] I believe its benefit in minimizing hematoma development far outweighs any potential risks.

DIAGNOSIS

Patients with prosthetic patch infection may present with tenderness, swelling, and erythema of the neck. However, it must be emphasized that not only is infection following CEA uncommonly encountered, but many patients with this presentation, particularly in the acute or subacute setting, may have only a superficial wound infection without deep space or patch involvement. In the latter scenario, administration of broad-spectrum antibiotics and drainage of any localized superficial purulent collections should result in prompt clinical improvement.

If the patient with a prosthetic carotid artery patch fails to respond, as manifested by persistent fever and/or leukocytosis, increasing tenderness and swelling, or advancing erythema, one must have a high index of suspicion for involvement of the patch. A carotid duplex ultrasound may be informative. The presence of a pseudoaneurysm in this clinical setting is presumptive evidence of prosthetic patch infection, although as noted above only a minority of carotid pseudoaneurysms have been demonstrated to have an infectious etiology.[13] However, since the surgical management of a non-infected carotid prosthetic patch-related pseudoaneurysm is similar to that of an infected pseudoaneurysm, and since the diagnosis of infection often cannot be made until the involved graft and associated tissue have been resected, one must approach all carotid pseudoaneurysms as if they are infected. Other ultrasound findings suggestive of patch infection include lack of good tissue incorporation, particularly in the chronic or subacute presentation, as well as fluid and/or gas in proximity to the patch. Suture line bleeding is also presumptive evidence of patch infection.

In the absence of bleeding and if the patient is clinically stable, once the working diagnosis of a patch infection has been made one should proceed to urgent arteriography. Angiographic evaluation is important to confirm the presence of a pseudoaneurysm and also to plan the surgical strategy. For example, an unusually high carotid bifurcation or a very distal extent of the pathologic process might make achieving adequate distal arterial control tenuous, so one should be prepared to perform mandibular subluxation or other technical maneuvers at the time of exploration.[18] In addition, the extent and severity of ipsilateral and contralateral cerebrovascular occlusive disease, and the potential collateral circulation, is relevant information in the patient who at operation might require carotid ligation. Obviously, in the patient who presents with hemorrhage, prompt exploration will most likely preclude preoperative angiographic evaluation, although the information obtained from a rapidly performed duplex scan may be of value.

SURGICAL MANAGEMENT

The principles of management of vascular graft infection in general are clearly applicable to the patient who presents with a prosthetic patch infection, namely, complete excision of the infected foreign body, thorough soft-tissue debridement, vascular reconstruction with autogenous material, and the administration of organism-specific antibiotics. In the specific setting of carotid patch infection, one wants to plan the operation so as to minimize the potential period of cerebral ischemia. In many respects exploration of the neck in the patient with a suspected carotid patch infection is similar to that undertaken in the patient undergoing operation for recurrent carotid stenosis. Specifically, one should attempt to obtain proximal and distal exposure through clean and relatively uninvolved tissue planes. While the scarring and tissue incorporation of the previously operated carotid artery may be less severe in the patient with patch infection than encountered in the typical patient undergoing operation for restenosis, the tissues will be extremely friable, so adequate proximal and distal

arterial control prior to exploring the site of infection is absolutely mandatory. This is an especially crucial consideration in the patient with a pseudoaneurysm, in whom acute suture line disruption leading to frank hemorrhage or distal thromboembolism, may occur as a consequence of arterial manipulation.

Therefore, it is recommended that the skin incision extend well above and below the original incision so that the common carotid artery can be exposed and encircled with a vascular tape just above the clavicle and the internal carotid exposed distally at the apex of the neck under the digastric muscle. I would then administer systemic heparin, and proceed to clamp the internal and common carotid arteries in that order, before attempting to explore the infected site. Once the patient has been protected from distal cerebral embolization in this fashion, the area of infection can be directly unroofed. If there is a pseudoaneurysm, one can directly enter it to identify the disrupted patch at the base. The entire patch and its complete suture line should then be rapidly excised, and the interior of the artery carefully inspected. Unless the artery appears friable and prone to disruption, I would place an indwelling shunt for cerebral protection. One should not underestimate the potential technical difficulty in achieving a satisfactory arterial repair in the infected, inflamed wound, and the length of time that might be required. An indwelling shunt makes the rapidity of repair a less important concern. One may then expose the external carotid artery for clamping, if it is patent and back-bleeding.

It is axiomatic that aggressive arterial debridement be carried our before attempting reconstruction. In general this will include a several-millimeter rim of arterial wall around the entire circumference of the original suture line. The adequacy of this debridement should not be compromised in order to salvage sufficient artery wall to reconstruct the vessel with a new patch, since it is not unreasonable – and in some cases it is probably preferable – to excise the entire area and place an interposition vein bypass. The excised native artery wall, explanted patch, and, if present, pseudoaneurysm wall and clot should be sent for immediate Gram stain and bacterial culture.

Once the infected prosthesis and adjacent tissue have been excised, the surgical choices are either arterial ligation or reconstruction. The former option is mentioned only to condemn this strategy since it may be associated with a 50% chance of significant neurologic morbidity.[13,19,20] Rather, cerebral perfusion should be preserved either via a repeat patch angioplasty or by performing a common carotid to internal carotid artery bypass. Although there is some evidence that PTFE is more resistant to infection than Dacron, in my opinion no synthetic material should be used in this setting. Rather, autogenous vein, and preferably greater saphenous vein, should be employed either as a patch or as an interposition graft. The vein should be harvested from the groin since the development of aneurysmal dilatation and/or patch rupture has almost universally been associated with the use of vein harvested from the ankle region.[21,22]

The decision to perform a repeat patch angioplasty as opposed to placing an interposition graft should be predicated upon the condition of the artery at the site of infection, the degree of surgical debridement of the vessel required, the extent of the surrounding contamination as assessed grossly at exploration, and the results of the intraoperative Gram stain. If the vessel appears diffusely friable, or if a major portion of the wall must be excised, resection of the involved artery in its entirety and placement of a vein bypass is the preferred option. One potential advantage of performing an interposition graft is that it should allow the construction of the proximal and distal anastomoses in relatively cleaner tissue planes remote from the primary septic focus. A straight shunt can be placed through the vein graft prior to constructing the anastomoses, both to maintain cerebral perfusion as well as to stent the anastomoses during their construction. The external carotid artery can be sacrificed.

A significant issue which I would factor into the decision to place a formal bypass graft is the responsible bacterial species. Although definitive culture results will not be available until one or more days postoperatively, the presence of Gram-negative organisms on Gram stain should militate toward placing an interposition bypass graft with proximal and distal anastomoses remote from the original patch site. This position is based upon the documented increased virulence and resistance of some Gram-negative species, such as *Pseudomonas aeruginosa*, and their potential to digest autogenous venous tissue through the elaboration of exogenous proteases.[23,24] The presence of an abscess is another relative indication for bypass.

Irrespective of the method of arterial reconstruction elected, monofilament suture, such as polypropylene, should be employed. Every effort should be made to identify the relevant cranial nerve anatomy in the scarred and inflamed wound so that wide soft-tissue debridement can be safely carried out. The reconstructed vessels should be covered, either by primary wound closure or with a rotational muscle flap (see below), depending upon the operative findings. A soft, closed suction drain should be left in proximity to the repair site. If the infected patch has been completely resected, post-operative antibiotic irrigation through the drain is probably not necessary, although this strategy has been advocated by some.[14] Finally, the patient should receive a protracted period of organism-specific antibiotics postoperatively. The optimal duration of antibiotic therapy is clearly not known. Recommendations have varied from 3 to 6 weeks of intravenous therapy, with consideration of lifelong antibiotic suppression if the original patch was salvaged.[14,16] In my opinion, if the prosthetic material and involved vessel were completely excised and a satisfactory autogenous reconstruction was performed, based upon our experience with peripheral prosthetic bypass graft infection, a 3-week period of intravenous antibiotic therapy, with another 3 weeks of oral drug administration, should be sufficient, although I am unaware of any conclusive scientific data to support this.

Rotational Muscle Flaps

One of the more innovative developments in the management of localized vascular infection has been graft coverage with a rotational muscle flap, whereby a muscle bundle is mobilized from a clean bed, and based on a pedicled arterial blood supply independent of the site of infection.[25–27] In addition to its obvious mechanical benefit of providing soft-tissue coverage, there is a growing body of experimental evidence suggesting that well-vascularized muscle tissue, perhaps by delivering a high level of antibiotics and immunocompetent cells to or by raising the oxygen tension in the infected wound, may actually promote eradication of the infectious process.[28–30]

Although muscle flaps have frequently been used for carotid artery coverage after radical head and neck cancer surgery,[31] and although there is growing experience supporting the efficacy of rotational muscle flaps to treat prosthetic graft infection in diverse anatomic sites in the body,[25–27] there has been limited experience with this approach in treating vascular infection in the neck. In a series of 18 patients who underwent muscle flap coverage of 21 infected prosthetic grafts at the Johns Hopkins Hospital, there was 1 case of an infected subclavian–carotid–carotid Dacron graft salvaged with rotational muscle flap coverage.[26] In another report, 2 patients with infected PTFE carotid patches underwent coverage with pectoralis major muscle flaps with salvage of the original patch.[15]

The role, if any, of rotational muscle flap coverage in the management of the patient with a carotid prosthetic patch infection will need to be determined by further clinical study. There are two potential situations in which this approach might be of benefit. As noted in the report of Zacharoulis et al., coverage of the infected carotid patch with a rotational muscle flap might allow salvage of the original patch and thus obviate the necessity for arterial reconstruction.[16] This approach should not be considered in the patient who presents with a pseudoaneurysm, bleeding, or other evidence of patch suture line disruption. It may be reasonable to consider rotational muscle flap coverage in the patient who presents with patch infection with a relatively low virulence organism, such as Staphylococcus epidermidis without compromise of suture line integrity, especially in the presence of confounding technical limitations such as high carotid bifurcation/patch making reconstruction problematic. In most cases I would still favor

complete patch excision and autogenous repair. This view is predicated upon the concern that residual/recurrent infection of a carotid patch might result in acute suture line hemorrhage, which could cause devastating neurologic – as well as hemodynamic and respiratory – sequelae.

On the other hand, based upon our experience utilizing muscle flaps to treat peripheral prosthetic graft infection, it is not unreasonable today to excise the infected patch, perform an autogenous reconstruction, and then use a well-vascularized muscle flap for coverage to maximize the chance for eradication of the infection and complete healing. I would seriously entertain this combined treatment in the patient with a virulent infection, such as in the presence of multiple organisms, especially Gram-negative species, or in the patient who presents with a significant neck abscess. The pectoralis major and sternocleidomastoid are the most appropriate muscles for patch coverage in the neck.[32] If the muscle is rotated with its overlying skin as a myocutaneous flap, immediate closure is achieved, whereas if the muscle only is mobilized, it provides an excellent bed for application of a split-thickness skin graft to complete closure.

CONCLUSION

No two patients presenting with infection involving prosthetic material in the vascular system are exactly alike. Our ability to eradicate infection completely in any individual patient will depend upon a number of factors, such as the prosthetic material involved, the nature and concentration of the responsible organisms, and the host's immunologic reserve. The current chapter has outlined an approach to the potentially serious complication of carotid prosthetic patch infection, founded upon sound surgical principles, and which can be expected to be successful in the majority of cases. On the other hand, it is well known that graft infection may linger indolently for protracted periods of time, only to reappear months or years later. Therefore, any patient undergoing surgical treatment of this rare complication of CEA will require lifelong clinical and duplex ultrasound follow-up.

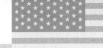

REFERENCES

6 Lord RSA, Raj TE, Stary DL, Nash PH, Graham AR, Goh KH. Comparison of saphenous vein patch, polytetrafluoroethylene patch, and direct arteriotomy closure after carotid endarterectomy. Part I. Perioperative results. *Journal of Vascular Surgery* 1989; **9**: 521–529.

7 Ouriel K, Green RM. Clinical and technical factors influencing recurrent carotid stenosis and occlusion after endarterectomy. *Journal of Vascular Surgery* 1987; **5**: 702–706.

8 Schultz GA, Zammit M, Sauvage ZR et al. Carotid artery Dacron patch angioplasty: a 10-year experience. *Journal of Vascular Surgery* 1987; **5**: 475–478.

9 Myers SI, Valentine RJ, Chervu A, Rogens RL, Bowers EL, Clagett GP. Saphenous vein versus primary closure for carotid endarterectomy: long-term assessment of a randomized prospective study. *Journal of Vascular Surgery* 1994; **19**: 15–22.

10 Perler BA, Ursin F, Shanks U, Williams GM. Carotid Dacron patch angioplasty: immediate and long-term results of a prospective series. *Cardiovascular Surgery* 1995; **3**: 631–636.

11 Thompson JE. Complications of carotid endarterectomy and their prevention. *World Journal of Surgery* 1979; **3**: 155–165.

12 Rosenthal D, Archie JP JR, Garcia-Rinaldi R et al. Carotid patch angioplasty: immediate and long-term results. *Journal of Vascular Surgery* 1990; **12**: 326–333.

13 Branch CL, Davis CH Jr. False aneurysm complicating carotid endarterectomy. *Neurosurgery* 1986; **19**: 421–425.

14 Graver LM, Mulcare RJ. Pseudoaneurysm after carotid endarterectomy. *Journal of Cardiovascular Surgery* 1986; **27**: 294–297.

15 Mora W, Hunter G, Malone J. Wound infection following carotid endarterectomy. *Journal of Cardiovascular Surgery* 1981; **22**: 47–49.

16 Zacharoulis DC, Gupta SK, Seymour P, Landa RA. Use of muscle flap to cover infections of the carotid artery after carotid endarterectomy. *Journal of Vascular Surgery* 1997; **25**: 769–773.

17 Raptis S, Baker SR. Infected false aneurysms of the carotid arteries after carotid endarterectomy. *European Journal of Vascular Surgery* 1996; **11**: 148–152.

18 Fisher DF, Clagett GP, Parker JL et al. Mandibular subluxation for high carotid exposure. *Journal of Vascular Surgery* 1984; **1**: 727–733.

19 DeBakey ME, Crawford ES, Morris GC, Cooley DA. Patch graft angioplasty in vascular surgery. *Journal of Cardiovascular Surgery* 1962; **3**: 106–139.

20 Lougheed WM, Elgie RG, Barnett HJM. The results of surgical management of extracranial internal carotid artery occlusion and stenosis. *Canadian Medical Association Journal* 1966; **95**: 1279–1293.

21 Eikelboom BC, Ackerstaff RGA, Hoeneveld H et al. Benefits of carotid patching: a randomized study. *Journal of Vascular Surgery* 1988; **7**: 240–247.

22 O'Hara PJ, Hertzer LP, Krajewski LP, Beven EG. Saphenous vein patch rupture after carotid endarterectomy. *Journal of Vascular Surgery* 1992; **15**: 504–509.

23 Geary KJ, Tomkiewicz ZM, Harrison HN et al. Differential effects of Gram-negative and Gram-positive infections on autogenous and prosthetic grafts. *Journal of Vascular Surgery* 1990; **11**: 339–347.

24 Bandyk DF, Esses GE. Prosthetic graft infection. *Surgical Clinics of North America* 1994; **74**: 571–590.

25 Perler BA, Vander Kolk CA, Manson PM, Williams GM. Rotational muscle flaps to treat prosthetic graft infection: long-term follow-up. *Journal of Vascular Surgery* 1993; **18**: 358–365.

26 Perler BA, Vander Kolk CA, Dufresne CA, Williams GM. Can infected prosthetic grafts be salvaged with rotational muscle flaps? *Surgery* 1991; **110**: 30–34.

27 Mixter RC, Turnipseed WD, Smith DJ Jr et al. Rotational muscle flaps: a new technique for covering infected vascular grafts. *Journal of Vascular Surgery* 1989; **9**: 472–478.

28 Mehran RJ, Graham AM, Ricci MA, Symes JF. Evaluation of muscle flaps in the treatment of infected aortic grafts. *Journal of Vascular Surgery* 1992; **15**: 487–494.

29 Dacey LJ, Miett TO, Huntsman WT et al. Efficacy of muscle flaps in the treatment of prosthetic vascular graft infections. *Journal of Surgical Research* 1988; **44**: 566–572.

30 Chang N, Mathes SJ. Comparison of the effect of bacterial inoculation in musculocutaneous and random-pattern flaps. *Plastic and Reconstructive Surgery* 1982; **70**: 1–9.

31 Leemans CR, Balm AJM, Gregor RT, Hilgers FJM. Management of carotid artery exposure with pectoralis major myofascial flap transfer and split-thickness skin coverage. *Journal of Laryngology and Otology* 1995; **109**: 1176–1180.

32 Mathes SSJ, McGrow JE, Vasconez LO. Muscle transposition flaps for coverage of lower extremity defects. Anatomic considerations. *Surgical Clinics of North America* 1954; **54**: 1337–1354.

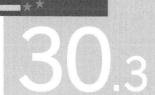

30.3 Editorial Comment

Because of the fortunate rarity of prosthetic carotid patch infection, only anecdotal case reports guide surgeons in its management. The most important management factor is prevention. This requires obsessional attention to aseptic technique, routine use of prophylactic antibiotics, careful hemostasis, and early recognition and management of wound complications. Prompt and uneventful wound healing with minimal neck edema and inflammation should be expected in every CEA and any deviation should prompt concern and increased vigilance. Early postoperative wound complications, such as those relating to drainage hematoma, and persistent edema, should be evaluated urgently with duplex ultrasound prior to any local wound exploration. Drainage of any carotid wound abscess or hematoma should not be undertaken without the input of a vascular surgeon.

Wherever possible, the surgeon should have some idea as to how high the dissection is likely to extend. Much of this information will come from duplex ultrasound, although it may be helpful to perform angiography. In practice, however, the urgency of clinical presentation will determine whether the luxury of preoperative investigation is possible. In some situations, it will be useful to have made arrangements for subluxing the mandible to facilitate distal access. This is not something that is readily possible once the operation is underway. Both authors have highlighted how important it is to ensure proximal control of the common carotid artery (just above the clavicle), and that direct dissection through the infected wound is dangerous. Although it would be preferable also to secure distal internal carotid artery control through uninfected tissues, in practice this is rarely possible because of the dense inflammatory reaction in the upper reaches of the neck. The use of inflated balloon catheters with three-way taps is otherwise invaluable in controlling hemorrhage from the external and internal carotid arteries whilst dissection proceeds.

The principles underlying the management of carotid patch infection are no different from those involving infections of prosthetic material elsewhere. All infected tissues should be debrided and the arterial edges trimmed back. Swabs and tissue should be taken for bacteriologic studies to guide appropriate antibiotic therapy postoperatively. Both authors emphasize the importance of using autogenous tissue for repairing the artery. The choice

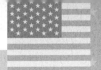

between using a patch or bypass graft will invariably reflect personal experience. However, bypass grafts are prone to developing stenoses and should be surveyed by duplex postoperatively. If there is any question concerning the viability of overlying tissues, it may be necessary to consider fashioning a rotational flap, although in practice this is not usually necessary. If, having considered all available options, it then becomes impossible to perform a reconstruction, the surgeon may have to consider carotid ligation. This is a difficult decision to make at the best of times, but may be facilitated by having access to TCD. Any patient with a proven patch infection requires long-term clinical and duplex surveillance, as recrudescence of infection can occur some years later.

Index

Abbreviations used: CCA, common carotid artery; ICA, internal carotid artery; MCA, middle carotid artery.

A

Abscess in prosthetic patch infection, 384–385
ACAS, *see* Asymptomatic Carotid Atherosclerosis Study
Accessory nerve injury, 207, 210, 215–216
ACST, *see* Asymptomatic Carotid Surgery Trial
Admission to hospital, same-day, 354–355
β-Adrenoceptor-blockers, coronary artery disease patients undergoing carotid endarterectomy, 176
Age
  cost-effectiveness of endarterectomy and, 76–77, 79
  perioperative (endarterectomy) risk and, 151, 152, 153, 158–159, 160, 163
  see also Longevity, anticipated
American College of Cardiology on perioperative cardiovascular risk predictors, 166
American Heart Association
  on perioperative cardiovascular risk predictors, 166
  on staged vs synchronous procedure in combined carotid/coronary disease, 48, 49, 51
Anaesthesia, *see* General anaesthesia; Locoregional anaesthesia
Aneurysmal disease, intracranial, imaging determining presence, 87
Angina, referral to cardiologist, 167–168
Angiography, *see* Computed tomographic angiography; Contrast angiography; Magnetic resonance angiography
Angioplasty (carotid)
  balloon/percutaneous transluminal, 315–330

advantages (potential), 315
current practice/technical aspects, 324–325
evidence for/historical aspects, 317–318, 322–324
future prospects, 318, 320, 325–327
hazards (potential), 315–316
of restenosed vessel, 373
patch, *see* Patch angioplasty
Angioplasty (coronary), balloon/percutaneous transluminal, endarterectomy and timing of, 164–165, 167
Angioscopy, completion, 303–304, 313, 336
Anterior and posterior circulation, relation between, 61–63
Antibiotics, prophylactic, with prosthetic patches
  in prevention of infection, 389
  in replacement of infected prosthetic patch, 385, 391
Anticoagulant drugs, 183, 188
  asymptomatic disease, 187
  peri-/intraoperative, 231–232, 234, 239–240, 242
  postoperative, 232, 240, 243
  preoperative, 237, 238
Anticonvulsants, postoperative, 335
Antihypertensives, 183
  perioperative (endarterectomy) risk and use of, 153
  postoperative, 335–336, 351
Antiplatelet therapy, 182–183, 234, 242
  peri-/intraoperative, 231, 234, 239
  postoperative, 242
    early, 232, 346
    long-term, 232–234, 240
    preoperative, 230–231, 237–238
Antiplatelet Trialists' Collaboration, 237
Antithrombin deficiency, 156
Antithrombotics, 230–243
  peri-/intraoperative, 231–232, 239–240
  postoperative

early, 232, 240, 348
  long-term, 232–234, 240
  preoperative, 230–231, 237–238
Anxiety/restlessness with local anaesthesia, 194, 196–197
Aortic atheroma, emboli from, coronary bypass patients, 51
Arrhythmias, referral to cardiologist, 168
Arterial haemorrhage, uncontrolled, 291
Arteriography, contrast, *see* Contrast angiography
Aspirin, 182–183, 187, 242
  in Casanova trial, 20
  dipyridamole and, *see* Dipyridamole
  postoperative
    early, 232
    long-term, 232–234, 240
    preoperative, 237–238
  in TIA patients, 183
  in Veterans' Administration asymptomatic disease trial, 21
Assessment
  intraoperative, *see* Monitoring
  preoperative, 25
    neurological, 139–148, 180
Asymptomatic Carotid Atherosclerosis Study (ACAS), 16–17, 21
  cost-effectiveness of endarterectomy, 70, 71, 75–76
  patch closure reducing restenosis rate, 281
Asymptomatic Carotid Surgery Trial (ACST)
  Europe/UK, 17, 21
  Veterans' Administration, 16, 20–21
Asymptomatic disease
  abandoning endarterectomy with distal extension in, 287
  brain scans, 130, 133, 137, 187
  cost-effectiveness of endarterectomy, 69–70
  defining, 15
  medical management, 187–188
  neurological assessment not required, 142
  randomized trials, 15–24

Asymptomatic restenosis, 368
Atheroma
    aortic, emboli from, coronary bypass
        patients, 51
    carotid, posterior tongue of, see
        Tongue of carotid plaque/atheroma
Atheromatous disease, diffuse,
    295–296
Atrial fibrillation, anticoagulants, 183
Auricular nerve, greater, injury, 216
Awake testing, 299–300
    shunts and, 205

B
B-mode ultrasound and pulsed Doppler,
    see Duplex scans
Balloon, protective (in carotid
    angioplasty), 316–317
Balloon angioplasty, see Angioplasty
Balloon test occlusion, 124–125
Baroreceptors, carotid, blood pressure
    and, 172
Basilar artery, symptoms relating to,
    143
    carotid surgery with, 57–65
    see also Vertebrobasilar symptoms
Beta-blockers, coronary artery disease
    patients undergoing carotid
    endarterectomy, 176
Bifurcation, carotid
    cranial nerve anatomy around, 208,
        213
    geometry, 262
    redundancy, 257–259
    transposition, 39
Bifurcation disease
    contrast angiography, 103
        as gold standard for severity
        classification, 90
    MR angiography, 103
Bleeding, see Haemorrhage
Blindness, monocular, neurological
    assessment and, 142
Blood flow, see Flow; Flow surface
Blood pressure
    abnormal, see Hypertension;
        Hypotension

management, 183–184, 188, 190,
    335–336, 351, 355–356
Brain imaging, preoperative, 129–138
    asymptomatic disease, 130, 133,
        137, 187
Bupivacaine (Marcain), 195
Bypass graft
    carotid, 257, 259–260
    coronary artery, as staged vs
        synchronous procedure in
        combined carotid/coronary
        disease, 46–56, 164, 166–167,
        172–173, 320

C
Calcified plaque, ultrasound problems
    with, 85, 86, 98
Cardiology, see Heart
Cardiovascular mortality, see Mortality
Cardiovascular symptoms,
    postoperative, prevention, 232–234
Carotid artery
    anatomical variants, imaging,
        125–126
    common, see Common carotid artery
    contralateral/non-operated, see
        Contralateral carotid artery
    disease
        combined with coronary disease,
            see Coronary artery disease
        distal/high, see Distal carotid
            disease
        extent, imaging in assessment of,
            86–87
        non-bifurcational, contrast
            angiography, 124
        proximal, see Proximal disease
        recurrent, see Restenosis
        residual, see Residual disease
        see also Occlusion; Stenosis
    external, endarterectomy, 260
    internal, see Internal carotid artery
    middle, see Middle carotid artery
Carotid Artery Stenting versus
    Endarterectomy Trial (CASET),
    318
Carotid Artery Surgery Asymptomatic

Narrowing Operation vs Aspirin
    (Casanova) trial, 20
Carotid bulb, disturbed flow, causes,
    262–263
Carotid Revascularization
    Endarterectomy versus Stent Trial
        (CREST), 318, 325–327
Carotid Surgery for Ischaemic Stroke
    study, 40
Casanova (trial), 20
CASET (trial), 318
CASIS (trial), 40
CAVATAS (trial), 318, 319, 320, 324
Cerebral artery
    anterior, clinical syndromes
        associated with occlusion of, 143
    middle
        clinical syndromes associated with
            occlusion of, 143
        MR angiography, 106
Cerebral embolism, focal, 337–338
Cerebral ischaemia, see Ischaemia and
    entries under Ischaemic
Cerebral monitoring, see Monitoring
Cerebrovascular (intracranial vessel)
    disease
    imaging determining presence, 87,
        106, 112–114, 135
    occlusive, see Occlusion, cerebral
        vessels
Cervical sympathetic plexus injury,
    210
Cholesterol levels, management, 184,
    186
Chronic obstructive pulmonary disease,
    159
Circle of Willis, 62
    colour duplex, 288
    patient presentation and importance
        of, 57–58
Circulation
    collateral, see Collateral circulation
    posterior and anterior, relation
        between, 61–63
Clamping/cross-clamping
    hypoperfusion/unconsciousness with,
        193, 197

in infected prosthetic patch
  replacement, 385
shunts during, see Shunts
vagus nerve damage, 214
Clinical effectiveness and cost-
  effectiveness, 67
Clinical trials, see Trials
Clopidrogel, 183
Closure, see Patch angioplasty closure;
  Primary closure
Coagulopathies, 156–157, 160
Cochrane Group/Collaboration
  regional vs local anaesthesia in
    endarterectomy, 194–195
  shunting, 246
Cognitive dysfunction in early stages of
  dementia, 140
Coiling, 257
Collateral circulation
  functional assessment, 62
  recruitment, imaging determining,
    87, 106
Colour duplex scans, see Duplex scans
Common carotid artery (CCA)
  abandoning endarterectomy of, 288
  bifurcation, see Bifurcation
  in bypass grafts, 260
  exposure, 266
  steps and shelves, 265
Communicating artery, posterior
  clinical syndromes associated with
    occlusion of, 143
  visualisation, 62
Comparative trials vs randomized trials
  in symptomatic disease, 9
Completion angioscopy, 303–304,
  313, 336
Complications (perioperative/surgery-
  related)
  cardiac, see Heart
  of general anaesthesia, patient
    selection and, 202–203
  neurological, see Neurological
    deficit/complications
  of patch angioplasty closure,
    265–266, 273, 275–276,
    384–395

in randomized trials in symptomatic
  disease, 6, 7
Computed tomographic angiography,
  122, 130
  with vertebrobasilar symptoms, 63
Computed tomography, 129–138
  asymptomatic disease, 130, 133,
    137, 187
  cost considerations, 67
  preoperative, 25, 129–138
  spiral, 294
  unusual/unexpected pathology on, 129
  see also Single photon emission
    computed tomography; Xenon CT
Congestive heart failure, referral to
  cardiologist, 167
Consciousness, sudden loss, 145
Contralateral/non-operated carotid
  artery
  disease progression, 362
  surveillance, 364
Contrast (conventional)
  angiography/arteriography, carotid
    (incl. digital subtraction), 118–128
  collateral flow assessed by, 87
  comparisons with other imaging
    methods, 103–106, 111
  cost considerations, 67, 92
  decision-making and, 287, 294
  disadvantages/safety considerations,
    87–88
  indications, 119–120, 123–124
  intraoperative, 308, 310
  operating without, 92–95
  plaque composition, 111–112
  with postoperative neurological
    deficits
    assessment of preoperative
      angiogram, 344
    postoperative angiogram, 343
  stenosis measurements, 9–10, 85,
    90, 101, 118–119
    inter-/intraobserver variability,
      103–104
Contrast (conventional)
  angiography/arteriography, coronary,
    in endarterectomy patients, 173

Convulsions (seizures), postoperative,
  335–336
Coronary angiography, endarterectomy
  patients, 173
Coronary angioplasty, percutaneous
  transluminal, endarterectomy timing,
  164–165, 167
Coronary artery disease
  combined carotid and, 167–168
    staged vs synchronous procedure,
      46–56, 164–165, 167–168,
      172–173, 320
  in endarterectomy patients
    evaluation and management,
      175–177
    incidence, 173–174
Cost
  imaging, 67, 92, 114–115
  reduction
    early discharge and, 67, 352, 356
    endarterectomy, 67–68
Cost-effectiveness, 66–81
  analysis/assessment, 66–67, 73–75
  clinical effectiveness and, 67
  impact of key variables, 76–78
  patch closure, 280–281
  postoperative care and, 350–359
Cranial extent of endarterectomy, 255
Cranial nerve damage (and its
  minimization), 206–218
  with expected high disease, 225, 226
  with unexpected high disease, 220,
    222
Cranial vessel disease, see
  Cerebrovascular disease
Crescendo transient ischaemic attacks,
  as emergency surgery indication, 28,
  30
CREST (trial), 318, 325–327
Cross-clamping, see Clamping

D
Dacron patch, 276, 384
  duplex scanning through, 309
Death, see Mortality
Dementia, cognitive dysfunction in early
  stages of, 140

Dextran (incl. low-molecular-weight dextran)
  intraoperative, 239, 242–243
  postoperative, 232, 340, 346
Diabetes
  management, 184, 190
  perioperative (endarterectomy) risk and, 156, 160
  restenosis risk, 279
Diffuse atheromatous disease, 295–296
Digastric muscle division in high disease, 225–226
Digital subtraction angiography, see Contrast angiography
Dipyridamole and aspirin
  postoperative long-term, 233, 234
  preoperative, 183, 231
Discharge from hospital, see Hospital
Disease, pre-existing, operative risk and, 149–163
Distal carotid disease (high lesions), 219–228
  expected at operation, 219–220, 224–227
  unexpected at operation, 220–223
    abandoning endarterectomy, 287–288, 294–296
    posterior tongue of plaque/atheroma, see Tongue of carotid plaque/atheroma
Distal end-point with endarterectomy, optimal, 255–272
Distal limits of plaque, imaging assessing, 86, 219
Doppler ultrasound (incl. transcranial and supraorbital Doppler), 122
  collateral flow assessed by, 87, 106
  as guide to disease activity, 15–16
  intraoperative (in endarterectomy), 39, 294–295, 304–305, 308, 313, 336
    cross-clamping and shunting and, 245–246, 247, 253–254, 302
    embolization diagnosis, 300, 301, 302
    thrombosis diagnosis, 302, 336

intraoperative (in infected prosthetic patch replacement), 385
postoperative, with neurological deficit, 337, 339, 340
preoperative, 25, 120
  MR angiography complementing, 106
  with vertebrobasilar symptoms, 62
  see also Duplex scans
Drains, postoperative, 389
Drug therapy, thrombosis prevention, see Antithrombotics
Duplex scans (incl. colour duplex), 25, 85–98
  comparisons with other imaging methods, 104–106
  cost, 67, 114–115
  contrast angiography following evaluation with, 122
  decision-making and, 286–287, 288, 293–294
  distal disease determination, 86, 219
  imaging algorithm including use of, 114–115
  indications for preoperative use, 94, 118
  intraoperative, 310, 313
    historical aspects, 309
    technique, 309
  limitations, 119–120
  MR angiography complementing, 106, 120, 123, 123–124
  operating only with, 92–95
  operating without, 87–88·
  postoperative, 350
    with neurological deficit, 337, 339
    in surveillance, 268, 362–364, 367, 369
  stenosis assessed via, 85–86, 91, 119
    accuracy and reliability, 119
  with vertebrobasilar symptoms, 62

E

Echocardiography, indications, 181–182
ECST, see European Carotid Surgery Trial

EEG, 300
  in cross-clamping and shunting, 245, 254
    general anaesthesia, 199, 250–251, 251, 252
    regional anaesthesia, 251
Electroencephalography, see EEG
Electronic devices and magnetic resonance imaging, 124
Emboli/embolism (and embolization), 5, 299
  angioplasty-related risk, 315–317
  from aortic atheroma, coronary bypass patients, 51
  cardiogenic, stroke or TIA due to, 181
  cerebral, focal, 337–338
  diagnosis, 300, 301–302
  middle carotid artery, see Middle carotid artery
  stroke due to, 299, 333, 340
    management, 340
  see also Thromboembolic symptoms; Thromboembolism
Emergency endarterectomy, 25–35
End-point, distal, optimal (with endarterectomy), 255–272
Endarterectomy, 191–330
  abandoning, 286–297
    with locoregional anaesthesia, 197
    optimizing outcome, 296
  anaesthesia, see General anaesthesia; Locoregional anaesthesia
  angioplasty compared with, 318, 324
  in combined coronary/carotid disease, as staged vs synchronous procedure, 46–47, 164–165, 167–168, 172–173, 320
  cost reduction, 67–68
  distal disease, see Distal carotid disease
  emergency, 23–35
  eversion, 39, 260–261
  flow surface optimization, 255–272
  imaging before, see Imaging

indications, pre-1985, 19
intimal flaps/fragments, *see* Intimal
    flaps and fragments
with non-hemispheric or
    vertebrobasilar symptoms, 57–65
plane, optimal, 255–256,
    271–272
postoperative care, *see* Postoperative
    management
preoperative assessment, *see*
    Assessment
procedure, 25–26, 191–330
    Heidelberg, 39–40
    with local anaesthesia, 195–197
prophylactic, before major surgery,
    17–18
quality control, 261, 300–301
reoperation after
    imaging considerations, 126
    for restenosis, *see* Restenosis
of restenosed artery, 373, 377–379
risk with, *see* Risk
selection for, *see* Selection
stenting compared with, 318, 324
technical defects, 264–266
thinned zone, excessively, 259
timing, *see* Timing
trials, *see* Trials
unique aspects, 171–173
urgent, 25–35
Endovascular intervention, 315–330
Epilepsy, focal, interpretation, 140
Erythrocyte sedimentation rate, 180
ESPRIT study, 183
European Carotid Surgery Trial (ECST)
    collaborative group (inc. MRC), 3–4,
    298
    cost-effectiveness analysis, 69
    ICA stenosis measurement, 102
    patient selection, 6
    perioperative complications, 6, 7
    stroke risk, 3–4, 17
    timing of surgery, 230
European Stroke Prevention Study,
    second, 183, 231
Eversion endarterectomy, 39, 260
Eversion plication, 258–259, 267

Evoked potentials, somatosensory,
    intraoperative, 39, 300
Exercise thallium-201 myocardial
    scintigraphy in cerebrovascular
    disease patients, 173
External carotid artery
    endarterectomy of, 260
    management during endarterectomy,
    265

F
Facial nerve injury, marginal
    mandibular branch, 207, 210, 216
Factor V Leiden (activated protein C
    resistance), 156, 156–157
Fibrinogen levels, elevated, 186–187
Fibrosis of artery secondary to
    recanalized old thrombus distal to
    critical stenosis, 295
Fitting (seizures), postoperative,
    335–336
Flaps, rotational muscle, with prosthetic
    patch infection, 391–392
Flow (blood), carotid
    disturbed, causes, 262–263
    low, tightly stenotic lesion of ICA with
        underfilling secondary to,
        294–295
    restoration (in surgery), embolization
        following, 301
    velocity, *see* Velocity
    see also Haemodynamics
Flow surface optimization with
    endarterectomy, 255–272

G
Gaseous embolization, 301
Gender
    angioplasty and stenting efficacy and,
    326–327
    endarterectomy risk, 151, 158
General anaesthesia, 193–205,
    250–251
    advantages, 193
    disadvantages, 193–194
    evidence for benefit of regional
        anaesthesia over, 193–205

shunts, 193–194, 250
    operation without, 250
    selective, 193–194, 199,
        250–251
Glossopharyngeal nerve injury (and its
    avoidance), 207, 210, 215
    expected high disease, 226
    unexpected high disease, 222
Glycaemic control, 184, 190
Graft, vein, *see* Vein graft
Greater auricular nerve, injury, 216

H
Haematological causes of cerebral
    ischaemia, 144
Haematoma, wound, 351
    infection and, 389
    local anaesthesia and, 194
Haemodynamic stroke, 338
Haemodynamics, 262
    in endarterectomy, 171–172
        haemodynamic failure during
            cross-clamping, risk prediction,
            245
        technical defects affecting,
            265–266
    see also Flow
Haemorrhage/bleeding
    intracranial, 335, 339, 348–349
    in prosthetic patch infection, 385
    uncontrolled, 290–291
Haemostasis, intraoperative, 239–240
Heart, 164–179
    carotid surgery-related risk to, 149,
        164–179
        classification of risk, 165–166
        incidence of cardiac morbidity and
            mortality, 174–175
        prediction of risk, 164–165
    cerebral ischaemia relating to
        problems in, 144
    congestive failure, referral to
        cardiologist, 167
    coronary disease, *see* Coronary artery
        disease
    echocardiography, indications,
        181–182

Heart (*cont'd*)
  ICU admission relating to, 356
  preoperative evaluation, 164–179
  surgery, prophylactic endarterectomy before, 17–18
  surgical mortality relating to, *see* Mortality
Heidelberg experience, 38–40
Heparin
  intraoperative, 231–232, 234, 239, 242
  preoperative, 238
  thrombocytopenia induced by, 156, 157, 232
High carotid disease, *see* Distal carotid disease
High-dependency unit, 351
HMG-reductase inhibitors (statins), 184, 186
Home, patient instructions for care at, 359
Homocysteinaemia, 187
Hospital
  length of stay/discharge, 351–352
    cost relating to, 67, 352, 356
    early discharge contraindicated, 356, 358–359
    early discharge indicated, 356
    same-day admission, 354–355
Hyperfibrinogenaemia, 186–187
Hyperlipidaemia, *see* Lipid, elevated
Hyperperfusion syndrome, 335, 339
Hyperplasia, neointimal, 361, 362, 371
Hypertension, 351, 355, 356
  management, 183–184, 188, 190, 351, 355, 356
  perioperative occurrence, 171, 172, 188
  perioperative risk (in endarterectomy) in patients with, 151, 153, 159
Hypoglossal nerve injury (and its minimization), 207, 209, 214–215
  with expected high disease, 225
  with unexpected high disease, 220
Hypoplasia, *see* `String sign'

Hypotension
  in endarterectomy, 171, 172
  management, 188, 351, 355
Hypoxia and hypoperfusion with cross-clamping, 193, 197
Hysteroscope, luminal thrombus detection, 303–304

I

Iatrogenic cranial nerve damage, *see* Cranial nerve damage
Imaging (predominantly preoperative), 25, 85–138
  algorithm, 114–115
  cost considerations, 67, 92, 114–115
  decision-making based on, 286–287, 293–294
  as guide to disease activity, 15–16
  with vertebrobasilar symptoms, 62–63
  see also specific modalities
Infarction
  cerebral
    lacunar, clinical syndromes associated with, 143
    recurrent, after previous stroke, 145
  myocardial, previous, referral to cardiologist, 168
Infection, prosthetic patch, 276, 280, 384–395
  diagnosis/presentation, 384, 385, 389–390
  incidence, 388
  initial management, 384–385
  operative management, 385–386, 390–391
  prevention, 388–389
Inflammatory disorders of vessels, *see* Vasculitis
Injury, cranial nerve, *see* Cranial nerve damage
Innominate artery, surgical decision-making with disease of, 288
Intensive care unit, 350, 351, 355–356

Internal carotid artery (ICA)
  distal disease, *see* Distal carotid disease
  eversion endarterectomy, 36, 260–261
  eversion plication, 258–259, 267
  narrow distal, *see* `String sign'
  proximal
    ligation, *see* Ligation
    redundancy, 257
    tightly stenotic, with underfilling secondary to low flow, 294–295
  pseudo-occlusion, MR angiography, 100
  small, restenosis risk, 361
  stenosis, degree
    NASCET vs ECST in measurement of, 102
    University of Washington criteria in stratification of, 91
  thrombosis, transcranial Doppler in detection of, 336
Interposition vein graft with infected prosthetic patch, 385, 391
Intimal flaps and fragments, 308–309
  repair/removal, 256
  restenosis risk, 361
  unrepaired, 308–309
Intracranial extent of endarterectomy, 255
Intracranial haemorrhage, 335, 339, 348–349
Intracranial vessel disease, *see* Cerebrovascular disease
Investigations, 180–182
  routinely performed, 180
  selectively performed, 180–182
Ischaemia
  cerebral, differential diagnosis, 143, 144
  myocardial, peripheral vascular surgery and risk of, 150–151
Ischaemic attacks, transient, *see* Transient ischaemic attacks
Ischaemic heart angina, referral to cardiologist, 167–168

Ischaemic injury, cerebral, 129
Ischaemic stroke see Stroke

J
Javid shunt, 246, 247
Joint Study of Extracranial Artery
  Occlusion, 37–38

K
Kidney failure, 157–158, 160
Kinking, 257, 271
  patching causing, 265–266

L
Lacunar infarction, clinical syndromes
  associated with, 143
Large vessel (macrovascular) disease
  brain scans, 130
  stroke or TIA in, 181
Laryngeal nerve injury
  recurrent, 207, 208–209, 214
  superior, 207, 209, 214
Leicester monitoring protocol, 304
Life expectancy, see Longevity,
  anticipated
Ligation (proximal ICA), 291
  with infected prosthetic patch, 391
Lipid, elevated (hyperlipidaemia)
  medical management, 184, 186, 190
  restenosis risk, 279–280
Locoregional anaesthesia, 172,
  193–205, 251, 355
  abandoning endarterectomy under,
    197
  advantages, 194
  disadvantages, 194
  evidence for benefit over general
    anaesthesia, 193–205
  shunts, selective/clinical, 197, 203,
    205
  technique, 195–197
Longevity, anticipated (and life
  expectancy)
  cost-effectiveness and, 76
  patient selection for randomized trials
    in symptomatic disease based on,
    12

Loupe magnification, 255
Luminal diameter measurements,
  contrast angiogram, 9–10, 85
Lung disease, 159, 160

M
Macrovascular disease, see Large
  vessel disease
Magnetic resonance angiography,
  99–117, 122–123, 128,
  130
  advantages, 102–103, 123
  anatomical variants on, 125–126
  asymptomatic disease, 130, 187
  in clinical practice, 106
  comparisons with other methods,
    103–106, 111
  costs, 114–115
  decision-making and, 294
  disadvantages, 88, 99–101
  duplex scans combined with, 106,
    120, 123, 123–124
  imaging algorithm including use of,
    114–115
  inter-/intraobserver variability,
    103–104
  intracranial disease assessment,
    106, 112–114
  reoperation (endarterectomy) and,
    126
  stenosis (and its measurement),
    85–86, 99, 101
    intra-/interobserver variability,
      103–104
  technical
    considerations/principles/theory,
      99, 108–109
  with vertebrobasilar symptoms, 63
Magnetic resonance imaging
  disadvantages/problems with, 124
  as guide to disease activity,
    15–16
  preoperative, 32
Mandible, subluxation (MS) or
  disarticulation
  in expected high disease, 219,
    224–225

in infected prosthetic patch
    replacement, 386
  in unexpected high disease,
    physiologic subluxation, 227–228
Mandibular branch of facial nerve,
  marginal, injury, 207, 210, 216
Marcain, 195
Marginal mandibular branch of facial
  nerve, injury, 207, 210, 216
Massachusetts General Hospital,
  urgent/emergency endarterectomy at,
  31–33
Medical conditions affecting operative
  risk, 149–163
Medical management, 140, 180–190
  endarterectomy patients, 188
    with coronary artery disease, 176
  neurological assessment in, 180
  in trials, 139
  optimal, 180–190
Medical Research Council, see MRC
Medicolegal aspects of neurological
  assessment, 140–141
Microvascular disease, see Small vessel
  disease
Middle carotid artery (MCA)
  embolism into, 288, 289
    detection, 302, 336, 339
    management, 339
  flow velocity, see Velocity
  management, 339
  occlusion (incl. mainstem and branch
    occlusion), 337
    detection, 336, 337–338
    management, 338
  thrombus extending into, 288
Migrainous phenomena, interpretation,
  140
Molt mouth prop, 227
Monitoring, intraoperative (incl.
  cerebral/neurological monitoring),
  298–312
  with cross-clamping, methods, 193,
    197, 199, 245–246, 247, 250,
    253–254
  failure to reduce operation-related
    stroke, 298

Monitoring, intraoperative (cont'd)
history, 308–309
role, principles underlying,
299–300
see also specific methods
Monocular blindness, neurological
assessment and, 142
Morbidity
with restenosis, 367–368, 375–376
surgical
cardiac morbidity, 174–175
patient selection for randomized
trials in symptomatic disease
based on, 12
Mortality, surgical
cardiac/cardiovascular mortality,
174–175
prevention, 230, 234
patient selection for randomized trials
in symptomatic disease based on,
12
MOTSA (multiple overlapping then slab
acquisition), 110, 110–111
MRC trials/funded trials
CAVATAS, 318, 319, 320, 324
ECST, see European Carotid Surgery
Trial
Multiple overlapping then slab
acquisition, 110, 110–111
Muscle flaps, rotational, with prosthetic
patch infection, 391–392
Myocardial infarction, previous, referral
to cardiologist, 168
Myocardial ischaemia, peripheral
vascular surgery and risk of,
150–151
Myocardial scintigraphy in
cerebrovascular disease patients,
173
Myoglossus muscle paralysis, 215

N

NACPTAR, angioplasty study,
322–323
NASCET, see North American
Symptomatic Carotid Endarterectomy
Trial

Neck
haematoma, see Haematoma
hostile, 286
Neointimal hyperplasia, 361, 362, 371
Nerve damage, see Cranial nerve
damage
Neuroimaging, see Brain imaging
Neurologic Event Severity Scale,
Massachusetts General Hospital
urgent/emergency endarterectomy
and, 31–33
Neurological deficit/complications,
333–349
anaesthetic technique and, 200
classification/categorization, 342
management, 333–349
Neurological status
monitoring in surgery, see Monitoring
perioperative (endarterectomy) risk
and, 153, 159–161
postoperative, 351
preoperative assessment, 139–148,
180
New England Medical Center, patient
guidance on postoperative care after
endarterectomy, 359
New York University Medical Center,
locoregional and general anaesthesia
compared, 201, 202
North American Percutaneous
Transluminal Angioplasty Register,
angioplasty study, 322–323
North American Symptomatic Carotid
Endarterectomy Trial (NASCET), 4,
38, 298
aspirin, postoperative, 232
ICA stenosis measurement, 102
patient selection, 6
perioperative complications, 6

O

Occlusion (and occlusive disease),
carotid
imaging determining presence,
85–86
and differentiation from high-grade
stenosis, 111

MCA, see Middle carotid artery
test occlusion, 124–125
see also Pseudo-occlusion;
Subocclusion
Occlusion (and occlusive disease),
cerebral vessels
clinical syndromes associated with,
143
imaging determining presence, 87
Ocular symptoms (incl. retinal
ischaemic symptoms/events)
brain scan, 129
neurological assessment, 140
not required, 142
Ophthalmic artery, flow reversal,
transcranial Doppler, 106
Oxfordshire Community Stroke Project,
37

P

Patch angioplasty closure, 263, 264,
265, 267, 271, 273–285
duplex scanning through patch, 309
primary closure compared with,
273–274, 280–282, 285
problems and complications,
265–266, 273, 275–276,
384–395
prosthetic patch, see Prosthetic patch
rationale/indications, 273, 384
repeat, 385–386, 391
restenosed artery, 373, 379
selective patching, 275, 285
vein patch, see Vein patch
Patients
admission/discharge, see Hospital
information on postoperative care
after endarterectomy, 359
in local anaesthesia
anxiety/restlessness, 194,
196–197
setting up, 196
preoperative assessment, 25
selection, see Selection
Percutaneous transluminal coronary
angioplasty, endarterectomy timing,
164–165, 167

Peripheral vascular disease
  referral to cardiologist, 168
  surgery for, perioperative risk,
    150–151
Pharmacotherapy, thrombosis
  prevention, see Antithrombotics
Plaque, carotid
  calcification, ultrasound problems
    with, 85, 86, 98
  characteristics/morphology
    contrast angiography, 111–112
    duplex scanning, 87
    MR angiography, 111–112
  distal limits, imaging assessing,
    86–87, 219
  posterior tongue of, see Tongue of
    carotid plaque/atheroma
Plasma viscosity, 180
Platelet inhibitors, see Antiplatelet
  therapy
Plication, eversion, 258–259, 267
Polytetrafluoroethylene (PTFE) patch,
  276, 384
  duplex scanning through, 309
Positron emission tomography with
  vertebrobasilar symptoms, 63
Posterior circulation, relation between
  anterior and, 61–63
Posterior communicating artery, see
  Communicating artery
Postoperative management, 26,
  331–398
  planning, safety and cost-
    effectiveness in, 350–359
  surveillance in, see Surveillance
Pre-existing medical conditions affecting
  operative risk, 149–163
Pre-medication in local anaesthesia,
  194, 196
Preoperative assessment, see
  Assessment
Primary closure, 263–264, 267, 282
  patch closure compared with,
    273–274, 280–282, 285
Prosthetic patch, 265, 276, 285
  complications, 276, 280
  infection, see Infection

Protection balloon, 316–317
Protein C
  activated, resistance (factor V
    Leiden), 156, 156–157
  deficiency, 156
Protein S deficiency, 156
Proximal disease
  endarterectomy in, 256
    abandoning, 288
  imaging assessing extent, 86
Pruitt/Pruitt—Inahara shunt, 246, 247
  in infected prosthetic patch
    replacement, 385
  in unexpected high disease, 220,
    221, 288
Pseudoaneurysm with infected
  prosthetic patch, 389
Pseudo-occlusion of ICA
  causes, 294
  MR angiography, 100
PTFE patch, see Polytetrafluoroethylene
  patch
Pulmonary disease, 159, 160

Q
Quality-adjusted life years and cost-
  effectiveness, 66, 67, 76, 77, 81
Quality control, 261, 300–301

R
Radioisotope scans, myocardial, in
  cerebrovascular disease patients,
  173
Radiology, see Imaging
Randomized trials
  of angioplasty, 318, 324
  in asymptomatic disease, 15–24
    clinical practice and impact of,
      21–23
  of patching vs primary closure,
    273–274, 280–282, 285
  of shunting, 246
  of stenting, 318, 324
    future, 318, 319, 325–327
  in symptomatic disease, 3–14
    retrospective and comparative trials
      vs, 9

Reconstruction methods
  in endarterectomy, 263–264
  in prosthetic patch infection,
    385–386, 390–391
  not possible, 386
Recovery room stay, 355–356
Recurrent laryngeal nerve injury, 207,
  208–209, 214
Regional anaesthesia, see Locoregional
  anaesthesia
Renal failure, 157–158, 160
Reoperation after endarterectomy, see
  Endarterectomy
Residual disease/stenosis, 264–266
  detection, 304, 310–311
Respiratory disease, 159, 160
Restenosis, 278, 360–362
  definition, 360–361
  intervention/reoperation, 362, 368,
    371–383
    recommendations, 379–380
    results, 379
    stents, 320, 324–325
    techniques, 373, 377–379
  morbidity/natural history, 367–368,
    375–376
  pathology, 376–377
  pathophysiology, 361–362
  prevention, 230, 234
    aspirin $\pm$ dipyridamole, 233,
      234
  rates/incidence of, 278–280, 361,
    367, 371, 375–376
    angioplasty and, 317
    patch closure and, 274–275, 278,
      281
  risk factors/aetiology, 278–280, 361,
    371, 376–377
Retinal ischaemic symptoms and
  events, see Ocular symptoms
Retraction devices with mandibular
  subluxation, 227
Retrospective trials vs randomized trials
  in symptomatic disease, 9
Reversed staged procedure in combined
  carotid/coronary disease, 51,
  53–54

Risk, operative (intra-/postoperative in
    endarterectomy)
  of cardiac complications, see Heart
  medical conditions affecting,
      149–163
  of stroke, see Stroke
Risk factors (in vascular disease)
  management, 183–184, 186, 190
  for restenosis, 278–280, 360, 371,
      376–377
Rotational muscle flaps with prosthetic
    patch infection, 391–392

S
Safety and planning of postoperative
    care, 350–359
Saphenous vein
  bypass using, reversed, 258, 260
  patch using, 263, 276, 384
    randomized trials, 282
Scintigraphy, myocardial, in
    cerebrovascular disease patients, 173
Sedation in local anaesthesia, 194
  oversedation, 194, 196
Seizures, postoperative, 335–336
Selection (for surgery/endarterectomy)
  in combined coronary/carotid
    disease, staged vs synchronous
    procedure, 46–47
  cost-effectiveness in, see Cost-
    effectiveness
  general anaesthesia-related
    complication rate and, 202–203
  randomized trials in symptomatic
    disease, 5–7, 12
Sex, see Gender
Shelves, common carotid, 265
Shortening of carotid, 257, 257–259,
    267
Shunts, carotid, 244–254
  designs/types, 246–247
    in unexpected high disease, 220,
      221, 228
  in general anaesthesia, see General
    anaesthesia
  indications/contraindications/predicti
    ng need, 244–254

in infected prosthetic patch
    replacement, 385
  integrity, ensuring, 302–303
  in locoregional anaesthesia, 197,
      203, 205
  neurological deficits with, incidence,
      342–343
  selective shunting, 193–194, 199,
      250
Single photon emission computed
    tomography (SPECT)
  preoperative, 32
  with vertebrobasilar symptoms, 63
Sinus in prosthetic patch infection,
    384–385
Siphon lesions, 86, 112
'Slim sign', see 'String sign'
Small vessel (microvascular) disease
  brain scans, 130
  stroke or TIA in, 181
Smoking cessation, 19, 184
Somatosensory evoked potentials,
    intraoperative, 39, 300
SPECT, see Single photon emission
    computed tomography
Spectral broadening in arterial stenosis,
    91
Spinal accessory nerve injury, 207,
    210, 215–216
Spiral CT, 294
SPIRIT study, 183
Staged procedure in combined
    carotid/coronary disease, 46–56,
    164–165, 167–168, 320
  reversed, 51, 53–54
Statins (HMG-reductase inhibitors),
    184, 186
Stenosis, 85–86
  asymptomatic, see Asymptomatic
    disease
  high-grade/critical
    differentiation from occlusion,
      111
    thrombus distal to, see Thrombus
  measuring, 9–10
    contrast angiography, see Contrast
      angiography

duplex scans, see Duplex scans
  MR angiography, see Magnetic
    resonance angiography
  NASCET vs ECST, 102
  recurrence, see Restenosis
  residual, see Residual disease
  symptomatic, see Symptomatic
    disease
  thresholds/guidelines for surgery,
      14
  tightly stenotic lesion of ICA with
    underfilling secondary to low flow,
      294–295
Stents, 315–330
  advantages (potential), 315
  evidence for/historical aspects,
      317–318, 322–324
  future trials, 318, 319, 325–327
  protective (in carotid angioplasty),
      316–317
Steps, common carotid, 265
'String sign'/'slim sign' (narrow distal
    ICA incl. hypoplasia), 119
  heparinization, 238
  surgical decision-making, 288,
      289–290, 294, 296
Stroke (predominantly ischaemic
    stroke), 36–45
  acute/acute severe, 37–38
    as emergency surgery indication,
      26–27
    neurological assessment,
      143–144
  completed
    preoperative brain scans,
      133–134, 137–138
    timing of endarterectomy after,
      36–45
  established, as emergency surgery
    indication, 27
  ipsilateral, rate during medical
    management of carotid disease,
    cost-effectiveness and, 77–78
  late stroke risk, 360
  medical management, 180–184,
      188
  natural history of, 36–37

non-disabling, 37, 38
perioperative and
    postoperative/surgery-related, 37,
    299, 333, 334–340
    anaesthesia technique and,
        199–200
    cost-effectiveness and risk of, 78
    in European Carotid Surgery Trial,
        3–4, 17
    in North American Symptomatic
        Carotid Endarterectomy Trial,
        10–11, 16, 17
    patching and incidence of,
        273–274
    prevention, 298–312, 336–340
    see also Monitoring
    treatment, 334–336
permanent, prevention, 230
previous, recurrent infarction after,
    145
progressing (in evolution), 37
    as emergency surgery indication,
        27, 30
    preoperative brain scans,
        134–135
restenosis leading to, 367–368
transient, as emergency surgery
    indication, 27
unusual causes, 180, 181
Stump pressure, determination with
    cross-clamping, 245
Styloid fracturing in high disease,
    225–226
Subclavian artery, 62
    disease, 61–62
Subocclusion, carotid, decision process,
    288–289
Superior laryngeal nerve injury, 207,
    209, 214
Surgery (non-carotid surgery), major,
    prophylactic endarterectomy before,
    17–18
Surveillance, postoperative,
    360–370
    clinical effectiveness and cost-
        effectiveness of, 68
Sutures, tacking, 256, 264, 271

Symptom(s)
    cardiovascular (endarterectomy
        patient), prevention,
        232–234
    as guide to disease activity, 15–16
    neurological
        atypical, 145
        interpretation, 140, 145, 337
        non-hemispheric or vertebrobasilar,
            carotid surgery with, 57–65
    ocular, see Ocular symptoms
Symptomatic disease
    abandoning endarterectomy with
        distal extension in, 287
    randomized trials, 3–14
Synchronous procedure, combined
    carotid/coronary disease, 46–56,
    172–173
Syncope, 145
Syphon disease, imaging determining
    presence, 86

T
Tacking sutures, 256, 264, 271
Technical defects, 264–266
    monitoring for, see Monitoring
Thallium-201 myocardial scintigraphy
    in cerebrovascular disease patients,
    173
Theron protection balloon, 316–317
Three-dimensional MR angiography,
    99, 109
    disadvantages, 102
Three-dimensional reconstruction, 294
Thrombocytopenia, heparin-induced,
    156, 157, 232
Thromboembolic symptoms on
    operated side, prevention, 232–234
Thromboembolism, venous, prevention,
    230
    see also Emboli; Thrombosis
Thrombolysis, 188, 345
Thrombophilias, 156–157, 181
Thrombosis (and thrombus), 303–304
    distal to critical stenosis
        acute/freshly layered thrombus,
            295

chronically layered thrombus, 295
    recanalized old thrombus, fibrosis
        of artery secondary to, 295
intraoperative/on-table, 299, 333
    detection, 302, 336
    in MCA, 288
    postoperative, 302, 333, 339
        in endarterectomy zone, detection,
            303–304
        prosthetic patch-related, 276
    prevention, see Antithrombotics
    stroke due to, 299, 333
        management, 338–340
Ticlopidine, 182, 231
Time-of-flight sequence, 109
Timing of surgery (incl. endarterectomy)
    completed stroke and, 36–45
    European Carotid Surgery Trial,
        230
    randomized trials in symptomatic
        disease and, 4–5
Tongue of carotid plaque/atheroma,
    posterior, in unexpected high disease,
    220–221, 256–257
    abandoning endarterectomy,
        287–288
Transcranial Doppler ultrasound, see
    Doppler ultrasound
Transient ischaemic attacks (TIAs)
    brain scans, 133, 137
    crescendo, as emergency surgery
        indication, 28, 30
    medical management, 180–184, 188
    neurological assessment not required,
        142
    unusual causes, 180, 181
Transient stroke as emergency surgery
    indication, 27
Transposition of carotid bifurcation, 39
Trauma, cranial nerve, see Cranial
    nerve damage
Trials (of surgery)
    comparative, 9
    neurological assessment in (pre-
        treatment), 139
    randomized, see Randomized trials
    retrospective, 9

Trickle flow on MR angiography, 99, 100

U

Ultrasound, *see* Doppler ultrasound; Duplex scans; Echocardiography
University of Washington criteria in stratification of degree of ICA stenosis, 91
Urgent endarterectomy, 25–35

V

Vagus nerve injury (and avoidance), 206–208, 213–214
  with unexpected high disease, 220
  see also branches
Vascular disease
  cerebral ischaemia caused by, 144
  peripheral, *see* Peripheral vascular disease
Vasculitis
  cerebral ischaemia associated with, 144
  stroke or TIA in, 181

Vein graft
  for bypass, *see* Bypass graft
  interposition, with infected prosthetic patch, 385, 391
Vein patch, 263, 265, 267–268, 275–276, 285, 384
  randomized trials, 281–282
  replacing infected prosthetic patch, 384, 391
Velocity (blood flow)
  interpretation of intraoperative data, 309
  in MCA, 336
    decision-making with uncontrolled haemorrhage and, 291
    emboli and, 302
    shunts and, 303
Venous haemorrhage, uncontrolled, 290–291
Venous thromboembolism, prevention, 230
Vertebrobasilar symptoms, 145
  carotid surgery with, 57–65
  see also Basilar artery

Veterans' Administration Cooperative Study for carotid endarterectomy
  in asymptomatic disease, 16, 20–21
  in symptomatic disease, 11–12
Viscosity, plasma, 180
Vision, neurological assessment and monocular loss of, 142

W

Warfarin
  postoperative, 243
  preoperative, 238
Warfarin in TIA/stroke patients, 183
Wound haematoma, *see* Haematoma

X

Xenon CT with vertebrobasilar symptoms, 63